LANGUAGE DEVELOPMENT

Foundations, Processes, and Clinical Applications

Brian B. Shulman, PhD

Dean
School of Health and Medical Sciences
Seton Hall University
South Orange, NJ

Nina C. Capone, PhD

Department of Speech-Language Pathology
School of Health and Medical Sciences
Seton Hall University
South Orange, NJ

JONES AND BARTLETT PUBLISHERS

Sudbury, Massachusetts

BOSTON   TORONTO   LONDON   SINGAPORE

World Headquarters

Jones and Bartlett Publishers
40 Tall Pine Drive
Sudbury, MA 01776
978-443-5000
info@jbpub.com
www.jbpub.com

Jones and Bartlett Publishers Canada
6339 Ormindale Way
Mississauga, ON L5V 1J2
Canada

Jones and Bartlett Publishers International
Barb House, Barb Mews
London W6 7PA
United Kingdom

Jones and Bartlett's books and products are available through most bookstores and online booksellers. To contact Jones and Bartlett Publishers directly, call 800-832-0034, fax 978-443-8000, or visit our website www.jbpub.com.

Substantial discounts on bulk quantities of Jones and Bartlett's publications are available to corporations, professional associations, and other qualified organizations. For details and specific discount information, contact the special sales department at Jones and Bartlett via the above contact information or send an email to specialsales@jbpub.com.

The authors, editor, and publisher have made every effort to provide accurate information. However, they are not responsible for errors, omissions, or for any outcomes related to the use of the contents of this book and take no responsibility for the use of the products and procedures described. Treatments and side effects described in this book may not be applicable to all people; likewise, some people may require a dose or experience a side effect that is not described herein. Drugs and medical devices are discussed that may have limited availability controlled by the Food and Drug Administration (FDA) for use only in a research study or clinical trial. Research, clinical practice, and government regulations often change the accepted standard in this field. When consideration is being given to use of any drug in the clinical setting, the health care provider or reader is responsible for determining FDA status of the drug, reading the package insert, and reviewing prescribing information for the most up-to-date recommendations on dose, precautions, and contraindications, and determining the appropriate usage for the product. This is especially important in the case of drugs that are new or seldom used.

Production Credits

Publisher: David Cella
Associate Editor: Maro Asadoorian
Production Director: Amy Rose
Senior Production Editor: Renée Sekerak
Production Assistant: Jill Morton
Senior Marketing Manager: Barb Bartoszek
Associate Marketing Manager: Lisa Gordon

Manufacturing and Inventory Control Supervisor: Amy Bacus
Photo Research Manager and Photographer: Kimberly Potvin
Cover Design: Kristin E. Parker
Cover Image: © Sergey Lavrentev/ShutterStock, Inc.
Composition: Shawn Girsberger
Printing and Binding: Malloy, Incorporated
Cover Printing: Malloy, Incorporated

Library of Congress Cataloging-in-Publication Data

Language development : foundations, processes, and clinical applications / edited by Brian B. Shulman and Nina C. Capone.
    p. cm.
  Includes bibliographical references and index.
  ISBN-13: 978-0-7637-4723-7
  ISBN-10: 0-7637-4723-8
  1. Language acquisition. 2. Child development. 3. Children--Language. 4. Communicative disorders in children. I. Shulman, Brian B. II. Capone, Nina C.
  P118.L264 2009
  401'.93--dc22

                        2008045995

6048
Printed in the United States of America
13 12 11 10 09   10 9 8 7 6 5 4 3 2 1

Dedication

This book is dedicated to the memory of my father,
Millard Shulman, who, along with my mother Eleanor,
taught me to always ask questions and encouraged me to work as hard
as I could to achieve the goals I set out for myself.

—Brian B. Shulman

I dedicate this text to my clinical and academic mentors:
Karla McGregor, Margaret Aylesworth, June Campbell,
Susan Mulhern, Ann Oehring, Kathleen Blenk, Cis Manno,
Eve Reider, and Ned Mueller.

—Nina C. Capone

Together, we dedicate this book to the students who will take
the knowledge contained in these pages and apply it to
the children whose lives they will influence through
evidence-based language assessment and intervention.

Contents

Foreword *xiii*

Preface *xvii*

About the Authors *xix*

Contributors *xxi*

1 Language Assessment and Intervention: A Developmental Approach 1
Nina C. Capone, PhD

Objectives 1
Introduction 1
What Is Language? 2
Receptive versus Expressive Language 6
Stages of Communication 7
Who Is the Speech-Language Pathologist? 8
Background History 10
Spontaneous Language Sampling 11
Formal Testing 12
A Developmental Approach to the Clinical Practice of Speech-Language Pathology 15
Case Studies 21
Key Terms 33
Study Questions 33
References 33

2 Child Development 35
Theresa E. Bartolotta, PhD, and Brian B. Shulman, PhD

Objectives 35
Introduction 35
Cognitive Development 36

Motor Development   40
Social–Emotional Development   41
Linguistic Development   43
Assessment of Young Children   46
Clinical Applications of Developmental Assessment   50
Key Terms   52
Study Questions   52
References   53

3   Historical and Contemporary Views of the Nature–Nurture Debate:
A Continuum of Perspectives for the Speech-Language Pathologist   55
Sima Gerber, PhD, and Lorain Szabo Wankoff, PhD

Objectives   55
Introduction   55
Nature, Nurture, and Interactionist Views   59
The Science of Child Development in 2008: Broader Perspectives   84
Conclusion: How to Use This Information as a Lifelong Student of Language
   Disorders   86
Key Terms   88
Study Questions   88
References   88

4   Hearing and Language Development   95
Deborah R. Welling, AuD

Objectives   95
Introduction   95
Anatomy and Physiology of the Peripheral Auditory System   96
The Process of Normal Auditory Development   102
Assessment of Hearing in the Pediatric Population   108
Hearing Impairment   113
Interventions for Hearing Loss   117
Language Development Typical of the Hearing-Impaired Population   123
Case Studies   129
Summary   131
Key Terms   132
Study Questions   132
References   133

5 Social–Emotional Bases of Communication Development   135
Carol E. Westby, PhD

Objectives   135
Introduction   135
Underpinnings of Social Competence and Language   136
Communicating with Others   144
Factors Affecting Social–Emotional Aspects of Communication   151
Assessing Social–Emotional Bases for Communication   157
Philosophy of Intervention for Social–Communicative Deficits   167
Conclusion   170
Key Terms   171
Study Questions   171
References   171

6 Gesture Development   177
Nina C. Capone, PhD

Objectives   177
Introduction   177
Defining Gesture Types   178
The Emergence of Gesture   180
Gesture Reflects the Child's Mental Representations   182
Gesture Reflects the Child's Readiness to Learn   184
Gesture Input to the Child   187
The Function of Gesturing   189
Children with Language Learning Impairments   190
Final Thoughts for the Clinician   192
Summary   193
Key Terms   193
Study Questions   193
References   194

7 Early Semantic Development: The Developing Lexicon   197
Nina C. Capone, PhD, William O. Haynes, PhD, and Kristy Grohne-Riley, MA

Objectives   197
Introduction   197
Preparing the First Year: Perlocutionary Stage   198
Intent to Communicate: Illocutionary Stage   198
The First Word: Locutionary Stage   199
A Preponderance of Nouns   202

Expressive versus Referential Word Learners   205
Innate Biases Make Word Learning Efficient   206
The Emergent Coalition Model of Word Learning   208
Learning a Word   209
An Associationistic Account of Lexical–Semantic Representations   210
Naming Errors of Overextension and Underextension   211
Naming Errors   212
Working Memory   215
Later Lexical Development   216
Summary   217
Key Terms   218
Study Questions   219
References   219

8 Speech Sound Disorders: An Overview of Acquisition, Assessment, and Treatment   225

Lynn K. Flahive, MS, and Barbara W. Hodson, PhD

Objectives   225
Introduction   225
The Speech Mechanism   226
Phonemes   227
Speech Sound System Development   230
Acquisition   230
Phonological Deviations   234
Suppression of Phonological Processes   236
Phonological Awareness   237
Evaluation of Children with Speech Sound Disorders   239
Treatment   244
Case Studies   248
Summary   249
Key Terms   250
Study Questions   250
References   250

9 Morphology   255

Theresa E. Bartolotta, PhD, and Brian B. Shulman, PhD

Objectives   255
Introduction   255
Definition   256
Morphological Development   256

Clinical Applications: Examination of the Case Studies   266
Summary   268
Key Terms   269
Study Questions   269
References   270

10 The Development of Grammar   271

Patricia J. Brooks, PhD, and Liat Seiger-Gardner, PhD

Objectives   271
Introduction   271
The Development of Grammar in Typically Developing Children   272
The Development of Grammar in Late Talkers   279
The Development of Grammar in Children with Specific Language Impairment   281
Summary   289
Key Terms   289
Study Questions   290
References   290

11 Comprehension of Language   297

Amy L. Weiss, PhD

Objectives   297
Introduction   297
Studying Language Comprehension in Young Children   298
What Is Language Comprehension?   300
Measuring Children's Language Comprehension   317
Case Studies   323
Summary   325
Key Terms   326
Study Questions   326
References   327

12 The Transition to the School-Age Years: Literacy Development   329

SallyAnn Giess, PhD

Objectives   329
Introduction   329
The Foundations of Literacy: The Emergent Literacy Period   330
Stage Theories of Reading Development   333
The Self-Teaching Hypothesis   335
Early Literacy: The Transition to School   336

Early Identification of Later Reading Disabilities   341
Case Studies   343
Summary   344
Key Terms   345
Study Questions   345
References   345

13 Multicultural Perspectives: The Road to Cultural Competence   349
Luis F. Riquelme, MS, and Jason Rosas, MS

Objectives   349
Introduction   349
Terminology   351
Culture   352
Cultural Competence   354
Bilingualism: Perspectives in the United States   356
Case Study   357
Cultural Variables Affecting the Assessment and Intervention Process   358
Linguistic Variables Affecting the Assessment and Intervention Process   361
Language Development: Bilingual Perspectives   362
Developmental Similarities and Differences Between Simultaneous-Bilingual and
   Monolingual Children   364
Collaborating with Interpreters/Translators   365
Improving Cultural Competence in Assessment   367
Treatment Considerations   371
Summary   372
Key Terms   373
Study Questions   374
References   374

14 Children with Language Impairment   379
Liat Seiger-Gardner, PhD

Objectives   379
Introduction   379
Primary Language Impairment   382
Secondary Language Impairment   392
Assessment Procedures for Children with Language Impairments   397
Intervention Strategies for Children with Language Impairments   400

Summary   405
Key Terms   405
Study Questions   406
References   406

15 Communication Development in Children with Multiple Disabilities: The Role of Augmentative and Alternative Communication   413

Melissa A. Cheslock, MS, Andrea Barton-Hulsey, MA, Rose A. Sevcik, PhD, and Mary Ann Romski, PhD

Objectives   413
Introduction   413
Communicative Profiles of Children with Multiple Disabilities   415
The Role of Augmentative and Alternative Communication in Language
  Development   419
Challenges for Successful AAC Communication in Developing Language   424
Navigating the Challenges: Foundations for Implementation of Augmented Language
  Intervention   429
Summary   440
Key Terms   441
Study Questions   441
Recommended Readings   442
References   442
Appendix 15-A: Case Study 1: Speech-Language Evaluation   447
Appendix 15-B: Case Study 2: Speech-Language Evaluation   451
Appendix 15-C: Case Study 3: Speech-Language Evaluation   456

Glossary   459

Index   487

Foreword

As a student of speech-language pathology, I became interested in the subject of language and language acquisition because of the mystery of it all. Learning about and realizing the power of language intrigued me. Recognizing that language can take you from the here and now, and transport you to the past, to the future, and to imaginary places; realizing that just by saying a word, a curse could be delivered or—a more pleasant thought—a promise could be made; and appreciating that while an act, or the absence of an act, could break a promise, merely saying the words "I promise" creates a bond of intention between two people fascinated me and propelled me into the study of language development and childhood language disorders. As I progressed in my study of language, I marveled more and more at authors of fiction who are masters of figurative language and symbolism, and I contemplated with wonder those authors of nonfiction who use language to describe events that upon reading become shared events between the author and the reader.

As a young child listening to fairy tales, few words stirred my imagination as much as my mother reading, "Once upon a time, there was . . .". As a child, I began to love going to plays, just to have words and actions envelop me for a few captivating hours. As a young teenager, I spent hours on the phone talking with my best friend about everything within our universe. It was our conversations that bonded us—talking about our plans for the future and dissecting every detail of the events of joy and disappointment in junior high and senior high.

I lived in a college town with four universities nearby. Often when famous individuals were invited to speak at these universities, my parents took me to hear them so I would be exposed to scholarly leaders. While I may not have understood much of what was said at these events, I was struck by the occasion, by the fact that these were people with thoughts and words, and that it was important to get "dressed up" to go to auditoriums, churches, or banquet rooms to hear them speak about their experiences and their views.

Later in the mid-1960s, as editor of my high school newspaper, I took my journalistic responsibility quite seriously, conscious that my fellow students and I were creating a manuscript of our words and our thoughts. I wrote editorials to persuade, to pontificate (yes, I may have been a little pompous), and to motivate. As a high school and college student in the 1960s, language was amazing! Phrases such as "The New Frontier," the "War on Poverty," and "We shall overcome" were galvanizing. During the era of activism, words, phrases, and language were vehicles of social, political, and economic change. Language is very powerful.

Thus, with my love for language, as a graduate student of speech-language pathology, I became fascinated with studying the processes of language acquisition. As children develop, they progress through the stages of language acquisition without formal instruction and without the benefit of systematic explicit tutelage. The outcome of their marvelous developmental journey is the acquisition of a phonological system, extensive semantic and grammatical systems that convey a myriad of thoughts and communicative functions, the ability to comprehend the language of others, and the capacity to perform executive functions. In literate cultures, children also acquire the milestones of literacy acquisition. Children begin with reflexive vocalizations to which their caregivers give meaning and reply as though there was communicative intent on the part of the baby. This social dance, replete with vocalizations and gestures, over the course of months evolves into intentional communication with a phonology, vocabulary, syntax, and pragmatics that correspond to the young one's linguistic community. This occurs around the globe, in all cultures, and across all socioeconomic circumstances. Given that our world is a social, economic, technological, and commercial village, an understanding and respect for all cultures, languages, and peoples is a requisite for all professionals.

Every year new information, new theories, and new evidence are published about development to explain the complexities that create and facilitate the language acquisition process. Language and communication are the products of a biological, developmental, and environmental synchrony of various systems, which together produce a linguistically capable and literate human being. This text examines these systems, including the role of biology, child development, and the linguistic input that abounds in the child's environment. In addition to responding to the biology and linguistic interplay, intentional well-formed communication develops when there is efficient hearing and appropriate social–emotional development. The authors who have contributed to this text provide the latest research and perspectives on language development among neurotypical children.

Concern for children who reveal difficulty with the language learning process brings many people to the discipline of communication sciences and disorders. An ever-expanding awareness of typical language learning processes is the foundation for assessment and intervention for young children with language learning disabilities. This book begins and ends with an awareness of our roles with and responsibilities to children who are challenged in learning to communicate—children whose phonology systems, vocabularies and concept development, syntactic systems, and understanding of language need the expertise of communication disorders specialists if they are to improve. This text bridges biological, environmental, technological, and professional venues to advance the development of professionals and children alike.

Noma Anderson, PhD
Professor, Department of Communication Sciences and Disorders
Florida International University
2007 President, American Speech-Language-Hearing Association

Preface

We welcome you to this introduction to language development. Students have their own reasons for wanting to understand how children learn language to effectively communicate with their parents, caregivers, peers, and others. Some of you may be interested in pursuing a profession that deals with children who have difficulty learning language. Others may have a niece or nephew, son or daughter, or cousin who sparked your interest in understanding this developmental challenge. For whatever reason you have chosen to take this path, prepare yourself: *The journey is exciting!*

This text, which was written, in part, by us and, in part, by some of our valued colleagues (and friends!), delineates the typical course of language development within the clinical context of language assessment and intervention. Teachers, speech-language pathologists, early childhood educators, psychologists, and linguists are just some of the professionals who study and/or work with the children we describe in our book.

Whenever we work with children, it is important to understand language development so that we can understand each child's strengths and challenges in communication. In addition, to work with children who have language and communication difficulties, we must understand each child's delays in the context of what we term "typical" development. There are a number of *special* chapters. Chapter 1 provides a clinical model that enables us to developmentally approach assessment and treatment of language impairments in children. Our book also places a child's language and communication development in the context of his overall development. The child's cognitive development (Chapter 2) and emotional development (Chapter 5), as well as the nature–nurture factors of language development (Chapters 3 and 4), are also discussed.

Chapter 13 focuses on cultural diversity and its connection to children learning more than one language within the multicultural communication context. As we all know, the number of culturally and linguistically diverse individuals in the United States continues to increase annually.

This text also juxtaposes the gains made by children who follow the "typical" developmental course with the delays experienced by children who are not necessarily keeping pace with their peers of the same age. Chapter 1 introduces three primary case studies: a child who is developing typically and two children who vary from typical development. In subsequent chapters, you will discover that these three case studies are explored further, from a variety of perspectives. Be on the lookout for additional case studies, some of which appear in Chapter 15. These case studies specifically relate to the use of augmentative and alternative communication with severely language-impaired children. Moreover, Chapter 14 is dedicated to a discussion of children with language impairment.

Whatever your reason for learning about language and communication development, our text presents a broader understanding of this complex developmental phenomenon. Understanding language development helps us to understand each child as an individual and to elucidate the individual child's needs within communication contexts.

We would like to express our sincere appreciation to our contributors: Theresa E. Bartolotta, Andrea Barton-Hulsey, Patricia J. Brooks, Melissa A. Cheslock, Lynn K. Flahive, Sima Gerber, SallyAnn Giess, Kristy Grohne-Riley, William O. Haynes, Barbara W. Hodson, Luis F. Riquelme, Mary Ann Romski, Jason Rosas, Liat Seiger-Gardner, Rose A. Sevcik, Lorain Wankoff, Amy L. Weiss, Deborah R. Welling, and Carol E. Westby. These nationally and internationally recognized experts share our view of the importance of linking information on language and communication development to the clinical process. The fact that these contributors represent diverse backgrounds, clinical experiences, and theoretical orientations has clearly strengthened our book.

We also extend thanks to those scientists and mentors who taught us to always ask questions and encouraged us to continually search for answers. We encourage you, our students and colleagues, to take the information we present here and to continue to ask clinically relevant questions that affect how members of our field describe, assess, and treat the challenges some children face in language and communication development. It is important to never assume that any solution is the best or only answer: *Inquiry is the key to learning, and clinical inquiry must never end in the face of the children we service.*

Brian B. Shulman, PhD
Nina C. Capone, PhD

About the Authors

BRIAN B. SHULMAN, PhD

Brian B. Shulman is dean of the School of Health and Medical Sciences at Seton Hall University in South Orange, New Jersey. Dr. Shulman received his doctor of philosophy and master of arts degrees, both in speech-language pathology, from Bowling Green State University (Ohio). His bachelor of arts degree in speech-language pathology is from the State University of New York College at Cortland.

Dr. Shulman holds the rank of professor in the Department of Speech-Language Pathology at Seton Hall University. He is a Board-Recognized Specialist in Child Language (BRS-CL) as conferred by ASHA's Specialty Board on Child Language. A Fellow of the American Speech-Language-Hearing Association (ASHA), Dr. Shulman has made numerous invited presentations to professional groups at international, national, state, and local levels. He has also served in a number of leadership positions within ASHA, including being Chair of ASHA's Board of Division Coordinators (BDC), serving as a member of ASHA's Council for Clinical Specialty Recognition, and being co-chair of two ASHA annual conventions. Dr. Shulman recently completed a three-year term as ASHA's nationally elected Vice President for Speech-Language Pathology Practice. In that role, he identified national issues, monitored the emergence of new areas of practice, addressed concerns of the work setting, and monitored and facilitated ASHA activities designed to promote all practice settings.

NINA C. CAPONE, PhD

Nina C. Capone is an associate professor in the Department of Speech-Language Pathology at Seton Hall University. Dr. Capone earned a bachelor of arts degree from Boston University (1990); her master's degree (1997) and PhD (2003) were conferred by Northwestern University.

Dr. Capone has held clinical positions at the Children's Seashore House (Philadelphia), Children's Memorial Hospital (Chicago), Bright Futures Early Intervention Clinic (Evanston, Illinois), and the Westchester Institute for Human Development (Valhalla, New York). Clinically, Dr. Capone evaluates and treats children with language, speech, and feeding delays. She has extensive experience in the area of pediatric dysphagia. She holds a Certificate of Clinical Competence from the American Speech-Language-Hearing Association and maintains her professional license.

Dr. Capone is the director of the Developmental Language and Cognition Lab at Seton Hall University. In her research, she investigates the relationship between semantic learning and lexical expression as well as the relationship between gesture and language development. She has been published in the *Journal of Child Language* and the *Journal of Speech, Language, and Hearing Research*. She has presented at both national (American Speech-Language-Hearing Association) and international conferences (International Association for the Study of Child Language, Symposium for Research in Child Language Disorders, Early Lexical Acquisition). Dr. Capone is also a reviewer for the *Journal of Speech, Language, and Hearing Research*, and has been an expert guest reviewer for three journals: *Brain and Language, Gesture,* and *Developmental Science*.

Since joining the faculty at Seton Hall University, Dr. Capone has been awarded a university Researcher of the Year Award and a Provost's Faculty Scholarship Award. She teaches several courses that cover the following topics: language development, language disorders, phonological and other speech disorders, early intervention, and pediatric dysphagia. In addition, Dr. Capone mentors undergraduate, master's, and doctoral-level students.

Contributors

Theresa E. Bartolotta, PhD
Associate Dean, Division of Health Sciences
School of Health and Medical Sciences
Seton Hall University

Andrea Barton-Hulsey, MA
Speech-Language Pathologist
Georgia State University

Patricia J. Brooks, PhD
Professor of Psychology, College of
 Staten Island
Graduate Center
The City University of New York

Melissa A. Cheslock, MS
Speech-Language Pathologist
Georgia State University

Lynn K. Flahive, MS
Instructor/Clinic Coordinator
Miller Speech and Hearing Clinic
Texas Christian University

Sima Gerber, PhD
Associate Professor, Queens College
The City University of New York

SallyAnn Giess, PhD
Speech-Language Pathologist
Orange Unified School District, California

Kristy Grohne-Riley, MA
Assistant Professor, School of Allied Health
 and Communicative Disorders
Northern Illinois University

William O. Haynes, PhD
Professor Emeritus, Department of
 Communication Disorders
Auburn University

Barbara W. Hodson, PhD
Professor, Communication Sciences and
 Disorders
Wichita State University

Luis F. Riquelme, MS
Director, Riquelme & Associates
Assistant Professor, Clinical Speech-
 Language Pathology
New York Medical College

Mary Ann Romski, PhD
Regents Professor, Department of
    Communication
Georgia State University

Jason Rosas, MS
Speech-Language Pathologist, Beth Israel
    Medical Center (NY)
The Graduate Center
The City University of New York

Liat Seiger-Gardner, PhD
Assistant Professor, Department of Speech
    and Hearing Sciences
Lehman College and The Graduate Center
The City University of New York

Rose A. Sevcik, PhD
Professor, Department of Psychology
Georgia State University

Lorain Szabo Wankoff, PhD
Assistant Professor, Queens College
The City University of New York

Amy L. Weiss, PhD
Professor, Department of Communication
    Disorders
University of Rhode Island

Deborah R. Welling, AuD
Associate Professor and Acting Chair,
    Department of Speech-Language Pathology
Seton Hall University

Carol E. Westby, PhD
Language/Literacy Consultant
Albuquerque, New Mexico

CHAPTER 1

Language Assessment and Intervention: A Developmental Approach

Nina C. Capone, PhD

OBJECTIVES

- ◆ Define language and its five domains
- ◆ Introduce the clinical process of language assessment and intervention
- ◆ Understand the importance of developmental milestones

INTRODUCTION

This chapter introduces the clinical process of language assessment and intervention within a developmental framework. Language assessment (evaluation) includes understanding a child's history of development relative to normal developmental milestones as well as the child's functional communication (e.g., conversation) and performance on formal tests. A thorough evaluation of the child can determine whether a delay or disorder exists, and whether the delay/disorder is specific to language or involves multiple areas of development (e.g., cognition, motor skills). The clinician can also hypothesize about the child's prognosis in terms of gains to be made with and without intervention (treatment).

Knowledge of milestones across developmental domains is essential for the speech-language pathologist. The developmental milestones that children pass through provide a set of expectations for the clinician about what children should be doing as they age. The clinician uses these milestones to evaluate the child's performance and functioning and compare it with that of same-age peers. Knowledge of developmental milestones can then guide the clinician in how best to educate parents and to make referrals to other professionals.

Comparing the child's current level of functioning with what is expected for his or her age or cognitive level can also help the clinician in determining whether intervention is warranted. If intervention is appropriate, then the first phase of intervention is to determine the appropriate goals for the client. Goals are the behaviors or skills that the clinician helps the child in learning. They are determined by the developmental milestones that the child should progress to next and by the component skills needed to achieve a more complex milestone. For example, following directions requires the child to attend to the speaker, to understand the vocabulary used in the direction, and to decode the grammar. When the clinician is well grounded in the normal progression of development, he or she can determine the appropriate treatment goals, appropriate activity level to target the goals, and the types of scaffolding to provide the child as part of therapy.

Development is predictable. Milestones emerge in a predictable sequence, and they emerge or are mastered within a timeline that is consistent for most children. For example, most children speak their first word around their first birthday, combine words around their second birthday, and soon thereafter acquire grammatical endings such as the present progressive verb form (e.g., the -ing in eating). Although development varies across children, most of them achieve milestones within a predictable age range. For example, although most children speak their first word at 12 months, clinicians consider a range of 11 to 13 months for achieving this feat to be typical.

Across areas of development there is also a predictable relationship between skills. Developmental skills fall under the broad areas of motor development (gross motor, fine motor) and cognitive development (play, gesture, memory, attention). Observation in one skill area builds the clinician's expectation about the level of development in other skill areas. For example, some gesture milestones predict language milestones, and motor, play, and language skills develop in parallel. For instance, children walk and say their first word around the same time. Pointing gestures precede first words, and when the child is combining words, he or she is also likely to be combining play schemes.

This chapter introduces the process of evaluation and intervention within a developmental framework. First, it reviews the definition of language and the criteria for becoming a speech-language pathologist. Second, it provides a table of major developmental milestones. Each of the remaining chapters of the text is dedicated to providing more detailed information about each developmental area. Third, it delineates the process of evaluation and intervention. Three case studies are introduced in this chapter and then referenced throughout the rest of the text as the various authors discuss specific areas of development. Authors will reference these case studies in three ways. First, information already present in the case studies may relate directly to a discussion. Second, additional analyses may be suggested for these hypothetical clients. Third, future performance in development can be predicted for each case as authors discuss skills at older age levels.

WHAT IS LANGUAGE?

The American Speech-Language-Hearing Association (ASHA) defines language as a complex and dynamic system of conventional symbols that is used in various modes for thought and communication (ASHA, 1982, p. 1). A variety of symbols express language—for example, the sound symbols heard in speech, the written symbols seen in text, the manual symbols seen in signed languages, and the iconic symbols seen on some augmentative communication devices. Therefore, language is separable from the modality of communication that an individual uses to express himself or herself and to understand others. Everyone in a given community must agree on the same set of symbols for communication to be successful. This need for consistency leads to the "conventional" part of the definition. Language as a dynamic system means that language systems evolve and change over time. For example, new vocabulary is added to a language with new technology, as in the case of *e-mail, text messaging,* and *blogging.*

Language is a rule-governed behavior, a characteristic that allows it to be generative. Each language has a set of rules that make what is expressed socially appropriate and grammatical within a culture. This set of rules also ensures that communication is successful. For example, the English rule is that subject pronouns are always expressed with the exception of the imperative. In contrast, in Italian, the subject pronoun can be deleted with multiple verb tenses because case and number are also marked by the verb ending. That language is generative means that there are infinite possibilities in what is said and understood. As a consequence, individuals can express and understand sentences that they have never heard before. They rely on the rule system to generate novel grammatical and socially appropriate sentences in a given language.

Language is described by at least five separable domains: pragmatics, semantics, phonology, morphology, and syntax. These separable domains can be grouped into the form (phonology, morphology, syntax), content (semantics), and use (pragmatics) rules of a language.

The form of the language comes from the sound system (phonology) and the grammar system (morphology and syntax). It is the structural aspect of the language. Phonology is the sound system of the language. It is the smallest unit of language that overlays meaning onto the motor movements of speech. Clinicians use a special notation—the International Phonetic Alphabet (IPA)—to describe the sounds of a language. IPA differs from the orthographic symbols that you are reading now. For example, even though the word *go* consists of two letters and the word *dough* is made up of five letters, each has only two phonemes (i.e., sounds): /g/ and /o/, and /d/ and /o/, respectively. The sound change in /g/ to /d/ from *go* to *dough* is what signals a change in word meaning. However, /g/ and /d/ on their own do not have meaning.

Morphology is the smallest unit of language that expresses meaning. Two types of morphemes are distinguished: bound and free. Bound morphemes must be attached to a root word. Root words are free morphemes because they can stand on their own. Consider three examples: *dogs, walks,* and *walked.* Each of these words contains two morphemes. The word *dog/s* contains the free morpheme *dog* and the bound morpheme plural *s.* In this instance, the morpheme plural *s* has the meaning of "more than one." Similarly, the third person singular verb conjugation *s* and the past tense *-ed* in *walk/s* and *walk/ed*, respectively, indicate when an action occurred. The *s* indicates the action is currently happening and the *-ed* indicates that the action is finished. Even though these morphemes carry meaning, they cannot occur on their own: They are bound to a root word. In contrast, the phoneme /s/ in *soap* expresses no meaning except in how it functions to differentiate the word from other words such as *rope*.

A further distinction made for morphemes is that bound morphemes can be inflectional or derivational. The morphemes just discussed are inflectional morphemes; they indicate the tense of verbs. Tense refers to the timing of an action (present, past, and so on). Derivational morphemes include prefixes (e.g., *re-*, *un-*) and suffixes (e.g., *-ness*, *-ly*). Derivational morphemes change the word class of the root morpheme. For example, the morpheme *-ness* changes the word *happy* from an adjective to a noun, *happiness*.

Syntax is the sentence-level structure of language that marks relationships between words and ideas. This domain includes rules for constructing different types of sentences, such as declaratives, interrogatives, negatives, passives, and other complex sentences with conjoined or embedded clauses. See **Table 1-1** for examples of each sentence type. The structure of phrases also falls under the purview of the syntactic domain. Syntactic rules also dictate our choice of words and the order in which those words occur. For example, in English, adjectives are expressed in the noun phrase (e.g., *the friendly dog*) but negation occurs in the verb phrase (e.g., *I am not feeding the friendly dog*; *I did not feed the dog*). The negative *not* cannot occur in the noun phrase and must be placed between the auxiliary (*am*) and the main verb (*feed*). In English, it is ungrammatical to say *Not, I am feeding the friendly dog*. English also requires a "dummy" *do* verb to be inserted if an auxiliary is not already present. In the second example, *I did not feed the dog*, the affirmative is *I fed the dog*. When this sentence is negated, the *do* verb (*did*) must be used. These sorts of rules fall under the syntactic domain of language. Much of what we understand about the theory and rule system of syntax comes from Noam Chomsky's theory of Universal Grammar (for a review, see Shapiro, 1997).

Semantics is the meaning system of language. It can include the meaning expressed by single vocabulary items (e.g., *dog* = noun, animal, four legs, barks, canine, domesticated) or the proposition expressed by vocabulary items in combination (e.g., *mommy shoe* = the shoe belongs to mommy; *shoe mommy* = a request for the child's shoe). Semantics actually consists of two distinct types of information: lexical and conceptual. Lexical information is the word form that includes the phonological composition of the word, where the word form is referred to as a lexeme. The conceptual information is the meaning associated with the lexeme. For example, the word *dog* comprises three phonemes in sequence /d/, /ɔ/, /g/, which together are expressed as the lexeme /dɔg/. The meaning of dog may include four legs, having a tail, barking, and being a domesticated animal. Children need to develop both lexical and conceptual

TABLE 1-1 Examples of Sentence Types	
Sentence Types	**Example**
Declarative	My sister walks the dog.
Interrogative	Who is walking the dog?
	What is my sister doing?
Negative	My brother does not walk the dog.
Passive	The dog was fed by my brother.
Conjoined	My brother and sister take turns walking the dog.
	My brother feeds the dog and my sister walks the dog.
Clausal Embedding	My sister walks the dog that lives next door.
	It is our dog that my brother feeds, not our bird.

information of words as well as the link between the two so that they can express and understand language successfully.

Pragmatics refers to how we use the form and content of language. Pragmatic behaviors may include the intention that an utterance or gesture conveys, the way in which we use and understand body language, the social appropriateness of an utterance, and the process of ensuring the appropriate amount of information is provided to a listener. For example, a toddler may point to a cookie and say *gimmie*, or he may say *want cookie*. In both instances, the intent of the communication is the same—the child wants the mother to give him the cookie—even though the form of that communication differs. In the first instance, the pointing gesture indicates the object; in the second utterance, the word *cookie* indicates the object. The pragmatic aspect of both utterances is the intention, to request. As another example of pragmatics, rules govern how one varies the language that is used with various listeners. That is, we do not use the same kind of language when speaking to a professor, a supervisor, or a stranger as we do with a parent, a sibling, or a friend. If we were to speak to all of these individuals similarly, one or more could be offended or made to feel uncomfortable.

Another aspect of pragmatics includes how much information is provided to the listener. The information given to a listener has to be sufficient without giving too little or too much information. For example, a speaker cannot use a pronoun (*he*) without having already identified to whom *he* is referring. As another example, speakers must introduce a topic of conversation. If a friend approached you and stated, *"I told the mechanic to rotate my tires,"* you should think this odd. According to pragmatic rules, we generally make greetings first and then introduce a topic. Further, we introduce a topic and then expand on details. In fact, we have some language conventions for acknowledging when we violate a rule such as this (e.g., *Oops, I changed lanes*, or *Sidebar*, or *I'm changing topics*). Violations in pragmatics often can be the source of humor between friends. Conversely, they can be problematic when the speaker has no awareness of these rule violations and when they are pervasive in disrupting communication. This problem often arises with children who have language learning delays.

Nonverbal behaviors such as eye contact and body gestures also fall under the domain of pragmatics. Nonverbal behaviors communicate information, as the pointing example given earlier illustrates. Consider the message received if a friend says to you, *"It is fine that you forgot to call me."* If the friend says this but also averts her eye gaze and has an angry tone in her voice, then the nonverbal aspects of this communication let you know the friend is not happy with you. Even though the form of the language expressed understanding, the nonverbal behaviors of eye contact and vocal tone did not. In contrast, if that friend says the same sentence but has a casual tone to her voice, then you can assume that no offense occurred. As with the other domains of language, pragmatic rules for nonverbal behavior must be learned, and these rules differ cross-culturally. Thus it is particularly important for clinicians to fully understand the pragmatic rules (as well as other rule systems) of the language and culture of their clients.

RECEPTIVE VERSUS EXPRESSIVE LANGUAGE

For communication to be successful, language must be produced as well as understood. The ability to understand or comprehend the domains of language is referred to as *receptive language*. The ability to produce or speak (sign, write, etc.) language is referred to as *expressive language*. Following a direction such as "Give me your cup" requires the child to understand individual words (*give, cup, me, your*) as well as the relationship between those words. Therefore, knowing which cup the child needs to perform the action is dependent on the child understanding the possessive pronoun in combination with the noun. It is the child's cup—not the mother's cup—that needs to be given. If the child throws the cup on the floor instead of handing it over to the mother, he may understand that "cup" is somehow involved in what was said to him, but might not understand the word "give" or the relationship between what he was supposed to do (the action of giving) and the goal of that action (to the mother).

In another example, if you show a child a picture of one shoe and a picture of two shoes and ask the child to show you *the shoes* (versus *the shoe*), she should be able to point to the picture of two shoes if she understands the plural *s* morpheme. If the child does not understand the plural morpheme, then she will randomly point to either picture.

The child's ability to comprehend a certain level of language often precedes the child's ability to produce the same language. This phenomenon is observed in both typically developing and language-delayed children. A child may follow a direction correctly but may not produce the same sentence until many months later. Some children with language impairments exhibit more expressive language than understanding of language; this is not typical in most children's development.

STAGES OF COMMUNICATION

Three stages of communication have been described: perlocutionary, illocutionary, and locutionary.

The *perlocutionary stage* refers to the unintentional stage of communication. During this stage, the infant produces behaviors such as burping or vocalizations that have no intended message. This stage typically occurs before approximately 8 to 10 months of age, although children who demonstrate delays in development may remain in this stage longer. These vegetative or unintentional behaviors are often responded to by adults as if they were intentional communicative acts. The infant may burp and the mother responds, *"Oh, you're full!"*, or the infant may vocalize a sustained /a/ and the father responds, *"Oh, you have something to say?"* These adult responses help the child to learn language and to gain a sense of what intentional communication gets them—namely, attention and the meeting of needs. It establishes turn-taking interactions, which is also a vehicle for caregivers to provide the child with models of language.

At approximately 10 months of age, the typically developing infant begins to use gestures and nonlinguistic vocalizations (e.g., jargoning) intentionally to communicate. For example, the child may request a cup by pointing to it. This intentional communication without the use of words is referred to as the *illocutionary stage* of communication.

Soon after, at approximately 12 months of age, the infant produces his first word and enters the *locutionary stage* of communication. This phase is characterized by intentional communication expressed with words. It is the linguistic (and metalinguistic) stage of communication.

Some behaviors observed during the perlocutionary and illocutionary phases of communication are referred to as prelinguistic skills. They include gestures, eye contact, joint attention, and turn-taking behaviors. The prelinguistic skills of eye contact, joint attention, and taking turns during an interaction are the building blocks of successful communication and language learning. If a child is not looking at you, attending to the activity, and able to take turns, then she will miss your language models and will not imitate what you have said or done. Imitation is another skill the infant needs to have to learn language. Some children who demonstrate delays in language learning do not engage in these prelinguistic behaviors. If this is the case, then these behaviors are appropriate goals of intervention.

The locutionary phase of communication development can be divided into two types of skills: linguistic and metalinguistic. The term *linguistic* (or language) has already been defined. Language develops throughout the lifespan. Development of some domains is largely completed by eight years of age (e.g., phonology), whereas other domains (e.g., semantics) continue to develop into adulthood.

The term *metalinguistic* refers to the child's ability to think and talk about language. This skill is necessary if one is to understand the language used in humor, riddles, and metaphors, for example. These kinds of higher-level language uses are often part of academic instruction, social communication, and cultural phenomena (e.g., advertising). Other examples of metalinguistic skill include a child's ability to identify the first or last sound in a word, to express a rhyming word, to explain why a joke is funny, and to define a word. These tasks require the child to consciously analyze and manipulate language. Proficient reading and writing skills are also considered metalinguistic skills.

WHO IS THE SPEECH-LANGUAGE PATHOLOGIST?

Speech-language pathologists are professionals who are trained in the assessment and treatment of disorders in the areas of speech (articulation, voice, fluency), language, cognition, and eating/swallowing. Speech encompasses the respiratory, laryngeal, velopharyngeal, and oral-motor movements that express language. Speech-language pathologists are also actively involved in elective services, such as training non-native speakers of English to reduce their primary language accent or facilitating gender-preferred speech-language patterns for transgender individuals.

Speech-language pathologists are typically licensed by their state and certified by ASHA. ASHA is the national organization that regulates the professional practice of speech-language pathologists and audiologists. Speech-language pathologists and audiologists are required to earn a graduate degree in speech-language pathology or audiology, respectively; complete a nine-month supervised clinical fellowship after their graduate degree; and pass a national examination (Praxis examination).

Referral to a speech-language pathologist occurs when a parent, teacher, or pediatrician is concerned that a child is delayed in meeting speech, language, or feeding milestones. For example, children begin combining words around their second birthday. Parents may notice that their child is not yet expressing phrases such as *mommy go* at this time even though their child's peers are doing so. Parents typically consult with their child's pediatrician and are then referred to a speech-language pathologist for an evaluation. A referral to an audiologist should also be made at this time to rule out a hearing loss. Sometimes the speech-language pathologist will first screen the child's hearing. If the child does not pass the hearing screening, the speech-language pathologist can then refer her to an audiologist for a complete evaluation.

When a speech-language pathologist first speaks with a concerned parent, s/he asks some general questions regarding the child's development to determine whether an evaluation is ap-

a 10-month-old infant, not the skills of a 12-month-old. The issue of correcting a child's age is important in determining whether a child is delayed, because the child acquires new skills and meets milestones quite rapidly in the first two years of life. Recall that the child typically says his first word at 12 months but will probably not have words at 10 months. A chronological 12-month-old who has an adjusted age of 10 months would not be considered delayed if he has not yet spoken his first word. It is common clinical practice to stop adjusting a child's age for prematurity after two years of age (chronological age).

SPONTANEOUS LANGUAGE SAMPLING

Analysis of a spontaneous language sample is critical to assessing the functional use of language skills for communication. Functional communication refers to the child's ability to use each language domain to communicate successfully in her everyday experiences. Analysis of the spontaneous language sample is considered a formal analysis because performance can be compared to same-age peers.

TABLE 1-2	Examples of Typical and Remarkable Events Reported in the Background History	
Background History	**Typical Events**	**Remarkable Events**
Prenatal	Child was born at term after 38 to 40 weeks' gestation, weighing 6 pounds, 3 ounces	Child was born prematurely, prior to 38 weeks' gestation
Birth	Child was born without difficulty	Child incurred loss of oxygen during the birthing process due to breech birth presentation
Medical/Health	Child has had no ear infections	Child has incurred multiple episodes of otitis media (ear infections)
Developmental	Child sat at 6 months, and walked and said first words by 12 months	Child walked at 15 months and is not yet saying first words at 18 months
Education	Child has not received special services for development	Child received early intervention services
Family History	No history of speech-language disorders is reported for family members	Members of child's family have been diagnosed with speech or language disorders (e.g., dyslexia)

The clinician can collect a spontaneous language sample by structuring a developmentally appropriate interaction. For younger children, the clinician can have developmentally appropriate toys available on a mat and include a developmentally appropriate storybook with pictures. For older children, the clinician can prepare appropriate topics of conversation about academic, social, hobby, vacation, and sports topics. A sample of the child's language is elicited under these conditions and recorded during the assessment. Later, the clinician can transcribe and analyze the child's language from the video/audio tape.

Most formal analyses require a sample of 100 utterances that are continuous and considered representative of the child's communication. Oftentimes the child's middle 100 utterances are analyzed because this section of the sample is thought to be most representative of the child's skills. That is, this part of the sample occurs after the child has gotten comfortable with the new environment but before he feels fatigued; at this point, the child tends to show his best colors. The same sample can be used to analyze each language domain.

The book *Guide to Analysis of Language Transcripts* (Retherford, 2000) provides a description of several analyses of semantics, morphology, syntax, and pragmatics. In addition, the manual provides normative data and interpretation of results. Two examples of common spontaneous language analyses used in clinical practice are the *mean length of utterance* (MLU) and the *number of different words* (NDW). The MLU is a syntactic measure of utterance length, in morphemes. The NDW is a semantic measure of how many different vocabulary words the child uses. Formal analyses of discourse and narrative samples are also available (e.g., Applebee's System of Scoring Narrative Stages; Applebee, 1978). The clinician's knowledge of developmental milestones is used in analyzing the language and cognitive behaviors observed in the spontaneous interaction. The authors of the various chapters in this text will discuss spontaneous language analyses further.

FORMAL TESTING

Formal tests have been developed to survey a child's skills in a variety of areas. Formal tests allow the clinician to calculate a raw score by adding the points for accuracy. When administering a formal test, the clinician determines the level of skills that the child has, known as the *basal* level of performance, and the upper limit of what the child can accomplish, known as the *ceiling* level of performance. This range from basal to ceiling determines the raw score. The raw score, which is the number of correct items on the test, is statistically converted to a normative scoring system. This normative score is already calculated for the clinician in tables provided in the test's manual.

Two examples of normative scoring systems are the *standard score* and the *percentile*. They are categorized as "normative-referenced" tests because a specific child's performance is compared to a sample of children used to provide a summary of typical (or "normal") development.

The standard score has a mean score and a standard deviation from the mean. For most tests, the mean score is 100 and the standard deviation is 15 points. Thus a score that falls within the range of either 85–100 or 100–115 is considered to be within one standard deviation of the mean; a score that falls within the range of either 70–85 or 115–130 is considered to be within two standard deviations of the mean; and so forth. By current clinical standards, a score that falls within the range of 85–115 is considered typically developing performance. Some subtests of a formal test will use a mean of 10 and a standard deviation of 3 (i.e., typical performance range is a standard score in the range of 7–13). The clinical convention currently used to identify children with a language delay is standard scores that fall below one standard deviation of the mean (i.e., a standard score below 85, or below 7 on an individual subtest).

A percentile score is based on 100% of children sampled and is best understood as how a child performs relative to how many children perform above her and how many children perform below her. For example, if a child's raw score places her at the 90th percentile for her age, then 10% of the children at the same chronological age performed better and 89% of same-age children performed more poorly. Using percentile scores, children who fall below the 10th percentile are generally identified as having a delay in the area of development being tested. The standard score of 85 and the 10th–15th percentile roughly coincide. Therefore, whether the clinician uses a standard score or a percentile score should not affect the child's classification as exhibiting a delay in language development.

One benefit to using a standard score or a percentile score is that the child's performance can be compared across formal measures of language and cognitive functioning because many formal tests use these types of normative scoring systems. The child's performance can be characterized as within normal limits (low average, average, high average) or outside of normal limits (above average, below average, or delayed). There is a broad range of skill levels that characterizes a child who falls within normal limits. For example, approximately 68% of the population of same-age peers falls within one standard deviation of the mean and approximately 95% of the population falls within two standard deviations of the mean.

Another type of formal test is the criterion-referenced test. The criterion-referenced test determines how many skills a child has at a certain age level. The skills surveyed are determined by the normal sequence of developmental milestones. When making a decision regarding the type of formal tests to administer and the normative scores to report, the clinician must be familiar with the governing body's criteria for eligibility of services. For example, in the early intervention system, a child's eligibility for speech-language services is determined by individual states. For preschool, primary school, and secondary school settings, individual school districts determine those criteria.

Formal tests of language can sample a variety of language domains, or they can test a particular language domain or skill in-depth. Formal tests that sample a variety of language domains provide the clinician with a general language score. For example, the *Preschool Language Scale, Fourth Edition*, (PLS-IV; Zimmerman, Steiner, & Pond, 2002) tests the child's comprehension and production of a variety of language domains. Two subtests are part of the PLS-IV: Auditory Comprehension and Expressive Communication. The PLS-IV is a normative-referenced test administered to children ages birth to 83 months. All domains of language are sampled on this test. For example, on the Auditory Comprehension subtest, an item at the 24- to 29-month-old age level samples a child's understanding of action words. The child is presented pictures and is asked: *Look at all of the children. Show me the child who is* _____. The clinician then fills in the blank with six actions (e.g., sleeping, eating) and the child must point to the correct pictured action. Children are credited with accuracy if they are correct for four of the six actions. By contrast, on the Expressive Communication subtest, an item at the 30- to 35-month-old age level samples the child's expression of plural *s*. The child is shown a set of pictures (babies, horses, blocks) and the clinician asks about each individually: *What are these?* The child needs to respond to only one of the three pictures accurately to be credited with expressing plural *s*.

The *Rossetti Infant–Toddler Language Scale* (RITLS; Rossetti, 1990) is a criterion-referenced test used to survey the development of children from birth to 36 months of age. The RITLS surveys skills across several skill areas, including interaction/attachment skills, pragmatic skills, gesture skills, play skills, receptive language skills, and expressive language skills. Children are scored as having a percentage of skills achieved under each skill area at each age level. For example, if a child demonstrates four of the five possible skills sampled, he is credited with 80% of the skills at that age level.

There are also formal tests that assess a single domain of language. These tests provide the clinician with a richer picture of the skills in a particular domain. For example, the *Peabody Picture Vocabulary Test, Fourth Edition*, (PPVT-IV; Dunn & Dunn, 2007) is a test of receptive vocabulary. The child is presented with a four-picture array and must identify the correct picture when the clinician says a word label. This test assesses the size of the vocabulary that the child comprehends.

The *Expressive Vocabulary Test* (EVT; Williams, 1997) is a test of expressive vocabulary. The child is presented with a series of single pictures and asked to name each one. This test assesses the size of the vocabulary that the child expresses.

The *Goldman–Fristoe Test of Articulation, Second Edition*, (GFTA-2; Goldman & Fristoe, 2000) is a test of expressive phonology. The child is presented with a series of single pictures and is asked to name each one. These pictures are different from those used in the EVT because the pictures that make up the GFTA are meant to elicit each consonant or vowel sound of English in different word positions (i.e., initial, medial, final). For example, the phoneme /g/ is tested through naming *girl, wagon,* and *frog.* Sound production is also tested in consonant clusters and diphthongs. Consonant clusters occur when two consonants are spoken together with no intervening vowel (e.g., /st/ in *stop*), and diphthongs occur when two vowels are spoken together with no intervening vowel (e.g., /aɪ/ in *eye*).

It should be emphasized here that formal tests, alone, should never form the sole basis for a speech-language pathologist's determination of a child's performance and subsequent intervention. If they must be used to determine a child's eligibility for services, the formal test data generated must be compared to data obtained through other assessment measures including, but not limited to, spontaneous language sampling.

A DEVELOPMENTAL APPROACH TO THE CLINICAL PRACTICE OF SPEECH-LANGUAGE PATHOLOGY

Knowledge of developmental milestones is critical to the practice of speech-language pathology. Clinicians survey several areas of development during an evaluation to understand the child's overall development. Understanding the child's language development within the broader context of the child's overall development enables the clinician to make a more reliable diagnosis, to make hypotheses about why a child may be delayed in language development, to predict the child's prognosis is for making gains, and to plan an appropriate course of intervention.

The developmental areas that clinicians may observe include gross and fine motor skills, gesture, play, and other areas of cognition, in addition to language abilities. The clinician may not use a published test to formally assess each of these areas. For example, the child's mother may report a delayed milestone, or the clinician may observe the child during the evaluation to be falling behind in a motor milestone (e.g., an eight-month-old child who is not yet sitting up). A referral to a physical therapist for a gross motor evaluation would be appropriate. Therefore, an informal observation of the child's skills outside of speech and language domains can lead the clinician to make the appropriate referrals to other professionals.

Assessment

In the context of assessment, if the clinician can gain a sense of the child's cognitive and motor development prior to the language assessment, then he or she can plan appropriate tests and activities for the evaluation. Similarly, if the clinician has a solid footing in developmental milestones, then he or she can make informal observations at the start of the evaluation session and alter the protocol if necessary. Careful planning of the language evaluation (as well as the ability to adapt quickly to the unexpected!) ensures that the diagnosis, prognosis, and plan for intervention are valid and reliable.

For example, if the clinician knows ahead of time that a five-year-old client has the cognitive functioning of a much younger stage of development, then he or she knows that some formal tests used with five-year-olds cannot be administered to this child. Instead, the clinician may choose a formal test that surveys a broader age range so that skills at all possible age levels are available for testing. If the six-year-old child is functioning more in line with a 30-month-old child's level of cognition, then the spontaneous language sample would be elicited using toys that are more appropriate for the latter age level. By contrast, it would be inappropriate to elicit a language sample using a story retell context because a child functioning at this age may not understand the task. An inappropriate context of analysis would not elicit a valid level of language skills, because the most representative sample of what the child could accomplish would be missed.

It follows, then, that the evaluation is not simply a listing of the things that the child cannot accomplish, but rather should include a profile of the child's strengths and achieved milestones. By including the child's strengths *and* weaknesses, the clinician presents the child in a broader developmental context and capitalizes on what the child can do to facilitate further development. It is also important for parents to be counseled about their child's strengths.

The clinician who is facile with his or her knowledge of developmental milestones can accommodate a child during the evaluation and make observations about techniques that may scaffold the child to the next skill level. A scaffold is formally defined as something to raise or support. In clinical practice, a scaffold refers to the support given a child that facilitates the next skill level. Scaffolds may include a model of a skill for the child to imitate (e.g., words, phrases, play schemes, gestures), or providing cues (multimodal hints) such as saying "Listen" while touching the child's shoulder to gain his attention prior to giving a direction. Any special accommodations that the clinician makes during the evaluation must be included in the evaluation report.

The clinician can also set aside time after testing for trial treatment activities. During this period, the clinician assesses the child's response to scaffolding of a few behaviors. Again, because the clinician will only know the child's areas of delay through the evaluation, he or she must be comfortable with developmental milestones so as to know what to target during trial treatment activities. The child's resulting performance is reported in a section of the evaluation report entitled "Trial Treatment."

The scaffolds to which the child responds (e.g., preparatory sets, cues, prompts, models) are considered by the clinician in his or her final analysis of the child's language development. The clinician's knowledge of the child's developmental level and knowledge of typical developmental milestones dovetail as the clinician begins to plan the child's intervention and to hypothesize about the child's prognosis for gains to be made with intervention. For example, if the child produces two-word combinations but is not marking early grammatical morphemes, the clinician will model simple sentences with present progressive verbs (e.g., *dancing*) because the grammatical morpheme *-ing* is expected to emerge next in development. If a 30-month-old child does not produce two-word combinations spontaneously but can imitate combinations when the clinician models them, the child may be at the cusp of that level of language development. Such a child would have a better prognosis of making this gain than the child who is not yet pointing or the child who is not yet able to imitate one- or two-word combinations. The latter child would first need to achieve the precursor gesture and imitation milestones.

The clinician who is knowledgeable about developmental milestones will be able to determine whether a child demonstrates development that is considered typical for her chronological (or adjusted) age, whether the child is delayed in skills, or whether the child demonstrates development that is atypical. Atypical behaviors are not seen as part of the typical course of development. For example, if a 25-month-old child speaks in only a few one-word utterances, this level of achievement is typical of a 12- to 18-month-old child and can be considered delayed expressive language development. However, if this same child is not exhibiting gesture or communicative eye contact, and/or joint attention, or if the child says more then she understands, then the clinician may consider this level to be atypical because eye contact and joint attention are present at the earliest stages of infancy. Also, we know that comprehension precedes production of language in typical development.

Knowledge of developmental milestones across skills areas helps the clinician determine whether a delay is specific to one area of development or whether it involves multiple areas of development. After the evaluation is completed, the speech-language pathologist must integrate, analyze, and interpret the child's history and performance on formal testing, spontaneous communication analyses, and trial treatment. Based on the clinician's interpretation, he or she makes a diagnosis, develops a statement regarding the child's prognosis for gains to be made with (or without) intervention, and recommends the appropriate course of action for intervention.

Even though a child may come to the evaluation as a result of concerns related to language development, the clinician may discover that the child has other areas of concern not previously identified. For example, the child may present with a voice disorder, issues with hearing, or motor development delays. Appropriate referrals to other professionals can be made for evaluation of motor, medical, or other cognitive/emotional concerns. These professionals may include a developmental pediatrician, neurologist, psychologist, audiologist, physical therapist, or occupational therapist.

If multiple areas of development are delayed, then the clinician can make hypotheses about which types of goals need to be set for intervention, taking into account the fact that skills in some areas of development are precursors to skills in other areas of development. For example, a child who is not yet sitting up, crawling, or standing may have difficulty exploring objects and the environment. These sensory-motor experiences are the building blocks for early semantic learning and set the stage for many parent–child interactions in which language is modeled and practiced.

Also, prognostic statements can be made based on the known relationships that exist between areas of development. For example, the child who demonstrates a delay in just expressive language is thought to have a better prognosis than the child who has a delay in the expressive language, receptive language, gesture, and play domains. Likewise, the child who demonstrates delays in more general cognitive functions (e.g., mental retardation) would not be expected to achieve the same level of gains even with intervention as the child who has an intelligence quotient that is within average range.

The assessment process not only leads to a diagnosis, prognosis, and recommendation for intervention, but it also allows the clinician to provide parent education regarding the typical course of development and where their child falls within that framework. The clinician who is facile with developmental milestones is better able to counsel parents about their child and the appropriate expectations caregivers should have for the child.

Setting Goals and the Intervention Process

After the evaluation is complete, the clinician writes a summary of his or her findings in an evaluation report. In some cases, the child may simply need to be monitored over time. If intervention is warranted, however, goals to be targeted in intervention are specified. The overarching goal of intervention is to facilitate development to age-expected or cognitively appropriate levels. Goals are the target behaviors the clinician will facilitate in the intervention process. The target behaviors are those behaviors that the child must evolve next in development and/or the component skills necessary to reach a particular milestone. In our example of the 30-month-old child who is not yet marking morphemes, an appropriate goal for intervention is that the child will begin marking present progressive verbs ending *-ing* in two-word combinations (e.g., *mommy eating*). The present progressive is one of the first morphemes to emerge in toddlerhood, so this makes it the appropriate target for therapy. A goal such as marking copula *to be* in short sentences would not be appropriate at this time, as copulas are not mastered until later in the preschool years.

Three types of goals are developed by the clinician: long term, short term, and session objectives.

+ Long-term goals relate to broadest areas of development or the end product of therapy. For example, a long-term goal might be "The child will demonstrate developmentally appropriate expressive language skills to support functional communication within academic and social contexts." Success in moving toward the long-term goal does not generally include a percentage of accuracy measure, but rather tends to be measured within the functional context of daily living.

+ Short-term goals are the smaller steps taken to achieve the long-term goal. Short-term goals are meant to be accomplished within weeks to months of setting them. For example, a short-term goal may be "The child will produce grammatical morpheme -ing in two- to three-word combinations within play-based activity at least 80% of the time." The target behavior in this case is -ing. Limiting the linguistic complexity to a phrase of two to three words is another type of scaffolding the clinician must consider.

+ Goals set for a particular treatment session are known as session objectives. A session objective is the smallest step taken to achieve the short-term goal (and ultimately the long-term goal). A session objective may be "The child will produce grammatical morpheme -ing in two-word combinations when provided an immediate verbal model and tactile cue by the clinician in 80% of trials." Here, we see that a richer scaffolding (a model and a cue) is provided initially because it will provide the child with the best opportunity to elicit and practice the behavior. As the child gains some mastery over producing the behavior, the clinician can reduce the scaffolding, thereby increasing the child's independence in communication. We would expect this level of independence at a short-term goal interval.

Keep in mind that the session objective and the short-term goal are benchmarks that lead to the accomplishment of the long-term goal. The prognosis for gains to be made toward meeting session objectives, short-term goals, and long-term goals is dependent upon several factors, including the severity of the language impairment, any concomitant disorders, and the family's and child's motivation to participate in intervention.

Once a set of long-term goals, short-term goals, and session objectives have been determined, the child is ready to embark on the intervention process. During this process, the clinician meets with the child for guided learning and practice. Within the therapy sessions, the clinician continues to use his or her knowledge of development to structure the expectations of the child and the therapeutic environment. As with the assessment process, the appropriate choice of toys, activities, and other materials is critical to the child's success in therapy. The clinician must choose materials that are within the child's developmental functioning so as not to overwhelm the child. The focus of the clinician should be to isolate the skill of difficulty as much as possible. If the child is having difficulty producing present progressive verb tense and the -ing form of the verb is targeted during an activity, then the child should work only toward imitating the verb form. If an activity is too complex, the child will use his learning resources to complete the activity as well as to learn the language form. This dual goal may overwhelm the child, such that he may not be successful.

The new clinician should clearly understand the difference between a goal, any therapeutic scaffolding, and the activity used to target the goal in an intervention session. The *goal* is the language behavior or milestone that the clinician targets during the therapy session (e.g., produce present progressive verb tense *-ing*). The *therapeutic scaffolding* includes models, cues, prompts, feedback, preparatory sets of information, structuring of the amount of language that the child must produce, and any environmental modifications. The *activity* is what the child and clinician engage in to practice the target goal behavior (e.g., playing Go Fish, reading a story and retelling it, playing with miniature toy figures or PlayDoh). The activity is neither the goal nor is it the scaffold. It is common for young clinicians who are just learning to navigate the clinical process to confuse these three concepts

Scaffolding can take many different forms. A verbal model is an exact demonstration of what the clinician wants the child to do. For example, if you want the child to produce the possessive *s*, then you might take 10 opportunities during a play activity with Sesame Street figures to model *Ernie's car*, *Bert's car*, *Cookie Monster's car*, and so forth. Always give the child plenty of time to process your model and imitate you. Perhaps the child will repeat *Ernie car*, without the possessive *s*. In such a case, the child may need an extra scaffold to make the target morpheme more salient. One scaffold could be a tactile cue. With a tactile cue, the clinician might say *Ernie's car* while running her finger along the child's hand while producing the possessive *s*. The tactile cue will highlight the important aspect of the language in a second sensory modality, making it more salient for the child. For older children, more verbal cues and prompts would be appropriate because such children should have reached a level developmental level and be able to understand them.

In the previous example, the clinician provided a model of the possessive *s* within a phrase—not a sentence or in conversation. Controlling the amount of language surrounding the target scaffolds the child because having more language around the target increases the difficulty of perceiving and producing it.

Feedback as a scaffolding tool helps children see, hear, or feel their own behavior as they practice. Some feedback tools include a mirror, an iPod with microphone, or a video recorder. Perhaps the clinician audio-records the child's practice. After each trial, the clinician and the child can then listen to the child's responses together, and the child can determine which trials were accurate or in error. This type of activity would be appropriate for an older child.

Understanding developmental milestones will help the clinician decide which types of cues, prompts, and feedback are appropriate for the child. When a goal is first introduced, the clinician's intention is to provide the most scaffolding needed for a child to produce the behavior. Having the correct level of scaffolding ensures the child practices the accurate behavior or skill as often as possible. It is important to remember that the clinician wants the child to have good practice on most, if not all, of the trials administered.

Accuracy may be measured using one of several conventions, including a percentage of trials (i.e., number of accurate productions ÷ total number of trials administered; 7/10 = 70%), or a frequency count within an interval of time (e.g., 5 times within a 10-minute activity). If the child is not achieving more than 50% accuracy with a goal, then the child is practicing the incorrect behavior just as much (or more) than the desired behavior. This 50% accuracy marker relates to chance levels of performance, as determined statistically. When the child is less than 50–65% accurate, the clinician must reassess the scaffolds, his or her expectations of the child, and the complexity of the activity being used. One option may be for the clinician to increase or change the type of scaffold provided to the child, or to train component parts to the goal. Over time, the scaffolds should be faded away so that the child becomes independent in his skills.

Another part of the intervention process is parent training and a home program. Education of the child's parents and other caregivers is ongoing and essential for the child to generalize what she is learning in therapy to her daily living environments (e.g., home, school, playground).

CASE STUDIES

Three case studies are referred to throughout this text to illustrate the discussions of the various topics in language development. Johnathon, Josephine, and Robert are toddlers who were evaluated because their mothers were concerned about their language development. Each evaluation report reviews the child's background history, clinical findings, diagnosis, prognosis, and recommendations.

Although Johnathon's mother expressed concern regarding her son's development, the evaluation found him to demonstrate typical language development (TD). In contrast, Josephine and Robert each show a language delay. Josephine's delay is characterized predominately by a delay in expressive language, whereas Robert's delay is more encompassing, including delays in receptive and expressive language as well as delays in gesture and play domains. Josephine is considered to have a better prognosis for outgrowing her language delay because she has strengths in receptive language, play, and gesture development. Research shows that children with strengths in these areas tend to fare better than children like Robert, who show delays in the expressive and receptive language, gesture, and play domains. Josephine is referred to as a late bloomer (LB), and Robert is referred to as a truly late talker (LT).

The idea to be noted here is that although both Josephine and Robert demonstrate delayed language development at their evaluations, their prognosis for developing age-appropriate language by later in the preschool years differs. Children who demonstrate language delays like those experienced by Robert are more likely to have persistent language delays into the preschool years and beyond. By four years of age, children like Robert are more likely to be diagnosed with specific language impairment (SLI).

JOHNATHON (TD)

Sex: Male
Age: 25 months

SIGNIFICANT HISTORY

Johnathon is a 25-month-old boy who was referred to this appointment to assess the status of his speech and language development. His mother was concerned that Johnathon was not yet formulating sentences and questioned his vocabulary development. Johnathon's *prenatal/birth* history was unremarkable. He was born at term weighing 8 pounds, 4 ounces. *Medical* history was fairly unremarkable, with the exception of one ear infection at 12 months and occasional colds. *Developmental* milestones were met in a timely manner. For example, he sat without support by 6 months and walked by 12 months. *Speech-language* history was fairly unremarkable, with first words emerging by 12 months. Johnathon was recently combining words. He followed age-appropriate directions, including those without contextual support (e.g., "Bring me your bottle"). Johnathon ate a full-textured diet. He was enrolled in a daycare program three mornings each week. He was described as interactive and enjoyed playing with a variety of toys. *Family* history was negative for speech-language disorders.

CLINICAL PROCEDURES

Tests

MacArthur Communicative Development Inventory (MCDI)
Rossetti Infant–Toddler Language Scale (RITLS)

Other

Play-based interaction
Spontaneous speech-language sample
Oral mechanism exam

CLINICAL FINDINGS

General Observations
Johnathon was a pleasant and interactive boy. He readily entered the playroom with his mother and separated without difficulty to explore the room. Breaks in attention generally occurred when a task was more difficult for him to complete such as those considered more appropriate for an older toddler.

Play

Johnathon's play skills were typical of same-age peers. He demonstrated play skills most typical of a 21- to 24-month-old, with skills continuing to emerge at the 24- to 27-month-old levels on the RITLS. Johnathon used most toys appropriately and chose toys selectively. He readily linked functional play schemes around familiar themes (e.g., doll play) and was observed to use objects symbolically (e.g., he put a toy key to his ear to represent a telephone).

Nonverbal Communication

Johnathon demonstrated communicative eye contact, turn-taking ability, and joint attention during the evaluation. Gestural communication was a strength for him. He demonstrated the prelinguistic gesture sequence of showing, giving, and pointing to objects and often combined these with spoken utterances.

Receptive Language

Johnathon responded to environmental sounds and to his name. His attention to verbal requests and comments was inconsistent only when commands were considered more advanced for his age. His performance on the RITLS was most typical of a 21- to 24-month-old toddler with a scatter of skills up to 24- to 27-month age levels. He completed single-step commands (familiar and novel) and chose familiar objects from an array of objects. More complex commands (e.g., two requests with one object, two-step related directives) were followed with gesture cues. His mother reported that Johnathon understands new words rapidly.

Expressive Language

Johnathon's performance on the RITLS was most typical of a child 21 to 24 months of age, with a scatter of skills up to the 24- to 27-month-old age level. For example, Johnathon used new words, combined words, and produced a self-referent. He was just beginning to use many action words and relate personal experiences. Johnathon used language to fulfill a full range of communicative functions. For example, he initiated interactions verbally with adults, responded to adult utterances, and requested assistance from adults in his environment. On the MCDI, Johnathon's mother reported him to have 212 words, which placed him at the 30th percentile for his age. His use of early developing morphosyntax was also considered to be at the 30th percentile for his age (e.g., *-ing*, plural *s*).

Phonology

Johnathon was at least 60% intelligible to this unfamiliar listener. His intelligible utterances were predominately single words and word combinations. Attempts at longer utterances resulted in reduced articulatory precision. Jargon was heard infrequently.

His phonological repertoire included a full repertoire of stop, nasal, and glide sound classes as well as the early-developing fricatives /h/ and /f/. Consonant substitutions were considered developmentally appropriate (e.g., /θ/ for /s/, reduced lingual tension of /r/). Johnathon produced a full repertoire of singleton vowels and occasional diphthongs. His syllable shape repertoire was predominately restricted to open syllables (CV /maɪ/, VCV /odɛ/, CVCV /wowo/). However, final consonants were emerging. The following phonological processes were heard and considered developmentally appropriate: cluster reduction, stopping of later developing fricatives (/s, z, θ, ð/).

Oral–Motor Examination
Structure, function, and sensation of the oral–facial musculature appeared to be sufficient to support speech and language development.

DIAGNOSIS AND PROGNOSIS

Johnathon is a pleasant 25-month-old toddler who presents with receptive and expressive language skills that are consistent with a child his age. Play, oral-motor, gesture, and attention skills appear to be age appropriate and sufficient to support continued language development.

RECOMMENDATIONS

Results from this evaluation were discussed with Johnathon's mother today. Speech-language intervention is not warranted at this time. Johnathon's mother was educated and counseled regarding typical cognitive and language development. She was encouraged to return to this clinic for reevaluation if at any time she was concerned about subsequent stages of Johnathon's language development. She was agreeable.

JOSEPHINE (LB)

Sex: Female
Age: 22 months

SIGNIFICANT HISTORY

Josephine is a 22-month-old girl who was referred to this appointment due to continued concerns about her limited expressive vocabulary. Josephine's *prenatal/birth* histories were unremarkable. She was born at term weighing 7 pounds, 2 ounces. *Medical/health* history was significant for pneumonia at 19 months and two ear infections since that time. She had known allergies to dust and mold. Josephine's *hearing* was recently evaluated and found to be within normal limits. *Developmental* milestones were reached in a timely manner (e.g., sat at 6 months, walked at 11 months).

Josephine's *speech-language* development was remarkable for limited vocalizations during infancy, including little babbling. Her first word was delayed until 15 months, and her mother believed Josephine to have a small vocabulary for her age. Her primary means of communication were gesturing and attempting to produce phoneme sequences that marked two syllables, but these utterances did not approximate known words. Marking two syllables was a recent accomplishment. Her mother stated that Josephine did not readily imitate words and had isolated instances of accurate word production, but the latter behavior was inconsistent. Josephine was beginning to demonstrate frustration with communication breakdown. Her strengths appeared to be in the domains of play and receptive language. Josephine followed two-step directions that required her to leave the immediate context (e.g., "Go to the family room and get your diaper"). Josephine ate a full diet at the time of this evaluation.

Josephine was evaluated for speech and language previously by her state's early intervention program. Results revealed a delay in expressive language. She was subsequently enrolled in language therapy, once weekly for the past two months. Josephine was otherwise cared for by her mother in the home. *Family history* was negative for speech-language disorders.

CLINICAL PROCEDURES

Tests

MacArthur–Bates Communicative Development Inventories (CDIs)
Rossetti Infant–Toddler Language Scale (RITLS)

Other

Play-based interaction
Spontaneous speech-language sample
Oral mechanism exam

CLINICAL FINDINGS

General Observations

Josephine was a delightful and interactive child who readily transitioned to the playroom without difficulty. She regulated her behavior well and showed age-appropriate attention to all tasks.

Play

Josephine's play development was well within normal limits (WNL) for her age. She demonstrated a scatter of skills up to at least the 27- to 30-month age level. For example, she readily performed many related activities during play, and she selectively chose and used toys appropriately. Josephine engaged in spontaneous doll play (e.g., covered the doll with a blanket; fed it a bottle, a spoon, and miniature food items; hugged it), and she pretended to talk on the phone and to write. She demonstrated symbolic play such as blowing on food during pretend cooking activity.

Nonverbal Communication

Josephine demonstrated the prelinguistic skills of communicative eye contact, joint attention, and turn-taking throughout the evaluation. She often used prelinguistic gestures (show, give, point) and iconic gestures (e.g., hand under cheek to indicate sleeping) to communicate and engage the clinician. Her performance on the RITLS was considered well WNL. Pragmatic skills were limited only by her sparse expressive language. However, nonverbal aspects of pragmatic development were WNL.

Receptive Language

Josephine's comprehension of language was well WNL with a scatter of skills up to at least the 24- to 27-month age level. For example, at this age level Josephine understood the concept of *one* and recognized family member names. At her age level (21–24 months), she chose one object from a group of five, and followed novel and two-step related commands. She understood new words rapidly by her mother's report. She readily responded to her name.

Expressive Language

Compared to her receptive language abilities, Josephine's expressive language was significantly delayed. On the RITLS, she presented with skills most typical of the 9- to 12-month age level. However, Josephine did not readily engage in spoken imitation or consistently use spontaneous vocalization, babble, or jargon, which typically emerges during that stage of development. The use of routine carrier phrases such as "Ready, get set" facilitated her expression (i.e., /go/). She was not yet using adult-like intonation or using words rather than gesture to communicate. Her strengths were that she used early phonemes (/t, d, n/), woke with a communicative call, shook her head "no" (and "yes"), and combined gesture and vocalization to communicate (12- to 15-month age level). By her mother's report on the MCDI, Josephine had seven words in her expressive vocabulary, which is most typical of a 12-month-old at the 50th percentile and consistent with her RITLS performance.

Phonology

Josephine's spontaneous vocalizations were limited in number and were less than 50% intelligible. Given her few spontaneous vocalizations, her phonological repertoire was judged to include the consonants /b, d, g, n, m, j, s, tʃ, ʔ/, the vowels /a, ə, ɪ, o, u/, and the diphthongs /aʊ, aɪ/. Her syllable shape repertoire included C /s/, CV /do/, CVC /nʌm/, CVCV /daga/, CVCVV /dagaʊ/. She occasionally produced brief periods of redublicated babble (e.g., /nanoməʔoʊ/). In addition, she produced a prolonged /s/ while playing; /h/ was elicited through playful, nonspeech imitation. Meaningful productions of /g/ were fronted (/do/ for /go/).

Oral-Motor Examination

Structure, function, and sensory aspects of the mechanism appeared to be within functional limits (WFL) and sufficient to support speech development. For example, Josephine presented with neutral jaw posture at rest, good lip rounding for /u/ in spontaneous utterances, and tongue tip elevation for the production of alveolar phonemes /d, n/.

DIAGNOSIS AND PROGNOSIS

Josephine is a delightful 22-month-old who demonstrates a mild to moderate delay in expressive language and a moderate delay in speech sound development. Her expressive language delay is characterized by limited vocalizations including babbling, jargoning, or word approximations; a small vocabulary; and a delay in combining words. Her speech sound delay is characterized by a phonological and a syllable shape repertoire that are smaller than expected, particularly in terms of her vowel repertoire. Other aspects of language and cognition (prelinguistic skills, receptive language, and play) are well within normal limits.

Prognosis is good that Josephine will outgrow her expressive language delay given her established prelinguistic skills, strong play and receptive language abilities, reliance on gesture to communicate, and ability to imitate gestures. Of concern are her restricted vocalizations and limited imitation of speech, particularly given her good imitation of gestures.

RECOMMENDATIONS

1. Continue to enroll Josephine in speech-language therapy through her state's early intervention program. It is recommended that intervention goals target parent education and training of language facilitation techniques (e.g., recasts,

expansion, parallel talk). These techniques can be used throughout the day with Josephine during functional activities.

2. Reevaluate Josephine's speech and language skills through this clinic in 12 months to assess her progress toward age-expected milestones.

ROBERT (LT)

Sex: Male
Age: 27 months

SIGNIFICANT HISTORY

Robert is a 27-month-old boy who was referred to this appointment to reassess the status of his speech and language development. Robert's *prenatal/birth* history was significant for maternal pre-eclampsia and cesarean section delivery at 31 weeks gestation. He was admitted to the neonatal intensive care unit for 3 months after birth. *Medical* history was remarkable for heart murmur, VSD (Ventricular Septal Defect—s/p repair), hypothyroidism (Synthroid prescribed), gastroesophageal reflux (Prevacid prescribed), asthma (Pulmacort and Xopanex prescribed), and failure to thrive. History was negative for ear infections but *audiological testing* revealed questionable unilateral hearing loss in the left ear. An audiological reevaluation was planned for within 6 months.

Developmental milestones were delayed for motor, speech-language, and feeding development. For example, walking was delayed until 17 months (adjusted age), and at the time of this evaluation he was not yet eating a full diet of textured foods. *Speech-language* history was remarkable for a delay in speaking first words (18 months, adjusted age) and he was not yet combining words. He followed simple directions (e.g., "Sit down"), but his mother believed Robert to have limited attention skills for his age.

Robert had a history of *early intervention*. At the time of this evaluation, he had received physical therapy, occupational therapy, and speech-language therapy through an early intervention program. Robert was enrolled in a daycare program five days each week. He was described as happy and enjoyed playing with other children. *Family* history was remarkable for an uncle diagnosed with specific language impairment as a child.

CLINICAL PROCEDURES

Tests

MacArthur–Bates Communicative Development Inventories (CDIs)
Rossetti Infant–Toddler Language Scale (RITLS)

Other

Play-based interactions
Spontaneous speech-language sample
Oral mechanism exam

CLINICAL FINDINGS

General Observations

Robert was an interactive and pleasant boy who readily entered the playroom with his mother. Consistent with his mother's report, Robert presented with limited attention skills for his age. He became easily excitable and disorganized in his behavior. His attention and behavior were more typical of a child approximately 12 months of age. For example, he did not remain engaged in a play activity for very long but preferred to wander around the room or hide under the table. Robert was motivated to interact with adults and imitated adult models. These behaviors were strengths for him.

Play

Robert's performance on the RITLS revealed established play skills at the 9- to 12-month age level, with a scatter of emerging play skills up to the 21- to 24-month age level. His play was characterized predominately by banging/shaking objects and relational play (placing objects within each other). Functional use of objects was emerging, but functional play schemes were not part of his established play repertoire. Robert engaged in simple games, and he showed an emerging ability to perform actions with objects (e.g., throw a ball) and imitate adult actions (e.g., put a key in a door). He was not yet pretending with stuffed animals or dolls.

Nonverbal Communication

Relative to Robert's other skills, his prelinguistic communication was a strength for him. His gesture performance was most typical of a 9- to 12-month-old child on the RITLS, with a scatter of skills up to the 21- to 24-month-old level. He consistently demonstrated communicative eye contact, joint attention, and turn-taking behaviors (both verbal and nonverbal), as well as prelinguistic gestures (e.g., showing objects, giving objects, pointing, requesting). He used gesture to satisfy basic needs (e.g., nods head "no," leads caregiver to desired object, indicates diaper is wet).

Receptive Language

On the RITLS, Robert's comprehension skills were most typical of a 9- to 12-month-old child, with a scatter of skills up to the 21- to 24-month age level. For example, he responded to simple commands (e.g., "Give me"), responded to requests to say words, and chose two objects from an array of objects. However, he did not show interest in pictures, identify body parts, or follow commands that required him to complete two actions with an object. Robert demonstrated inconsistent attention to his name. He was also inconsistent in attending to gesture cues meant to scaffold his comprehension of spoken language.

Robert had difficulty attending to formal tests of receptive vocabulary, so the MCDI: Words and Gestures test was used informally to survey his comprehension of vocabulary. His performance on the MCDI revealed a receptive vocabulary of at least 194 items across a variety of categories, including clothing, household items, people, and descriptive words. This vocabulary size is considered typical of toddlers 18 to 24 months of age (normative range = 150–500 words; Miller & Paul, 1995).

Expressive Language

On the RITLS, Robert's expressive language was assessed to be most typical of a 9- to 12-month-old, with a scatter of skills up to the 15- to 18-month age level. His spontaneous vocalizations were predominately characteristic of reduplicated babbling and emerging variegated babbling (e.g., /mamamo/, /mimɪ/). Robert was not yet jargoning consistently or producing words within jargoned utterances. He was not yet combining pointing with words. Robert used fewer than 10 intelligible words during this session, but those expressed were for imitation (e.g., /nɛ/ for *night-night*) or for spontaneous naming (e.g., /o/ for *telephone*). His mother reported an expressive vocabulary of 14 words. His expressive vocabulary included 2 sound effects/animal sounds (i.e., *baa, uh oh*), 2 vehicles (*bus, car*), and several toy and routines items (*night-night, hi, bye*). Early developing morphemes (e.g., *-ing*) and early word combinations were not observed or reported (normative age range for emergence = 18–24 months).

A strength for Robert was his motivation to use spoken vocalizations to interact with others for a variety of pragmatic functions, including protest, response, initiation, and labeling. However, he was not yet engaging in adult-like dialogue or taking turns in conversation. He relied on gesture and vocalizations instead of words.

Phonology

Robert was less than 25% intelligible. His sound and syllable shape repertoires were most typical of a child 12 to 18 months of age. His phonological repertoire included a restricted set of consonants (/m, n, p, b, d, j, l, v, ʔ/), vowels (/i, ɪ, ɛ, e, ʌ, ʊ, o, a/), and a diphthong (/aʊ/). The following phonemes were not heard: /t, k, g, f, æ, u, ɔ, ɔɪ/. With immediate verbal models, the diphthong /aɪ/ was elicited in *night-night*. Robert's syllable shape repertoire was restricted to simple open syllables such as CV, V, VCV, and CVCV (e.g., /ba/, /o/, /ʌda/, /mimɪ/). Robert attempted to imitate words heard in conversation today. His attempts were largely accurate for simple syllables, with the exception of slight vowel distortions or diphthong reductions (e.g., /ba/ for *bye*) and final consonant deletions (e.g., /opɛ/ for *open*). Spontaneous productions of multisyllable words resulted in phonological simplifications (e.g., /o/ for *telephone*).

Oral–Motor Examination

Structure, function, and sensory aspects of the mechanism appeared to be largely within functional limits to support continued speech and language development, with the exception of reduced range of facial–labial movements for rounded phonemes and slightly reduced strength of facial–labial muscles for full and consistent bilabial plosion.

DIAGNOSIS AND PROGNOSIS

Robert is a delightful and engaging 27-month-old who demonstrates mild to moderate delays in speech as well as receptive and expressive language development. In addition, other cognitive areas that affect speech and language development present as delayed, including play, gesture, and attention skills. His speech, language, gesture, and play development are most typical of a 12- to 15-month-old child, with a scatter of emerging abilities up to the 21-month age level. His speech delay is characterized by reduced intelligibility owing to a small phoneme and syllable shape repertoire, and to a lesser extent by some subtle oral–motor weakness. His expressive language delay is characterized by a small expressive vocabulary, no jargon or use of jargon with words, and delay to combine words. His receptive language delay is characterized by inconsistent attention to spoken language, a small vocabulary, and limited comprehension of age-level directions.

Robert is at risk for continued speech and language delays given his delays in comprehension, play, and gesture. Prognosis for gains to be made with speech-language therapy appears to be good because his established prelinguistic social skills and his motivation to imitate adult models. Ongoing assessment of his attention development, auditory processing skills, and questionable hearing loss will need to be made to determine the etiology of his comprehension performance.

RECOMMENDATIONS

It is recommended that Robert continue to be enrolled in speech-language therapy. A play-based approach to intervention is most appropriate for him. Gesture and multimodal cueing will facilitate imitation (verbal and nonverbal) and development in a variety of skill areas (speech, language, play). Robert's attention, auditory processing skills, and questionable hearing loss should be continually assessed to determine how each contributes to his comprehension performance. Goals of speech-language intervention should include the following:

Long Term Goal 1: Robert will demonstrate developmentally appropriate attention skills to support continued social–emotional, cognitive, and language development.

- *Short Term Goal 1:* Increase intervals of sustained attention to objects, activities, and books.

Long Term Goal 2: Robert will demonstrate developmentally appropriate play skills to support continued social–emotional, cognitive, and language development.

- *Short Term Goal 1:* Expand Robert's play repertoire to include object exploration, cause–effect toys, and functional play schemes.
- *Short Term Goal 2:* Expand Robert's play repertoire to include symbolic play schemes and linking of play schemes for pretend play.

Long Term Goal 3: Robert will demonstrate developmentally appropriate receptive language skills to support functional communication and pre-academic development.

- *Short Term Goal 1:* Facilitate Robert's ability to direct attention to language spoken to him.
- *Short Term Goal 2:* Expand Robert's receptive vocabulary of words that are part of his daily routines.
- *Short Term Goal 3:* Increase comprehension of unfamiliar one-step directions that include identification of objects.

Long Term Goal 4: Robert will demonstrate developmentally appropriate expressive language skills to support functional communication and pre-academic development.

- *Short Term Goal 1:* Increase expressive vocabulary for functional communication that includes naming and requesting. Initial vocabulary targets should be organized around themes such as animals, body parts, house hold items, doll play, and vehicles.
- *Short Term Goal 2:* Establish use of personal identification by name (*Robert*) and early pronouns (*me, mine*).
- *Short Term Goal 3:* Establish Robert's ability to combine words that express early semantic relations.

- *Short Term Goal 4:* Establish Robert's ability to produce early developing morphemes to mark present progressive tense (*-ing*) and spatial relations (*in, on*).

Long Term Goal 5: Robert will demonstrate developmentally appropriate speech intelligibility to support functional communication and pre-academic development.

- *Short Term Goal 1:* Expand Robert's phonological repertoire to include velar stop consonants (/k, g/), alveolar stop /t/, and early-developing fricatives (/f, h/).
- *Short Term Goal 2:* Expand Robert's syllable shape repertoire to include closed syllable shapes (CVC, CVCVC, VC).

KEY TERMS

assessment	phonology
background history	pragmatics
evaluation	scaffolds
formal testing	semantics
functional communication context	speech-language pathologist
intervention	spontaneous language sampling
language	syntax
milestones	treatment
morphology	

STUDY QUESTIONS

- ✦ Define language and its five domains.
- ✦ What are the procedures of a language evaluation?
- ✦ How do clinicians use their knowledge of developmental milestones in the clinical practice of speech-language pathology?
- ✦ Compare and contrast long-term goals, short-term goals, and session objectives.
- ✦ What are some scaffolds that a clinician might use in language therapy?

REFERENCES

American Speech-Language-Hearing Association (1982). *Language.* Retrieved January 15, 2008, from www.asha.org/policy.

Applebee, A. (1978). *The child's concept of a story: Ages 2 to 17.* Chicago: University of Chicago Press.

Dunn, L. M., & Dunn, D. M. (2007). *The Peabody Picture Vocabulary Test,* 4th ed. Bloomington, MN: NCS Pearson.

Fenson, L., Marchman, V. A., Thal, D. J., Dale, P. S., Reznick, S., & Bates, E. (2006). *MacArthur–Bates Communicative Development Inventories*, 2nd ed. Baltimore: Brookes.

Goldman, R., & Fristoe, M. (2000). *Goldman–Fristoe Test of Articulation*, 2nd ed. Circle Pines, MN: American Guidance Services.

Miller, J.F., & Paul, R. (1995). *The clinical assessment of language comprehension*. Baltimore, MD: Brooks Publishing.

Retherford, K. (2000). *Guide to analysis of language transcripts*, 3rd ed. Eau Claire, WI: Thinking Publications.

Rossetti, L. (1990). *The Rossetti Infant–Toddler Language Scale*. East Moline, IL: LinguiSystems.

Shapiro, L. (1997). Tutorial: An introduction to syntax. *Journal of Speech, Language and Hearing Research, 40,* 254–272.

Williams, K. (1997). *Expressive Vocabulary Test*. Circle Pines, MN: American Guidance Services.

Zimmerman, I. L., Steiner, V. C., & Pond, R. E. (2002). *Preschool Language Scale*, 4th ed. San Antonio, TX: Psychological Corporation.

CHAPTER 2

Child Development

Theresa E. Bartolotta, PhD, and Brian B. Shulman, PhD

OBJECTIVES

+ Describe developmental milestones across multiple domains (cognition, motor, social–emotional, linguistic)
+ Discuss assessment of child development in natural environments
+ Review clinical tools for developmental assessment of children
+ Describe clinical applications of developmental assessment to language development

INTRODUCTION

This chapter introduces the developmental milestones achieved by children across multiple domains in the early years of life. It reviews each domain (cognitive development, fine and gross motor development, social–emotional development, language development) separately to define and describe significant achievements in each area. While clinicians must certainly have an understanding of each domain, the domains interact in an important way, so that achievements in one area result in growth in another area. For example, once a child learns to pull to standing and begins to explore the environment, the child is exposed to new stimuli, which in turn can enhance cognitive and language development. It is not a coincidence that typically developing one-year-old children learn to walk and use their first words at approximately the same time. Likewise, when a child experiences a delay in one area, the effects on other areas can be quite profound. For example, if a child has a diagnosis of cerebral palsy and, therefore, does not begin to walk until near the second birthday, the child's exposure to stimuli in the environment may be quite limited. This child's knowledge of the world may be affected because of limitations in opportunities to learn as a result of physical delays, which then influences the words to which the child is exposed and eventually begins to use.

This chapter begins with a review of key milestones in cognition, motor development (gross and fine), social–emotional achievements, and language development (including prelinguistic and early linguistic behaviors). It then reviews assessment in the child's natural environment using observation of the child combined with interview of parents or significant adults in the child's life. Clinical tools for developmental assessment that are commonly used by early childhood practitioners of differing backgrounds (speech-language pathologists, early childhood teachers, developmental psychologists) are described as well. The case studies are revisited with an eye toward the developmental information that might be gleaned from each assessment. In short, we consider how skills or delays in motor, cognitive, or social–affective development may influence the language development of each child.

COGNITIVE DEVELOPMENT

Cognitive development refers to the progressive and continuous growth of perception, memory, imagination, conception, judgment, and reason; it is the intellectual counterpart of one's biological adaptation to the environment (Nicolosi, Harryman, & Kresheck, 1989). Cognition also involves the mental activities of comprehending information and the processes of acquiring, organizing, remembering, and using knowledge (Owens, 2008). This knowledge is subsequently used for problem solving and generalization to novel situations.

Many theories have been proposed regarding how children learn about their environment and how cognitive development proceeds. One of the significant theorists in this area, Jean Piaget, viewed the child as an active participant in the learning process. He considered that new learning took place as the child interacted with the environment and with other people. According to Piaget, cognitive development is based primarily on four factors: maturation, physical experience, social interaction, and a general progression toward equilibrium (Piaget, 1954). Piaget's theories have withstood the test of time, and more recently have been considered in new light with regard to the effort that a child makes in learning language. For example, Bloom and Tinker (2001) have proposed a model for language development that suggests language emerges out of complex developments in cognition, social–emotional development, and motor skills. This model ties in nicely with what Piaget suggested more than 50 years ago—namely, that the child learns by acting on the environment (and with others). In other words, what begins as *sensorimotor* activity gradually transforms into *complex, abstract* thought.

For Piaget, cognitive or intellectual development is the process of restructuring knowledge. The process begins with a cognitive structure, or a particular way of thinking. This way of thinking is based on what the child currently knows or has experienced. As the child encounters a novel experience, *disequilibrium* is created. The child must compensate for this disturbance and solve the conflict between what he currently knows and his new experience. Piaget referred to this process as *adaptation* (Piaget, 1954). All organisms must adapt in response to changes in the environment, and it is through this process of adaptation that a child integrates new information.

Two aspects of the adaptation process are key: assimilation and accommodation. *Assimilation* refers to the child's attempts to incorporate new stimuli into existing cognitive schemas (structures). For example, suppose a child is familiar with dogs because there is a German shepherd at home, and then she encounters a poodle. The child is able to assimilate the features of the poodle into the cognitive schema she has for *dogs* because the poodle and the German shepherd share a number of core features. Thus, as the child encounters varied breeds of dogs in her life, she recognizes the common aspects that these animals share and incorporates the new features into her cognitive schema for *dogs*. This strategy allows the child to integrate and organize new information and assists in development of categories.

When a child encounters a new stimulus that does not fit into his existing cognitive schema, his cognitive processes undergo the process of *accommodation*, whereby new schemes are developed to integrate the new information. Thus, if a child encounters a donkey for the first time, he may initially try to incorporate this new animal into his cognitive schema for *dogs*. Of course, the donkey is a vastly different type of animal and cannot be integrated into the *dog* schema, so a new schema is created. As each of these adaptations in cognition is made, the child is continuing on his path to maintain equilibrium with the environment.

Multiple theories have been put forth regarding the process of cognitive development and the relationships between cognition and language. It is clear that cognition, at least initially, precedes language development, and many cognitive aspects are prerequisites to language development. The relationship between cognition and language likely grows more interdependent over time, as growth in one area fuels growth in another area. Although Piaget's theory of the stages of cognitive development in young children did not answer all questions about cognition in early childhood, his descriptions of cognitive achievements in childhood can help us understand other aspects of the child's behavior, including the acquisition of milestones in language development.

In observing children, Piaget noticed patterns in their responses to intellectual tasks. Children of similar ages responded in ways that were, at the same time, remarkably similar and yet remarkably different from adult responses and expectations. Likewise, children at different ages had their own characteristic way of responding (Labinowicz, 1980). **Table 2-1** illustrates the four cognitive developmental stages categorized by Piaget.

The first two stages of cognitive development, the sensorimotor and preoperational periods, are collectively termed the *preparatory, prelogical stages*. Likewise, the concrete and formal operational stages are collectively termed the *advanced, logical thinking* stages. Each individual stage, however, is characterized by specific developmental milestones.

Beginning at birth and extending to age two years, the child coordinates his physical actions. This stage is termed the sensorimotor period. The child's behavior, while primarily motoric, is described as *preoperational* and *preverbal*; there is no conceptual thought, although

TABLE 2-1	Piaget's Stages of Cognitive Development	
Stage	**Age Range**	**Summary**
Sensorimotor	Birth to 2 years	At the start of this period, the child is totally reflexive and reacts to stimuli in the environment. Sensory input results in a motor action—for example, sucking in response to stimuli on the face or cheek. Through repeated exposure, the child learns that a bottle provides nourishment and begins to suck in response to the sight of the bottle. The child then begins to take a more active role in the feeding situation and attempts to hold the bottle and then self-feed. By the end of this period, most reflexes are inhibited and the child's actions are deliberate and purposeful.
Preoperational	2–7 years	In this stage, the development of language and cognition are closely linked. The child's growing vocabulary and language skills allow for development of complex play skills and a greater use of social language, reflected in development of complex story telling. As the stage progresses, the child begins to understand that others share different viewpoints and begins to develop a sense of time. The child can think about things and events that aren't immediately present.
Concrete	7–11 years	As this stage progresses, the child begins to develop abstract thought and the ability to make rational judgments. Accommodation greatly increases here. The child can mentally manipulate information and problem-solve in a more sophisticated, though still concrete way.
Formal	11–15 years	Here cognition is fully developed. Now an adolescent, this person is able to consider multiple points of view when problem solving. Thought is more abstract and the adolescent can incorporate principles of logic.

Sources: Ginsburg & Opper (1988); Labinowicz (1980).

what begins as the infant's reflexive behavior evolves into intellectual behavior by the end of the sensorimotor period. The amount of cognitive growth that occurs during this stage is quite extraordinary. For that reason, Piaget subdivided the sensorimotor period into six stages (**Table 2-2**). Because of our interest in early cognitive and language development, it is important to look closely at these six stages, as the foundations of communication behavior are formed in this period. It also gives us a good opportunity to examine the close links between the various aspects of cognitive, motor, and linguistic development. As you review Table 2-2, consider how

TABLE 2-2   Piagetian Stages of the Sensorimotor Period: Birth to 2 Years of Age

Stage	Age Range	Features
Reflexive	Birth to 2 months	A child interacts with the environment purely through reflexes such as sucking, looking, or grasping.
Primary Circular Reactions	2–4 months	A child begins to coordinate sensory input and new motor patterns. For example, child may accidentally suck his thumb and enjoy the sensation. He later repeats the action.
Secondary Circular Reactions	4–8 months	Input–output patterns (schemas) become more complex and externally focused. A child may put a toy in his mouth repeatedly to trigger a response in the environment.
Coordination of Reactions	8–12 months	Intentional behavior is evident in this stage. A child will also combine schemas to achieve a desired effect. A child will imitate the behavior of others. A child will recognize that objects have particular qualities (e.g., a rattle is shaken, a ball is thrown).
Tertiary Circular Reactions	12–18 months	A child will explore new ways to achieve purposes. For example, the child may knock over a container to access something inside. The child is usually beginning to walk, and has great access to new aspects of the environment. Words also emerge, which give the child great power and control in this stage as communication is more sophisticated (e.g., child can request an object using the name, instead of having to retrieve it physically).
Early Representational Thought	18–24 months	Expanding language skills gives the child more ability to control the environment. The child can now talk about events and things that are not present using words. For example, a child can request "cookie" when none are in sight.

Sources: Ginsburg & Opper (1988); Labinowicz (1980).

each developmental milestone is marked by integrated changes in motor and communicative skills. This ideal progression is especially important to remember when we study children who do not follow a typical developmental path. Difficulties in one area, such as motor development can, therefore, affect communication or other developmental domains.

During the preoperational stage, ranging from two to seven years, the child is able to represent action through thought and language. His intellectual development at this stage is called *prelogical*. As the child matures and enters the advanced, logical thinking stages, he develops the ability to apply logical thought to concrete problems such as *reversibility* (the ability to follow a line of reasoning back to where it began), *seriation* (the ability to mentally arrange elements in a series according to value, size, or any other criterion), and *classification* (the act of grouping objects according to their similarities). As the child enters Piaget's formal operations stage of cognitive development, he begins to develop an ability to solve both verbal and scientific problems. Abstract thought and logical reasoning dominate the intellectual growth of the child at this final stage of cognitive development.

Later in this chapter, we will discuss assessment of cognitive skills. The professionals most often involved in assessment of cognitive skills in young children include psychologists, developmental pediatricians, and teachers.

MOTOR DEVELOPMENT

When we talk about motor development, we usually consider gross motor and fine motor skills. *Gross motor* skills refers to movements involving large muscles, such as trunk muscles used for sitting upright and leg muscles used for walking. Smaller muscles, such as those in the fingers or tongue, are used for *fine motor* tasks, such as writing or talking, respectively. The professionals who are most often involved in the assessment of motor skills in children include physical and occupational therapists.

The major motor development achievements of the first 18 months of life are highlighted in **Figure 2-1**. The data presented in this figure are based on an international, longitudinal study of more than 800 healthy children (WHO Multicentre Growth Reference Study Group, 2006).

As you study Figure 2-1, consider ranges of ages during which skills are expected to emerge. For example, the skill of walking can be expected to emerge anytime between 8 months of age and 18 months of age, with the median age expected to be 12 months. That is a wide window during which this skill may emerge. Thus a child who is not walking at 14 months is not necessarily impaired in gross motor development, although she should be evaluated carefully by an appropriately trained specialist who could assess evidence of other skills involving gross motor development. As can be seen from Figure 2-1, some gross motor skills should emerge earlier in development, such as crawling, walking with assistance, and then standing alone. If these skills are not yet present in a 14-month-old child, there may be greater cause for concern.

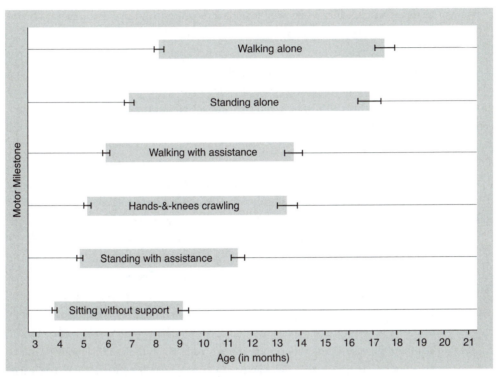

FIGURE 2-1   Windows of achievement for six gross motor milestones.
Source: WHO Multicentre Growth Reference Study Group (2006). WHO motor development study: Windows of achievement for six gross motor development milestones. *Acta Paediatrica Supplement, 450,* 86–95.

The value of using a scale that displays windows of achievement is that we can ask the question, "Which motor milestones should a child of a particular age have reached?" If the child is not demonstrating one or more of those skills, then perhaps careful reassessment or referral to a knowledgeable professional should begin.

SOCIAL–EMOTIONAL DEVELOPMENT

Social–emotional development in children is most often evaluated by psychologists and teachers. A child must be interested in socializing and communicating with others to be an effective communicator. Consequently, difficulties with social interaction can profoundly impair communication; indeed, this problem is one of the hallmark features of autism (Gerber, 2003).

In early infancy, we are most concerned with a child's connectedness with his world. This connectedness is initially expressed through nonverbal modes, such as eye contact and facial expression. The infant will produce a behavior that elicits a reaction in the environment. The infant will respond to this reaction, thereby resulting in learning. For example, in the first month of life, a baby will smile reflexively. There is no evidence that the smile is of itself a planned action. In response, adults in the environment will usually react in a positive manner, using exaggerated vocalizations and laughter. Over time, the infant learns that the smile elicits a very positive reaction from others. Thus, between two and seven months of age, we see the emergence of a social smile, which is a purposeful act. Its development is evidence that learning has taken place for this young child.

A key behavior that is of interest to those who work with young children is the ability to achieve and then maintain self-regulation. Development of regulatory capacity evolves from control of physiological responses to control of emotional state and attention (National Research Council & Institute of Medicine, 2000)—in other words, the child's ability to maintain *homeostasis*, or to keep everything in balance. When infants are first born, they have little regulatory capacity beyond keeping their physiological responses in balance, such as body temperature, heart rate, and respiration. These behaviors are not under the baby's volitional control. Initially, responses to stimulation in the environment are not under the baby's control, but rather occur automatically, leading them to be called *reflexive* responses. For example, an infant will startle in response to a noise or will begin to suck in response to a touch on the cheek. As the infant matures, these reflexes are integrated as the infant's ability to *self-regulate* (i.e., control the body) grows over time. The ability to self-regulate is very helpful to the learning process and is related to the adaptation process described by Piaget's theory of cognitive development.

All humans are bombarded with sensory input almost constantly. Our bodies are exposed to visual, auditory, tactile, and olfactory stimuli, as well as changes in temperature, motion, and balance. We must make decisions about how and when to respond to each of these stimuli. As we mature, we learn to ignore certain stimuli and to pay attention to others. This ability to discriminate between stimuli, and then determine which to ignore (or suppress) and which to attend to, is at the core of regulatory development.

Sleep–wake cycles are good examples of the development of regulation. In the first month of life, infants sleep many hours per day. They awaken briefly to feed and then fall asleep again for just a few hours. This pattern continues throughout the day and night, and results in parents who are constantly tired. After the first few weeks of life, the infant is able to maintain the awake state for a longer period of time, which provides the baby with an opportunity to observe and learn from her environment. The time during which the infant remains awake lengthens. Although the sleep periods lengthen, they decrease in number. This is an example of the development of regulation for the sleep–wake cycle. The result is a rested, alert baby and happy, rested parents! Now consider what happens when a baby is not well or has symptoms of "colic" (where the baby cries for hours at a time): Both baby and adult become dysregulated in this scenario and, as a result, are less attentive to and appreciative of stimuli.

Infants have a preference for faces, and it is through this preference that they establish the foundation for early social relationships with others. Children establish imitation skills by studying others in their environment. This practice begins as imitation of facial expressions (such as smiles) and then develops into imitation of more complex behaviors, such as actions on objects (e.g., throwing a ball, emptying a container), specific motor patterns (e.g., clapping, dancing), and eventually speech and language development. A strong social–emotional foundation is key to the development of verbal language behavior.

LINGUISTIC DEVELOPMENT

Other chapters in this text will cover the nuances of speech and language development in significant depth. Our purpose in this chapter, however, is to summarize the acquisition of major language milestones and to discuss the interaction of these behaviors with cognitive, motor, and social–emotional development. **Table 2-3** summarizes key communicative (linguistic) behaviors and links them with social–emotional milestones.

In the first two months of life, infants make sounds for limited purposes. They may cry to seek assistance, usually for fulfillment of a physical need such as hunger or other discomfort. When they are calm and in a regulated state, they may make pleasure sounds; these noises may sound like vowels, but are not yet true speech sounds. Nevertheless, these *quasi-resonant nuclei* may form the basis for later sound-making.

As the infant approaches three to four months of age, he produces cooing sounds, which approximate a single syllable consisting of a consonant and a vowel. The child's production of different vowels also increases and diversifies. Sometime after four months of age, the infant begins to babble, which consists of production of strings of consonant–vowel productions. Initially these vocalizations will consist of repetitions of the same sound pattern over and over (e.g., *ba-ba-ba*). As time goes on, the variety of sounds used in one string will vary, and the babble becomes more complex (e.g., *ba-ta-ba-taba-ti-ba-ti*).

Intonation, volume, and pitch begin to vary, too. As the infant approaches 9 to 10 months of age, this vocal pattern is called jargon. At this time, adults will report that the baby seems to be speaking a true language, except without true words. The jargon is often accompanied by gestures and body movements, as well as changes in facial expression. All of these developmental behaviors prepare the child to eventually use true words, first by themselves, and then in strings of longer and longer phrases.

Sometime around 10 to 12 months of age, the first word emerges. The first word is typically an approximation of the true word, in that the child must produce a simplified version

TABLE 2-3	Acquisition of Communication and Social–Emotional Milestones	
Age Range	**Communication**	**Social–Emotional**
Birth to 1 month	Reflexive smile	Homeostasis
	Crying	Self-regulation and interest in environment
	Cooing	
2–7 months	Selective attention to faces	Attachment formation with significant others
	Discriminates between faces	
	Social smile	Has a "falling in love" look with others
	Development of mutual eye gaze	
	Imitates some sounds	
	Responds to name	
	Smiles and vocalizes to mirror	
	Can make basic wants and needs known to influence environment	
7–12 months	Obeys some commands	Expresses different emotions
	Speaks one or more "words"	Takes turns with others
	Imitates inflections, rhythms, facial expression	Realizes he can have an effect on the environment
	Babbles	
	Develops jargon	
12–24 months	First true words and phrases	Develops independence
	Tries to "tell" stories	Engages in interactive play with adults
	Vocabulary growth spurt around 18 months	
	Begins two-word combinations	

Sources: Ginsburg & Opper (1988); National Research Council and Institute of Medicine (2000); Owens (2008).

because he cannot say all of the sounds in the right sequence. For example, *bottle* might be first said as *ba* or *baba*. Adults will recognize these first word attempts (or babbles) as true words and reinforce the child's attempt to speak, usually with much excitement. The child may repeat the word over again as a result of the adult's excitement. This is an example of the importance of a strong social bond in the development of communication skills.

Another development that will occur typically before the first birthday is imitation of adult speech. This seems to be both a word-learning strategy and a social bonding strategy for the child. Imitation serves many purposes for a young child learning to communicate. For instance, it is a way for the child to experiment with words, as adults will provide feedback to the child based on how appropriate the child's word choice was. It is also a way for the child to engage in a "conversation" with the adult, without requiring the child to have a large expressive vocabulary. Consider the following exchange between a 15-month-old child and her parent while walking in the park:

Parent: Oh, look at the bird! (points to a bird pecking at the ground)
Child: Ba. (gestures toward the bird)
Parent: Oh, do you like the bird? Isn't it pretty? I think it's eating. Look at it eat!
Child: A. (while looking at the bird)
Parent: That's right, it's eating.
Parent: Oh, it's going bye-bye. (points to the bird and waves as it flies away)
Child: Ba. (waves)

This brief exchange is a rich example of conversation as a word-learning experience and social opportunity for a young child. The child participates in an event (watching a bird) while hearing a noun (*bird*), a descriptor (*pretty*), and action words (*eat, eating, going, bye-bye*). The simultaneous exposure to an event linked with words provides an opportunity for the child to learn the meanings of words, thereby building both comprehension and vocabulary. Through use of imitation, the child is also able to participate in a verbal exchange with the parent or caregiver, over several turns, while using very few sounds or words.

Bloom and Tinker (2001) have proposed a three-component model of language development, termed the *intentionality model*, which emphasizes the impact of *engagement* (social and emotional development) and *effort* (cognitive development) in the process of language acquisition. In this model, the child's responsiveness to the environment, and his social connectedness to others, establishes for the child what is relevant to learn and what the motivation to learn is. The concept of cognitive effort concerns the work that is required in actively learning about the world. A child must be socially connected to the world and motivated to learn more about the world to figure out how to communicate with others. Thus the intentionality model brings together the components of cognition and social–emotional development and unites them with language in a clear way.

In this section, we have discussed the complex nature of development in young children and highlighted the interaction between various developmental domains (cognition, motor, social–emotional, and linguistic). Consideration of this interaction is important when assessing a child's development. In the next section, we highlight developmental assessment processes and review commonly used assessment tools for young children.

ASSESSMENT OF YOUNG CHILDREN

When a clinician wants to evaluate a young child's development, he or she should focus on four important factors: who, where, when, and how. Let's consider each in turn.

Who refers to the individuals involved in the evaluation process. An evaluation may be accomplished by a team of professionals (the preferred approach) or it may be carried out by one professional working independently (a less preferred, yet common approach). The personnel involved may vary based on which concerns are expressed about a child and how the referral process is initiated, for example. A parent may worry that a child is not yet talking at the age of 18 months and, after consulting with the child's pediatrician, be referred to an early intervention agency for assessment. These agencies, which are typically funded by state and/or federal governments, employ teams of professionals to evaluate children between birth and three years of age; if needed, they may also provide specialized interventions and instruction to children with disabilities and their families.

An alternate scenario arises when a child who is suspected of having a speech or language delay is referred to a speech-language pathologist for evaluation. This is often a very effective way to begin a developmental assessment, because the speech-language pathologist is trained to evaluate a child's overall development as well as focus critically on the acquisition of communication skills. If the speech-language pathologist suspects that a child may have a problem that affects areas of development other than (or in addition to) communication, the family can be referred to other specialists (such as physical or occupational therapists) or to early intervention teams for assessment.

Whether the child is being evaluated by one professional or a team of professionals, it is crucial that a parent (or caregiver, if a parent is not available) be included as part of the evaluation team. The parent can interpret the child's behavior; make the child feel comfortable and safe, thereby helping the child maintain a sense of balance and regulation; and engage the child in activities that will demonstrate specific skills for the evaluators to observe. The young child may be hesitant to interact with strangers and may not be able to display his best skills in an evaluation setting. However, in the presence of a familiar adult, the child may be able to play and socialize and display a range of skills.

Where refers to the setting of the assessment. For the birth-to-three population, U.S. federal guidelines require that children be assessed in their "natural" environment. This approach allows the evaluators to observe how the child interacts in typical situations using objects or toys that are familiar to the child. Evaluations most frequently occur in homes, daycare environments, or schools.

When refers to the timing of the assessment. Ideally, evaluations occur when a parent or other adult first raises a concern to a pediatrician or other knowledgeable professionals. Early diagnosis of developmental problems is known to lead to improved outcomes for children

(National Research Council & Institute of Medicine, 2000). Even if professionals' assessment determines that a child does not qualify for intervention services because the delay is quite small, they can still provide a family with suggestions to maximize the child's development growth and eliminate the need for any further concern.

How refers to the assessment tools that are used and the way they are administered. Information is collected about young children using three major assessment strategies:

- Direct *elicitation*, in which an evaluator asks a child to perform a task (e.g., running, stacking blocks, or imitating words)
- *Observation*, in which a child is given materials and the evaluators observe what the child does independently (e.g., the actions a child performs when given a doll, a truck, or a book)
- *Interview*, in which a familiar adult is asked a series of questions, usually about a skill that cannot be directly observed in the assessment setting (e.g., toileting, sleep patterns, or what occurs when the child is angry)

A large number of assessment tools are available for child development professionals to use when evaluating young children. The tools described here represent a selection of published, well-regarded tools that are currently used to evaluate young children. The first four tools measure communication skills specifically; the remaining tools evaluate children across multiple developmental domains. All of these tools may be administered by individual professionals (speech-language pathologists, teachers, psychologists, or other developmental specialists) or by professionals working in teams. They are most effectively used when administered in the presence of a parent or other knowledge adult, in a setting familiar to the child, using materials or toys familiar to the child. Refer to the manual that accompanies each tool for appropriate guidelines on administration.

Communication and Symbolic Behavior Scales

The *Communication and Symbolic Behavior Scales* (CSBS) (Wetherby & Prizant, 1993) is a standardized, norm-referenced test that can be used with children, from birth through the preschool years, who are at risk for communication difficulties. It can be administered by a speech-language pathologist or other child development professional in approximately one hour, using natural play routines or other typical adult–child interactions. As part of this assessment, a parent or caregiver completes a questionnaire that gleans information about the child's typical behaviors. The child is subsequently observed in structured play situations that are, ideally, videotaped to eliminate the need for examiners to take notes during the assessment. The child's language skills and use of symbols (i.e., gestures, facial expressions, and play) are then scored on the CSBS rating scales. Of value to examiners is a videotaped tutorial that provides training on the scoring system.

Child development professionals can use the CSBS to determine the degree of a child's communication impairment, identify areas of strength and need, and plan for intervention programs. The child's CSBS scores can then be used to chart progress as the child moves through an intervention program.

Rossetti Infant–Toddler Language Scale

The *Rossetti Infant–Toddler Language Scale* (RITLS; Rossetti, 1990) is a popular criterion-referenced measure that is used by speech-language pathologists to assess communication skills in the birth-to-three population. The RITLS, which is available in English and Spanish (Latin American dialect) versions, assesses interaction–attachment, pragmatics, gesture, play, and language comprehension and expression in children who may be at risk of communication impairment. It can be administered using a combination of observation, elicitation, and parent report of behaviors. A parent questionnaire can be completed in advance of the evaluation session to alert the examiner to areas of potential concern. Results of the RITLS are displayed on a graph in three-month intervals, highlighting the areas of strength and concern for a child. The manual now provides severity rating guidelines, which assist examiners in reporting the findings to parents and caregivers and can help in the development of intervention programs. The RITLS can also be readministered periodically to chart a child's progress over time.

Receptive–Expressive Emergent Language Test

The *Receptive–Expressive Emergent Language Test, Third Edition*, (REEL-3; Bzoch, League, & Brown, 2003), is a norm-referenced tool that evaluates a child's receptive and expressive language and vocabulary usage based on results of a caregiver interview. This assessment tool is designed to identify children through age three who have language impairments or other disabilities that result in impaired language skills. The REEL-3 can be administered in less than one hour and has proven to be a valid, reliable measure of language skills.

MacArthur–Bates Communicative Development Inventories

The *MacArthur–Bates Communicative Development Inventories* (CDIs), *Second Edition*, (Fenson, Marchman, Thal, Dale, Reznick, & Bates, 2006), is a norm-referenced tool, available in English and Spanish, that is used to measure language and communication skills of children between the ages of 8 and 37 months. Parents or caregivers complete standardized report forms that measure words, gestures, and sentences used by young children. The forms are then scored by a speech-language pathologist or other professional, with the entire process taking less than one hour. Guidelines on interpretation of scores and development of intervention programs are provided.

As discussed earlier, children are often evaluated by a team of professionals as part of an early intervention assessment. Many tools are available for professionals that measure multiple developmental domains in children. Some states or agencies may require that teams use only certain tools. Here we profile three commonly used tools that measure developmental skills in young children.

Hawaii Early Learning Profile

The *Hawaii Early Learning Profile* (HELP; Parks, 1992) comprises a series of curriculum-based assessments that measure cognitive, linguistic, gross and fine motor, social, and self-help skills in children between birth and six years of age. It is *not* a standardized tool, but rather provides a developmental sequence of skills across multiple domains that are used by professionals to identify needs of children, track growth and development of skills, and plan for intervention based on areas of need. The HELP tool is completed by professionals and parents working together in a naturalistic assessment setting. HELP: 0–3 is intended for use with the infant–toddler population, and HELP: Preschool is used for evaluation of children between three and six years of age.

Learning Accomplishment Profile

The *Learning Accomplishment Profile* (LAP) system (Chapel Hill Training-Outreach Project, 2004) is a series of screening and assessment tools that are used to measure developmental skills in children from birth through five years of age. The LAP, which is available in both English and Spanish versions, measures language, cognition, social–emotional, and fine and gross motor skills and is commonly used by preschool teachers or members of early intervention teams. A core feature of the LAP program is a set of curriculum guides that can be used in classrooms as well as in homes with individual children. For the birth-to-three-year population, the *Early Learning Accomplishment Profile* (Chapel Hill Training-Outreach Project, 2001) is designed to provide an early diagnosis of developmental difficulties that may require in-depth evaluations by specialized professionals.

Battelle Developmental Inventory

The *Battelle Developmental Inventory, Second Edition,* (BDI-2; Newborg, 2005), is a norm-referenced, developmental assessment tool for children from birth through age 7 years, 11 months. Like the other developmental tools described in this section, it measures personal–social, adaptive, motor, communication and cognitive ability. The BDI-2 screening test can be administered in less than 30 minutes and can be used to identify those children who should receive comprehensive assessments because of concerns about developmental abilities. This tool is administered by interviewing a parent or caregiver about a child's development. The results of the BDI-2 can also be used to identify targeted activities to help children reach developmental milestones.

CLINICAL APPLICATIONS OF DEVELOPMENTAL ASSESSMENT

When we examine the case studies, we see that the MBCDI and the RITLS are used to evaluate the language development of all three children (Johnathon, Josephine, and Robert). The "Significant History" section of each evaluation reports a concern about an aspect of communication development for each child.

JOHNATHON (TD)

Johnathon's mother was concerned that he was not yet using sentences and thought his vocabulary might be limited. Johnathon (the TD case), who was 25 months old at the time of his evaluation, met his developmental milestones in a timely manner. We see that there are no concerns regarding motor or cognitive skills, or even early language development. Johnathon used his first words at 12 months. His play skills were described as varied, and there were no reports of social or sensory difficulties.

When we review the results of the evaluation, we see that Johnathon's skills fall within the 21- to 27-month range. This is typical achievement for a child who is developing according to accepted norms. As discussed earlier in the chapter, there is a developmental window during which skills are expected to emerge. Johnathon's window of development for all his skills is solidly clustered within a few months on either side of his chronological age of 25 months. The findings of the evaluation were that Johnathon's skills were typical for his age and that he was not a candidate for intervention. The speech-language pathologist who conducted the evaluation spent time with Johnathon's mother, educating her regarding typical cognitive and language development. A speech-language pathologist might also provide examples of activities that could be used in daily activities to strengthen and expand Johnathon's play behavior and vocabulary skills.

JOSEPHINE (LB)

Josephine (the LB case) did not demonstrate such a well-balanced window of development as did Johnathon. At age 22 months, she was described as meeting her motor milestones on time, but her speech and language development was mildly delayed. In infancy, she did not use the range of vocalizations that were expected and her babbling was limited. Josephine used her first words at age 15 months, which is slightly delayed. At age 22 months, she was just producing two-syllable units—a skill that should be acquired much earlier in the second year of life. The emergence of two-word phrases is expected at this age, but the syllables she was making were not clearly words.

On the MBCDI and RITLS, Josephine's play behavior, nonverbal communication, and expressive language skills were all within close range of her age level (24–30 months). However, her expressive language skills were typical of a 9- to 12-month-old child, as she did not yet imitate words or use varied vocalizations such as babbling and jargon. Her window of development is quite large and demonstrates a moderate gap between expressive language and her other skills.

Based on this finding, it was recommended that Josephine be enrolled in speech and language intervention through an early intervention program. A critical part of the intervention will be parent education and training so that Josephine's communication skills can be maximized.

ROBERT (LT)

Robert (the LT case) has a more complex presentation than the other two children. At age 27 months, Robert's significant history is lengthy and complex. He has a history of health problems that includes premature birth and cardiac, thyroid, digestive, respiratory, and growth issues. He has been diagnosed with a possible hearing loss in one ear. Developmental milestones are delayed for motor, communication, and feeding skills.

Think back to our earlier discussion of the importance of the infant's ability to develop homeostasis and self-regulation in the early months of life. Robert was hospitalized for three months after birth, during which time he underwent cardiac surgery and received multiple medications. The lingering effects of this early difficult period in his life cannot be discounted. Robert's ability to develop social bonds with caregivers was likely affected as well.

At the time of the evaluation, Robert was able to follow some simple directions, but his mother was concerned about his attention skills. Recall the intentionality model of language acquisition proposed by Bloom and Tinker (2001). They emphasized the interaction between cognitive effort, social–emotional development, and language skills—and there are concerns in Robert's history about all three of these areas. A review of Robert's test results indicates that his skills are widely scattered; his window of development is very large. His play skills are solidly within the 9- to 12-month level but there is a scatter of emerging skills up to the 21- to 24-month level. His development is not proceeding in an orderly, systematic way. His nonverbal communication and receptive and expressive language skills are all solidly observed within the 9- to 12-month range, with scatters up to 24 months in some areas.

Robert's strengths are his happy demeanor and his interest in playing with other children. He also enjoys interacting with adults and imitated the adults during the evaluation. This is a good prognostic indicator, in that imitation may be a helpful strategy to use in intervention.

The finding of the evaluation was that Robert presented with a speech and language impairment as well as delays in cognitive, play, and attention skills. As a result, it was recommended that he be enrolled in intervention activities. Because he enjoyed play with others, a play-based approach that could capitalize on his strengths was recommended. An important issue to consider is his suspected hearing loss. It will be important that Robert's hearing be reassessed to determine its impact (if any) on his ability to attend and learn. It is important that Robert be provided with every opportunity to obtain the maximum benefit from all of his daily interactions as he works hard to engage with the world and acquire successful communication skills.

KEY TERMS

cognition   gross motor skills
fine motor skills   social–emotional development

STUDY QUESTIONS

+ Describe the processes of learning that occur when a child encounters a new object. Give an example, and speculate about how the child integrates the new information about the object into her existing knowledge about the world.
+ Describe the processes of learning that occur when a child hears a new word, including how the child integrates that knowledge into his existing vocabulary.

- What skills are required for a child to engage in a game of patty-cake with an adult? At what age would this skill be acquired?
- Learning to walk and talk occur at roughly the same time in a child's development. Describe how you think these processes are related, and how change in one aspect of development might influence change in another.

REFERENCES

Bloom, L., & Tinker, E. (2001). The intentionality model and language acquisition: Engagement, effort, and the essential tension. *Monographs of the Society for Research in Child Development, 66*(Serial No. 267).

Bzoch, K. R., League, R., & Brown, V. L. (2003). *Receptive–Expressive Emergent Language Test*, 3rd ed. Austin, TX: PRO-ED.

Chapel Hill Training-Outreach Project. (2001). *Early Learning Accomplishment Profile*. Lewisville, NC: Kaplan Early Learning Company.

Chapel Hill Training-Outreach Project. (2004). *Learning Accomplishment Profile*, 3rd ed. Lewisville, NC: Kaplan Early Learning Company.

Fenson, L., Marchman, V. A., Thal, D. J., Dale, P. S., Reznick, S., & Bates, E. (2006). *Macarthur–Bates Communicative Development Inventories*, 2nd ed. Baltimore: Brookes.

Gerber, S. (2003). A developmental perspective on language assessment and intervention for children on the autistic spectrum. *Topics in Language Disorders, 23*(2), 74–94.

Ginsberg, H. P., & Opper, S. (1988). *Piaget's Theory of Intellectual Development*, 3rd ed. Englewood Cliffs, NJ: Prentice-Hall.

Labinowicz, E. (1980). *The Piaget primer: Teaching, learning, teaching*. Menlo Park, CA: Addison-Wesley.

National Research Council & Institute of Medicine. (2000). *From neurons to neighborhoods: The science of early childhood development*. Washington, DC: National Academy Press.

Newborg, J. (2005). *Battelle Developmental Inventory*, 2nd ed. Itasca, IL: Riverside.

Nicolosi, L., Harryman, E., & Krescheck, J. (1989). *Terminology of Communication Disorders: Speech-Language-Hearing*, 3rd ed. Baltimore: Williams & Wilkins.

Owens, R. E. Jr. (2008). *Language Development: An Introduction*, 7th ed. New York: Pearson Education.

Parks, S. (1992). *Hawaii Early Learning Profile*. Palo Alto, CA: VORT.

Piaget, J. (1954). *The construction of reality in the child*. New York: Basic Books.

Rossetti, L. (1990). *The Rossetti Infant–Toddler Language Scale*. East Moline, IL: LinguiSystems.

Wetherby, A. M., & Prizant, B. M. (1993). *Communication and Symbolic Behavior Scales*. Baltimore: Brookes.

World Health Organization Multicentre Growth Reference Study Group. (2006). World Health Organization motor development study: Windows of achievement for six gross motor development milestones. *Acta Paediatrica Supplement, 450*, 86–95.

CHAPTER 3

Historical and Contemporary Views of the Nature–Nurture Debate: A Continuum of Perspectives for the Speech-Language Pathologist

Sima Gerber, PhD, and Lorain Szabo Wankoff, PhD

OBJECTIVES

+ Explore the continuum of the traditional "nature–nurture" debate as it relates to the acquisition of language
+ Understand the historical impact of the nature–nurture perspective on the field of speech-language pathology
+ Describe a contemporary model of language acquisition within the broader science of child development
+ Propose a perspective on using theories of language acquisition to guide the assessment of and intervention for children with language disorders

INTRODUCTION

In this chapter, we start the discussion with our shared interest in the amazing moment when a child says his first word or, in the case of children with language delays and disorders, the disappointing and unexpected moment when he does not. This is a defining time in the child's life, and in the life of his parents. The child who begins to talk at 12 months or so sees in the delighted faces of his caretakers that he has accomplished something extraordinary in this ordinary achievement. The parents of this child, in turn, experience the magic of knowing what their baby is thinking and feeling through his use of words.

The scenario is quite different for the child and his family when the first word is not spoken when expected; again, life will change. The child may experience the anxiety or frustration that naturally arises when there is a disconnect between what one knows and what one can express; the child may also sense his caretakers' concern as they wonder what has happened to the precious first words and perhaps begin to question, in worrisome ways, if their child is "normal."

Who are these children who do not speak when we might expect them to? In reality, they represent a continuum, including those children who are initially indistinguishable from their peers, aside from their late start in talking, and who will ultimately move on to typical functioning. The continuum also includes those children who will struggle throughout their lives with developing a linguistic system and with communicating. Distinguishing those children at the extreme ends of the continuum is not difficult; however, our understanding of the developmental components that have been affected in any particular child and the interplay between and among these components can be a challenge to disentangle.

While students of speech-language pathology traditionally begin their study of language development with an exploration of the nature–nurture debate, for many of the children they will work with, there is little debate. Most often, the parents have provided the "good enough" input that we assume is needed to activate language learning. Given this fact, we turn to the possibility that this child has come to the world with some disruptions in the biological endowments that lead to talking.

As an example, one of the authors of this chapter saw an 18-month-old child who had many developmental concerns. Timmy was experiencing delays in the following areas:

- Motor development, including difficulty standing, walking, and holding his body upright when sitting
- Emotional development, including a restricted range of affect and few reciprocal interactions
- Language development, including no single words, few sounds, and questionable comprehension
- Social-communication development, including few intentions expressed and minimal responsiveness to others
- Play development, including a limited range of interests in toys and objects

In Timmy's case, the absence of words was merely one of a rather complex composite of developmental derailments. Naturally, the questions Timmy's parents asked were the logical ones: Why wasn't he talking? How could they help him begin to talk? What would Timmy be like when he was five?

For those of us interested in helping children and parents experience the joys of shared communication, we begin our assessment and subsequently develop an intervention plan by trying to discover what separates the talking child from the nontalking child or, in some cases, the communicating child from the noncommunicating child. As we observe the child's interactions, we typically pose a first set of global diagnostic questions that will help us understand the underpinnings of the child's delay:

+ Does the child have the sensory abilities to learn language?
+ Does the child have the motor coordination skills needed to produce speech?
+ Does the child have the range of ideas and knowledge that serve as the foundations for language?
+ Does the child have the social interactive and affective capacities that lead to language?

If the answer to certain questions is "no"—for example, "She doesn't hear well enough to learn language"—we can begin the intervention process by providing the child with what she needs (e.g., hearing aids or a cochlear implant) and be confident that this is an appropriate starting point for accelerating the child's process of language learning. When the challenges are more pervasive—for example, limited social-affective capacities—the intervention process becomes less clearly defined. Nonetheless, our starting point for any child is our understanding of her developmental needs and the formulation of an initial program, which will require time and collaboration on the part of the child's educators, therapists, and, to a great extent, her parents.

Although some children we see will have identified biological, neurological, or sensory deficits, Timmy did not. His hearing was within normal limits, his neurological evaluation was unremarkable, and his genetic testing was negative. The possibility that his difficulties had biological underpinnings was inferred from the developmental derailments described previously and the absence of any environmental explanations for his delays.

Because there were significant concerns about Timmy's range of ideas and his social-affective capacities raised concerns, Timmy's speech-language pathologist began to formulate questions about his strengths and challenges in early capacities that are prerequisites for language acquisition. In some ways, these questions take us to the behavioral manifestations of the developmental capacities introduced in the four questions listed earlier and are posed with the hope that they will lead to determining intervention priorities based on the child's individual profile:

+ Can the child extract information from the world around him/her, processing what s/he sees and hears?
+ Can the child plan and execute the movements required for producing speech (i.e., for respiration, phonation, resonance, and articulation)?
+ Can the child learn from his/her interactions with the world and generalize beyond his/her immediate experience, create meaning at symbolic levels, and integrate new learning?
+ Can the child form social–affective relationships with his/her caretakers and other significant others in his/her life that are rooted in engagement, which include shared attention, intentionality, and reciprocity?

+ Can the child learn the rules of the language that govern the development of a linguistic system (i.e., phonological, syntactic, semantic, pragmatic)?

With our beginning answers to these questions and our initial hypotheses in place, we can start to shape the child's world of interactive, play, and linguistic experiences in a way that we hope will facilitate the induction of the form, content, and use of language.

As we consider the status of the nature–nurture debate in 2008, the contemporary science of child development informs this discussion in interesting new ways. In fact, this science suggests that the nature–nurture question as it relates to child development is obsolete. As Siegel (1999) suggests, "[T]here is no need to choose between brain or mind, biology or experience, nature or nurture. These divisions are unhelpful and inhibit clear thinking about an important and complex subject: the developing human mind" (p. xii).

Speech-language pathologists, whether they have articulated it or not, have always believed that experience has the power to shift the direction of development and, by inference, the child's developing neurological system. We now have evidence from contemporary science that supports the claim that experience affects brain architecture—which is welcome news to parents and educators alike. In fact, Siegel (1999) speaks of the neurobiology of interpersonal experiences and the way in which the structure and function of the brain are shaped by these experiences: "human connections shape the neural connections from which the mind emerges" (p. 2). Knowing the elements of experience that lead to further learning and healthy functioning translates immediately and significantly into the therapeutic interaction we facilitate with children who are experiencing atypical development.

As the science of the relationship between biology and experience becomes better defined, both new and seasoned students of speech-language pathology are obligated to periodically and frequently revisit what we know about the interaction between the contributions of the child's inborn capacities and the environmental influences that lead to the capacity to understand and produce language. We have come a long way from the unparalleled moment when Chomsky (1957) introduced the notion of the innate abilities that children bring to the task of learning language. As amazing as this moment was for students of child language, it was somewhat bewildering for those of us who wanted to help children who were not learning language naturally and/or easily. We wondered how to apply Chomsky's thinking, as we imagined what the implications of innate mechanisms were for language-disordered children.

The charge for this chapter is to review the traditional debate of nature–nurture and its impact on the world of speech-language pathology, present a model of language acquisition that is in sync with the best thinking in the science of language acquisition, and recast the nature–nurture debate within the contemporary science of child development. Specific examples of nature, nurture, and interactionist perspectives are reviewed as we consider their impact on our understanding the profiles of, the assessment of, and the treatment of children with language disorders. As we integrate what we have learned from these various discussions, we will keep Timmy and his parents in mind, imagining what a sound and scientific approach to systematically, yet naturally, facilitating his language development might look like.

NATURE, NURTURE, AND INTERACTIONIST VIEWS

The study of theories of language development is considered pro forma for undergraduate and graduate students in speech-language pathology. Theories of language acquisition are considered central to the education of the future speech-language pathologist for several reasons. First, theories that are *descriptively adequate* provide the student of language development with clues about what language knowledge is. The theoretical model provides an outline of what is learned by children when they acquire language. In fact, theories of language acquisition can predict the facts of development by providing a list of principles that guide development. Second, theories of language development that have *theoretical adequacy* will account for not only the facts of language development, but also the mechanisms of language learning—that is, "how" language is learned (Bohannon & Bonvillian, 2005).

Traditionally, the theoretical approaches that are typically included in accounts of language occupy different positions on a continuum with regard to how much emphasis is placed on the internal wiring of the child (i.e., the child's given *nature*) versus the environmental input that the child receives (i.e., *nurture*). The nature argument presumes that the organism (in this case, the child) comes heavily "wired" to perform the awesome task of acquiring language. The rationalist philosophy from the works of Descartes (1960/1637) and Plato (1960) underlies this nativistic psychology or nature argument for language learning. In contrast, John Locke's (1960/1690) empiricist philosophy underlies behaviorist psychology, or the nurture argument, which relies primarily on observable, environmental factors to explain language development. In contrast to these two views, an interactionist approach to language development focuses not only on structures and mechanisms internal to the child, but also on the powerful influence that experiential and social factors have in concert with unobservable mental faculties. For the interactionist, the focus is placed on both the process of acquisition (how language is learned) as well as the structure of the organism learning language.

These paradigms of language acquisition have influenced the work of speech-language professionals in many ways. Interestingly, by tracing the chronology of events for the nativistic, behavioral, and interactionist approaches to the development of language, we can begin to understand how the trends in modern language science have evolved over time, how they have been influenced by past paradigms, and, ultimately, how they have affected the profession of speech-language pathology over the last 50 or so years. Different paradigms and their differing perspectives will be described as they relate to two questions:

+ What children acquire when they acquire language
+ Which processes account for how children acquire language

Nature: Rationalist Paradigm

Transformational Generative Grammar—Chomsky	1957; 1965
Biological Bases	1960s–present
Developmental Psycholinguistics	1960s–present
Government Binding—Principles and Parameters—Chomsky	1980s
Minimalist Program—Chomsky	2000s
A Contemporary View—Pinker and Jackendoff	1990s–present

According to the rationalist philosophy, which gave rise to the nature perspective, the processes of the human intellect (e.g., sensation, perception, thinking, and problem solving) are characterized by principles of organization. These processes of cognition are qualitatively different from the fairly disorganized events that occur in the observable world. The organizing principles and processes that characterize cognitive structures are said to enable humans to make sense of events in the world. From this perspective, speaking and understanding language are considered fundamentally human traits that are biologically determined. In contrast, reading and writing require extensive metalinguistic abilities and are learned with much more effort and repetition, typically in a school setting (Catts & Kamhi, 2005; Sakai, 2005).

Transformational Generative Grammar—Chomsky

Within the nature perspective, linguistic formulations of language development, such as those proposed by Noam Chomsky, are central. The early versions of Chomsky's Transformational Generative Grammar (1957; 1965) described the innate knowledge that enables the native speaker to produce a potentially infinite number of novel utterances. Chomsky's goal was for his theory to have descriptive adequacy (i.e., to adequately describe human language knowledge) as well as explanatory adequacy (i.e., to adequately describe how the child acquires language).

Chomsky's Transformational Generative Grammar (1957; 1965) and then Government Binding, also known as Principles and Parameters (Chomsky, 1982), were elaborate descriptions of the native speaker-hearer's language knowledge of the components of language: syntax, semantics, and phonology. In the syntactic component, which was central to the Transformational Generative Grammar, the underlying level of meaning of an utterance was represented by the deep structure, whereas the superficial form of an utterance (the syntactic form that we hear or produce) was represented by the surface structure. Chomsky utilized the tools of structural linguistics to represent the form of deep and surface structures with phrase structure rules or tree diagrams through constituent analyses. In the syntactic component, the deep structures and surface structures of particular sentences were linked through a series of transformations that were captured and represented by transformational rules.

According to Chomsky's (1965) early view, the child brought a language acquisition device (LAD) armed with linguistic universals to the task of language learning. Each native speaker–hearer of a language appeared to possess a wealth of knowledge about his or her "grammar." (The linguist used the term "grammar" in the descriptive sense to denote the systematic knowledge that language users possess.) Chomsky termed this knowledge *linguistic competence*. In his account of language acquisition, the LAD was said to enable children to develop a language system fairly rapidly. This language system was sufficiently complex and generative, allowing children to create a potentially infinite number of novel utterances. This capacity was termed *linguistic creativity*, an ability which every native speaker-hearer clearly possessed (Chomsky, 1957; 1965).

Chomsky's description of language acquisition, according to Transformational Generative Grammar, suggested that the child's innate LAD armed with language universals could explain not only the rapidity and uniformity of the language acquisition process, but also the complexity of the language knowledge that is acquired (Chomsky, 1982; 1988). Early formulations argued that children were endowed with formal and substantive linguistic universals, such as the three components of the grammar (e.g., syntax, semantics, and phonology) and categories or units of language (e.g., parts of speech or phonological features) (McNeil, 1970). Later accounts described the innate capacities as inherent biases or constraints that empowered children to treat linguistic input in particular ways (Wexler, 1999). Thus children learning English might be listening for word order to signal grammatical relations, whereas children learning Hungarian might be listening for noun inflections for that information (Berko-Gleason, 2005; Slobin, 1979).

According to Transformational Generative Grammar and Principles and Parameters accounts of language acquisition, the child operated as a mini-linguist. That is, the child utilized not only the universal features that languages have in common, but would ultimately establish the parameters that make his particular language unique. As the child accrued more and more examples of his own language, he could generate hypotheses about how his language works, and these hypotheses would eventually be either confirmed or disconfirmed. Ultimately, the child was said to intuit a finite set of generative rules—that is, rules with the capacity to generate and understand a potentially infinite number of novel utterances.

Biological Bases

Although Chomsky was among the first to suggest that humans possess linguistic knowledge at birth, the psychologist Eric Lenneberg (1967) provided much of the groundwork for the view that language is biologically based. He argued that language, like walking but unlike writing, shows evidence of the following properties:

+ *Little variation within the species.* Lenneberg argued that all languages are characterized by a system of phonology, words, and syntax.
+ *Specific organic correlates.* Lenneberg argued that like walking but unlike writing, there is a universal timetable for the acquisition of language. He suggested that critical periods exist for second-language learning as well as for rehabilitation after language loss due to injury or insult to brain function.
+ *Heredity.* According to Lenneberg, even with environmental deprivation, the capacity for language exists—although it might be manifested in the use of signing, as seen in hearing-impaired individuals.
+ *No history within species.* Lenneberg argued that because we have no evidence for a more primitive human language, language must be an inherently human phenomenon (Lenneberg, 1967).

Recent arguments for the biological basis of language typically refer to data in several related areas. These include cerebral asymmetries for speech and language; critical periods for speech and language development; speech perception processes in infancy; central nervous system development; and genetic evidence from speech and language disorders research (Sakai, 2005; Werker & Tees, 1984). Furthermore, over the last 30 years, investigators have combined basic research in first language acquisition with research in brain imagery to understand how children become multilingual (Lust, 2007).

Those who argue for the biological basis of language cite data on cerebral asymmetries that are present even at birth in areas of the brain that are critical for language functioning. For example, the Sylvian fissure is longer and the planum temporal is larger on the left side of the brain than on the right side in the majority of fetal and newborn brains. Furthermore, the degree of asymmetry appears to increase as the brain matures, whereas plasticity of the brain decreases over time (Sakai, 2005).

Evidence for a critical period for language learning has traditionally come from studies of individuals who have experienced cerebral damage and language impairments after puberty. Rehabilitating the loss of language that occurs prior to puberty has typically been found to be less challenging than when this loss occurs after puberty (Sakai, 2005). Similarly, a critical period for language learning is often cited as evidence that second languages are easier to acquire before puberty than after. Finally, in the unique case of a child named Genie who was not exposed to language early in life, great difficulties in the acquisition of morphology and syntax were noted (Curtiss, 1974).

Findings from now-classic studies in infant speech perception have lent tremendous support for the nature thesis. In the original work, Eimas, Siqueland, Jusczyk, and Vigorito (1971) demonstrated that the sucking patterns of infants were modified as speech sound stimuli were changed. Infants as young as one month old could perceive the distinctions between /b/ and /p/ in the syllables [ba] and [pa]. Interestingly, the studies that followed this seminal work demonstrated that babies can make finer phonetic discriminations at 6 months of age than they can at 10 months when their experience with their own language is more extensive (Trehub, 1976; Werker & Tees, 1984).

The most recent and compelling evidence supporting a biological basis for language comes from findings that newborns adjust their high-amplitude sucking to preferentially listen to speech as compared to complex nonspeech analogues. In a study by Vouloumanos and Werker (2007), infants were presented with isolated syllables of human speech contrasted with nonspeech stimuli that controlled for critical spectral and temporal parameters of speech. With similar stimuli, it had previously been demonstrated that infants as young as two months of age preferred listening to speech. In the Vouloumanos and Werker (2007) study, newborn babies, who were one to four days old, demonstrated a similar bias for listening to speech when their contingent sucking responses to speech and nonspeech sounds were compared.

Arguments for the biological basis for speech and language also find support in the research on the growth and development of the central nervous system in the early years of life. These developments include massive increases in brain weight, the formation of myelin sheaths on the axons, and increases in the number of neuronal connectors in the cortex during the first years of life—all of which correlate with advancements in language abilities. Finally, data from genetic studies that show strong patterns of inheritance for family members of children with specific language impairment also provide support for proponents of a biological basis of language development (Sakai, 2005).

Developmental Psycholinguistics

Since the 1970s, research in psycholinguistics has provided further data to support the "nature" position. Utilizing the scientific method for empirical research, psycholinguists have systematically examined the concepts that grew out of Chomskian linguistics. Through their work, the field of psycholinguistics was born, and systematic studies of child and adult language processing proliferated. Psycholinguistic investigations described how language knowledge is used as well as how the language acquisition process takes place (Bever, 1970; Bransford & Franks, 1972; Brown, 1973; Fodor, Fodor, Garrett, & Lackner, 1974; Gleitman, Gleitman, & Shipley, 1972).

In an effort to describe how children ultimately acquire linguistic competence (i.e., intuitive knowledge of the rules of their language), child language researchers collected language samples and derived the rules that children appeared to be using even at the earliest stages of language development. Language data was analyzed and researchers attempted to establish the word classes that children were using by determining the position and distributional frequencies with which the words occurred in the samples, known as "pivot grammars" (Braine, 1963). Other researchers performed in-depth analyses of the emergence and use of grammatical morphology, describing the gradual acquisition of 14 grammatical morphemes (Brown, 1973; deVilliers & deVilliers, 1973).

As mentioned previously, nativistic notions about child language development changed over time. In response to the earlier Chomskian accounts of language knowledge, researchers in the early 1960s studied the emerging grammar of the young child while focusing on syntactic rules. In the late 1960s and early 1970s, however, Semantic Generativists focused on the role of semantics in language and language learning (Fillmore, 1968). Thus developmental psycholinguistic research shifted from an interest in syntax to an interest in the semantic knowledge that supports the development of syntax. Young children's knowledge of underlying semantic relations (e.g., agent, action, and object) was viewed as the impetus for their developing grammar, because semantic relations typically occurred in predictable positions in sentences. For example, in the frequently used declarative sentence type, the agent occupies the initial position and is typically the grammatical subject of the sentence (Schlesinger, 1977).

With the advent of the work of developmental psycholinguists such as Lois Bloom (1970), semantics or the content of child language was considered key to determining the child's grammar. The importance of nonlinguistic context in interpreting the meaning of the child's language was emphasized. Further, the acquisition of semantic categories such as spatial terms, dimensional terms, and semantic features was investigated in an effort to understand the unfolding of the child's semantic knowledge (Clark, 1973).

Government Binding—Principles and Parameters—Chomsky

Government Binding Theory was formulated in its most comprehensive form by Chomsky (1982). This account of language described idiosyncratic parameters of particular languages as well as universal principles across different languages. The idiosyncratic patterns of particular languages were captured in the "parameters," which were set differently for different languages. For example, the fact that a particular language differs in the direction in which it embeds its clauses to form complex sentences (right or left branching) is captured in the parameter setting of the particular language (Leonard & Loeb, 1988).

Research in language development was also influenced by Chomsky's theory of Principles and Parameters. For example, as noted by Leonard and Loeb (1988), the following three sentences appear to be superficially similar in that all three italicized forms have an antecedent.

However, the forms in sentences 1 and 2 are anaphors and are bound by the governing category (they refer to the head noun), whereas the pronominal "they" in sentence 3 can refer to a noun outside of the governing noun.

1. The girls liked *each other*.
2. The boys hurt *themselves*.
3. The children knew *they* were naughty.

In language development, children's use of simple pronominals without antecedents (e.g., *Mark likes him*) precedes their use of anaphors or pronouns with antecedents. Sentences with pronominals, which refer to a noun outside of the head noun, are acquired later (Leonard & Loeb, 1988).

Cross-linguistic evidence in child language has been a rich source of data supporting Chomsky's theory, as discussed by Leonard and Loeb (1988). For example, unlike Japanese- and Mandarin Chinese–speaking children, English-speaking children find the following sentences to be of increasing difficulty:

1. David fell to the ground when he reached the finish line.
2. When David reached the finish line, he fell to the ground.
3. When he reached the finish line, David fell to the ground.

In English, the branching direction parameter is set for right branching, where subordinate material typically occurs after the main clause, as in sentence 1. In Japanese and Mandarin Chinese, a left branching setting is required, so that subordinate material will typically occur first, as in sentences 2 and 3. Thus speakers of Japanese and Mandarin Chinese will have little difficulty recognizing referentially dependent forms or pronominals that precede the referents for which they stand (as in sentences 2 and 3) . By comparison, English-speaking children will be slower in acquiring left-branching sentences (Leonard & Loeb, 1988).

Minimalist Program—Chomsky

Most recently, Chomsky has presented his current theory as the "Minimalist Program" (Chomsky, 2002). As Pinker and Jackendoff (2005) suggest, Chomsky has scaled down his Extended Standard Theory (Chomsky, 1972) and Government Binding Theory (Chomsky, 1982) to create a "parsimonious" and "elegant" theory that is truly minimalist in its description of what the language faculty is (p. 219). In this version of his theory, Chomsky has reduced the language faculty to its narrowest form and has excluded information that had previously been incorporated on semantics, morphology, phonology, and grammatical relations. The minimalist commitment to including only the barest of necessities in the theory dictates only the inclusion of a level of representation for meaning, a level of representation for sound, and a recursive element called "merge" that provides the mechanism for joining words or phrases. This element accounts for the linguistic novelty of productions for native speaker-hearers and young children.

A Contemporary View—Pinker and Jackendoff

Pinker and Jackendoff (2005) maintain that this minimalist view is inadequate because it ignores 25 years of research in the areas of phonology, morphology, syntactic word order, lexical entries, and the connection of a grammar to language processing, all of which are critical for a theory of language acquisition.

Pinker and Jackendoff (2005) address more challenging questions, such as "What is included in the language faculty?", by arguing that the language faculty is an adaptation for the communication of knowledge. This specialized language faculty triggers the development of linguistic knowledge that uses at least four different mechanisms for conveying semantic relations: hierarchical structure, linear order, agreement, and case. According to these authors, the four mechanisms are sometimes used redundantly. In arguing against the Minimalist Program, Pinker and Jackendoff suggest that how the specialized language faculty is characterized must be based on existing research, not on a program or theory that is incompatible with the facts.

In the more recent incarnations of the "nature" paradigm, Pinker (2006) addresses the question, "What are the innate mechanisms necessary for language learning to take place?" Certain cognitive accomplishments, such as the representational function, are known prerequisites for language to unfold. Furthermore, metacognitive control or executive functioning to monitor the incoming stimuli, the motor output, and the learning that takes place is assumed. Finally, individuals must operate with an unfolding theory of mind as the "language instinct" or the language faculty does its work.

Despite the impact of nature arguments of language acquisition, the limitations of this view are worth noting. For example, contrary to earlier findings, recent evidence suggests that caretakers do respond to the language errors of youngsters, including the syntactic ones (Saxton, Galloway, & Backley, 1999). Furthermore, the assumption that language acquisition is essentially completed by four or five years of age has not been supported, nor has the critical period been clearly identified (Hulit & Howard, 2002). Finally, the notion that language is acquired through a species-specific LAD is controversial, as research into animal communication raises the question of whether language is fully unique to humans (Pinker, 1984).

Modern-day cognitive scientists continue to examine the relative contributions of cognitive prerequisites, preexisting language faculty, and the role of exposure or the experiences of the infant (Kuhl, 2004; Gopnick & Meltzoff, 1986; Clark, 2004). Based on the evidence gathered so far, it appears that the "nature" argument alone is not sufficient to explain the child's accomplishment in developing language. Rather, the relative importance of an innate language faculty versus environmental influence continues to be viewed as controversial.

Implications from a Nature Perspective: Understanding, Assessing, and Treating Children with Language Disorders

From the "nature" perspective, the assumptions about children who fail to develop language typically include the possibility that the child is experiencing deficits in the following areas:

+ The language faculty that the child brings to language learning
+ The language processor that the child brings to language learning
+ The ability to convert linguistic input into meaningful information that will enable the child to construct a grammar (Leonard, 1992)

In fact, these possibilities are considered most relevant to the discussion of children who are referred to as having a Specific Language Impairment (SLI). Such children seem endowed with many of the developmental capacities that are necessary for learning language, yet fall behind their typically developing peers in the acquisition of a linguistic system, in particular, the acquisition of the morphosyntactic rules of the grammar. In fact, children with SLI often have less well-developed morphosyntactic systems than younger children with comparable Mean Length of Utterance (MLUs), and these differences persist over time. Of interest here is the explanation that the grammatical limitations are based in the underlying grammatical representations. An extended optional infinitive account (Rice, Wexler & Cleave, 1995) and more recently, an agreement-tense omission model (Wexler, Schutze, & Rice, 1998) have been proposed as explanations for these grammatical problems

In terms of the assessment of and intervention with children with language impairments, the "nature" hypotheses led the way for many of the hallmarks of the clinical work of a speech-language pathologist. For example, assessing children's language to describe their knowledge of the rules of the grammar, particularly in terms of morphology and syntax, was clearly an outgrowth of the work of the linguists and psycholinguists of the time. Determining children's mean length of utterance and measuring their linguistic progress relative to this parameter (rather than relative to their chronological age) revolutionized our thinking about the stages and expectations of language acquisition. The use of samples of spontaneous language as the data to determine children's linguistic knowledge and intended meanings can also be attributed to the methodology learned from linguistic inquiry. These assessment goals and procedures brought our clinical evaluations into a new era and have had a lasting impact on our evaluation protocols.

In reference to intervention for children with language challenges, following the introduction of the "nature" perspective, goals of therapy were written based on inferences about what children needed to learn about the rules of their language and what they were ready to learn given their stage of language acquisition. The focus of these goals was clearly on syntax and, less frequently, on the semantics of language. Typical intervention goals addressed the child's lexicon, morphological elements, and syntactic structures that represent the foundations of the linguistic system.

Emphasis on expanding the child's length of utterance, the use of various sentence types, and the use of Brown's 14 grammatical morphemes took center stage in the intervention process.

In reference to strategies of language intervention, the notion of enhancing the processing of the informative elements in the linguistic signal also can be traced to our interpretations of the work of the "nature" perspective. For example, increasing the salience of the linguistic input would include using prosodic and syntactic bootstrapping techniques. Prosodic bootstrapping refers to the placement of target elements at the end of the utterance for greater salience (e.g., *Yes, she is* to emphasize the copula form); syntactic bootstrapping refers to teaching a particular verb form in several linguistic contexts to heighten the varied syntactic uses of the form (e.g., She *pushed me; Who pushed her?; Don't push*) (Nelson, 1998).

Despite the undeniable impact of linguistic theory on the field of speech-language pathology, a clear limitation that followed us into the present is this theory's more narrow focus on language form. Given that many children who experience difficulties in learning language are challenged in areas such as the development of the precursors to language, cognitive development, and social–affective development, interventions must often override attention to the structure of the language. Nonetheless, by embracing the thinking of linguists, the work of speech-language pathologists moved into the realm of linguistic science.

Nurture: Behaviorist Paradigm

Classical Conditioning	early 1900s
Operant Conditioning	1950s–present
Mediational Models	1960s–1970s

The impetus for the nurture argument in learning and language was the "blank slate" philosophy of John Locke (1960/1690). This empiricist approach eventually gave rise to behaviorism in psychology. According to this perspective, explanations of behavior rely only on observable phenomena; in the most radical version of this position, no inferences regarding internal, unobservable events are made. Thus researchers and theoreticians who focused on the impact of the environment targeted primarily observable and measurable events to explain development.

Classical Conditioning

Classical conditioning was associated with the twentieth-century Russian physiologist Pavlov (1902). In his most famous experiment, a dog was presented with food along with the ringing of a bell. After repeated pairings of the two, the dogs would salivate upon hearing the bell even before the meat powder was introduced. Through classical conditioning, an association (a conditioned response) was formed between the bell and salivation; this association had not previously existed. While the meat powder was termed the "unconditioned stimulus," the bell became the "conditioned stimulus." Salivation was the "unconditioned response" to the meat powder and the "conditioned response" to the bell. The phenomenon of stimulus generalization was observed as well. That is, although the conditioned response would fade or become extinguished with time, before its extinction, some salivation could be elicited by similar bells (Cairns & Cairns, 1975; Pavlov, 1902). Pavlov's classical conditioning paradigm introduced the world of psychology to the concepts of stimulus, response, paired association, and stimulus generalization.

Operant Conditioning

The paradigm of operant conditioning, including the notion of a verbal operant such as "tacts" (naming behaviors) and "mands" (commands), was developed by B. F. Skinner (1957). Proponents of this "nurture" view argued that although environmental stimuli were not always identifiable, the frequency of certain behaviors or antecedent behaviors could be increased if positive reinforcers (or consequences) were contingent upon the targets.

The principles of operant conditioning were derived from and based on observations made and data collected in animal laboratories. For example, if a rat in a cage received reinforcement with pellets of food for its bar pressing (i.e., bar pressing that was initially accidental), the frequency of its bar pressing was found to increase. Also, the type of response could be shaped through a schedule of reinforcement of successive approximations to the target stimulus.

In these views, explanations for the acquisition of speech and language relied heavily on the role of imitation as well as paired associations between unconditioned stimuli (e.g., food or a bottle) and unconditioned responses (e.g., physiological vocalizations). Invoking principles of classical conditioning, phonological productions or vocalizations would be the conditioned responses to the caretaker's vocalizations (i.e., conditioned stimuli) that had been paired with the unconditioned stimuli (e.g., food or bottle).

The law of effect (i.e., the intensity and frequency of a response will increase with reinforcement, a principle of operant conditioning) was utilized to explain the acquisition of the production of words. Language acquisition was viewed as the result of gradual or systematic reinforcement of desirable or target behaviors. Thus, initially, gross approximations of the target (e.g., any vocalization at all), would be reinforced. According to this view, parents would teach children language through both imitation training of words and phrases as well as the shaping of phrases and sentences through successive approximations of adult-like speech.

From the perspective of conditioning, the sentence was described as a chain of associated events. Each word would serve as the response to the preceding word and the stimulus to the following word. According to the argument, grammatical categories and various sentence types could be learned through contextual generalization. In this explanation, children would generalize grammatical categories based on word position (Braine, 1966).

Mediational Models

Because stimulus–response approaches were reserved for describing and explaining observable phenomena, behaviorists became more creative in their attempts to invoke explanations of unobservable phenomena. For example, by the 1960s, mediational models (Mowrer, 1960) were being developed to help explain how the acquisition of meaning could be accounted for in behavioral terms. Meaning was described as the internal response that had become paired with an initial response to an object or event. In turn, a word was a conditioned stimulus that had become paired with some event or person. Ultimately, the word or the conditioned stimulus could come to elicit a conditioned response or a meaning response.

As with the "nature" theories, "nurture" explanations had some limitations. Although selective reinforcement and paired associations could account for certain aspects of sound and word learning, relying solely on principles of behaviorism to explain the acquisition of language knowledge proved inadequate. Stimulus–response explanations could not begin to describe or explain the development of the complex system of language knowledge that the young child acquires in such a short amount of time. Behaviorists were challenged to account for unobservable meaning knowledge, utterance novelty and complexity, and the rapidity with which language was typically acquired. Critics argued that parents more typically would give children feedback about their inaccuracies in meaning rather than about their inaccuracies in syntax.

While mediational models and left-to-right probabilistic models (Staats, 1968) were developed to explain the acquisition of meaning and sentence novelty in stimulus–response terms, their explanations did not prove convincing. Nevertheless, although the behavioral, mediational, and left-to-right probabilistic models did not effectively account for unobservable and complex language knowledge, behavioral psychology did make valuable contributions to psychology in general and to the speech-language pathology field in particular.

Implications from a Nurture Perspective: Understanding, Assessing, and Treating Children with Language Disorders

Given the constructs of the "nurture" theories, these concepts ultimately added little to our understanding of the underlying origins of language disorders in children. Nevertheless, the impact of the behavioral paradigm on assessment and intervention has been pervasive in our field.

In reference to assessment protocols, the emphasis on observation of behavior, data-driven descriptions, quantification, and measurement began to define speech-language pathologists' evaluation of language. The use of standardized, formal tests for identifying deficits in all areas of language became, and has continued to be, the anchor of speech and language evaluations. In addition, principles from this approach have been used in IDEA legislation and its amendments. For example, legal documents such as the individualized education plan and individual family service plan must be generated for children with special needs, including those with language disorders, to assure that these children receive the assessments and services to which they are entitled. These documents identify goals, which are written in terms of observable behaviors, specify mandates for treatment, indicate performance criteria for achieving goals, and clarify the context in which the target behavior is to be elicited. The primary concern is to quantify behavioral change so as to document the treatment efficacy of the intervention used. In this sense, the construct of assessment expanded to include not only the initial evaluation of the child, but also periodic, data-driven reevaluations to determine the extent of the child's progress and learning relative to previously established goals.

The "nurture" paradigms have had a profound impact on speech-language interventions. From both a historical perspective and a contemporary one, the use of behavioral programs such as applied behavioral analysis and variations of this methodology has defined a great deal of the work done within the speech-language pathology field. More than 40 years of research generated from this perspective has documented treatment efficacy in the training of children with communication and language impairments.

During the 1960s and 1970s, language training programs were developed under the aegis of the stimulus–response psychology model (Gray & Ryan, 1973). Many of these programs were characterized by the use of constructs from classical and operant conditioning, including the identification of antecedent and consequent events, specification of the desired response, determination of effective reinforcers, implementation of schedules of reinforcement, and use of strategies such as imitation, shaping, successive approximations, prompting, modeling, and generalization. While behavioral approaches to intervention vary, their common characteristics include highly structured contexts, adult-directed operant conditioning procedures, and reliance on preset curricula.

Applied behavior analysis (ABA) introduced by Lovaas (1977) was an outgrowth of the operant conditioning paradigm and has continued to be a popular approach to enhancing language development, particularly for children on the autistic spectrum. In ABA, an individualized treatment program is developed for each child. Based on the child's strengths and weaknesses, a curriculum focusing on skills such as matching, imitation, play, and receptive and expressive language is developed. Variations of Lovaas' ABA method include the Natural Language Paradigm and Pivotal Response Treatment (Koegel & Koegel, 2006) which focus on motivation and the child's self-initiations.

Finally, in reference to generalization, criticisms of behavioral approaches have often centered around the child's difficulty using his newly learned behaviors in the contexts of his daily life. Milieu or incidental teaching was designed to address this issue by using naturally occurring learning contexts and child-initiated topics as the content of the interaction in an attempt to enhance generalization (Warren & Kaiser, 1986).

As Nelson (1998) suggests, the irony of using behavioral approaches for language intervention was "that language seems to be too complex a system for some children to master on their own, but breaking it down into manageable pieces does not make it simpler so much as different" (p. 61). Nonetheless, the use of structured approaches to language intervention has held tremendous appeal for speech-language pathologists and policy makers who are attracted to the science underlying evidence-based practice. The significant incongruity between the foundational principles of the "nature" arguments (role of the child's inborn capacities) and the "nurture" arguments (role of the child's environment) has presented a dilemma for clinicians who are looking to theoretical paradigms to govern their work. This need for rapprochement of conflicting ideologies has been, and continues to be, a frequently revisited theme in clinical intervention.

Interactionist: Cognitive Interactionist Paradigm

Information Processing Models   late 1800s–present

Cognitive-Constructivist Models   early 1900s–present

Interactionist models of language development can be discussed relative to two paradigms: cognitive interactionist (Information Processing and Cognitive-Constructivist) and social interactionist (Social-Cognitive; Social-Pragmatic; Intentionality Model). Within each of these paradigms, various perspectives can be described, all of which presume that the child brings some preexisting information to the task of language learning and that her environmental input plays a significant role in her language development. The specifics of what the child brings to language learning and how the environment interacts with these innate capacities varies within these views. While they are grouped together as interactionist views in this section, the implications of each perspective for speech-language pathologists are dealt with separately to reflect the unique contribution each has had on the discipline.

Information Processing Models

In a historical description of information processing approaches to language, Klein and Moses (1999) note that in the late nineteenth century and early twentieth century, Broca and Gall were among the first researchers to try to locate language functions in the brain. The connection between brain function and language was studied in victims of brain injury due to stroke, in patients with traumatic war-related injuries, and, ultimately, in children with language disorders and learning disabilities. Descriptions of brain function and modes of language processing as well as perceptual–motor aspects of childhood language disorders were described by Cruickshank (1967) and Johnson and Mykelbust (1967).

An information processing model of language was eventually developed by Osgood (1963). Osgood's model identified the modalities that were said to underlie language functioning—namely, visual and auditory memory, auditory discrimination, visual association, visual reception, and auditory closure. Traditional information-processing accounts of language development described language processing as a series of steps that were said to occur consecutively or serially, where the steps included attention, sensation, speech perception, lexical search, syntactic processing, and memory storage (Cairns & Cairns, 1975).

More recent information-processing accounts of language, which are sometimes referred to as "connectionistic," describe parallel processing rather than serial processing of language. According to this view, networks of processors are connected and several operations or decisions may occur simultaneously (Bohannon & Bonvillian, 2005). These multilayered networks of connections function to interpret linguistic input from the exemplars provided to them. The statistical properties of syntactic forms determine their rate of acquisition, and cues that consistently signal particular meanings should be acquired first.

Research reported by Bates and MacWhinney (1987) and MacWhinney (1987) has offered support for this view by using data from the acquisition of several languages, including French, English, Italian, Turkish, and Hungarian. For example, Turkish children, whose language has an extremely reliable case-marking system, master case considerably sooner than word order, which has often been considered a universal cue to sentence meaning over other cues (Bohannon & Bonvillian, 2005; Slobin & Bever, 1982).

Critics of the connectionist model include those who question the paradigm on theoretical grounds. While information processing networks might provide neat explanations for describing linguistic rules, they resemble biological systems only superficially (Berko-Gleason, 2005; Fodor & Pylyshyn, 1988; Sampson, 1987). Most importantly, these connectionist accounts omit any mention of social interaction.

Implications from an Information Processing Perspective: Understanding, Assessing, and Treating Children with Language Disorders

Clearly, the information processing perspective, in attempting to explain the origins of childhood language disorders, supports the view that the child has difficulty processing the information necessary for learning a language. In fact, this perspective resonates in contemporary thinking which claims deficits in information processing and executive functioning underlie language-learning disabilities.

In terms of language assessment, the models described earlier served as the impetus for the development of many tests that continue to be used widely by speech-language pathologists. For example, the Illinois Test of Psycholinguistic Abilities (ITPA) developed by Osgood (1963) reflected the notion of different levels of language functioning (e.g., receptive, expressive, and associative) and different modalities of language (e.g., verbal, auditory, and visual). The idea of discrete components of processing that can be isolated, tested, and ultimately remediated is a familiar construct in contemporary practice. Use of formal language testing continues to be the accepted protocol for securing speech and language services for children suspected of having language-learning difficulties. The proliferation of speech and language testing materials in the last 40 years reflects this practice. In fact, the ITPA-3 (Hammill, Mather, & Roberts, 2001), a revision of the earlier test, speaks to the continuing interest in this approach to language assessment.

In reference to treatment, many speech-language pathologists support the use of intervention programs that reflect the belief in processing mechanisms as the underpinnings for language learning. Consider the prevalence of auditory processing programs such as *Fast ForWord* and auditory integration training. The premise of these programs is that the child's difficulty in processing auditory signals has contributed to disruption in the child's comprehension and/or production of language. Viewed from a somewhat different perspective, language intervention programs designed to facilitate the child's development of executive functions such as organization, memory, and retrieval reflect the notion that discrete language functions underlie language learning and can be remediated if deficient, resulting in improved language performance.

Information processing models have had far-reaching effects on the field of communication disorders. Our clinical wisdom tells us that this is a productive approach to take with some children who have language-learning difficulties. Even so, the idea that this perspective describes the challenges faced by *all* children with language disorders and, therefore, represents the approach to be taken with *all* children would be criticized from within the clinical world of speech-language pathology as well as from more contemporary research findings about the relationship between processing and language acquisition (Gillam et al., 2008).

Cognitive-Constructivist Models

Jean Piaget, a Swiss biologist who referred to himself as a genetic epistemologist, became fascinated with the acquisition of knowledge and the "activity" of the body and mind that lead to intellectual growth (Flavell, 1963). His keen observations of children as they engaged in exploration, play, and problem solving provided the data for his model of functional invariants:

- *Adaptation*, which consists of assimilation and accommodation (i.e., the mechanisms for the acquisition of knowledge)
- *Schemas*, or mental structures, which corresponded to consistencies in the infant's or child's behaviors or actions
- *Assimilation*, which occurs when a child applies a mental schema to an event, and which embodies play, exploration, and learning about the environment

+ *Accommodation,* which occurs as a result of the child's new experience with an object,
event, or person, and which embodies the child's ability to incorporate the new information, resulting in changes in the child's mental schemas (Piaget, 1952)

From a Piagetian perspective, learning is accomplished throughout the lifespan by active
participation of infants, children, and adults. For example, children pursue their goals and
interests while their mental schemas are adapted to new experiences. Children were said to
direct their own learning as they encountered new experiences and challenges during their ongoing interactions in the world (Flavell, 1963).

Piaget (1952) noted that there were qualitative differences in how children would respond
to external events over time. These qualitative differences were captured in his account of
developmental stages from birth until formal, scientific operational thought, the cornerstone of
scientific inquiry.

In the realm of language development, the traditional Piagetian view maintains that a direct relationship exists between cognitive achievements and later linguistic attainments. More
specifically, Piagetian theory predicts that cognitive prerequisites for early word learning, in
the sensorimotor period (i.e., the first two years of life) include concepts of object permanence,
intentionality, causality, deferred imitation, and symbolic play (Piaget, 1955).

Critics of Piagetian theory and neo-Piagetians have questioned several of Piaget's
assertions. For example, researchers report that certain accomplishments, such as imitation
of tongue movement, occur much earlier than Piaget reported. Other researchers believe that
the systematic evolution of mental structures does not explain development because there is
wide variation in when these accomplishments are attained by children beyond the differences accounted for in Piaget's concepts of horizontal and vertical decalage. Finally, some
neo-Piagetians argue that with training, children can accomplish cognitive tasks that they
do not discover on their own. This performance contradicts Piaget's assertion that cognitive
achievements are the result of the child's independent mental activity.

Implications from a Cognitive-Constructivist Perspective: Understanding, Assessing, and Treating Children with Language Disorders

Given the relationship between cognition and language presented by Piaget, the notion that
children with language disorders might be exhibiting language delays because of their cognitive
deficits took center stage. The nature of language disorders was now reconsidered from this perspective with an eye toward identifying the cognitive prerequisites to language, from birth through
early childhood, as the potential source of the disruption in language learning. In addition, the fact
that language was just one of a number of symbolic behaviors paved the way for considering language impairments as a reflection of a symbolic disorder rather than a language disorder alone. In
fact, this period marked the beginning of a new line of inquiry relative to the cognitive abilities of

children with specific language impairment. The possibility that these children might have unrecognized cognitive deficits led to a reconsideration of what was meant by "normal" cognition and to a new arena for studying the relationship between cognition and language (Johnston, 1994).

This view of the cognitive underpinnings to language found a place in the assessment protocols used by speech-language pathologists in a number of ways. First, assessment of the sensorimotor stages of development was now included in language evaluations as clinicians began to assess children's abilities in areas such as object permanence, means-end behavior, and causality. Second, children's play itself was seen as a rich source of information about their ideas and schemas as well as their overall cognitive achievements. The use of developmental paradigms to systematically assess stages of play became a central component of language evaluations and is considered by many to be the heart of the assessment process (Westby, 1980; Westby, 2000). The interest in children's symbolic capacity, rather than language alone, moved the assessment process beyond children's rules of language to the potential foundations for their thinking and, therefore, talking.

In reference to intervention, Piaget's theories and the subsequent applications of these theories to the study of language acquisition had a tremendous impact on both the goals and the contexts of language intervention. For example, the repertoire of goals typically began to include cognitive behaviors such as the sensorimotor developments mentioned earlier. The notion that children must acquire a broad foundation of ideas and world knowledge prior to talking gave speech-language pathologists license to facilitate development in areas other than language.

The importance of children's developmental stage, rather than just their chronological age, was emphasized as intervention was planned according to what was developmentally appropriate for each child's cognitive stage. Furthermore, the emphasis on play as both a goal and a context of therapy represented another distinct shift in focus away from linguistic goals and structured, adult-directed interactions. The view that children were active learners in their developmental processes led speech-language pathologists to encourage children to interact more freely with toys and objects as they explored the world and learned through this exploration. Although the relationship between cognition and language was delineated, the exact nature of this relationship—including the particular cognitive prerequisites to language—was not necessarily agreed upon. Nonetheless, the idea that cognition supports language acquisition and that the two are integrally related throughout the developmental process shifted and broadened the work (and play) of the speech-language pathologist.

Interactionist: Social Interactionist Paradigm

Social-Cognitive Models	mid-1900s–present
Social-Pragmatic Models	mid-1900s–present
Intentionality Model	2001

Social-Cognitive Models

Other developmental interactionists who have influenced the language learning research include Vygotsky (1986) and Bruner (1975; 1977). Vygotsky believed that children's cognitive development resulted from interaction between children's innate skills and their social experiences with peers, adults, and the culture in general. In addition, Vygotsky is well known for his description of the "zone of proximal development"—that is, the area between what a child can accomplish independently and what he can accomplish with another person who has greater knowledge, experience, or skill in the area. When collaborating on a task, the child and the adult engage in a dialogue that is then stored away by the child for future use as "private speech." According to Vygotsky, when language emerges in the form of private speech, it can be used as a tool to guide and direct problem-solving and other cognitive activities.

Similarly, Bruner's work (1975; 1977) was pioneering relative to social interactionist theories of language acquisition. Bruner (1977) suggested that when caregivers and their infants engage in joint referencing, they share a common focus of interest that ultimately contributes to language acquisition. Three mechanisms (indicating, deictic terms, and naming) serve to establish joint reference between a caregiver and baby, essentially laying the groundwork for "cracking the linguistic code" and providing entry into the language acquisition process. For example, when "indicating," the caregiver will use gestural, postural, or vocal means to get the baby's attention. With time, these indicators become more conventional symbols as the caregiver adjusts his or her communication to the level of the child. If the child reaches for an object that the caretaker is holding or if the child looks at the caretaker, the child is likely to receive an enthusiastic response from the adult. When the child begins to use gestures and vocalizations to show, point, or give objects, the caregiver will typically respond verbally, vocally, or gesturally to the child. When using "deictic terms" (e.g., *here, there, this, that, you, me*) with changing referents, caregivers incorporate spatial and contextual cues to assist children in comprehending this terminology. "Naming" occurs when the child can associate a label with a referent, which is accomplished receptively before it is accomplished expressively.

Bruner also introduced the notion of "scaffolding" as one way in which caregivers facilitate language learning and dialogue. Caregivers are said to adjust the degree of linguistic and non-linguistic support that they offer to children as they are learning language. For example, as the young child becomes more verbal, the caretaker will typically need to provide less nonverbal cuing during conversation (Bruner, 1975; Bruner, 1977).

In contemporary social-cognitive research, children are said to possess a unique capacity that enables them to learn language by interpreting the intentions of those who interact with them. Social cognitive views, such as that advocated by Paul Bloom (2000), suggest that children learning language need at least a primitive theory of mind to enable them to adequately interpret the intentions of others. Children's requisite cognitive abilities allow them to process information, while their preformed concepts for entities in the world serve as the basis for word learning and language development. While helpful adults might accelerate or assist in the process of word learning, as long as children can infer the referential intentions of others, no other social support is necessary. Tomasello, Carpenter, and Liszkowski (2007) support the view that children's inference of intentionality is critical for word and language learning.

According to Tomasello (2003), pointing gestures are an important part of the system of shared intentionality. Prior to language use, pointing not only establishes joint attention, but serves to influence the mental states of others by attempting to influence how another thinks, feels, and acts (Tomasello, Carpenter, & Liszkowski, 2007; Goldin-Meadow, 2007). In support of this view, Goldin-Meadow (2007) suggests that pointing at 14 months is a better predictor of lexical vocabulary than the speech of the caretaker. Pointing serves the child by not only drawing attention to the self, but to the objects that he finds interesting enough to communicate about. The child's use of pointing or gesture with words also helps him segue into syntax. For example, "children combine pointing gestures with words to express sentence-like meanings ('eat' + point at cookie) months before they can express the same meanings in word + word combination ('eat + cookie')" (Goldin-Meadow, 2007, p. 741).

From the perspective discussed here, language use originates from shared attention and the interpretation of intentionality. The basic processes that explain language learning in this view are the understanding of intentions and children's general cognitive abilities, including pattern abstraction and category construction. Owing to their unique social capabilities, human infants learn to interpret the communicative intentions of others, communicate their own intentions, and utilize their cognitive resources to create language knowledge that is both interpersonally driven and intrapersonally developed.

Social-Pragmatic Models

Pragmatics in linguistic theory has traditionally been concerned with the functions of language, speaker–listener roles, conversational discourse, and presupposition. Research in the pragmatics of language originated in the work of Austin (1962) and Searle (1969). In terms of the functions of adult language, linguists identified three types of speech acts: perlocutions, illocutions, and locutions. *Perlocutions* referred to how listeners interpreted the speaker's speech acts; *illocutions* referred to the intentions of the speaker; and *locutions* referred to the meanings expressed in the utterance.

In describing how intentionality develops in young children, Bates, Camaioni, and Volterra (1975) used this paradigm of functional categories. During the perlocutionary stage, which was said to extend from birth to nine months, the child's actions and behaviors are given communicative intent by the caretaker. For example, the caretaker might interpret a baby's cooing as a sign of happiness or contentment. The illocutionary stage (8 to 12 months) marks the period of time when children first produce their truly intentional behaviors, either vocally or gestur-ally. Gestures such as showing, giving, or pointing, perhaps accompanied with vocalizations, are typically used. During this time, children are said to produce the nonlinguistic precursor to the declarative referred to as the protodeclarative (e.g., gesturing or vocalizing to point out an object or event) as well as the nonlinguistic precursor to the imperative referred to as the protoimperative (e.g., gesturing or vocalizing to request an object or an event). The third stage, referred to as the Locutionary Stage (12 months of age), is characterized by the use of words produced with gestures to convey specific meanings and intentions.

A pragmatic approach to child language was taken by Halliday (1975), who described the functions of his son Nigel's nonlinguistic communication. These functions included satisfying needs, controlling the behaviors of others, interacting, and expressing emotion and interest. With his first words, Nigel could explore and categorize things in his environment, imagine or pretend, and inform others of his experiences.

John Dore (1974; 1975) identified the primitive speech acts of children at the one-word stage of language (e.g., labeling, answering, requesting an action, requesting an answer, calling, greeting, protesting, repeating/imitating, and practicing) as well as the speech acts of children at multiword stages of language development. Beyond such speech acts, research in the area of pragmatics addressed the child's knowledge of presupposition (Greenfield & Smith, 1976) and the child's understanding of conversational protocol, including topic control and conversational turn-taking (Bloom, Rocissano, & Hood, 1976).

One of the research topics that grew out of social-pragmatic views of language was the nature of the adult input to babies and young children. Since the 1970s, researchers in child language have noted that adults speak differently to very young children than they do to other people. These patterns, which have been referred to as "motherese," are characterized by ut-terances that are shorter in length, simpler in grammatical complexity, and slower in rate of speech. Also typical of motherese is the use of fewer verbs, fewer tense markers, and vocabulary that is less diverse and more concrete (Phillips, 1973; Snow, 1973; 1978; 1999).

In a similar vein, more recent studies have described child-directed speech (CDS) as con-textually redundant and perceptually salient. Because most CDS refers to the here and now (i.e., codes an ongoing action or activity within the child's view), it is contextually redundant (Akhtar, Dunham, & Dunham, 1991; Tomasello, 1988). In terms of perceptual salience, CDS typically has an overall higher fundamental frequency, exaggerated stress, a wider range of in-tonation, more distinct pausing, and, as noted earlier, an overall slower rate (Lund & Duchan, 1993). Researchers suggest that the vocal and grammatical parameters of the primary linguistic data that are provided by the caretaker make semantic, syntactic, phonological, and pragmatic information more accessible to the young infant, who is innately wired to receive this informa-tion. Findings from a number of studies have suggested that infant-directed speech facilitates segmentation of the speech stream, which in turn leads to the discovery of phonemes and words (Saffran, Senghas, & Trueswell, 2001; Kuhl, 2004; Thiessen, Hill, & Saffran, 2005).

It should be emphasized that although CDS has been found in many different cultures and languages throughout the world (e.g., Chinese, Arabic, Spanish, Marathi, and Comanche), CDS is not used to the same extent in all communities (Golinkoff & Hirsh-Pasek, 2000). For example, in the findings reported by Brice-Heath (1983), child-directed speech was not as prevalent in one of the Carolina Piedmont communities studied.

Implications from a Social-Cognitive and Social-Pragmatic Perspective: Understanding, Assessing, and Treating Children with Language Disorders

Some theories of language acquisition have had a profound impact on the study of specific populations of language-impaired children. For example, social-cognitive and social-pragmatic theories, which clarified the relationship between children's capacity for interaction and their capacity to learn to comprehend and produce language, spoke directly to the profiles of children with autistic spectrum disorders (ASD).

Clearly, children with autism present challenges in intentionality, as they often appear to be noncommunicative. In fact, the difficulty in reading these children's intentions set them apart from typically developing children and from other groups of children with language impairments. Based on social-cognitive and social-pragmatic views of language acquisition, speech-language pathologists working with children on the autistic spectrum began to broaden their understanding of why these children experienced such severe difficulties in the acquisition and use of language. Atypical behaviors, such as echolalia, were reconsidered. Using taxonomies of communicative intentions, the ground-breaking work of Prizant and Duchan (1981) as related to the functions of echolalia and delayed echolalia opened the door for considering that the "inappropriate" behaviors of children with ASD were, in fact, communicative and intentional, albeit in unconventional ways.

Many taxonomies of pragmatic development that focused on nonlinguistic aspects of communication also contributed to expanding the understanding of the nature of communication impairments in children whose deficits went far beyond their linguistic systems. The emphasis on gesture, facial expression, body language, eye gaze, presupposition, and listener perspective as foundations of communicative competence helped us to more accurately describe many children's challenges in language. These taxonomies were eventually adapted for use in assessment as the functions of language, the forms that were used to express these functions (nonlinguistic and linguistic, conventional and unconventional), and the longitudinal patterns of development in functions and means were analyzed. Simultaneously, taxonomies of conversational skills that addressed speaker–listener roles, topic control, and topic expansion (Prutting & Kirchner, 1987) were included in the battery of assessment tools as the evaluation of language expanded beyond morphology and syntax.

These theories of language also had a dramatic effect on the interventions used with children with language disorders. Expanding the repertoire of language intervention goals to prelinguistic and nonlinguistic domains of communication and recognizing all the categories of pragmatics as potential targets of therapy marked a shift that allowed speech-language pathologists to more accurately address the nature of many children's language and communication impairments. Beyond children with autism, other groups of language-disordered children were identified who demonstrated problems in pragmatics—for example, children whose difficulties in language use resulted from their difficulty with language formulation. As a consequence, speech-language pathologists began to consider new parameters of language use and the "obligations" of the language user. Intervention goals were generated that embraced prelinguistic precursors to language, functions of language, conversational skills, adjacency and contingency, discourse genres, communication repair, listener adaptation, and, to some extent, the social-emotional underpinnings of the pragmatics of language. Finally, an interest in the language and conversational skills needed for successful peer interactions emerged primarily as a result of social-cognitive and social-pragmatic models of language.

Intentionality Model

We end this section on interactionist views of language acquisition with a contemporary model that reflects an integrated perspective on the developmental language process. This model has particular resonance and relevance for understanding, assessing, and treating children with language disorders. Further, models of this type hold great promise for the speech-language pathology discipline because they provide the kinds of expansive paradigms that anchor our clinical work in the breadth and depth of typical development.

In 1978, Bloom and Lahey proposed a theory of language acquisition that revolutionized the work of speech-language pathologists. This view of language as the integration of form (phonology, morphology, syntax), content (semantics), and use (pragmatics) was subsequently translated into assessment and intervention paradigms (Lahey, 1988). The resulting "map" of language development, which traced the child's expression of ideas from single words to complex sentences, provided speech-language pathologists with developmental information that was at once organic, dynamic, and grounded in typical development.

More recently, Bloom and Tinker (2001) have enhanced the original model, embedding the development of form, content, and use into two broader developmental domains, *engagement* and *effort*. These authors suggest that the study of language has often resulted in the isolation of a particular aspect of language in an effort to investigate and study it. They remind us that "we need to consider what it means when we take the units of language out of the very fabric of the child's life in which they are necessarily embedded" (p. 4); "Somehow the child has to be kept in the picture as the major player, as the agent of the practices that contribute to the acquisition process" (p. 5). These concerns resonate with speech-language pathologists, who have the awesome task of isolating units of language so as to increase their saliency during the intervention process and, at the same time, trying to connect this process to "the very fabric of the child's life" (p. 4).

Bloom and Tinker's model suggests that a child's intentionality contributes to her development in two ways. First, the child's actions in the world (sensorimotor actions, emotional displays, play, and speech) as well as her acts of interpretation and expression of language lead to the development of new representations or the mental contents of her mind. Second, the child's participation in a social world depends on and is promoted by these acts of expression and interpretation between the child and her caregiver.

The child's agency is a central theme in this model and is critical for those speech-language pathologists who hope to borrow from models of typical acquisition to inform models of intervention. In this formulation, the child perceives, apprehends, and constructs intentional states. As the child expresses these states and interprets others' intentional states from their actions and their words, new intentional states and representations are formed. Intentional states include *psychological attitudes* (e.g., beliefs, desires, feelings) directed toward *propositional content* (e.g., persons, objects, and events in the world). Thus the intentionality model speaks to the interaction between two domains of development, affect and cognition, in the young child. The child's expression of his intentions is realized through emotion, play, and speech.

Although the intentionality model might be envisioned as a psychological model, Bloom and Tinker suggest that it embraces the social and cultural world of the child as well. Their treatment of the social world resides in the child's representations of others in his mind. The interaction of the child with the physical and social world and the effects of these interactions on his development lead us to consider this model as one example of the interactionist view of development.

One component of the intentionality model (**Figure 3-1**) is *engagement*, which refers to "the child's emotional and social directedness for determining what is relevant for learning and the motivation for learning" (Bloom & Tinker, 2001, p. 14). Here, Bloom and Tinker are referring to the intersubjectivity that develops between the child and her parent, which serves as the foundation for the child's relatedness to other persons throughout life. The relationship

FIGURE 3-1   The intentionality model.
Source: Intentionality Model appearing in Bloom, L. & Tinker, E. (2001). *The intentionality model and language acquisition.* Monographs of the Society for Research in Child Development, *66* (4), 267.

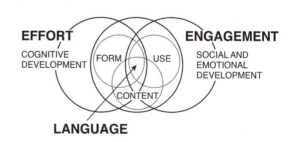

between the child and her caregivers, the child's relationships to objects and events, and her relationships in the physical world all contribute to the child's development of engagement.

The component of *effort* refers to the cognitive processes and the work it takes to acquire language. Early discussions of language acquisition emphasized the ease of learning to talk, as evidenced by the fact that children had accomplished most of this task by age three years. In contrast, Bloom and Tinker (2001) underscore the effort and resources that are required to integrate the various dimensions of expressing and interpreting language. The complexity of these tasks is captured when considering that

> expression, at a minimum, requires the child to construct and hold in mind intentional state representations, retrieve linguistic units and procedures from memory, and articulate words and sentences. For interpretation, at a minimum, the child must connect what is heard to what is already in mind, recall elements from memory that are associated with prior experiences of the words, and form a new intentional state representation. (Bloom & Tinker, 2001, p. 15)

Effort can also be understood in terms of the complexity of what children are learning simultaneously. For example, children are learning to interpret and express intentions at the same time that they are learning about the world, their emotional lives, and the emotional lives of significant others. In this view, the child's cognitive resources are a very real part of the acquisition process and will help us to understand what he can and cannot do at different points in time. The implications of this concept for thinking about children with challenges in speech, language, and communication are immediately apparent as we imagine the additional drain on resources that must be experienced when aspects of learning are limited by neurological, psychological, and emotional disruptions.

Implications from the Intentionality Model: Understanding, Assessing, and Treating Children with Language Disorders

Using Bloom and Tinker's (2001) intentionality model, disorders of language can be addressed relative to the area or areas of language that are compromised, rather than from a categorical or etiological framework. The advantage of using Bloom and Tinker's perspective is that we can begin to view challenges in language from two dynamic developmental domains—effort and engagement. Children with primary problems in effort and those with primary problems in engagement can be distinguished from one another, and the resulting impact of these derailments on the development of form, content, and use can be considered. In the spirit of Bloom and Lahey (1978) and Lahey (1988), language-disordered children would be classified on the basis of the areas of language and language-related developments that might be considered strengths and challenges, rather than using etiological categories such as specific language impairment, mental retardation, autistic spectrum disorders, and so forth.

For individual assessments of children, Bloom and Tinker's (2001) intentionality model is invaluable. Developmental models of language, which are both broad and integrated, offer speech-language pathologists a rich paradigm from which to assess language in a way that will lead directly to intervention. Using the intentionality model, they can specify which of a number of developmental areas—social, affective, and cognitive—require attention prior to or simultaneously with the attention given to components of language. Assessment based on this thinking leads to more holistic intervention goals and procedures, as the interrelationship between and among the developmental components is recognized and the use of developmental sequences and processes is prioritized (Gerber, 2003).

Although Bloom and Tinker's model does not offer a packaged set of intervention plans, it anchors the work of speech-language pathologists in a perspective that embraces many of the models of language acquisition that have been discussed in this chapter. The clinician who begins the treatment of any particular child with an integrated understanding of the processes and products of typical language acquisition and then combines this knowledge with an inherent understanding of the interpersonal relationships within which these processes and products unfold will be ready to meet the challenges and joys of facilitating each child's comprehension and production of language.

THE SCIENCE OF CHILD DEVELOPMENT IN 2008: BROADER PERSPECTIVES

A contemporary review of the science of language acquisition would not be complete without a discussion of the most recent perspectives on the science of early child development. Since 2000, a number of reports have been published that reflect the work of the National Scientific Council on the Developing Child. This interdisciplinary team of scientists and scholars has addressed what the biological and social sciences "do and do not say about early childhood, brain development, and the impact of intervention programs" (National Research Council & Institute of Medicine, 2000, p. 2). The status of the nature–nurture debate comes across loud and clear in the findings and recommendations of this group, as the interactionist view is presented in the most contemporary framework.

The Council's analysis of decades of data from a small number of intensive child development programs supports the assumption that it is possible to improve many outcomes for "vulnerable children;" however, it also demonstrates that many programs have not yielded beneficial results. Several of the findings from this analysis of cutting-edge neuroscience, developmental-behavioral research, and program evaluation are particularly relevant to the nature–nurture issue in language acquisition. The review presented in this section puts the topic of language acquisition into a broader scientific and developmental context and serves as another source for intervention implications.

Early experiences determine whether a child's developing brain architecture provides a strong or weak foundation for all future learning, behavior, and health. (National Research Council & Institute of Medicine, 2000, p. 3)

Among the many conclusions that have been drawn from this finding is that a need exists for earlier intervention programs for children at risk. Early intervention has the potential to influence the child's brain circuitry—once again speaking to the interaction between nature and nurture. For speech-language pathologists, this finding supports the benefits provided by early, finely tuned adult input and well-designed interactive experiences and sets the stage for honing the experiences that the young child with language difficulties will receive. For vulnerable children, the plasticity of the brain and the windows of opportunity in early childhood are the keys to ensuring intensity of services and parental participation in the intervention plan.

In fact, the world of communication disorders has a long history of supporting early and intensive intervention for children with developmental delays. Contemporary studies aimed at identifying prelinguistic markers of language and communication disorders speak to the urgency of earlier identification, which will then lead to earlier intervention (Wetherby et al., 2004). Similarly, our growing awareness of the role of the parent–child relationship will, hopefully, result in paradigm shifts relative to the determining who the participants are during language intervention sessions (Longtin & Gerber, 2008).

The interactive influences of genes and experience shape the architecture of the child's developing brain. (National Research Council & Institute of Medicine, 2000, p. 8)

In this view, genes dictate when specific brain circuits are formed, while experiences shape their formation. Children's inborn drive toward competence and their experience with responsive relationships motivate the developmental process and lead to healthy brain architecture. The "mutuality and reciprocity" typical in the "serve and return" nature of early interactions is key to children's development and, therefore, key in the construction of intervention goals and strategies. In typical development, a parent or caretaker can provide these opportunities for mutuality and reciprocity to the child, who is an eager and active participant in the process. For children who are developing atypically, the same interactive dance, which may be much harder to choreograph, must nonetheless be prioritized as a step toward shaping the architecture of the child's developing brain.

Brain architecture and the skills that come with development are built "from the bottom up," with simpler developments serving as the foundations for more advanced ones. (National Research Council & Institute of Medicine, 2000, p. 8)

Here, the take-home message for speech-language pathologists interested in language acquisition speaks to the importance of a developmental perspective for facilitating the comprehension and production of language. Using the terminology of brain architecture, "higher-level circuits build on lower-level circuits, and adaptation at higher levels is more difficult if lower-level circuits are not wired properly." Similarly, more complex skills build on simpler ones. While this hierarchy may seem self-evident, the implication of this multilayer structure for professionals developing intervention programs clearly sets the direction of the program content. An extensive understanding of the steps in development within any particular domain (language, affect, cognition) and a commitment to developmentally expanding the child's repertoire of skills is the logical implication of this finding.

Cognitive, emotional, and social capabilities are inextricably intertwined throughout the life course, and their interactive relationship develops in a continuous process over time. (National Research Council & Institute of Medicine, 2000, p. 10)

This finding presents one of the greatest challenges for professionals working with children who have developmental derailments. The implication here is that to provide the best experiences for promoting development, clinicians must think not only about their particular area of expertise, but also about the relationship and interrelationship of that area with other developmental domains. In fact, the most promising intervention programs are likely to be those that keep the interactive flow between and among developmental threads in view and plan for each goal with an eye toward the prerequisites and corequisites of that specific development. Prioritizing a particular area of development, such as language, while honoring the simultaneity and interconnectedness of the child's development in social, affective, cognitive, and regulatory domains presents an ongoing learning opportunity for clinicians.

CONCLUSION: HOW TO USE THIS INFORMATION AS A LIFELONG STUDENT OF LANGUAGE DISORDERS

How can a "student" of speech-language pathology embrace the most current thinking about language development and, at the same time, benefit from the long history of contributions made to our understanding of language acquisition and the influences of these contributions on the field of speech-language pathology? More specifically, how will we determine how to work and play with Timmy and what to encourage as a sound and scientific approach to facilitating his linguistic and communication development?

Before addressing Timmy's case, perhaps we should remind ourselves of the diversity in individual profiles of the children we have seen or will see over our careers. Although the authors of this chapter have seen many children with autism, language impairment, cognitive delays, and language-learning disabilities in their more than 30 years (each!) as speech-language pathologists, they would definitely say they have never seen the same child twice.

This diversity in and of itself gives us a first clue to answering the question, "How do I know when to use which theory or model of language?" "It depends" would have to be the honest and informed answer.

Understanding that each child's profile of strengths and challenges is a natural result of his biology and experience and the interplay between the two suggests that the possibilities are endless relative to the areas of development in which to support, enhance, facilitate, or teach. Perhaps for one child, the inability to learn the linguistic rules of the language will be the roadblock to further language learning; in such a case, understanding and addressing the perceptual, psycholinguistic, and pragmatic aspects of rule learning will be the charge to his speech-language pathologist. For another child, whose ideas about the world seem to be standing in the way of his development of greater comprehension and production of language, the notions of the child as an active learner of the sensorimotor, symbolic, and ideational underpinnings of language should be reviewed. For a third child, whose social–emotional affective development is derailed, emphasizing caretaker–child interactions, shared attention, reciprocity, and coconstruction of meaning would be an excellent starting point.

In the end, what would we advise the new or seasoned speech-language pathologist relative to the question of theories of language acquisition? For sure, each theory has some relevance to the larger puzzle of determining how it is that typically developing children come to comprehend and produce novel utterances with social savvy and an understanding of the interpersonal customs and constraints of their language. Given that reality, plus the fact that no one really knows why a particular child is having difficulty with language and communication, wise speech-language pathologists will keep their eyes and ears open and consider this topic to be a work in progress. Interestingly enough, although speech-language pathologists often think about borrowing from what is known about children who are typically developing, clinical findings about children with challenges in language acquisition and the paths to their progress will inform theories and models of language as well.

For Timmy, considering the range of delays and disruptions that he was experiencing, the speech-language pathologist would do best to encourage his parents to provide support in all aspects of development that relate to language and to find the kind of intervention that speaks to a cohesive, interdisciplinary, broad view of the factors that influence the ability to learn a linguistic system and the pleasures of communication. In fact, this is just what Timmy's parents did. For this child, the result was a very good one: Timmy progressed in his comprehension and production of language, his affective engagement and reciprocity, his social interaction, and his development of ideas. This comprehensive approach fit well with the parents' own philosophy of how to help their son, an aspect of intervention that should not be minimized. Today, Timmy is a three-year-old with lots to say and a growing sense of the joys of interacting. But should he meet additional challenges along the way, his speech-language pathologist would do well to go back to the theories of language acquisition and look yet again for clues to the nuances and mysteries of development and disorder.

KEY TERMS

Empiricist theories

Intentionality model

Interactionist theories

Language acquisition theories

Language assessment

Language intervention

Nature–nurture debate

Rationalist theories

STUDY QUESTIONS

- ✦ How does the traditional nature–nurture debate relate to the study of language acquisition?
- ✦ Describe how empiricist theories have influenced the field of speech-language pathology.
- ✦ Describe how nativistic theories have influenced the field of speech-language pathology.
- ✦ Describe how interactionist theories have influenced the field of speech-language pathology.
- ✦ Describe the components of Bloom and Tinker's (2001) intentionality model.
- ✦ With reference to a particular child, describe how this discussion of specific theories would affect your approach to assessment and/or intervention.

REFERENCES

Akhtar, N., Dunham, F., & Dunham, P. (1991). Directive interactions and early vocabulary development: The role of joint attentional focus. *Journal of Child Language, 18*, 41–49.

Austin, J. (1962). *How to do things with words.* London: Oxford University Press.

Bates, E. (1975). *Language and context: The acquisition of pragmatics.* New York: Academic Press.

Bates, E. Camaioni, L., & Volterra, V. (1975). The acquisition of performatives prior to speech. *Merrill-Palmer Quarterly, 21*, 205–216.

Bates, E. & MacWhinney, B. (1987). Competition, variation, and language learning. In B. MacWhinney (Ed.), *Mechanisms of Language Acquisition* (157–194). Hillsdale, NJ: Erlbaum.

Berko-Gleason, J. (2005). *The development of language.* Boston: Pearson Education.

Bever, T.G. (1970). The cognitive basis for linguistic structures. In R. Hayes (Ed.), *Cognition and development of language* (279–362). New York: Wiley.

Bloom, L. (1970). *Language development: Form and function in emerging grammars.* Cambridge, MA: MIT Press.

Bloom, L., & Lahey, M. (1978). *Language development and language disorders.* New York: John Wiley & Sons.

Bloom, L., Rocissano, L., & Hood, L. (1976). Adult–child discourse: Developmental intervention between information processing and linguistic knowledge. *Cognitive Psychology, 8*, 521–552.

Bloom, L., & Tinker, E. (2001). The intentionality model and language acquisition. *Monographs of the Society for Research in Child Development, 66*(4), 267.

Bloom, P. (2000). *How children learn the meaning of words.* Cambridge, MA: MIT Press.

Bohannon, J. N. III, & Bonvillian, J. D. (2005). Theoretical approaches to language acquisition. In J. Berko Gleason (Ed.), *The development of language* (230–291). Boston: Pearson Education.

Braine, M. D. S. (1963). On learning the grammatical order of words. *Psychological Review, LXX,* 323–348.

Braine, M. D. S. (1966). Learning the positions of words relative to a marker element. *Journal of Experimental Psychology, 72,* 532–540.

Bransford, J. D., & Franks, J. J. (1972). Sentence memory: A constructive vs. interpretive approach. *Cognitive Psychology, 3,* 193–209.

Brice-Heath, S. (1983). *Ways with words.* Cambridge, UK: Cambridge University Press.

Brown, R. (1973). *A first language: The early stages.* Cambridge, MA: Harvard University Press.

Bruner, J. (1975). The ontogenesis of speech acts. *Journal of Child Language, 2,* 1–19.

Bruner, J. (1977). Early social interaction and language acquisition. In R. Schaffer (Ed.), *Studies in mother–infant interaction* (271–289). New York: Academic Press.

Cairns, C., & Cairns, H. (1975). *Psycholinguistics: A cognitive view of language.* New York: Holt, Rinehart & Winston.

Catts, H., & Kamhi, A. (2005). *Language and reading disabilities.* Boston: Pearson Education.

Chomsky, N. (1957). *Syntactic structures.* The Hague: Mouton.

Chomsky, N. (1965). *Aspects of a theory of syntax:* Cambridge, MA: MIT Press.

Chomsky, N. (1972). *Studies on semantics in generative grammar.* The Hague: Mouton.

Chomsky, N. (1982). *Lectures on government and binding.* New York: Foris.

Chomsky, N. (1988). *Language and the problems of knowledge.* Cambridge, MA: MIT Press.

Chomsky, N. (1993). *Lectures on government and binding.* Berlin: Mouton de Gruyter.

Chomsky, N. (1995). *The minimalist program.* Cambridge: MIT Press.

Chomsky, N. (2002). The secular priesthood and the perils of democracy. In A. Belletti & L. Rizzi (Eds.), *Nature and language* (162–187). Cambridge, UK: Cambridge University Press.

Clark, E. (1973). What's in a word? On the child's acquisition of semantics in his first language. In T. E. Moore (Ed.), *Cognitive development and the acquisition of language* (65–110). New York: Academic Press.

Clark, E. (2004). How language acquisition builds on cognitive development. *Trends in Cognitive Science. 8,* 472–478.

Cruickshank, W. M. (1967). *The brain-injured child in home, school, and society.* New York: Syracuse University Press.

Curtiss, S. (1974). *Genie: A psycholinguistic study of a modern day "wild" child.* New York: Academic Press.

Descartes, R. (1960/1637). Discourse on method. In Staff of Columbia College (Eds.), *Introduction to contemporary civilization in the West* (812–837). New York: Columbia University Press.

de Villiers, J., & de Villiers, P. (1973). A cross-sectional study of the development of grammatical morphemes in child speech. *Journal of Psycholinguistic Research, 2,* 267–268.

Dore, J. (1974). A pragmatic description of early language development. *Journal of Psycholinguistic Research, 4,* 343–350.

Dore, J. (1975). Holophrases, speech acts, and language universals. *Journal of Child Language, 2,* 21–40.

Eimas, P., Siqueland, E., Jusczyk, P., & Vigorito, J. (1971). Speech perception in infants. *Science, 171,* 303–306.

Fillmore, C. (1968). The case for case. In E. Bach & R. Harmas (Eds.), *Universals in linguistic theory* (1–90). New York: Holt, Rinehart, & Winston.

Flavell, J. H. (1963). *The developmental psychology of Jean Piaget.* New York: D.Van Nostrand Co.

Fodor, J. A., Fodor, J. D., Garrett, M. F., & Lackner, J. R. (1974). Effects of surface and underlying clausal structure on click location. Research Laboratory of Electronics, Massachusetts Institute of Technology. *Quarterly Progress Report,* 113.

Fodor, J., & Pylyshyn, Z. (1988). Connectionism and cognitive architecture: A critical analysis. *Cognition, 28,* 3–71.

Gerber, S. (2003). A developmental perspective on language assessment and intervention for children on the autistic spectrum. *Topics in Langue Disorders, 23, 2,* 74–95.

Gillam, R. B., Loeb, D. F., Hoffman, L. M., Bohman, T., Champlin, C. A., Thibodeau, L., Widen, J., Brandel, J., Friel-Patti, S. (2008). The efficacy of fast for word language intervention in school-age children with language impairment: A randomized controlled trial. *Journal of Speech, Language, and Hearing Research, 51,* 97–119.

Gleitman, L. R., Gleitman, H., & Shipley, E. E. (1972). The emergence of the child as grammarian. *Cognition, 1,* 137–164.

Goldin-Meadow, S. (2007). Pointing sets the stage for learning language—and creating. *Child Development, 78*(3), 741–745.

Golinkoff, R. M., & Hirsh-Pasek, K. (2000). *How babies talk.* New York: Plume.

Gopnik, A., & Meltzoff, A. N. (1986). Relations between semantic and cognitive development in the one-word stage: The specificity hypothesis. *Child Development, 57,* 1040–1053.

Gray, B. B., & Ryan, B. (1973). *A language training program for the non-language child.* Chapaign, IL: Research Press.

Greenfield, P., & Smith, J. (1976). *The structure of communication in early language development.* New York: Academic Press.

Halliday, M. A. K. (1975). *Learning how to mean: Explorations in the development of language.* London: Edward Arnold.

Hammill, D., Mather, N., & Roberts, R. (2001). *Illinois Test of Psycholinguistic Abilities,* 3rd ed. Austin, TX: Pro-ed.

Hulit , L. M., & Howard, M. R. (2002). *Born to talk,* 3rd ed. Boston: Pearson Education.

Johnson, D. J., & Mykelbust, J. R. (1967). *Learning disabilities: Educational principles and practices.* New York: Grune & Stratton.

Johnston, J. (1994). Cognitive abilities of children with language impairment. In R. Watkins & M. Rice (Eds.), *Specific language impairments in children* (vol. 4, 107–121). Baltimore: Paul H. Brookes.

Klein, H., & Moses, N. (1999). *Intervention planning got children with communication disorders.* Boston: Allyn & Bacon.

Koegel, R., & Koegel, L. (2006). *Pivotol response treatments for autism.* Baltimore: Paul H. Brookes.

Kuhl, P. K. (2004). Early language acquisition: Cracking the speech code. *Neuroscience, 5,* 831–843.

Lahey, M. (1988). *Language disorders and language development.* New York: Macmillan.

Lenneberg, E. (1967). *Biological foundations of language.* New York: Wiley.

Leonard, L., (1992). The use of morphology by children with specific language impairment: Evidence from three languages. In R. Chapman (Ed.), *Processes in language acquisition and disorders* (186–201). St. Louis: Mosby.

Leonard, L., & Loeb, D. (1988). Government-Binding Theory and some of its implications: A tutorial. *Journal of Speech and Hearing Research, 31,* 515–524.

Locke, J. (1960/1690). An essay concerning human understanding. In Staff of Columbia College (Ed.), *Introduction to contemporary civilization in the West* (1010–1069). New York: Columbia University Press.

Longtin, S., & Gerber, S. (2008). Contemporary perspectives on facilitating language acquisition for children on the autistic spectrum: Engaging the parent and the child. *The Journal of Developmental Processes, 3 (1),* 38–51.

Lovaas, O. I. (1977). *The autistic child: Language development through behavior modification.* New York: Irvington.

Lund, N. J., & Duchan, J. F. (1993) *Assessing children's language in naturalistic contexts,* 3rd ed. Englewood Cliffs, NJ: Prentice-Hall.

Lust, B. (2007). *Child language: Acquisition and growth.* The Growth of Language. Cambridge: Cambridge University Press.

MacWhinney, B. (1987). *Mechanisms of language acquisition.* Hillsdale, NJ: Erlbaum.

McNeil, D. (1970). *The acquisition of language: The study of developmental linguistics.* New York: Harper & Row.

Mowrer, O. H. (1960). A stimulus-response analysis and its role as a reinforcing agent. *Journal of Comparative and Physiological Psychology, 65,* 251–260.

National Research Council & Institute of Medicine (2000). *From neurons to neighborhoods: The science of early childhood development.* Washington, DC: National Academy Press.

Nelson, N. (1998). *Childhood language disorders in context: Infancy through adolescence,* 2nd ed. Boston: Pearson Education.

Osgood, C. (1963). On understanding and creating sentences. *American Psychologist, 18,* 735–751.

Pavlov, I. P. (1902). *The work of the digestive glands.* Trans. W. H. Thompson. London: Charles Griffin.

Phillips, J. R. (1973). Syntax and vocabulary of mothers' speech to young children: Age and sex comparisons. *Child Development, 44,* 182–185.

Piaget, J. (1952). *Origins of intelligence in children.* New York: Int. Univ. Press.

Piaget, J. (1955). *The language and thought of the child.* Translated by M. Gabain. Cleveland, OH: Meridian.

Pinker, S. (1984). *Language, learnability, and language development.* Cambridge, MA: Harvard University Press.

Pinker, S. (2006). The blank slate. *General Psychologist, 41*(1), 1–8.

Pinker, S., & Jackendoff, R. (2005). The faculty of language: What's special about it? *Cognition, 95,* 201–236.

Plato. (1960). The republic. In Staff of Columbia College (Ed.), *Introduction to contemporary civilization in the West* (4–28). New York: Columbia University Press.

Prizant, B., & Duchan, J. (1981). The functions of immediate echolalia in autistic children. *Journal of Speech and Hearing Disorders, 46,* 241–250.

Prutting, C., & Kirchner, D. (1987). A clinical appraisal of the pragmatic aspects of language. *Journal of Speech and Hearing Disorders, 52,* 105–119.

Rice, M. L., Wexler, K., & Cleave, P. (1995). Specific language impairment as a period of extended optional infinitive. *Journal of Speech and Hearing Research, 38,* 850–863.

Saffran, J. R.., Senghaas, A., & Trueswell, J. C. (2001). The acquisition of language by children. *Proceedings of the National Academy of Sciences, 98*(23), 12874–12875.

Sakai, K. L. (2005). Language acquisition and brain development. *Science, 310,* 815–819.

Saxton, M., Galloway, C., & Backley, P. (1999). *Negative evidence and negative feedback: Longer term effects on the grammaticality of child speech.* Paper presented at the VIIIth International Congress for the Study of Child Language, San Sebastian, Spain.

Sampson, G. (1987). Review of *Parallel distributed processing: Explorations in the microstructure of cognition, vol. 1: Foundations,* by D. Rummelhart, J. McClelland, and PDP Research Group. *Language, 63,* 871–886.

Schlesinger, I. M. (1977). *Production and comprehension of utterances.* Hillsdale, NJ: Lawrence Erlbaum.

Searle, J. R. (1969). *Speech acts.* Cambridge, UK: Cambridge University Press.

Siegel, D. (1999). *The developing mind: How relationships and the brain interact to shape who we are.* New York: Guilford Press.

Skinner, B. F. (1957). *Verbal behavior.* Upper Saddle River, NJ: Prentice Hall.

Slobin, D. (1979). *Psycholinguistics,* 2nd ed. Glenview, IL: Scott, Foresman.

Slobin, D., & Bever, T. (1982). Children use canonical sentence schemas: A crosslinguistic study of word order and inflections. *Cognition, 12,* 229–265.

Snow, C. (1973). Mother's speech to children learning language. *Child Development, 43,* 549–565.

Snow, C. (1978). The conversational context of language acquisition. In R. Campbell & P. Smith (Eds.), *Recent advances in the psychology of language* (vol. 4a, pp. 253–269). New York: Plenum Press.

Snow, C. E. (1999). Social perspectives on the emergence of language. In B. MacWhinney (Ed.), *The emergence of language* (257–276). Mahwah, NJ: Erlbaum.

Staats, A. W. (1968). *Learning, language and cognition: Theory, research, and method for the study of human behavior and its development.* New York: Holt, Rinehart and Winston.

Thiessen, E. D., Hill, E. A., & Saffran, J. R. (2005). Infant-directed speech facilitates word segmentation. *Infancy, 7*(1), 53–71.

Tomasello, M. (1988). The role of joint attentional processes in early language development. *Language Sciences, 10,* 69–88.

Tomasello, M. (2003). *Constructing a language: A usage based theory of language acquisition.* Cambridge, MA: Harvard University Press.

Tomasello, M., Carpenter, M., & Liszkowski, U. (2007). A new look at infant pointing. *Child Development, 78,* 705–722.

Trehub, S. (1976). The discrimination of foreign speech contrasts by infants and children. *Child Development, 47,* 466–472.

Vouloumanos, A., & Werker, J. F. (2007). Listening to language at birth: Evidence for a bias for speech in neonates. *Developmental Sciences, 10*(2), 159–171.

Vygotsky, L. S. (1986). *Thought and language.* Trans. A. Kozulin. Cambridge, MA: MIT Press.

Warren, S. F., & Kaiser, A. P. (1986). Incidental language teaching: A critical review. *Journal of Speech and Hearing Disorders, 51,* 291–299.

Werker, J. F., & Tees, R. C. (1984). Cross-language speech perception: Evidence for perceptual reorganization during the first year of life. *Infant Behavior and Development, 7,* 49–64.

Westby, C. (1980). Assessment of cognitive and language abilities through play. *Language, Speech and Hearing Services in the Schools, 11,* 154–168.

Westby, C. (2000). A scale for assessing development of children's play. In K. Gitlin-Weiner, A. Sandgun, & C. Schaefer (Eds.), *Play diagnosis and assessment* (15–27). New York: Wiley.

Wetherby, A., Woods, J., Allen, L., Cleary, J., Dickenson, H., & Lord, C. (2004). Early indicators of autism spectrum disorders in the second year of life. *Journal of Autism and Developmental Disorders, 34,* 473–493.

Wexler, K. (1999). Maturation and growth of grammar. In W. Ritchie & T. Bhatia (Eds.), *Handbook of child language acquisition* (55–110). New York: Academic Press.

Wexler, K., Schutze, C., & Rice, M. L. (1998). Subject case in normal and SLI children: Evidence for the AGR/TENSE deletion model. *Language Acquisition, 7,* 317–344.

CHAPTER 4

Hearing and Language Development

Deborah R. Welling, AuD

OBJECTIVES

- Describe the structure and understand the functional differences between the conductive and sensorineural systems
- Have a basic understanding of the process of normal auditory development
- Have a basic understanding of different methods used in the assessment of the pediatric population
- Identify and describe the different characteristics of the various types of hearing loss
- Understand the treatment options available for different types of hearing loss
- Understand how each type of hearing loss affects speech and language development

INTRODUCTION

One of the most important ingredients for normal speech and language development is for the process of auditory development to occur normally as well. Unfortunately, a nearly endless list of events can cause hearing to be either temporarily or permanently impaired, thereby impeding the process of normal language development. Also, hearing loss can occur as the result of prenatal factors and be present from the time of birth, or it can occur at some later point. To make matters more complicated, hearing loss is not an "all or nothing" affair, with the only two options being that you either hear something or you do not. Rather, hearing ability can range from completely normal hearing to profoundly deaf, and anywhere in between.

This chapter introduces the normal anatomy and physiology of the ear, the process of normal auditory development, the ways in which a child's hearing is assessed, and the possible outcomes of such testing. It also investigates possible interventions for hearing-related problems—for example, hearing aids and cochlear implants. Finally, we discuss some of the speech, language, and other general learning-related characteristics of the various forms of hearing loss.

We conclude our "tour" of hearing and its role in language development by reviewing each of our case studies in light of the information presented in the chapter.

ANATOMY AND PHYSIOLOGY OF THE PERIPHERAL AUDITORY SYSTEM _____

The descriptions of the conductive (outer and middle ear) and sensorineural mechanisms (inner ear) that follow are simply meant as an introductory look at the basic structures of the peripheral auditory system and the way in which they work. The primary purpose of providing this information is to assist the reader in obtaining a fundamental understanding of the anatomy and physiology of the ear and to lay a foundation upon which the remaining concepts of this chapter can be built.

Anatomically speaking, the ear consists of three separate regions: the outer ear, the middle ear, and the inner ear. In terms of how the ear functions and performs its job, however, it can be separated into two regions or systems: the conductive system and the sensorineural system. For the purposes of the present discussion, we will discuss the ear on the basis of its functional or working divisions—that is, the *conductive mechanism* and the *sensorineural mechanism*.

The Conductive Mechanism

The conductive (mechanical) mechanism includes both the outer ear and the middle ear. In its normal state, this system is an air-filled environment. The conductive system as a whole (that is, the outer and middle ears as unit) has the job of gathering the sound (also known as acoustic energy) from the environment, converting the sound or acoustic energy into mechanical energy, and then delivering this mechanical energy to the inner ear (sensorineural mechanism).

Because the inner ear is a fluid-filled space as opposed to the air-filled space of the middle ear, this conductive function presents a challenge to the middle ear. The middle ear needs to overcome the resistance of the fluid; if it does not, the sound energy will not be effectively transmitted to the inner ear and the person will not hear properly. To visualize this difference between the air-filled middle ear and the fluid-filled inner ear, imagine swinging your hand through the air. Now imagine that you are trying to swing your hand through partially set gelatin. Quite obviously, you will use more effort when your hand is going through the gelatin than when it is going through the air. This analogy demonstrates the different resistance that characterizes the air-filled middle ear versus the fluid-filled inner ear.

The two main portions of the outer ear are the pinna (or auricle) and the external auditory canal (or meatus; also known as the ear canal). The pinna (**Figure 4-1**) is the object that sits on each side of our heads; this structure is made of cartilage and covered by skin. Some of the major landmarks on the pinna include the helix, antihelix, tragus, antitragus, concha (bowl-shaped portion), and lobule (earlobe).

The external ear canal (**Figure 4-2**) is a tube that is approximately 25 mm (roughly 1 inch) in length and approximately 7 mm in diameter. It starts at the pinna and extends all the way down to the *tympanic membrane* (eardrum). The outer one-third of the ear canal is cartilaginous and is a continuation of the cartilage of the pinna; the inner two-thirds of the canal are bony. The entire ear canal is covered with skin, which continues and forms the outermost of the eardrum's three layers.

The outer ear has several functions—some acoustic (sound related) and some non-acoustic (Yost, 2007). Contrary to the belief of some persons that the sole function of the pinna is to provide a place to hang earrings, the pinna does serve several acoustic functions, along with this decorative, "non-acoustic" one. First, the pinna acts as a collector and director of sound. The "collector" function is ac-

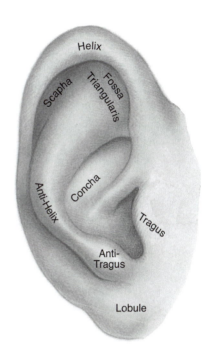

FIGURE 4-1   The pinna (auricle) of the ear.

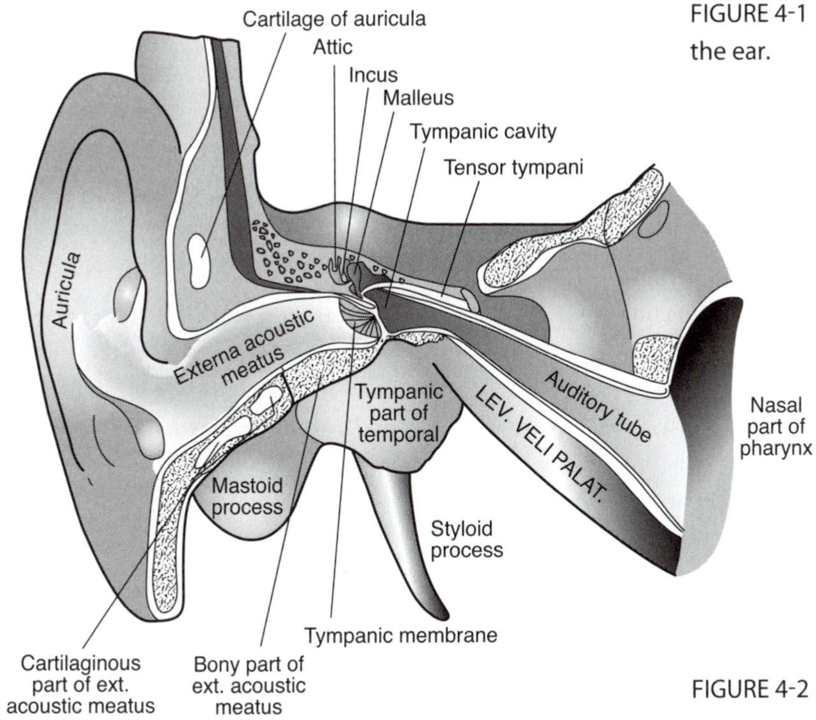

FIGURE 4-2   The ear.

complished by the cupped shape; it collects the sound and then directs it down toward the eardrum. In fact, cupping a hand around your ear in an attempt to improve your hearing actually will provide a small loudness boost in the sound level.

A second acoustic function of the pinna is that it helps in determining the location of the source of a sound, also known as *localization*. If you look at Figures 4-1 and 4-2 (or, better yet, examine your own pinna), you may notice that the ear is not a flat surface. Rather, it contains all kinds of nooks and crannies, or hills and valleys, to use another analogy. The way in which sound bounces off the various curves and grooves of the pinna provides information that the brain can use to determine the direction from which the sound is coming.

Another sound-related function performed by the outer ear is the result of the *resonance properties* of the outer ear structure, which enhance the sound in a particular portion of the frequency range. In other words, some frequencies are given a natural boost—a necessary action if the sound is to eventually reach the fluid-filled inner ear effectively. Specifically, both the pinna and the ear canal have a frequency where they tend to enhance the sound most effectively (resonant frequency). For the pinna, this frequency is approximately 2000 Hz; for the ear canal, it is approximately 5000 Hz. In real-life listening situations, this enhancement translates into a "boost" in the loudness of sound in the "treble" range. The "treble" range corresponds to some of the consonant sounds, so improvement in this area is most helpful for improving speech intelligibility.

In addition to serving these acoustic functions, the outer ear fulfills some non-sound-related roles. Most importantly, it protects the eardrum from direct injury. This feat is accomplished, at least in part, by the anatomy itself. Examine Figure 4-2 again, noticing that the ear canal does not form a straight horizontal line, but rather sits at an angle. Furthermore, it is characterized by curving and bending, and the inner two-thirds of the canal wall is made up of bone. The combination of these structural details helps protect the surface of the eardrum from injury.

Another non-acoustic function of the outer ear relates to cerumen (ear wax). This brownish waxy stuff found in the ear canal consists of the secretions of two types of glands (cerumenous and sebaceous), both of which are located in the outer one-third of the ear canal. The secretions act as a protective layer for the skin and tissue underneath, helping to prevent infections by trapping potentially harmful irritants. In addition, the wax serves a self-cleaning function by combining with dirt and sloughed-off (dead) skin cells. This normal process includes the forces of gravity, body heat, and the normal activities of chewing and speaking, which collectively cause the wax to gradually make its way to the opening of the ear canal.

Figure 4-3 depicts the middle ear. For this structure, the eardrum is the outermost (lateral) border, and the temporal bone (which contains the inner ear, among other structures) makes up the inner (medial) wall. Other important structures within the middle ear space

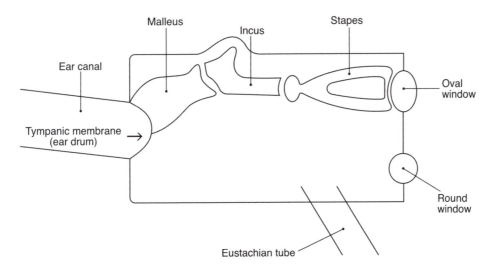

FIGURE 4-3   The middle ear space.

include the oval and round windows (on the medial wall), which make up part of the border to the inner ear; the eustachian tube (on the anterior wall), which provides a connection to the nasopharynx; and the three smallest bones in the human body—the malleus (hammer), incus (anvil), and stapes (stirrup), which are collectively known as the ossicular chain.

The eustachian tube connects the middle ear space to the nasopharynx (or throat). Among its purposes are the provision of air to the middle ear space and the equalization of the pressure between the middle ear and the outside atmosphere. Rarely are these functions more happily appreciated than when a person is going up in an airplane. Without the pressure equalization function of the eustachian tube, many people would be extremely uncomfortable.

The main objective of the middle ear system, however, is to *effectively* deliver the mechanical sound energy into the inner ear. To accomplish this goal, the middle ear system must first give a substantial boost to the mechanical energy when it gets to the middle ear. Recall that the fluid has higher resistance (also known as *impedance*) than air. If the boost in energy is not provided, this fluid will act as a barrier of sorts and prevent the efficient transmission of the sound. The greater resistance (impedance) of the fluid-filled environment as compared to the air-filled environment is known as an *impedance mismatch*. If the sound (mechanical energy) is not amplified when it gets to the middle ear, instead of the sound being transferred to the inner ear, there will be insufficient energy such that the sound will not get beyond the middle ear. Overcoming this impedance mismatch is accomplished by the *middle ear transformer function*, which requires a combination of factors.

The first factor affecting the middle ear transformer function is the size mismatch—that is, the size of the eardrum is much larger than the size of the stapes footplate (where the sound exits the middle ear and enters the inner ear). This size difference alone increases the sound pressure approximately 18-fold by the time it enters the inner ear. The second factor involved is the position of each of the ossicles in relation to the others; this varying placement creates a lever action that also increases the sound pressure. Lastly, the cone shape of the eardrum adds pressure to the sound energy being transmitted by the ossicular chain. These factors, which are collectively known as the transformer function, increase the sound by as much as 25 to 30 decibels (dB) by the time it reaches the inner ear. Without these factors working in unison, the sound energy would not be sufficient to reach the inner ear and a hearing loss would result.

The Sensorineural Mechanism

The sensorineural mechanism involves both the inner ear and the auditory nerve. The inner ear, in turn, houses both organs for balance (vestibular system) and structures concerned with hearing. For this introductory look at the ear, however, we will limit our discussion to the anatomy and physiology as they relate to the process of hearing only.

To quickly summarize the discussion of the ear's conductive mechanism, sound enters the outer ear as acoustic energy, is enhanced somewhat by the combined resonance characteristics of the outer ear (pinna resonance and ear canal resonance), reaches the eardrum, and then enters the middle ear, where it is amplified sufficiently so that it can overcome the impedance mismatch (difference in the properties of resistance) between the air-filled middle ear and the fluid-filled inner ear. The sound, in the form of mechanical energy, then reaches the junction of the stapes footplate in the oval window, where it is poised to enter the fluid-filled inner ear. It is the job of the sensorineural system to convert this mechanical (also known as vibratory) energy into an electrical impulse that will travel through the auditory nerve and be sent up to, and be used by, the brain. To see the path that the sound takes, refer to the arrows in **Figure 4-4.**

When the sound has crossed the threshold into the vestibule of the inner ear (see Figure 4-4), it is ready to enter the *cochlea*, which houses the *organ of Corti* (end organ of hearing). Figure 4-4 shows the cochlea partially uncoiled; in its normal state, however, the cochlea is coiled up like a conch shell. The name "cochlea" itself derives from the Greek *kokhlias* (meaning "snail screw") and *koklos* (meaning "spiral shell"). For a better understanding and visualization of this structure, imagine that we unroll the cochlea (**Figure 4-5**) to take a look at some of the significant structures—namely, the scala media (which houses the organ of Corti), the scala vestibuli above it, and the scala tympani below it. The top boundary of the scala media is Reissner's membrane; the bottom boundary is the basilar membrane. Both the scala ves-

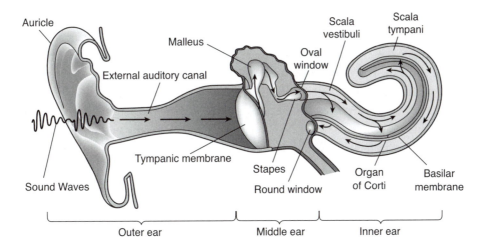

FIGURE 4-4   The outer, middle, and inner ear.

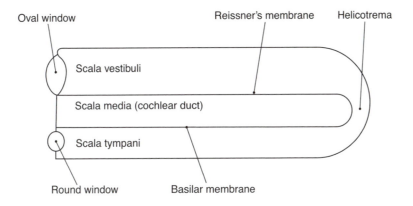

FIGURE 4-5   The cochlea uncoiled.

tibuli and the scala tympani are filled with perilymph, whereas the scala media is filled with endolymph. The endolymph and perilymph are both gelatinous-type fluids, though each has a unique chemical composition. The endolymph has high potassium content, for example, whereas the perilymph has high sodium content; this difference plays a significant role in the process of hearing.

Because the cochlea is completely filled with fluid, the sound that enters the inner ear as mechanical energy becomes a wave as it enters scala vestibuli. This wave, in turn, travels all the way around through the helicotrema and into scala tympani. The helicotrema is a passageway that permits communication between the scala vestibuli and the scala tympani.

The "traveling wave" of sound energy eventually causes displacement (movement) of the basilar membrane, as well as the organ of Corti sitting on top of it. Within the organ of Corti, it sets into motion the structures known as outer hair cells and inner hair cells. This movement of the outer and inner hair cells causes bending of the tops of these cells, a process referred to as a shearing action. At this point, the mechanical energy (sound) is converted into electrochemical energy. The shearing action causes the mixing of the sodium and potassium ions within the two fluids, which in turn leads to the electrical impulse that causes the auditory nerve to "fire." The resulting electrochemical reaction sends the information along the auditory nerve, which is then delivered to and used by the brain.

For a more detailed description of this process, the interested reader is directed to *The Auditory System: Anatomy, Physiology, and Clinical Correlates* by Musiek and Baran (2007) or *Fundamentals of Hearing: An Introduction* by Yost (2007).

THE PROCESS OF NORMAL AUDITORY DEVELOPMENT

The previous section profiled the normal anatomy and physiology of the auditory system. In this section, we explore how this system develops and matures. To do so, we first look at the prenatal period, which is where the story begins. We then proceed to the postnatal period and examine normal auditory behavior and auditory skills development.

Prenatal Auditory Development

The process of auditory maturation involves both the peripheral and central auditory pathways. That is, all of these structures need to function properly if a person is to detect, recognize, and process sound normally. We will begin by looking at what occurs during the prenatal period, as the literature now includes ample documentation of prenatal responses to sound (see, for example, Holst, Eswaran, Lowery, Murphy, Norton, & Preissl, 2005; Tye-Murray, 2004; Werner, 2003). The gestational time is, therefore, not only when the structures of the ear and auditory pathways are developing, but also when the fetus actually becomes aware of the presence of sound.

The ear starts developing very early in the prenatal period, beginning roughly during the third week of development (five weeks gestational age). At approximately weeks 26 to 28 of gestation, the human ear begins to function and the fetus starts to respond to sounds that originate from outside of the womb. As the gestational weeks pass, the ear develops enough for the fetus to respond to sound at even softer levels.

Interestingly, evidence suggests that the fetus is capable of more than just the mere detection of sound. Kisilevsky and her colleagues provide evidence that higher-order auditory perception (more than a mere awareness of sound's presence) begins before birth (Kisilevsky,

Hains, Jacquet, Granier-Deferre, & Lecanuet, 2004). Werner (2003) reports that during the last few weeks of pregnancy, the fetus is capable of not only hearing maternal speech while in the womb, but also recognizing some of what was heard after birth. In addition to the fetal response to the mother's voice (Kisilevsky et al., 2004; McMullen & Saffran, 2004), the fetus appears to learn about aspects of linguistic sound such as the prosody, rhythm, and intonation of the mother's native language (McMullen & Saffran, 2004). In fact, if a mother reads a rhythmic story to her fetus in the last few weeks of pregnancy, her newborn will recognize the story even if another woman reads it (Werner, 2003). This is a clear indication of more than a "mere awareness" of sound's existence and suggests the development of higher-order auditory perceptual ability prior to birth.

Postnatal Auditory Development

The gradual development of the auditory system that begins during the prenatal period continues after birth. Indeed, the auditory system does not become truly adult-like until a child reaches approximately 12 years of age. Because the subject of development of the auditory system is such an enormously complex topic, we cannot hope to cover it in full detail here. Instead, this section takes a very cursory look at auditory maturation for the infant and young child, as this process underlies the development of auditory behaviors and auditory skills levels.

At birth, the child is thrown into a sea of sound without having the ability to discern what is what; in fact, the child has the potential to be a native speaker of any language on the planet. From this "universe" of sound begins the normal process of language learning, and the child must start on the journey of figuring out what is important to listen to so as to become a competent communicator in his native tongue. From a bottom-up point of view, the first auditory maturational hurdle for the child to successfully "jump" is that of *encoding*. Sound encoding is a basic and essential skill whereby the ear and auditory pathway (in a bottom-up fashion) physically receive and code sound, and then send it on its way toward the brain for eventual interpretation. Sound encoding allows, for example, the perception and analysis of the acoustics of speech. In essence, the child learns that sound has meaning and that he can produce sound for the purpose of communication in his environment.

At this point in time, the infant is still listening in a nondiscriminatory way. For the development of normal language and processing skills to begin, it is essential that the infant learn to listen in a selective way. This extended learning process will continue through the preschool years and through the time the child is ready for school. In fact, it continues to be fine-tuned for an extended period after that point as well.

This aspect of speech perception initially may involve the infant selectively focusing on a specific feature of a sound. It may then involve the child's listening to complex speech. In later years, listening selectivity may involve aspects of listening that allow for understanding speech in a background of noise. While the child is expected to develop selective listening skills by the time she enters grade school, this skill actually continues developing as the child is exposed to unique and challenging listening situations. Nevertheless, even normally developing children can and do have more difficulty than adults when it comes to selectively listening, especially when the listening conditions are less than ideal.

An example of a situation that may prove more problematic for a child is one characterized by excessive background noise and/or reverberation. An abundance of literature documents the negative effects that background noise and reverberation have on children. In addition to noisy and reverberant conditions (like those found in the average classroom), children may encounter situations in which the speaker's face may not be visible. Each of these situations presents unique challenges to young children, who must learn to listen flexibly so that they can learn how to communicate effectively when they are thrust into those types of settings.

One final note about how noise and reverberation affect children's ability to hear, perceive, understand, and process the content of speech: Nonauditory effects may also play key roles. Detrimental nonauditory effects may, for example, include motivational and cognitive issues such as learned helplessness, poor problem-solving skills, low frustration tolerance, and low academic achievement (particularly when it comes to reading) (Bistrop, Haines, Hygge, MacKenzie, Neyen, & Petersen, 2002).

Auditory Behavioral Development

While their auditory systems are undergoing neuromaturational growth, children experience concomitant behavioral changes in the ways in which they react and respond to sound. This principle was demonstrated earlier in the prenatal section, which discussed how the fetus responds to sound at 26 to 28 weeks gestational age, several weeks later can respond to softer loudness levels, and eventually responds to rhythm and intonation. As a consequence, the way newborn infants and children respond to sounds is very different from the way adults tend to respond to the same sounds. In fact, maturation of the auditory system is manifest in a child's behavioral responses to sound as well as in the development of specific auditory skills levels.

The differences between the auditory behaviors of children and adults can be observed in a clinical setting—for example, by looking at the type of sound to which they respond best, the intensity (subjectively loudness) required to get a response, and way in which they do the responding. For instance, if the hearing sensitivity of an adult is being evaluated, the stimulus used would be a *pure tone* (an individual frequency of sound), and the adult would be expected to respond at a threshold level. *Threshold* here is defined as the softest level required for a person to just be able to detect the presence of the sound half of the time—that is, the level where 50%

of the time the person hears the sound and 50% of the time the person does not. Additionally, the adult would respond by raising a hand each time the sound was heard.

If a child were to be tested, the expectations would be very different from those for an adult. In fact, not only do the expectations differ from adult to child, but expectations for a younger child differ from those for the older child. With an infant from birth through approximately 7 months of age, the anticipated response pattern might include such behaviors as eye widening, startle, or a change in or cessation of activity. When the child reaches 7 months of age or so, we begin to see the addition of sound searching and sound localization behaviors. As a child approaches approximately 2½ to 3 years of age, the response pattern is expected to mature, thus enabling the child to respond by putting a ring on a dowel or dropping a block in a bucket each time she hears a sound. It is at approximately this age that the child begins to understand the connection between the sound stimulus and the required behavioral response.

The type of stimuli used would also quite likely be different. When performing behavioral testing in very young children (younger than 2 years), it may be necessary to use some form of a broadband stimulus—for example, speech or music. The typical "beeps" that adults associate with a hearing test are not of interest to the very young child. However, when the child reaches 2½ to 3 years of age, he may be developmentally ready to respond to the "beeps." The loudness level at which we would expect to see the responses would likely be the *supra threshold* level (a level that is louder than the "barely detectable" threshold level). The older the child, the lower (better) the response level, and hence the closer the child comes to the threshold level. The behavioral differences observed within the pediatric population are explored further in the assessment section of this chapter.

The observable differences between the auditory behaviors of adults and children are a testament to the process of auditory maturational development that begins in utero and continues well into the school-age years.

Auditory Skills Development

Just as neuromaturational changes are observable in auditory behaviors, so, too, are they observable in the child's development of specific auditory skills. Normal auditory skills development involves the acquisition of several individual components before the child can reach the ultimate and most difficult of the goals—namely, comprehension of linguistic and nonlinguistic sounds. The skills discussed in this section are covered in hierarchical fashion, with the simplest of the levels (detection) being presented first and the most complicated of the levels (comprehension of linguistic and nonlinguistic sounds) being presented last.

An important issue to be aware of in terms of the development of these skill levels is that they are not typically mastered in the "nice and neat" sequential hierarchy described in this section. Rather, a child may be mostly at one level, yet be able to perform some tasks at the next higher level. This "messiness" occurs because the child is constantly being bombarded with all manner of sound (e.g., speech, environmental) simultaneously. In essence, all speech, whether simple or complex (in addition to environmental sound), is thrown at the child at the same time, so all of the skills are targeted at the same time. It would be unreasonable to expect a child to acquire these skills in an orderly, sequential way when the information is being presented in a natural, somewhat random fashion. This interweaving may explain why a child can show abilities at one level while not having completely mastered the level below it. For example, the child may begin to exhibit "discrimination" of simple words, even though she has not fully mastered "detection" of some types of sound.

Another important issue is the fact that the "natural, somewhat random" language environment to which the child is exposed is not the only way the child can learn the auditory skills necessary for the development of language. A *bottom-up approach* to language learning may also be employed; in fact, it may be necessary. The issue of how best a child learns language typically becomes the subject of discussion when a child is not developing speech and language in the normal fashion, for whatever reason, and intervention of some sort is clearly in order. For this population, the bottom-up approach in a therapeutic setting may be beneficial—for example, with children who have hearing loss. It is most especially helpful with children who have additional handicapping conditions (Nevins & Garber, 2006), which 30% of all hearing-impaired children are reported to have (Tye-Murray, 2004). This directed and planned approach typically employs a linear presentation that moves in sequence from easiest to most difficult skills to develop. The therapist focuses on the child mastering one skill or skill level completely and then moves on to the next, more difficult level.

Many models have been proposed to describe the normal development of auditory skills. On the surface, it might appear that there is considerable variability among these models. A careful investigation, however, reveals that they are actually more similar than not, although some of the models go into more detail than others. The version presented here includes some of the most basic and essential components of auditory skills development; it is not intended to be an exhaustive list of all skills necessary to attain the ultimate goal of comprehension.

Detection Level

The *detection level* is the most basic level of sound awareness. It refers to the baby's ability to detect the presence or absence of sound in the environment. In the normal-hearing infant, this is a clear-cut and uncomplicated process. Unfortunately, with the hearing-impaired child, matters become more complex.

When a child sustains a hearing loss, the issue of amplification (or cochlear implant) must be considered first; subsequently, the issues of making sure that the child's device is functioning, and that it is being worn, become important. Even with appropriate and adequate amplification, the child's parents and/or caregiver must be diligent in exposing and directing the child to as much speech and as many sounds in the environment as possible.

Hearing-impaired children will have varying degrees of difficulty with this skill level (as well as the ones discussed in the following subsections), depending on the nature and severity of hearing loss sustained. There may be some sounds (particularly the lower frequencies) that the child hears and will respond to better than others (particularly the higher frequencies); this situation often arises when a child has a sensorineural hearing loss, for example (see the "Hearing Impairment" section).

Discrimination Level

The *discrimination level* is the next higher level in difficulty (but remember that these skill levels are not mutually exclusive). Children may still be developing some skills at the detection level even as they begin to develop some skills at the discrimination level. Within the discrimination level, however, skills will be learned in the same way as the other skill levels are learned—that is, in an easy to difficult order.

With the discrimination level, children first master discrimination of the *suprasegmental* aspects of language—for example, pitch, prosody, rhythm, stress, and inflection—before they master the *segmental* aspects. In fact, as described in the section on prenatal development, some evidence suggests that children respond to these suprasegmental aspects of sound before birth. As part of the development of this ability, a young child may be exposed to a parent expressing anger toward a sibling. The child may recognize the anger without needing to understand the entire dialogue that explains what the parent is angry about.

Later, children learn to respond to segmental aspects of speech, which include such elements as phonemes, morphemes, and syllables. This ability might be demonstrated by playing a "same/different" game using *dish* versus *car*, for example.

Identification Level

At the *identification level*, the child is able to identify or label an item; this ability can be shown by naming the item or pointing to it. To demonstrate this skill, a few items could be placed in front of the child—for example, a ball, a sock, a shoe, and a hat. You could then ask the child, "Where is the shoe?"

Auditory memory and later recall are essential ingredients for a child to function at the identification level and for the overall perception of speech in general. Another fundamental component of successful speech perception is *attention*, or the ability on the part of the child to focus in on the person speaking so as to understand the content and meaning of what is said. *Auditory closure* is yet another necessary skill; it can be defined as the ability to fill in a missing or misspoken part of a word or message. For example, if a phoneme is missing from a spoken word—for example, if the word is pronounced as /oa-meal / instead of /oatmeal/— auditory closure allows us to hear the word correctly. This latter skill is particularly useful in the hearing-impaired population.

Comprehension Level

The *comprehension level*—that is, the comprehension of sound and its meaning—is the ultimate goal of the hearing maturation process. Complete comprehension of speech and environmental sounds, in all settings, requires many individual skills and considerations, particularly when we consider the possibility of hearing impairments or auditory processing disorders. A full discussion of the multitude of functions and factors that determine a child's ability to understand and process spoken language is beyond the scope of this chapter, however. The interested reader is directed to the references list at the end of this chapter for other sources of information on this topic.

ASSESSMENT OF HEARING IN THE PEDIATRIC POPULATION

In the preceding section, we learned about the process of normal auditory development. One prerequisite for the development of these skills is to have normal hearing sensitivity. One of the most frequently asked questions when dealing with young children is "How do we go about testing a child's hearing?" A thorough discussion of the assessment of hearing sensitivity, even if limited to the pediatric population, is certainly beyond the scope of this chapter and textbook. To fully appreciate the sections that follow, however, a basic understanding of the pediatric evaluation process is in order.

Audiologic assessment of children bears a few similarities to the assessment process in the adult population, but for the most part is a very different affair. The similarity arises from the fact that we want to determine the person's hearing sensitivity and speech recognition ability in both populations. The difference reflects the fact that the testing process is somewhat different for each developmental level—for example, for newborns/infants, toddlers, preschoolers, school-age children, and so on. Some of these differences include the specific test procedure of choice, the types of responses expected, and the level of participation expected from the child, among other things. Children's capabilities will undoubtedly vary from one developmental level to the next; therefore, the examiner's expectations and the techniques employed to assess hearing must also vary. This section gives a very basic overview of the pediatric assessment process.

Assessment of Children from Birth to Six Months of Age

At one time, it was fairly common for hearing loss to go undetected until approximately 2½ years of age, or possibly earlier or later depending on the nature and severity of the impairment.

Sadly, this delay in diagnosis led to an unavoidable concomitant delay in speech, language, cognitive, and overall development that might have been minimized with earlier detection and intervention. In recognition of this and other related issues, the National Institute of Health (NIH) convened in 1993 and produced a consensus statement entitled *Early Identification of Hearing Impairment in Infants and Young Children*. This statement outlined recommendations for achieving universal newborn/infant hearing screening. Until its publication, only two states had enacted newborn hearing screening legislation: Hawaii in 1990 and Rhode Island in 1992.

In 2000, the Joint Committee on Infant Hearing (JCIH) of the American Speech-Language-Hearing Association (ASHA) produced a position statement titled *Principles and Guidelines for Early Hearing Detection and Intervention Programs*. The JCIH endorsed the position advocated by NIH—namely, early detection and intervention, with the ultimate goal to maximize linguistic and communicative competence and literacy development for children who are hard of hearing or deaf (ASHA, 2000). Its recommendations outlined guidelines for implementation of newborn screening, detection/confirmation of hearing loss, and intervention/follow-up related to hearing impairment. For complete details on the principles and guidelines for infant hearing screening programs, visit the ASHA's Web site (www.asha.org).

Two categories of assessment procedures that can be employed for hearing testing: *behavioral* and *electrophysiologic*. Either or both of these approaches may be employed, depending on the particular case.

A behavioral task is one that requires a response from a person. For example, with a behavioral task such as dropping a block or putting rings on a stick, children are required to make the connection between the auditory stimulus that they hear and the behavioral response of dropping a block or putting a ring on a stick. Newborn infants, quite obviously, are unable to comply with the demands of this type of behavioral task because they are not developmentally able to do so.

Electrophysiologic procedures do not require any active participation from the child. These tests are unaffected by any degree of sleep or arousal and are not negatively affected by sedation. Further, they can be performed on anyone, from pediatric patients to geriatric individuals. Therefore, electrophysiologic tests are the procedures of choice for screening hearing in the newborn infant population.

Some of the electrophysiologic procedures adopted for this purpose include *otoacoustic emissions* (OAE); *auditory brain stem response audiometry* (ABR) possibly with *auditory steady-state response* (ASSR); and *acoustic immittance measures* (*tympanometry* and *acoustic reflexes*). These noninvasive procedures are often used for the purpose of hearing screening in newborn infants. If the infant passes either the OAE or ABR test, then no further referral is made. If the child does not pass these tests, or if the child has other issues that are cause for concern, then a further referral for assessment is made. For a diagnostic assessment (as opposed to routine screening) of hearing sensitivity, clinicians typically use a test battery approach, applying as many of these procedures as possible. Put simply, a diagnosis of hearing impairment—or the determination that hearing sensitivity is normal, for that matter—should never be based on a single isolated test result.

In many hospital neonatal units, OAE testing is used as the initial screening procedure. This test is a quick, easy-to-administer, highly sensitive, and cost-effective procedure. OAE testing is based on the principle that a normal and healthy cochlea not only hears sound, but can also produce sound. Otoacoustic emissions can be either spontaneously present or evoked. With an *evoked* OAE, a sound is sent into the ear, and in response the ear produces a sound and sends it back out; this response can be recorded. By contrast, *spontaneous* OAEs, as the name suggests, are spontaneously present. However, because they are present in only a minority of the general population, no clinical diagnostic significance can be attached to them.

An abundant body of research has documented that evoked OAEs are not present in the setting of a damaged cochlea; therefore, the presence of an evoked OAE tells us that the cochlea is healthy. Nevertheless, because a hearing loss may still occur (however unlikely it may be) as a result of damage to a part of the auditory system that is farther along the auditory pathway than the cochlea, the presence of an OAE suggests a healthy cochlea only. Normal OAE responses are associated with hearing threshold levels no poorer than the level of a mild hearing loss (approximately 30 dB). When used in the pass/fail mode, OAE testing has an average pass rate as high as 90%; the 10% of babies who fail are referred for further testing.

In a two-stage screening process, the first test typically consists of OAE, to be followed by ABR testing (and possibility ASSR testing). Both the ABR and the ASSR are "evoked response" tests, meaning that sound is put in the ear with the goal of stimulating a response from the ear. This "evoked response" is then recorded. Whereas OAE testing looks at activity in the ear only as far as the cochlea, the ABR goes farther, examining the activity along the auditory nerve and brain stem pathways as well. During this test, surface (noninvasive) electrodes are placed on the baby's skull (forehead, vertex, and earlobes), and recordings are then made of the neuroelectrical activity that occurs when sound is presented to the ears.

The ASSR and the ABR differ from each other in terms of the type of sound stimulus each uses to evoke the response. Modulated pure tones, clicks, and tone bursts are all examples of different types of sounds that are available with these testing procedures. Each different type of sound stimulus (e.g., modulated pure tone, tone burst) gives potentially different information about the child's hearing ability. One major consideration in deciding which procedure to use—ABR or ASSR—is the degree of hearing loss suspected in the particular child. These choices are best made on a case-by-case basis.

The important question here is not which procedure is the best to use (ABR or ASSR), but rather how the two might be used together beneficially and which information each can add to the total hearing picture (Hall, 2005). Generally speaking, the ABR can provide frequency-specific information, which is necessary information for a person of any age in whom hearing loss is suspected. Also, this type of testing can accurately estimate levels of hearing sensitivity (thresholds) in people whose hearing falls within the normal to moderately impaired range. By contrast, the ASSR uses a different type of sound stimulus, which might provide even better frequency-specific information; it is particularly good at differentiating between severe and profound hearing impairment. Being able to make this distinction helps in deciding which intervention strategy may be the best option.

Acoustic immittance testing (also known as tests of middle ear function) includes both tympanometry and acoustic reflex testing; neither of these procedures is intended for use as a stand-alone test. Rather, these techniques should be used only in conjunction with the rest of the tests. Tympanometry and acoustic reflex testing should be done on every patient, of every age from pediatric to geriatric, whenever possible. These two procedures should not be limited to the birth to seven months of age population.

Tympanometry is not a measure of hearing, but rather provides an objective look at middle ear function (or middle ear dysfunction, as the case may be). During this test, a graph known as a tympanogram is created; it can be used to determine whether middle ear pathology is present (for example, an ear infection or punctured eardrum). Because tympanometry does not assess hearing sensitivity, it should be used in conjunction with the other hearing test results to differentiate the various types of hearing loss. It might also suggest whether a medical referral is necessary.

Acoustic reflex testing, which is also part of the immittance test battery, involves the recording of the stapedius muscle activity. The stapedius muscle (tendon) runs though the middle ear. When sound becomes too loud for a person, this muscle fires, and the ensuing muscle reflex activity can be recorded. The findings from this type of testing are used in conjunction with the audiologic assessment findings and provide valuable diagnostic information that may be helpful in determining the type of hearing loss and its severity.

Assessment of Children from 7 Months to 24–30 Months of Age

When the infant reaches approximately 6 to 7 months of age, she may be developmentally capable of being engaged in at least some behavioral procedures for hearing assessment. The results from these tests, in conjunction with the results obtained from the procedures previously, may be helpful in making a diagnosis of hearing impairment.

Visual reinforcement audiometry (VRA) is a technique that is quite often successful with infants from the age of seven months through about two years. Any child who is developmentally within the seven months to two years age range, regardless of chronological age, is an appropriate candidate for use of VRA. This assessment procedure makes use of toys that light up, sound, and the child's localization behaviors. It involves conditioning the child to search for the sound when it is heard. When the child hears the sound and localizes it, he is rewarded with the toy lighting up. Using this technique, it is possible to obtain a behavioral hearing test on a child in this developmental age range.

Assessment of Children from 30 Months to 5 Years of Age

When children reach 2½ years of age, and continuing until they are approximately 5 years of age, they can usually be engaged in some form of conditioned play techniques. For older children in this range, almost any form of a game can be employed. With younger children, games typically need to be modified into their simplest forms to find an activity that the child is developmentally capable of being engaged in with consistency and reliability. The game itself or the manner in which the child responds to it does not matter; the key consideration is simply that the child responds to the game consistently and reliably.

The goal of *conditioned play audiometry* (CPA) is to turn the hearing test into a listening game for the child. Almost any toy or game will do for this type of assessment. The idea is to condition the child to do something each time a sound is heard—for example, dropping a block, putting a ring on a stick, or putting a piece in a puzzle. Again, finding a task that the child can perform both consistently and reliably is the goal.

From age approximately five years onward, children should be more adult-like and should be able to complete a hearing test by using standard hand-raising responses. In other words, they should be capable of raising a hand each time a sound is heard.

Speech Recognition Assessment

A speech recognition assessment yields information that is essential to filling in the child's overall auditory picture. It should be performed as soon as the child is developmentally ready. Because such testing requires willingness and active participation from the child, however, children may have to be four or five years of age before they will participate.

The two measures that are relevant to our needs here are *speech recognition threshold* and *speech recognition score*. The speech recognition threshold is simply the very softest level that the child can recognize as speech 50% of the time; the speech recognition score represents the percentage of speech that is understood when the speech signal is made sufficiently loud for the child (this is a measure of the clarity of speech). This latter measure is a particularly vital piece of information because it is frequently an accurate predictor of the child's later potential functional abilities.

A variety of commercially available tools have been designed for this purpose, covering a range of developmental levels. The tests often make use of pictures, toys, and objects to which the child can point; for older children, there are word lists (appropriate for the kindergarten-age child) that the youngster is asked to repeat. The information obtained in this way is essential in planning and implementing an individualized program for the development of the child's auditory skills.

HEARING IMPAIRMENT

Now that we have learned about the many techniques that are used for testing children's hearing sensitivity, we should consider the possible results of those tests. This section identifies the various types of hearing loss, along with some of their more common etiologies and characteristics. The treatments and interventions for these disorders are discussed later in this chapter.

Three types of hearing loss are distinguished:

+ A *conductive hearing loss* is associated with damage in the outer and/or middle ear.
+ A *sensorineural hearing loss* is associated with damage to the inner ear and/or auditory nerve.
+ A *mixed hearing loss* is when both a conductive hearing loss and a sensorineural hearing loss are present at the same time.

Some children have a *unilateral hearing loss*, in which one ear has normal hearing and one ear has impaired hearing; the loss in such a case may be conductive, sensorineural, or mixed in nature.

Conductive Hearing Loss

As discussed earlier in this chapter, sound is collected by the pinna, sent down the ear canal to the eardrum, and then passed through the middle ear space. Adequate middle ear transfer function is essential for effective transmission of sound into the inner ear. When sound is not efficiently conducted through the outer/middle ear pathway (i.e., the conductive pathway), a conductive hearing loss results. Such a problem may occur (to name but a few causes) as a result of a blockage of wax, an infection or foreign body in the ear canal, a perforated eardrum, or the all-too-common ear infection. *Anything* that blocks or stops sound from being effectively transmitted through the outer and/or middle ear will cause a conductive hearing loss. By far, the most common etiology for conductive hearing loss in children is ear infection, also known as *otitis media*.

Otitis media is one of the most common diseases of early childhood. It is the nemesis of audiologists and speech-language pathologists alike—not to mention parents, childcare providers, and pediatric healthcare professionals. By the age of six years, nearly all children will have had at least one episode of otitis media, and perhaps as many as two-thirds of children will have had recurring episodes.

The suspicion or identification of otitis media in the preschool setting is mitigated by the fact that a significant percentage (perhaps one-third, or even more) of cases with otitis media will be asymptomatic. In one study of 302 children younger than four years of age, 40% of the children with acute otitis media never complained of, or had symptoms of, an earache. Fever was not present in 31%, and sleep was not disturbed in half of the children with acute otitis media (Pichichero, 2000). Obviously, if there is no pain, no fever, and there are no symptoms, there are no signs for the parent to pick up on. If the child is not verbally sophisticated enough to convey what she is experiencing (as is frequently the case with young children), the condition will go undetected. It is no surprise, then, that otitis media is a major cause of hearing loss and language delay in the preschool population.

Conductive hearing loss is usually characterized by a decrease in the loudness of sound, but the clarity of speech often remains intact. That is, there is typically no distortion of sound (a characteristic often seen in other types of hearing loss). Conductive hearing loss is very often medically and/or surgically treatable. When it results from a condition such as otitis media, its severity may fluctuate, with some days being either much better or much worse than others. This ever-changing hearing loss leads to very inconsistent responses and behaviors on the part of the child who has this type of disorder; one day the child may be very responsive, but the next day he may be quite unresponsive.

Sensorineural Hearing Loss

A sensorineural hearing loss occurs when damage to a structure within the inner ear and/or auditory nerve pathway (the sensorineural pathway) prevents the transmission of sound to the brain. Such a hearing loss may be the result of an almost unlimited number of causes, such as genetic, prenatal, and postnatal syndromes; diseases; and disorders.

According to the ASHA (2000), genetic (heredity) factors are believed to account for more than half of all cases of sensorineural hearing loss in children. Congenital (present at birth) causes that are common in children include prenatal infection (e.g., rubella or cytomegalovirus), prematurity, anoxia, and Rh-factor complications. The "acquired" category includes etiologies such as meningitis, measles, and mumps, among others.

Sensorineural hearing loss, unlike conductive hearing loss, involves a loss of sensitivity *and* (in most cases) a distortion of speech; this dual nature is a hallmark of this type of hearing loss. The amount of speech recognition difficulty varies not only from one person to the next, or from one particular hearing loss to the next, but also from day to day in the same person. It is this loss of clarity (or speech recognition loss) that frequently makes the fitting of a hearing aid in such cases a challenging task. Most hearing aids simply amplify sound, making it louder. When the child has a sensorineural hearing loss that is characterized by distortion of speech, however, the hearing aid may make the sound louder, but it will *not* make the sound clearer. Add in the noise and reverberation of the average classroom setting, and it is no wonder that children with this type of hearing loss have an enormously difficult task in trying to hear in these environments. Not surprisingly, some of these children are known to display such behaviors as falling asleep on their desks, complaining of headaches, and exhibiting other telltale signs of the difficulties they face on a routine basis.

A subcategory of sorts within the realm of sensorineural hearing loss is *high-frequency sensorineural hearing loss*. Many, if not most, cases of sensorineural hearing loss are characterized by hearing sensitivity being somewhat better in the lower frequencies but noticeably poorer in the higher frequencies. Lower-frequency sounds (think of the bass control on your stereo) include background noise, for example; in terms of speech and language, they often include sounds such as the vowel sounds. High-frequency sounds (think of the treble control on your stereo), by contrast, include consonant sounds, with the sibilants (e.g., /s/, /θ/, /ð/, /ʃ/, /f/) having the highest frequency content of the consonants. With a high-frequency hearing loss, the person's ability to hear high frequencies is not merely somewhat poorer; it is *much* poorer. At the same time, hearing for lower-frequency sounds often remains intact. For example, a hearing loss characterized as being "high frequency" may have normal hearing sensitivity for the lower-frequency background and vowel type sounds, while having profoundly impaired hearing for the higher-frequency consonant sounds.

Unfortunately for those children who have this type of hearing loss, the consonants tend to carry most of the meaning of speech. That is, if someone spoke and we could hear only the vowel sounds, we would not have any idea what the person was trying to say. Conversely, if we heard only the consonant sounds, we would have a very good idea of what was being said. As an example, suppose the only part of a word you hear someone say is the vowel sound /i/. The word the person is saying could be any one of perhaps hundreds or even thousands of words. Suppose now that you do not hear the vowel, but only the consonant sounds /p – n/. We have now narrowed down our list of possible words from perhaps hundreds or thousands, to perhaps only a handful at most.

Needless to say, high-frequency sensorineural hearing loss will typically result in the child having very poor speech recognition scores. We will address this issue further in a later section of this chapter.

No discussion of sensorineural hearing loss would be complete without saying a few words about the differences between "having a hearing impairment," "being profoundly deaf," and "being Deaf." The term "Deaf" with a capital "D" refers to the Deaf population and will be addressed later in this chapter. The distinction being made here between hearing impaired and deaf is a functional one; it has less to do with the degree of hearing impairment and more to do with the child's overall level of auditory functioning.

As suggested earlier, nearly all persons with sensorineural hearing loss, regardless of the degree of loudness loss (i.e., mild, moderate, severe, or profound), will experience some degree of speech clarity problems. Furthermore, the severity of the loss is not necessarily an indication of what the speech clarity is likely to be. In other words, those with mild degrees of hearing loss are not necessarily those with minimal speech understanding problems, and vice versa. Almost any combination of these two factors (loudness and clarity) is possible. When each affected individual is *appropriately* fit with hearing aids, it is certainly possible that the person with moderate hearing loss and poor speech clarity will function worse than the person with severe hearing loss but better speech clarity—recall that hearing aids simply make things louder, not clearer.

In conclusion, the distinction between hearing impaired and deaf is not solely an indication of the "degree" or severity of loudness loss. Rather, it indicates the person's *functional ability*, which is a consequence of many factors, of which "degree" of loudness loss is just one. Other factors determining a person's overall functional ability may include such characteristics as prelingual or postlingual onset of hearing loss, age of onset for postlingual losses, speech understanding ability, successful use of a hearing aid, speech reading skills, and cognitive abilities.

Mixed Hearing Loss

A mixed hearing loss exists when there is damage to both the conductive and sensorineural pathways at the same time. An example of this type of hearing loss is when a person with a congenital sensorineural hearing loss gets an ear infection. The sensorineural hearing loss *plus* the conductive hearing loss (from the ear infection) *equals* a mixed hearing loss. When we consider the vast array of conditions and factors that may result in a conductive or sensorineural hearing loss, we begin to realize the nearly limitless possible combinations of conditions that can create a mixed hearing loss. In light of the almost unlimited supply of etiologies of mixed hearing loss, presenting a discussion of "typical" etiologies and "classic" characteristics becomes nothing less than a daunting task. Rather than attempting this feat, this section looks at the most common cause of conductive loss and the most common cause of sensorineural loss and then considers the scenario in which they occur together.

Where children are concerned, genetic factors are believed to account for more than 50% of cases of sensorineural hearing loss. On the conductive side, the most common hearing loss is due to otitis media. This combination *possibly* represents one of the most likely scenarios for mixed hearing loss in children; that is, the "mixed hearing loss" child whom clinicians *might* be most likely to see is born with a sensorineural hearing loss and then gets an ear infection on top of it.

The characteristics of this particular mixed hearing loss largely depend on the underlying sensorineural pathology. Given that otitis media typically results in loudness loss only, it is most helpful to look at the sensorineural component, which dictates the speech clarity ability. The addition of the ear infection means that sounds have to be louder for the child; the percentage of the conversation that the child understands (assuming it is made louder to overcome the hurdles imposed by the ear infection) should remain the same as when the child had the sensorineural loss and no ear infection.

Unilateral Hearing Loss

A unilateral hearing loss (UHL) is simply a hearing loss that affects one ear only. It may be the result of conductive, sensorineural, or mixed pathology. The more severe the loss, the more difficulty the child is likely to have. However, the precise outcome depends on other factors as well.

Several characteristic areas of concern arise with the child with a UHL, including difficulty in the localization of a sound source (which may be cause for safety concerns for the young child) and difficulty hearing and/or understanding if the speaker is facing the bad ear as opposed to the good one. The factor that will likely be most damaging for all areas of learning and development is a background filled with noise or reverberant conditions. The amount of difficulty in understanding speech may range from mild to severe, depending on the hearing loss as well as the amounts of background noise and reverberation. Thus a child with a UHL may perform as well as a normal-hearing child or as poorly as a severely impaired child, depending on the particular conditions and circumstances.

INTERVENTIONS FOR HEARING LOSS

Given that the vast majority of all knowledge and learning (perhaps as much as 90%) occurs incidentally, applying the appropriate intervention for hearing loss becomes imperative. This section considers the available medical–surgical treatments, hearing aids, cochlear implants, and aural rehabilitation options for various types of hearing loss.

Medical–Surgical Treatments for Otitis Media

In keeping with the purpose of this book, which is to present the foundations and processes essential to language development, the issue of treatment or interventions for a conductive hearing loss, like that caused by otitis media, must be addressed. Generally speaking, otitis media is treated medically, surgically, or by both methods.

The most important action a speech-language pathologist can take when otitis media is suspected is to refer the child to the appropriate clinician. If the child is demonstrating symptoms of otitis media such as fever, earache, inconsistent responses to sound, and irritability, then the child should be referred to a medical doctor immediately. The physician, preferably an ear specialist, is a person who specializes in the medical treatment of diseases and conditions. If the child is suspected of having a hearing loss for an unknown reason, however, he or she should be referred to an audiologist—that is, a person who specializes in the diagnosis and treatment of hearing loss. If the audiologist's assessment reveals evidence of this type of middle ear pathology, a medical referral will then be made.

Once the child is referred to the physician, there are typically two ways that otitis media is treated, and the child may require either or both of these options. The first option is antibiotic treatment; the second possibility, especially when a child has chronic episodes with no relief from medication, is surgery. The purpose of the surgery is to drain the fluid that has built up during the episode of otitis media. During this procedure, tubes are inserted into the child's eardrum to allow air to flow into the middle ear space and keep the fluid from building up again. Assuming that treatment is successful, the conductive part of the hearing loss will be eliminated.

Of course, not all conductive hearing losses are attributable to otitis media. Hence, antibiotic treatment and tube surgery are not the only treatment options for conductive hearing loss. The particular medical and/or surgical treatment available for the child will depend on the particular pathology in question. The recommendation in such cases is to follow the path outlined earlier: If there is a suspicion of hearing loss that might be related to a medical concern, the child must be referred to a physician. If the concern is primarily one of impaired hearing (without suspected medical involvement), a referral to an audiologist is appropriate.

There is always the possibility that the conductive pathology in question cannot (or the patient is given the choice not to) be treated with medicine or surgery. In this event, the patient might be a candidate for a hearing aid.

Hearing Aids

A general rule of thumb is that the type of hearing loss for which individuals are most often fitted with a hearing aid is a sensorineural hearing loss. Nevertheless, there are two caveats to this rule of thumb. First, a hearing aid might also be an appropriate choice if is the person has a conductive pathology that cannot be treated by the physician. Second, some cases of sensorineural hearing loss cannot be helped with hearing aids. For the latter cases, as discussed in the following section, cochlear implants may be appropriate.

One of the most important facts to understand about a hearing aid is that it is not a panacea for all hearing problems. It does not restore hearing to "normal," and some of the most troublesome situations that the child will experience without a hearing aid will be the same ones that will be troublesome with the hearing aid. For example, classroom settings are especially problematic for children with a hearing loss because of the presence of noise and/or reverberation. In fact, classrooms may be difficult for normal-hearing children as well. Additionally, while hearing aids will make speech louder and more "accessible" to the hearing-impaired child, the speech message may still be unclear or muffled. This outcome reflects the impaired speech recognition skills associated with the hearing loss and explains why even the most effective possible hearing aid choice does not restore the child to "normal." This is true even if the child sustains what has been classified as a "mild" hearing loss.

The primary hearing aid style used in the pediatric population is the "behind-the-ear" (BTE) style hearing aid (**Figure 4-6a**). Other styles of hearing aids are also in use, albeit not for the pediatric population. The "in-the-ear" (ITE) style (**Figure 4-6c**) may be used for the older child, perhaps in the pre-teen or teenaged years. "In-the-canal" (ITC) hearing aids (**Figure 4-6d**) and "completely in-the-canal" (CIC) hearing aids (**Figure 4-6e**) are rarely used for children. One of the main reasons why these styles are not used in the pediatric population (and the ITE is used only in older children) has to do with the fact that these hearing aids are entirely custom molded. Each time the child grows, the entire hearing aid needs to be sent back and remade to refit the child; this happens quite often in young children. With the BTE-style hearing aid, only the earmold portion needs to be remade (see **Figure 4-6b**), and the hearing aid along with the old earmold remain with the child during this process.

The basic difference in the styles, other than appearance, relates to their tendency to produce *feedback*—also known as "that annoying whistling" that relatives and close friends of the hearing impaired person complain about. The larger the size of the hearing aid, the more power it can provide without producing feedback.

The basic components of a hearing aid (regardless of style) are the same: the microphone, the processing circuit(s), and the receiver. With the BTE model, the child also needs an earmold to couple the hearing aid to the ear. With the ITE, all of the components are internal. The amount of power and other electroacoustic requirements are based on the hearing loss and are determined by the audiologist for each child individually.

A question that is commonly asked about hearing aids is "Which is better—getting one hearing aid or two?" The answer to this question is not a simple one. The issue of one versus two hearing aids has very little, if anything, to do with the degree of hearing loss (mild versus severe, for example). Instead, having two hearing aids is the preferred choice whenever possible and regardless of degree of loss, because two hearing aids allow for balanced or stereo listening. This skill is crucial in being able to understand speech in noisy settings. However, there are also many reasons why using two hearing aids might not be advisable. This decision will be made by the audiologist on a case-by-case basis.

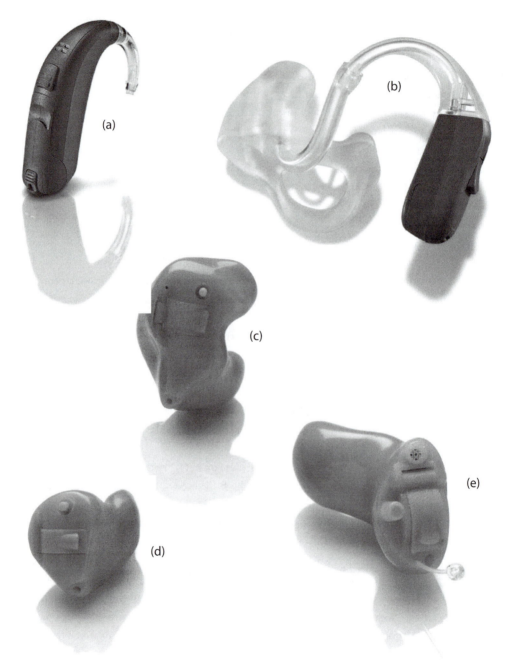

FIGURE 4-6   Hearing aids. (a) "Behind the Ear" model. (b) "Behind the Ear" model with ear mold. (c) "In the Ear" model. (d) "In the Canal" model. (e) "Completely in the Canal" model.
Source: Courtesy of Sonic Innovations, Inc.

The primary goal in selecting the most appropriate and effective intervention technique is always to maximize the auditory input that the child receives. Remember, the vast majority of learning occurs incidentally. Unfortunately, some children receive either no benefit or very minimal benefit from hearing aids, even with the most powerful devices. For these children, cochlear implantation might be a consideration.

Cochlear Implants

Cochlear implant technology was inspired by the desire to help those severely and profoundly impaired individuals who were unable to obtain any substantial benefit from conventional hearing aids. Cochlear implants research began about 30 years ago (in adults). The devices did not receive FDA approval in the United States for children 2 years of age until 1990, and for children 12 months of age until 2002.

A cochlear implant differs from a hearing aid in that it is not simply another device that makes sound louder. Rather, this device is implanted within the cochlea and provides the sensation of sound by electrically stimulating the auditory nerve.

The cochlear implant (**Figure 4-7**) contains an external microphone that looks like a BTE hearing aid. This microphone picks up all of the sound from the environment and sends it to the speech processor (**Figure 4-7a**). The speech processor then analyzes the sound and converts it into a digital sound signal, which in turn is sent to the transmitter. Internally (**Figure 4-7b**), the implant includes a receiver/stimulator and an electrode array. The sound is sent from transmitter to receiver, where the sound is converted into an electric impulse. This impulse is transmitted to the electrode array, which then stimulates the auditory nerve.

Not everyone with a severe or profound hearing loss is a candidate for a cochlear implant. In addition to having certain audiologic test results, a child must meet many other requirements to be considered a candidate for implantation. Some of these include (but are not limited to) having a functional auditory nerve, having no medical contraindications, having a family with realistic expectations, and being willing to work closely and reliably with the audiologist, speech-language pathologist, and other implant team members and professionals.

After all of the necessary assessments have been completed, the candidacy approved, and the implantation surgery performed, the process of rehabilitation for the child can begin. Rehabilitation starts four to six weeks post surgery, when the child is fit with the microphone and processor, and programming the implant begins for the individual child. The programming of the unit (referred to as mapping) is an ongoing process, as adjustments and reprogramming are frequently necessary, particularly with young children. Simultaneously with the ongoing mapping of the cochlear implant device, the child will undergo speech-language therapy, auditory (skills) training, counseling, and other interventions. Clearly, there is an extensive amount and variety of intervention with children who receive cochlear implants.

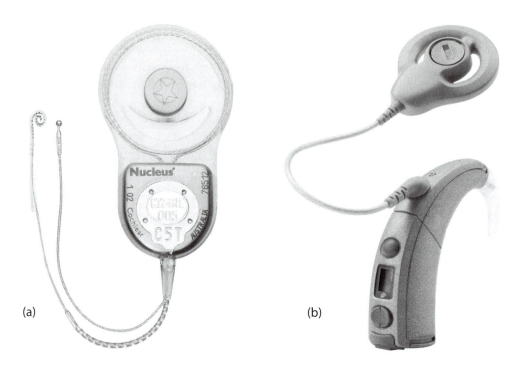

(a)   (b)

FIGURE 4-7   Cochlear implants. (a) Internal "implantable" components. (b) External components.
Source: Courtesy of Cochlear Americas, Inc.

Aural Rehabilitation

Aural rehabilitation (or habilitation, as the case may be) with a child begins with the evaluation process and must be tailored to the child's individual needs, taking into account all manner of details specific to the child. A comprehensive aural rehabilitation plan should examine and consider each of the following area for inclusion, which are based, in part, on the preferred practice patterns outlined by ASHA (2006):

- Ongoing audiologic evaluations to monitor the child's hearing status
- Selection, fitting, and ongoing monitoring of and follow-up with the appropriate device (i.e., hearing aid or cochlear implant) and with the child's functional ability while using it
- Parental education about the child's hearing loss; the care, use, and maintenance of the selected device; and educational choices for the child
- Parental counseling regarding the ramifications of the auditory, speech-language, and cognitive effects of the hearing loss on the child and the social–emotional effects on the child *and* other family members

+ Referral to the local board of education for child study team (educational) evaluation and determination of the appropriate preschool or educational setting (if appropriate)
+ Referral to other professionals as necessary
+ Referral to a speech-language pathologist for evaluation and intervention
+ Planning and implementation of an auditory training program to assist the development of essential listening skills (i.e., the developmental skill levels of detection, discrimination, identification, and comprehension)

Training for the development of auditory listening skills is an essential element of the aural rehabilitation program. Hearing-impaired children will move through the same stages of detection, discrimination, identification, and comprehension observed in normal-hearing children, but they typically need more assistance and perhaps more time to accomplish this development.

The child who has normal hearing and is developmentally normal acquires the skills necessary for normal spoken language in a natural environment with little or no special attention necessary. By comparison, the hearing-impaired child may need an intensive amount of additional assistance that a bottom-up therapeutic approach will provide. In a bottom-up approach, each of the skill levels is individually targeted with well–thought-out and well-planned activities; the child masters one skill before the therapist moves on and targets the next. For the severely to profoundly hearing-impaired child to develop normal speech and language skills, this individualized bottom-up approach is a necessary addition to the natural top-down–type environment.

LANGUAGE DEVELOPMENT TYPICAL OF THE HEARING-IMPAIRED POPULATION

Conductive/Otitis Media Population

As suggested previously in this chapter, by far the most likely conductive hearing loss in the pediatric population is that caused by otitis media (the common ear infection). Otitis media and the resulting "temporary and fluctuating" hearing loss that results are all too often underestimated. This infection is most prevalent between the ages of birth and three years, the time that is absolutely crucial for the development of language. This section provides an overview of the general and language-related effects of otitis media.

Some general characteristics have been identified among children who have a hearing loss as a result of otitis media, but one of the most frequently observed and most important of which to be aware is "inconsistent" behaviors and responses to sound. Children with this type of hearing loss might be quite responsive and communicative one day only to become very unresponsive the next day; this inconsistency reflects the fact that the hearing loss often fluctuates. Specifically, the way the child responds on any given day is directly related to the severity of the infection on that day: As the severity of the ear infection varies, so does the resulting degree of hearing loss. If a child is having a "bad hearing day" when you choose to screen or evaluate the child's language skills, the child may demonstrate unexpectedly depressed scores overall. This poor performance may have little to do with the child's true capabilities, but rather may indicate that the child did not understand the directions because he did not hear them properly. Be especially careful, before you perform a speech evaluation, to ensure that hearing has been evaluated and you are aware of any precautions (such as making sure the child can see you when you're speaking) that may be necessary for the results to be valid.

The fact that the child hears better on one day than another is not the only factor to be considered. Conductive hearing loss also affects language development in that the fluctuating hearing loss causes inconsistent sound input, which means that the language and general information input is inconsistent as well. As mentioned repeatedly in this chapter, the vast majority of learning occurs incidentally. If auditory input is inconsistent, not only will the child's awareness of and response to sound be inconsistent, but learning will be inconsistent as well. The output can be only as good as the input allows.

Children who experience otitis media often do not get all or any of the message the first time around. As a consequence, they may require frequent repetition and may not even be aware of someone speaking if the speaker is not within the child's range of vision. Such hearing-impaired children have a very difficult time following directions, are unable to attend to a story read-aloud, and have a tendency to use gesture rather than verbal expression to communicate. Undoubtedly, the latter preference is related to the concomitant speech and language difficulty.

When all of these factors are considered together, it becomes glaringly apparent that the seemingly "benign" episode of "temporary" hearing loss related to an ear infection is a rather costly episode indeed. The potential ramifications of these fluctuating episodes of ear infections with hearing loss must not be underestimated.

To understand the full implications, we should explore the link connecting the "temporary and fluctuating" hearing loss associated with otitis media to "specific" language-related deficits. Hearing loss related to otitis media with effusion (a specific form of the pathology) "has been hypothesized to disrupt children's ability to process language at a rapid rate, affecting both comprehension and production in phonology, vocabulary, syntax, and discourse" (Roberts & Hunter, 2002). While there is controversy in the literature on this issue, some points of consensus in this area have been achieved. For example, there is *some* agreement about a relationship between a history of otitis media in early childhood and later receptive and expressive language deficits. Also, a meta-analysis of prospective studies (Roberts, Rosenfeld, & Zeisel, 2004) revealed a significant negative correlation between children having episodes of otitis media with effusion (OME) and poorer language abilities, both expressively and receptively in preschoolers. Roberts and her colleagues did not, however, find a statistically significant correlation between OME and vocabulary, syntax, or speech.

Another example of how seemingly benign episodes of otitis media are not so "benign" (in fact, they may be anything but benign) arises in the area of auditory processing. There is overwhelming agreement and an abundance of information in the literature correlating recurring episodes of otitis media in early childhood with later auditory processing deficits. Inadequate auditory processing skills lead to impaired aural/oral language comprehension skills, among many other negative effects. Following is a list of the specific areas of auditory processing that may be affected, whether singly or in combination of these areas:

- Auditory discrimination
- Auditory attention
- Auditory figure/ground
  - Speech in noise
  - Selective listening
- Phonologic awareness
- Auditory closure
- Auditory sound blending (phonemic synthesis)
- Auditory segmenting
- Auditory memory
- Auditory association
- Decoding of speech
- Temporal processing
  - Temporal resolution
  - Temporal masking
  - Temporal ordering
  - Temporal integration

For additional information on this topic, readers are directed to publications by ASHA (1996) and Jerger and Musiek (2000).

Sensorineural Population

The language characteristics of the hearing-impaired and profoundly deaf (sensorineural) population are such a vast topic that we will hardly be able to scratch the surface of them in this text. Instead, because of space limitations, this chapter addresses oral language skills only. This is not a statement about a preference for oral versus manual communication. Rather, because this text focuses on oral language development, our discussion is limited to children who are using an aural/oral method of communication. Interested readers are encouraged to explore this topic further on their own.

Sensorineural hearing loss may vary from borderline or minimally impaired to profoundly deaf, or it may fall anywhere in between these two extremes. Hence, a child's speech and language abilities depend on how mild or severe the nature of the hearing loss happens to be for the individual. Additionally, other factors—for example, age when the hearing loss is identified, age when the child is fit with a hearing aid or cochlear implant, and cognitive abilities—will inevitably affect the overall language functioning of the individual.

In general, hearing losses that are either very mild or limited to an extremely narrow frequency range tend to be associated with relatively mild deficits in speech and language development. In fact, until the implementation of universal newborn hearing screening programs, this type of hearing loss might have gone undetected until later in life (and sometimes still does). Some, if not many, of these children may have been misdiagnosed as emotionally disturbed. An abundance of literature now illustrates the negative impact that such "mild" or "minimal" losses have, and these children clearly do benefit from intervention. From this point forward, however, we will focus on the language development of the more significantly impaired population.

Phonology and speech intelligibility among children with serious hearing impairments quite obviously will vary tremendously. A child will have a difficult time producing a particular speech sound that cannot be perceived. Therefore, the better the quality of the speech input heard by the child, the more intelligible the child's speech will be. Conversely, the more garbled the speech signal that the child receives, the poorer the child's intelligibility will be. This is one of the many reasons why it is imperative that a child be fit with the most effective means of amplification (hearing aid or cochlear implant) possible and that the device be worn consistently.

Let's first take a look at the child who has a more moderate degree of impairment. For example, the child with hearing loss in the mild to moderate/severe range typically has speech production errors comparable to those of normal-hearing children with articulation or phonological delays (Schow & Nerbonne, 2007). Such a child's overall intelligibility will largely depend on the child being fit with hearing aids that are as effective as possible at as early an age as possible.

Next, we consider the child who has a high-frequency sensorineural hearing loss. In this type of hearing loss (discussed in depth earlier in this chapter), hearing for the low-frequency sounds is much better than hearing for high-frequency sounds. This type of impairment will have a significant negative impact on the child's phonological development. The child will hear the vowel sounds rather well, but will not hear the consonant sounds well, if they are heard at all. The way the child speaks will reflect this difficulty, so the child might not be highly intelligible. The intelligibility level will vary depending on the child. That being said, such a child's production of vowel sounds and the lower-frequency consonants (such as /r/ and /l/) will be fairly intelligible, whereas her production of the higher-frequency sibilant sounds (such as /s/, /ɵ/, /ð/, /ʃ/, /f/) may be characterized by distortions, substitutions, and omissions.

Children with a high-frequency hearing loss will also experience speech recognition difficulties related to the fact that they hear mostly the vowel sounds and not the consonant sounds. Their speech recognition (understanding) is impaired just as their intelligibility is. Such children must have intervention at as early an age as possible (for example, a hearing aid, aural rehabilitation, or speech-language therapy) and very careful monitoring if they are to develop normal speech, language, and listening skills.

Now consider the more significantly hearing-impaired (severe to profound) population. An important caveat about this population is that the implementation of universal newborn hearing screening and the astounding advances in cochlear implant technology and candidacy have had an impressive impact on the lives of these children and their language learning potential. In fact, children who have been congenitally and/or prelingually deafened are now (often) being mainstreamed, when at one time they most likely would have wound up in a program for profoundly hearing-impaired individuals. The language potential and abilities of these children have vastly improved, albeit through the use of intensive rehabilitative intervention strategies. However, there remains a significant population that requires the special attention and interventions available only in a program for the hearing impaired.

Schow and Nerbonne (2007) discuss the results of a study done by Carney in 1986, which revealed that children with this level of hearing had approximately 20% intelligibility overall, with a range of 0% to 100%. In 1986, however, children were not even considered candidates for cochlear implantation. In fact, FDA approval for pediatric implantation was not received until 1990. The advent of this therapeutic option has no doubt had a tremendous impact on children's potential. Today, anticipated speech intelligibility is perhaps better considered in relation to the degree of hearing impairment *after* implantation rather than the severe to profound degree of loss *prior to* intervention.

The same consideration applies where language skills are concerned. As pointed out by Nevins and Garber (2006), the auditory access provided by the cochlear implant gives young, severely to profoundly deaf children the greatest potential to develop auditory skills in a naturalistic, albeit facilitated manner. They point out, quite correctly, that this process requires considerable therapeutic intervention. Thus how severely delayed the child's language is may be more closely correlated to the child's "functional auditory abilities" after intervention.

Language abilities will vary as greatly, just as speech intelligibility will. Children with significant sensorineural hearing loss will typically demonstrate difficulty in the areas of expressive and receptive language development. These deficits often lead to learning problems and lower academic achievement and therefore will negatively affect vocational choices. Clearly, both phonology and vocabulary are diminished in such cases. Hearing-impaired children develop their vocabulary more slowly and tend to learn concrete words more easily than abstract ones. They also demonstrate difficulty in grasping syntax and morphology. Indeed, one well-documented difference between how a hearing-impaired child and a normal-hearing child develop is in the rate at which they do it—the hearing-impaired child is obviously delayed.

Finally, children with hearing loss tend to comprehend and produce shorter and simpler sentence structures than do their normal-hearing counterparts. They have difficulty with the comprehension and production of complex sentences, as well as in the writing of such sentences. This is a clear testament to why children in the functionally profound (deaf) group have lower academic achievement and are more limited in vocational choices and social interactions. However, it bears repeating that with the advances in cochlear implant technology, severe to profoundly hearing-impaired children have a greater possibility of achieving their full potential, although tremendous amounts of intervention and effort are required to do so.

Unilateral Population

The diverse nature of unilateral hearing loss makes it difficult to typify the language characteristics of the population with this type of hearing impairment. Nevertheless, there are noteworthy research findings and key clinical and school setting observations to share.

In terms of language learning and the academic performance of unilaterally impaired children, the literature suggests a wide range of abilities and performance. Researchers tend to agree that the presence of a UHL potentially puts a child at a developmental disadvantage. Risk factors associated with an increased likelihood of delays or deficits include onset of the hearing loss at an early age, severe to profound degree of loss, and right UHL versus left UHL (Bess, 1986). Some specific examples of areas where children with UHL consistently perform more poorly include (lower) verbal IQ; (poorer) speech discrimination in noise; (poorer) language performance on the Token Test for Children (Klee & Davis-Dansky, 1986; Bovo, Martini, Agnoletto, Beghi, Carmignoto, & Milani, 1988; Bess & Tharpe, 1986; Lieu, 2004); and a variety of auditory, linguistic, and cognitive difficulties that appear to compromise educational progress (Bess, 1986). Finally, all of the literature reviewed is in agreement that as many as 35% of all children with UHL fail at least one grade in school, with many needing additional resource room assistance.

The literature makes clear that children with unilateral hearing loss may encounter very significant difficulties as a result of their hearing impairment. The old adage about "needing only one good ear" is absolutely not true. Children need normal hearing sensitivity in both ears, and a lot more on top of that. One normal-hearing ear will not be enough. Children with UHL must be carefully evaluated and receive regular monitoring of both hearing status and developmental progress (auditory, language, cognitive, and academic) when they start school.

A Note about Deaf Culture

Deaf with a capital "D" refers to the *Deaf culture* (or Deaf community), where being Deaf involves much more than just having a profound degree of hearing loss. This term does not refer to the audiologic category of profound hearing loss, because someone may be a member of the Deaf community without necessarily falling into that exact category. Likewise, someone with a profound hearing loss may have been educated in a mainstreamed setting; thus the person may not know sign language and may not be part of the Deaf community. The Deaf community may also include people with other degrees of hearing impairment who perhaps went to schools for deaf persons, children or close relations of someone who is Deaf, or even other professionals (interpreters, for example).

The Deaf community has its own culture, its own language (sign language), and its own accepted cultural norms. Hearing-impaired members of the Deaf community are, for the most part, isolated from the "hearing world." It is not surprising, therefore, that they have developed a separate and unique culture. This is the community with which these individuals identify and where they feel that they belong.

Historically speaking, the Deaf community on the whole has been against cochlear implant technology for their children. Indeed, in 1990, the National Association for the Deaf (NAD) came out with a statement against such devices. Members of the Deaf culture view cochlear implant technology for their children as being no different than the foot binding that occurred in ancient China—that is, this technology is seen as an assault on the people of their community. Historically speaking, one of the candidacy requirements for receiving a cochlear implant has been for the family to have the child enrolled in an aural/oral language learning approach. When we consider this fact, it is easy to understand how the Deaf community perceives cochlear implants as a threat to their culture. The proponents on each side of this issue remain fairly firm in their respective positions, but there has appeared to be some slight softening (or at least more open-mindedness) on both sides in recent years.

CASE STUDIES

JOHNATHON (TD)

Johnathon, a 25-month-old boy, is an example of a typically developing child. In terms of his auditory maturational level, Johnathan's responses to environmental sounds, his name, and attention to verbal requests demonstrate sound encoding and selective listening, as evidenced by his interpreting of the incoming sound and gleaning meaning from the ongoing speech.

Johnathon's development of auditory skill levels and his tendency to develop them in an overlapping manner—an approach typical of a normal-hearing child in a naturalistic environment—are also apparent. This child demonstrates evidence of (age-appropriate) detection, discrimination, identification, and even comprehension of linguistic and nonlinguistic sound, each in varying degrees (as is expected in the normally developing child). Specifically, Johnathon's report notes that his receptive and expressive language skills were demonstrated to be "most typical of a 21- to 24-month-old toddler, with a scatter of skills up to 24- to 27-month age levels."

In conclusion, Johnathon appears to be a classic example of a normally developing child. Based on his overall level of development and lack of significant history for recurring ear infections, there would be no audiologic or auditory recommendations for this child.

JOSEPHINE (LB)

Josephine is a 22-month-old girl who has been found to have a mild to moderate delay in expressive language development and a moderate delay in speech sound development. Significantly, she has a history of two known episodes of ear infections. Given that approximately one-third (or more) of all cases of otitis media are asymptomatic, it is quite likely that this child has actually had more than two episodes of ear infection or that the episodes were longer in duration.

Josephine's expressive language development, not surprisingly, is significantly delayed, as is her speech sound (phonological) development—also not a surprising finding in light of her history. Recall that the vast majority of learning occurs incidentally; if Josephine's input is inconsistent, then her output will be inconsistent as well. Phonological development, vocabulary, and discourse are some of the areas that have been observed to be adversely affected by episodes of otitis media. It appears that Josephine's current level of functioning is in agreement with what has been observed in children who have her type of history with ear infections.

In terms of Josephine's auditory behavior and skills development, her nonverbal and receptive language skills demonstrate that she has an understanding of encoding, is developing selective listening, and has reached age-appropriate levels in terms of detection, discrimination, identification, and comprehension. Given her prelinguistic skills, strong play and receptive abilities, and the fact that her recent hearing evaluation was within normal limits, her prognosis for overcoming this delay with early intervention is quite good.

ROBERT (LT)

Robert, a 27-month-old developmentally delayed child, has been enrolled in an early intervention program and is receiving physical, occupational, and speech-language therapies. An additional part of his history that is of great significance is a left unilateral hearing loss. This type of impairment puts Robert at risk of further delays in auditory, language, cognitive, and academic development. To have a better assessment of the impact that this hearing loss has already had and may potentially continue to have on his overall development, an audiologic reevaluation must be performed as soon as possible to determine the severity of the hearing loss in the left ear.

Robert's receptive and expressive language abilities are both delayed and are reported to be most typical of a 9- to 12-month-old child. Likewise, his nonverbal communication is judged to be typical of a 9- to 12-month-old child. While it seems highly unlikely that this delayed development is solely (or in major part) related to a unilateral hearing loss of any degree, its presence coupled with Robert's already delayed development might possibly have a synergistic effect. In other words, the resulting deficits that he may experience will very likely be greater than the deficits from a UHL alone or a speech/language delay alone.

Robert's hearing sensitivity and auditory level of functioning must be assessed and regularly monitored, and a program of aural/auditory rehabilitation needs to be carefully planned. Further, Robert may be a candidate for some form of amplification; this issue needs to be assessed during the rehabilitation planning process.

SUMMARY

This chapter covered a broad range of ear- and hearing-related concepts. The information provided here is not meant to be all inclusive, but rather serves as an introduction to the ear and its essential role in normal speech and language development. Damage to hearing can occur at any time from conception through birth and beyond. Numerous causes of damage to the ear and hearing mechanism may potentially result in hearing loss, leading to sensory deprivation for the child and an alteration in the normal process of development. Speech-language pathologists should have a full appreciation of the grave impact that the various types of hearing loss can potentially have on a child's speech, language, and overall learning processes.

KEY TERMS

Acoustic immittance measures

Acoustic reflex

Attention

Auditory brain stem response audiometry

Auditory closure

Auditory memory

Behavioral (procedure)

Bottom-up approach

Cochlea

Comprehension level

Conditioned play audiometry

Conductive hearing loss

Conductive mechanism

Deaf culture

Detection level

Discrimination level

Electrophysiologic (procedure)

Encoding

Feedback

Functional ability

High-frequency sensorineural hearing loss

Identification level

Impedance

Impedance mismatch

Localization

Middle ear transformer function

Mixed hearing loss

Organ of Corti

Otitis media

Otoacoustic emissions

Pure tone

Resonance properties

Segmental

Sensorineural hearing loss

Sensorineural mechanism

Speech recognition score

Speech recognition threshold

Suprasegmental

Suprathreshold

Threshold

Tympanic membrane

Tympanometry

Unilateral hearing loss

Visual reinforcement audiometry

STUDY QUESTIONS

+ List and briefly describe both the acoustic and nonacoustic functions of the outer ear.
+ Describe the middle ear transfer function and state why it is so important to the process of hearing.
+ List and briefly describe each of the auditory skill levels presented in this chapter.
+ What are the categories of hearing loss described in this chapter?
+ Briefly describe the typical language development characteristics of a member of the conductive/otitis media population.
+ Briefly describe the typical language development characteristics of a member of the sensorineural population.

REFERENCES

American Speech-Language-Hearing Association (ASHA). (1996). Central auditory processing: Current status of research and implications for clinical practice. *American Journal of Audiology, 5*(2), 41–54.

American Speech-Language-Hearing Association (ASHA). (2000). JCIH year 2000 position statement: Principles and guidelines for early hearing detection and intervention programs [position statement]. www.asha.org/policy.

American Speech-Language-Hearing Association (ASHA). (2006). Preferred practice patterns for the profession of audiology. www.asha.org/policy.

Bess, F. H. (1986). The unilaterally hearing impaired child: A final comment. *Ear and Hearing, 7*(1), 52–54.

Bess, F., & Tharpe, A. (1986). Case history data on unilaterally hearing-impaired children. *Ear and Hearing, 7*(1), 14–19.

Bistrop, M. L., Haines, M., Hygge, S., MacKenzie, D. J., Neyen, S., & Petersen, C. M. (2002). *Children and noise: Prevention of adverse effects.* Denmark, Copenhagen: National Institute of Public Health, Denmark. Retrieved August 14, 2007, from http://www.si-folkesundhed.dk/upload/noiseprevention.pdf.

Bovo, R., Martini, A., Agnoletto, M., Beghi, A., Carmignoto, D., & Milani, M. (1988). Auditory and academic performance of children with unilateral hearing loss. *Scandinavian Audiology Supplement, 30,* 71–74.

Gallaudet Research Institute. (1996). *Stanford achievement test, ninth edition: Form S, norms booklet for deaf and hard-of-hearing students.* Washington, DC: Gallaudet University.

Hall, J. W. (2005, August 20). Confirmation of infant hearing ability: Electrophysiologic techniques and interpretation. Retrieved August 14, 2007, from http://www.cms-kids.com/SHINE_Electrophys_Diag_11.PPT.

Holst, M., Eswaran, H., Lowery, C., Murphy, P., Norton, J., & Preissl, H. (2005). Development of auditory evoked fields in human fetuses and newborns: A longitudinal MEG study. *Clinical Neurophysiology, 116*(8), 1949–1955.

Jerger, J., & Musiek, F. (2000). Report of the consensus conference on the diagnosis of auditory processing disorders in school-aged children. *Journal of the American Academy of Audiology, 11,* 467–474.

Kisilevsky, B. S., Hains, S. M. J., Jacquet, A. Y., Granier-Deferre, C., & Lecanuet, J. P. (2004). Maturation of fetal responses to music. *Developmental Science, 7*(5), 550–559.

Klee, T. M., & Davis-Dansky, E. (1986). A comparison of unilaterally hearing impaired children and normal hearing children on a battery of standardized language tests. *Ear and Hearing, 7*(1), 27–37.

Lieu, J. E. (2004). Speech-language and educational consequences of unilateral hearing loss in children. *Archives of Otolaryngology, Head and Neck Surgery, 130*(5), 524–530.

McMullen, E., & Saffran, J. (2004). Music and language: A developmental comparison. *Music Perception, 21*(3), 289–311.

Musiek, F. E., & Baran, J. A. (2007). *The auditory system: Anatomy, physiology, and clinical correlates.* Boston: Pearson Education.

Nevins, M. E., & Garber, A. (2006). Auditory skill development. HOPE Online Library. Retrieved July 22, 2007, from www.cochlear.com/HOPE.

National Institute of Health (NIH). (1993). Early identification of hearing impairment in infants and young children [consensus statement]. *NIH Consensus Statement Online, 11*(1), 1–24.

Pichichero, M. E. (2000). Acute otitis media: Part 1. Improving diagnostic accuracy. *American Family Physician, 61*(7), 2051–2056.

Roberts, J., & Hunter, L. (2002, October 8). Otitis media and children's language and learning. *The ASHA Leader.* www.asha.org/about/publications/leader-online/archives/2002/.

Roberts, J. E., Rosenfeld, R. M., & Zeisel, S. A. (2004). Otitis media and speech and language: A meta-analysis of prospective studies. *Pediatrics, 113,* e238–e248.

Schow, R. L., & Nerbonne, M. A. (2007). *Introduction to audiologic rehabilitation,* 5th ed. Boston: Pearson Education.

Tye-Murray, N. (2004). *Foundations of aural rehabilitation: Children, adults, and their family members,* 2nd ed. Clifton, NJ: Delmar Learning.

Werner, L. (2003). Prenatal auditory stimuli: Truth, fiction or moot point? *Hearing Health, 19,* 2. Retrieved July 22, 2007, from http://drf.org/hearing_health/archive/2003/sum03_prenatalaudi_ex.htm.

Yost, W. A. (2007). *Fundamentals of hearing: An introduction,* 5th ed. San Diego, CA: Elsevier.

CHAPTER 5

Social–Emotional Bases of Communication Development

Carol E. Westby, PhD

OBJECTIVES

+ Describe the social/cognitive underpinnings of language and communicative competence
+ Explain the ways that child characteristics, disabilities, and environmental factors influence the development of social and communicative competence
+ Assess children's social–emotional and language bases for communicative competence
+ Describe a philosophy of intervention for social–communicative deficits

INTRODUCTION

Language acquisition involves three components: (1) the learning of well-formedness—that is, the rules of grammar (syntax); (2) the capacity to refer and to mean (semantics); and (3) communicative function or intent—that is, the ability to get things done with gestures and words (pragmatics). Without communicative intent, other aspects of language are meaningless. Some children appear to master syntax and semantics, but fail to use them for interactive communication. True language is a social activity, and a primary function of language is to sustain and maintain emotional attachments.

Each of these components of language is addressed in the three case studies introduced in Chapter 1. For all three children, the evaluator claims that aspects of pragmatics are the children's communicative strengths. The evaluator notes that all three children engage in joint attention, turn-taking, and prelinguistic gestures; furthermore, she also suggests that Josephine (the late bloomer) and Robert (the late talker) show strengths in these areas. Some children with developmental delays or language impairments, however, exhibit delays or disorders in these early pragmatic elements; in some cases, deficits in pragmatic aspects of communication are most delayed or different. Also, many children who initially appear to exhibit fairly typical pragmatic skills, despite delays or deficits primarily in syntax and semantics, later exhibit difficulties with social–emotional/pragmatic aspects of communication. Today increasing attention is being given to the early precursors of communicative intent and pragmatic communication skills, as well as to the long-term influences of both early and later differences is social–emotional development.

This chapter discusses the nature and development of social competence, including precursors to a theory of mind and the affective and social bases of communication. It also explores the development of communicative intent and social uses of language, factors affecting social–emotional aspects of communication, and methods for assessing and facilitating the social–emotional bases of communication and communicative competence.

UNDERPINNINGS OF SOCIAL COMPETENCE AND LANGUAGE

Elements of Social Competence

Social competence comprises three areas of social development that must function in an integrated manner: (1) secure attachment, (2) instrumental social learning, and (3) experience-sharing relationships.

Attachment refers to the affective tie of infants to their parents. Children who have secure attachment generally have parents who are highly attuned and responsive to them.

Instrumental social actions are those that are done to achieve a specific objective in a social setting—for example, requesting, seeking assistance, and pointing to an out-of-reach toy; following classroom behavior rules to get a reward; standing in line at McDonalds to get food; or asking for instructions to complete a class assignment. These actions are tied to external reinforcements. Children learn the relationship between communicative actions and specific results, and they associate these actions and consequences with specific settings and times in which they occur (e.g., requesting a snack at snack time).

Experience-sharing, the third element of social competence, involves the desire and skills to be a good reciprocal playmate, to value others' points of view, to develop friendships, and to conduct emotion-based interactions. Experience sharing occurs without concern for external rewards. It requires that participants constantly reference the emotional states and actions of their communicative partners and, in turn, base their own actions on their evaluations of their partners' behaviors.

These elements of social competence underlie the reason that children develop language to communicate. Children talk to maintain social contact, often for no other reason than to share an experience, feeling, or thought with another person (Bates, Bretherton, Beeghly-Smith, & McNew, 1982). This motivation for sharing reflects the need infants have to sustain "intersubjectivity"—that is, an interfacing of mind with other persons. *Intentionality* drives language acquisition, and intersubjectivity drives intentionality. Initially, this intersubjectivity reflects the child's experience of emotions. Gradually, however, children come to recognize others' experiences of emotions. Increasingly, this appreciation of intersubjectivity, or what has been termed a *theory of mind* (ToM), contributes to children's ability to predict behaviors of others and participate in effective social conversation (Bretherton, 1991; Bruner, 1986; Hewitt, 1994). Participating in discourse—and particularly discourse about past experiences—further promotes ToM and the ability to make appropriate inferences that are essential for appropriate social interactions and text comprehension.

ToM, or intersubjectivity, which underlies developing social and language competence, is influenced by *endogenous factors* within the child and *exogenous factors* in the environment. *Primary intersubjectivity* occurs early (when the child is 0–6 months of age) and reflects a system that promotes the infant's tendency to use and respond to eye contact, facial affect, vocal behavior, and body posture in interactions with caregivers. This primarily dyadic interactive phase of social development provides the information and experience that, in combination with cognitive maturation, allows infants to begin to develop representations of themselves and others as having both distinct and shared affective experiences. *Secondary intersubjectivity,* which involves conscious awareness of both self and others as sharing an experience, occurs between 6 and 18 months of age (Tomasello, 1995). The experience of secondary intersubjectivity has positive reinforcement value for the child and, therefore, contributes to ongoing motivation for social interactions.

Developing intersubjectivity is not possible without joint attention. This type of early engagement is integral to the development of the ability to understand others' thoughts, intentions, and feelings, and it reflects sensitivity to the reward values of sharing with others (Tomasello, 1995). *Joint attention* (JA) involves the integration of information about self-experience of an object or event with information about how others experience the same object or event. Infant joint attention predicts childhood cognitive and language outcomes and individual differences in childhood social interactive competence in typically developing children, at-risk children, and children with autism (Mundy & Arca, 2006).

Several types of joint attention develop in the 3- to 18-month period of infancy:

+ *Responding to joint attention (RJA):* The infant follows the direction of gaze, head turn, and or point gesture of another person.
+ *Initiating joint attention (IJA):* The infant uses eye contact and or deictic gestures (pointing or showing) to spontaneously initiate coordinated attention with a social partner. This communication is a type of protodeclarative. In other words, the infant is seeking interaction with another simply for the sake of sharing an experience.
+ *Initiating behavior requests (IBR):* The infant uses eye contact and gestures to initiate attention coordination with another person to elicit aid in obtaining an object or event. IBR is a protoimperative; it is used for less social but more instrumental purposes.

RJA is a type of primary intersubjectivity; IJA and IBR reflect secondary subjectivity. RJA and IJA serve social functions. The goals and reinforcement of RJA and IJA behaviors revolve around the sharing of experiences with others and the positive emotions that such early social sharing engender in young children. IJA and RJA are both related to later language development and social outcomes in the second and third years of life and to decreased risk of later disruptive behaviors (Mundy & Thorp, 2006). In contrast, high rates of IBR, which may reflect an impulsive and object-driven style of behavior, are associated with greater externalizing or disruptive behaviors in later life (Sheinkopf, Mundy, Claussen, & Willoughby, 2004).

Emergence of Language

Social–emotional development reflected in joint attention initially triggers or enables language; later, language becomes the medium though which children further develop social–emotional cognition that enables understanding of their social world and acquisition of their culture. It enables them to share and understand emotions, goals, and expectations (Bloom, 1990, 1993; Bretherton & Beeghly, 1982; Dunn, Bretherton, & Munn, 1987). Language acquisition cannot be understood by looking at only the child's cognitive and linguistic abilities because it is the child's emotional development that drives communication. Instead, language acquisition can only be understood by also looking at the social interactions or cultural settings in which language occurs (Bruner, 1983). To acquire language, children must be sensitive to the sound patterns and grammatical constraints of the language, to referential requirements, and to communicative intentions. Such sensitivity grows in the process of fulfilling certain general nonlinguistic functions—predicting the environment, interacting transactionally, getting to goals with the aid of another, and so on. Bruner has suggested that such functions must first be fulfilled by prelinguistic communicative means; only after these means reach certain levels will children generate linguistic hypotheses.

Because communication depends on effective interactions between infants and adults, we must understand what children and adults bring to interactive episodes and the way these interactions are organized.

What the Child Brings to Interactions

Infant Engagement Tools. Infants are born with endogenous processes that enable them to perceive people as being similar to themselves. This awareness is not based on facial features or movement, but rather on affective awareness. Legerstee (2005) proposed that infants are born with an affect sharing device (AFS) that has three components:

+ Self-referential processes that allow infants an awareness of their own mental states
+ Interpersonal awareness that allows infants to recognize the emotions of others
+ An innate sense of emotional attunement

The AFS enables infants to recognize whether their own emotions and the emotions of others are similar. Mirror neurons in the cortex may be implicated in this attunement process (Bertenthal & Longo, 2007). Mirror neurons respond similarly both when individuals initiate an action or experience an emotion and when they see the same action performed or the same emotion experienced by someone else (Schulte-Ruther, Markowitsch, Fink, & Piefke, 2007).

At approximately six weeks of age, infants can visually fixate on their mothers' eyes, hold the fixation, and widen their own eyes. This fixation results in the mother feeling a greater sense of connection with the infant. With this eye fixation, social play between infant and adult begins in earnest. Infants can not only seek out interaction, but also terminate interaction. They can gaze directly into the adult's eyes, can turn their heads slightly so that they see the adult out of the corner of their eyes, or can lower their heads and turn far enough away to totally avoid visual contact. These engagement–disengagement behaviors enable infants to control the amount of stimulation they desire (Schaffer, 1984; Stern, 1977).

By the end of the third month after birth, infants' mature motor control of gaze direction gives them complete control over what they see. With this ability, they can start or stop face-to-face interaction, because these interactions are built around mutual gaze. By looking at the mother, infants can start an encounter because the mother will look back. Children can continue the interaction by smiling or end it by averting their eyes or turning their heads away. Mutual gaze represents the turn-taking that is later seen in verbal conversation. In these early months, babies are learning the nonverbal basis of social interaction upon which language is later built. They are able not only to fixate on an object, but also to pursue it. In the second half of the first year, infants become interested in objects as their increasing motor abilities enable them to reach, grasp, and manipulate the objects in their world. Once this occurs, the mother–infant interaction becomes a triadic affair between the mother, infant, and object.

Infants younger than one week old can distinguish and imitate facial expressions such as happy, sad, and surprised (Meltzoff & Moore, 1977). Near the end of the first year, they are able to engage in social referencing—that is, they are able to perceive the link between a person's affect and the eliciting stimulus. Infants use this social referencing to make judgments about how to respond to a situation. They are particularly alert to a parent's indications of fear. By the end of the first year, child and parent engaging in ongoing co-referencing, each noting and responding to the emotional sharing of the other. These social–emotional characteristics lead infants to interact with adults in ways that are useful for language development.

All neurotypical babies exhibit these gaze and emotional expression behaviors. They do not, however, all respond in the same way to their social and physical environments.

Temperament. Each baby comes with its own personality or temperament. *Temperament* is defined as behavioral style, or the how of behavior. Temperament significantly determines the pattern of interactions infants experience with their environments, including what infants respond to and how they respond. Variations in infant temperament involve differences in general mood, in activity level, and in adaptability to changes in routine. Large differences also exist between babies in terms of the intensity of their responses, in their tendency to approach or withdraw from new experiences, in their persistence, in their distractibility, and in their sensitivity to stimulation.

Thomas and Chess (1977) described three temperamental patterns: *easy, slow-to-warm-up*, and *difficult*. Recently, more positive terms have been substituted for Thomas and Chess's original labels: *flexible, fearful*, and *feisty*. Flexible babies have a regular overall pattern. They accept new experiences readily, exhibit mild reactions to discomfort, and make smooth adjustments to changes in routines. Fearful babies share some of the same style of flexible babies, but tend to withdraw from new experiences. They will gradually adapt to new situations but need to be handled sensitively in the process. Such babies generally cannot be pressured into new experiences. Feisty babies are easily distressed. They express their likes—and much more often their dislikes—in no uncertain terms. They react forcefully and negatively to new experiences and to even minor changes in routine, and they show little or no consistency in their schedule. It is difficult for caregivers to predict the behaviors of these children.

Infants' temperaments are a major factor in determining the nature of the interactions that infants experience with significant people in their environment. What is essential for the best development of children is the existence of a "good fit" between infant and caregiver. Flexible babies, who are abundantly adaptable, can be reared by nearly anyone. Raising fearful and feisty infants takes more sensitivity and insight on the part of caregivers. Goodness of fit results when the expectations and demands of the environment are in accord with the child's own capacities, motives, and behavioral style. Poorness of fit occurs when dissonances between the two lead to incompatibility. An active, intense parent may be comfortable with an intense baby who cries vigorously with change. A parent who expects the infant to have a regular time routine and be able to tolerate changes in caregivers may be unnerved by a feisty baby and have no idea how to calm or interact with the child. Children with difficult temperaments can be perfectly normal children who can develop normal social behaviors, but their temperament does predispose them to developmental problems because their caregivers may not be able to establish effective communicative interactions with them.

Children's temperaments also influence the ways that mothers engage in reminiscing, or talking about past experiences (Laible, 2004). Mothers are more likely to elaborate when discussing a child's past behavior if they perceive that the child is high in effortful control. Mothers are better able to elaborate in reminiscing with children whose temperaments are easy or flexible, because such children are inclined to self-regulation and attention. In contrast, children with feisty temperaments may limit their mother's ability to effectively communicate with them when discussing the past. Laible (2004) noted that children ages three to five years whose mothers engaged in more elaborated discussion of past experiences displayed more behavioral internalization and higher levels of emotional understanding than children whose mothers did not elaborate in the same way.

Attachment. Children's attachments to their caregivers are influenced both by what the child brings to the interaction and, in many cases, by what the caregiver (typically the mother) brings to the interaction. Four types of caregiver–child attachments have been identified based on children's behavior in the "Strange Situation" (Ainsworth, Blehar, Waters, & Wall, 1978). With this assessment method, the caregiver brings the child into a playroom, leaves the room briefly, and then returns. Attachment categories are based on what the child does upon the caregiver's return:

+ Children with *secure attachment* protest the mother's departure and quiet promptly on the mother's return, accepting comfort from her and returning to exploration or play.
+ Children with *avoidant attachment* show little to no signs of distress at the mother's departure, a willingness to explore the toys, and little to no visible response to the mother's return.
+ Children with *resistant-ambivalent attachment* show sadness on the mother's departure and on the mother's return; they also show some ambivalence, signs of anger, or reluctance to "warm" to her, and they fail to return to play.
+ Children with *disorganized-disoriented attachment* seem to have no clear strategy for responding to their caregivers. They may at times avoid or resist approaches to the caregiver; they may also seem confused or frightened by her, or freeze or still their movements when she approaches them.

Mothers' communication with their children and the child's attachment to the mother have been shown to be related to the caregiver's own attachment history and his or her interpretation of that history (Main, 1996).

What Caregivers Bring to Interactions

Children set the tone for interactions, but caregivers determine what children learn about interactions within the culture.

Mainstream Caregivers. The majority of information regarding socialization of communication comes from studies of white, middle-class families. Most caregivers use a variety of behaviors to engage and maintain the interest of infants. When caregivers interact with infants, they often exaggerate their facial expressions in space and time. Caregivers may use an expression of mock surprise—opening their eyes wide, raising their eyebrows—and saying something like *oooooh* or *aaaaah* to signal a readiness to interact. They may move their heads from side to side or toward the infant. The facial expressions are slow to form and are then held. Caregivers may play with the speed and rate of these behaviors, speeding up and then slowing down. As the interaction continues, they may smile to indicate that the interaction is going well or they may use an exaggerated frown or pout when the interaction is running down or in trouble. The repertoire of facial exaggerations is limited, and a few patterns are repeated frequently. These facial exaggerations facilitate infant's abilities to read facial expressions (Stern, 1977).

Mainstream caregivers also tend to engage in baby talk (Snow & Ferguson, 1977). They simplify syntax, use short utterances, use many nonsense sounds, transform words (e.g., *pwitty wabbit* for "pretty rabbit"), raise vocal pitch, and exaggerate loudness and intensity of vocalizations—ranging from a whisper to a loud "pretend scary" voice. Sometimes the speech is sped up, and other times it is slowed down, elongating vowels on certain words—for example, *What a gooooooood little baby*. Pause times between utterances are also elongated, as though to allow time for the infant to respond. In essence, the caregiver appears to be shaping the infant's turn-taking behavior to the form necessary when the child becomes verbal. The mother also tends to repeat runs of interactions: *You're a pretty baby; you're such a pretty baby, you're the prettiest baby mommy has ever seen*. Many of these runs involve questions and answers, *Are you hungry? Are you? Huh? I think you are*. During each vocalization, the mother brings her head closer to the infant. Between questions, the mother moves away. Each question is accompanied by a distinct facial expression.

From the infant's birth, mainstream adults look for reasons for infants' behaviors and comment to the infants about possible intentions: *You're so hungry. You don't like beets. You want mommy to pick you up*. When adults view infants as intentional, they attempt to find the object or event (referent) that is triggering the child's behavior: *You're looking at your teddy bear. You want your bottle*. In so doing, adults guide children into referencing (labeling) and requesting behaviors.

As children develop the verbal ability to label and request, adults provide scaffolding questions to assist the children in producing more information. In mainstream homes, this scaffolding especially occurs during storybook reading, as in the following example:

Mother: Look!
Child: (touches picture)
Mother: What are those?
Child: (vocalizes a babble string and smiles)
Mother: Yes, they are rabbits.
Child: (vocalizes, smiles, and looks up at mother)
Mother (laughs) Yes, rabbit.
Child: (vocalizes, smiles)
Mother: Yes.

(Bruner, 1983, p. 78)

As children acquire the routine and begin to take over their pieces (e.g., labeling the picture), the adult ups the ante by asking a more complex question: *What's the rabbit doing?* Once the child labels the object and what it is doing, the caregiver ups the ante again: *Why is the rabbit is doing that? How does he feel about what he is doing?* Through these social exchanges, children come to understand how to take turns in conversations, maintain a topic, and provide information in their culture.

Cultural Variations in Caregiver–Child Interactions. Anthropological studies have made it clear that cultures differ in their child-rearing practices. Each culture has its own perspective on infant capabilities, who provides cares for infants, the types of interactions between adults and children, and the role of the infant and young child in the family. Because of these variations, people of different cultures respond to and interact with infants and young children in different ways (Field, Sostek, Vietze, & Leiderman, 1981; Greenfield & Cocking, 1994; Heath, 1983; Johnston & Wong, 2002; Lynch & Hansen, 2004; Nugent, Lester, & Brazelton, 1989; Rogoff, 2003; Vigil, 2002).

In particular, cultures tend to differ in terms of whether they are socializing children to become independent or to become interdependent. Cultures that socialize children toward *independence* promote *individualism*—that is, a focus on the individual; cultures that socialize children toward *interdependence* promote *collectivism*—that is, a focus on the group. Caregivers in individualistic cultures are more likely to follow the infant's lead in interactions. They follow the child's line of regard when establishing joint attention and are likely to label what they see the child looking at or to interpret what they think are the child's desires. In contrast, caregivers in collective cultures are more likely to expect the child to follow their line of regard and attend to the desire of the caregiver. In these instances, caregivers are more likely to give directives that children are to follow (Vigil & Westby, 2004).

Individualistic cultures tend to attribute intentional behavior to infants, whereas collectivistic cultures do not expect infants to exhibit intentional, goal-directed behavior. Heath (1983) reported that black working-class families in the North Carolina Piedmont area did not view infants as intentional and, therefore, did not see them as conversational partners. Because infants were not seen as being able to communicate, their cries and vocalizations were not systematically attended to. When adults do not see infants as intentional, they are unlikely to talk with infants, provide labels, or ask questions. When they do not see toddlers and young children as information givers, they are less likely to support them in their attempts to produce lengthy, topic-maintaining dialogues (Heath, 1983; Whiting & Edwards, 1988).

Because adults in mainstream cultures view infants' earliest behaviors as intentional, they label and give infants what they look at. Consequently, early communicative functions in these cultures are likely to include requesting and labeling. In cultures that do not view infants as intentional, one may find other early communicative functions. In the New Mexican Hispanic and Mexican American cultures studied by Briggs (1984) and Schieffelin and Eisenberg (1984), which did not perceive intentionality in infants, adults determined that the first words that should be used were polite and social words. Using the expression *dile* (say to him/her), adults gave children messages to repeat to someone else. What the adults told the children to say did not reflect the children's intentions, but instead reflected the adults' beliefs concerning how different individuals should be addressed.

Some cultures that believe that infants are not intentional also believe that children learn to talk primarily by observing others, rather than by engaging in talk with adults. In these environments, children are allowed to observe many adult interactions around them. They often begin talking by imitating words and phrases they hear. In these circumstances, children's first words are likely to be those that attract their attention. Heath (1983) observed that early language functions of black children in the North Carolina Piedmont region included bossing, cussing, fussing, begging, and comforting—not the early communicative functions reported for mainstream children.

The remainder of this chapter addresses the social–emotional bases of communication in mainstream children. Some principles are applicable to all children, but one must be alert to ways in which culture may affect the structure and functions of children's communications.

COMMUNICATING WITH OTHERS

Children's social communicative abilities develop in two directions. *Vertical development* refers to increasing hierarchical development associated with increasing age and cognitive understanding. *Horizontal development* refers to the range of abilities or communicative functions within a particular developmental level.

Vertical Development

Intentionality

Bates (1976) described three stages in children's emergence of pragmatic or intentional communicative behaviors: perlocutionary, illocutionary, and locutionary.

In the *perlocutionary* stage, from birth to approximately nine months, infants have a systematic effect on adults without intending to. Adults interpret infant's smiles, cries, and coos as though they were intentional, although they are not. The infant does not intentionally cry or smile to seek a response from an adult, yet adults talk to the infants as though the infant is being intentional: *Oh, you want mommy to sing that again*, or *You don't want any more carrots; mommy will take them away*. Perlocutionary behavior is sometimes referred to as functional communication. The infant's or child's behavior functions as a communication to adults, even though the child's behavior is not intentionally goal directed.

Around nine months of age, when infants are able to establish joint attention, they enter the *illocutionary* stage. Infants now use behaviors intentionally to gain the adult's attention. Many of these behaviors become conventionalized; that is, they are gestures that others would use (e.g., reaching, waving bye-bye). If a child wants a toy and his mother is not looking at it, he will point at the toy with his arm outstretched and index finger pointed, look toward the toy, then shift his gaze to his mother's face, then shift his attention back and forth. A cry or vocalization is deliberately used to get another's attention. The child may whine, then check whether the adult is attending. If not, the child may escalate the whine to a cry, but again may stop to check if the adult is attending.

During this stage, one observes what Bates (1976) considered precursors to language: the protoimperative (IBR) and the protodeclarative (IJA). The *protoimperative* is defined as the child's use of a means to cause the adult to do something. It grows out of the child's attempts to do something herself. Hence, the first protoimperatives (IBRs) involve instances of reaching and looking between the desired object and the event. Later the child may bring an object or toy to an adult, seeking assistance with operating it. For example, the child may recognize a music box, yet be unable to wind it herself. She brings the box to an adult, hands it to the adult, and then waits expectantly for the adult to wind it. By contrast, a *protodeclarative* (IJA) is defined as a preverbal effort to direct the adult's attention to some event or object in the world. Included here are showing objects and exhibiting oneself for the sole purposes of gaining attention. For example, a child may bring a toy to an adult simply to capture the adult's interest and attention.

Between 13 and 18 months of age, children enter the *locutionary* stage. During this phase of development, they begin to use conventionalized words to make things happen. The child who earlier pointed to the cookie now says, *cookie*; the child who simply handed the mother a toy to wind now says, *help*.

Referencing and Requesting

To engage in illocutionary and locutionary behavior, children must be able to *reference*—to refer to a person or object. People use referencing to manage and direct one another's attention by linguistic means. Initially the management of joint referencing is under the control of the adult. For instance, the caregiver highlights objects by moving them into the infant's view. Once the infant's attention can reliably be gained by showing objects, the caregiver begins to prepare the child for the object by calling the child's name or saying, *Oh, look*, or *See what I have*. Between 8 to 12 months of age, infants discover that the adult's speech signals the adult is looking at something and the infants begin to follow the adults' line of regard. By age 12 months, infants follow the adult's line of regard, search for an object, and, if they find none, they look at the adult's face again, and then again look outward. Shortly after this, the child begins to point.

Once pointing and consistent words appear, caregivers initiate *what* and *where* games (*What's this? Where did it go?*).

Once children can reference, they can request. This entails not only coordinating one's language with the requirements of action in the real world, but doing so in culturally prescribed ways. Bruner (1983) distinguished three types of early requests:

+ Request for an object
+ Invitation or request to an adult to share a role relationship in play or in a game
+ Request for supportive action in which the child tries to recruit an adult's skill or strength to help him achieve a desired goal

The caregiver's role is different in each of these requests. In the first type of request, the caregiver must figure out what the child wants; in the second, what the invitation is for; and in the third, what kind of help the child needs. Requests for visible and near objects occur before one year of age. Requests for remote or absent objects and for supportive action or assistance explode around 18 months, when children develop representational capacity.

Once children are using words to request absent objects and supportive actions, caregivers begin to enforce the cultural expectations for requests. Children are expected to really need the object or the assistance and not request something they can get or do for themselves. Requests should not require unreasonable demands from caregivers (e.g., *I can't go upstairs and get find your book now—I'm fixing dinner*) and the child must respect the voluntary nature of responses to requests (e.g., the caregiver requires the child to say *thank you* after the request is fulfilled). Certain requests are related to time, and can be fulfilled only within a particular time frame (e.g., *You can't have cookies before dinner*).

Verbal requests can be one of three types:

Direct requests: *Gimme that! More milk. Please pass the butter.*

Indirect requests: *Could you get that pencil? Why don't you close the door?*

Hints or nonconventionalized requests: *It's cold in here. I haven't gotten my allowance yet.*

Successful requesting requires that children gain attention, that their requests be clear and persuasive, that they maintain the desired or expected social relationships, and that they have strategies for making repairs when their request is not understood (Ervin-Tripp & Gordon, 1986). In addition, children must produce requests that recognize the following aspects:

+ The social status or the relative power of the speaker and the addressee
+ The intrusiveness of the request
+ Ownership/possession
+ Rights and obligations (Gordon & Ervin-Tripp, 1984)

In general, children are sensitive to roles, rights, and possessions by age two, knowing that they should be more polite when asking for something from someone older, when asking for something that is not their own, and when the person they are asking is not obligated to respond. They have limited awareness of intrusiveness before school age. Lawson (as cited in Ervin-Tripp & Gordon, 1985) reported that a two-year-old child used different forms of speech to her father, her mother, and children at nursery school depending on whether they were her own age or older. She used direct imperative requests to two-year-olds, and embedded requests or requests with tags such as *please* or *okay*.

Ervin-Trip and Gordon (1986) reported that 60% of two- and three-year-old children's requests to outsiders used politeness markers, whereas only 1% of requests to mothers and 14% to 24% of requests to other children were polite. These researchers suggested that children assume that mothers must be available for services, whereas older children and visitors do not have to be available. Requests for objects that belonged to others were usually polite even to mothers and siblings.

Two- and three-year-old children seldom provide justifications for their requests. A marked increase in justification of requests occurs around age four (e.g., *I need a red crayon cause mine is broke*). At this age, children begin to challenge adults' refusals of requests. They later use information gained from adults' reasons for their refusals to persuade adults of their needs, desires, or intents (e.g., *I'll eat all my dinner if I can have a Popsicle now*).

As children become sensitive to the social rules underlying requests, they produce more indirect and nonconventualized requests. Between ages four and eight years, children not only use politeness modifications for issues of status and rights, but also become sensitive to how their requests might intrude on the activities of others. Children understand direct and indirect requests during the preschool years, but comprehend nonconventualized requests or hints only when they reach approximately eight years of age. Conventionalized requests (directives and indirectives) can be learned as formulas; that is, caregivers can tell a child what to say in a particular situation. By comparison, nonconventionalized requests require greater cognitive and social knowledge.

Horizontal Development

Once children engage in illocutionary and locutionary behavior, they communicate a variety of intentions. A number of taxonomies have been developed to code communicative intents. The categories vary depending on the age of the children studied, the philosophical orientation of the researcher, and the degree to which discourse and social context are considered (Chapman, 1981). Taxonomies may classify gestures or language at the following levels:

+ *The utterance level.* Each utterance is coded based on what the speakers are doing at the moment. Are they labeling, requesting, warning, promising, or ordering?

+ *The discourse level.* In this taxonomy, the utterance is categorized according to its relationship to other utterances. Does the utterance initiate a conversation, maintain the
conversation, acknowledge another speaker, clarify an utterance, or terminate the conversation? Utterances coded at the utterance level can also be coded at the discourse
level. An utterance may function as a label at the utterance level and as a topic initiator
at the discourse level. At the discourse level, utterances may also be considered in terms
of how they manage the conversation. Does the utterance function to get a turn, hold
one's turn, or allow another person to take a turn?
+ *The social level.* The utterance can be placed in its social context. Language varies according to the setting and the roles of the participants in these settings. This is particularly true with politeness and argumentative behavior. How does the utterance function
to soften or strengthen the communication?

Communication in the illocutionary and early locutionary phases involves efforts to
regulate another's behavior for purposes of achieving a goal, seeking social interaction, or
establishing joint attention for the purpose of sharing information. **Table 5-1** presents communicative intents, coded at the utterance level, that have been reported during the illocutionary and early locutionary stages (Coggins & Carpenter, 1981; Dore, 1975; Halliday,
1975; Wetherby & Prizant, 1989). Communicative intentions in this stage can be gestures
or verbal utterances that serve to (1) regulate behavior, (2) engage in social interaction, and
(3) establish joint reference. In the table, items marked with an asterisk (*) generally appear
only in the locutionary period.

Even during the illocutionary stage, children are likely to use all three major functions. As
they move into the multiword locutionary stage, requests for social routines and showing decrease, whereas calling, requesting permission, acknowledging, requesting information, and requesting clarifications increase. Rate increases substantially between the early illocutionary and
multiword locutionary stages. Children display an average of about one act per minute during
the prelinguistic stage, two acts per minute in the one-word stage, and five acts per minute by
the multiword stage.

During the preschool years, communicative functions become less tied to the concrete
environment and more closely related to language referring to language. **Table 5-2** presents
Dore's schema (1978) for coding communicative functions for preschool-aged children.

TABLE 5-1   Early Communicative Intents

Behavioral Regulation

☐ Request for specific object — demands an object

☐ Rejection of an object — refuses an object

☐ Request for action — commands someone to perform an action (e.g., raises arms to be picked up)

☐ Protest of action — refuses an activity by someone

Social Interaction

☐ Greeting — gains attention, indicates notice of initiation or termination of activity (e.g., *hi, bye*)

☐ Request for social routine — initiates routines such as peek-a-boo or pat-a-cake

☐ Showing off — attracts attention

☐ Calling — gains attention of someone

☐ Acknowledging — indicates that the speaker's communication was received

☐ Requests permission — seeks approval to carry out an activity

☐ Personal — expresses moods or feelings

Joint Attention

☐ Transferring — places an object in another's possession

☐ Comment on an object — directs someone's attention to an object

☐ Comment on an action or event — directs someone's attention to an event

☐ Request for information — seeks information, explanations, or clarifications*

☐ Clarification — utterances used to clarify previous communication*

Generally appear only in the locutionary period.

TABLE 5-2	Communicative Functions in Preschool Children	
Requests	For information	Where's Michael going?
	For action	Get me some more paste.
	For acknowledgment	You know what?
Responses to Requests	Providing information	(Why isn't Karen here?) She's sick.
	Expressing acceptance, denial, or acknowledgment	Okay.
		You can't have it.
Descriptions of Past and Present Facts	Labeling or describing objects and actions	I'm eating my lunch. Anna spilled her milk.
	Describing properties and locations	My candle has lots of red paint on it. I put it in my cubbie.
Statements	Of facts or rules	It's not nice to grab.
		We have to share the wagon.
	Of explanations, reasons, or causes	Sara can't go swimming 'cause she's got a cold.
Acknowledgments	Recognizing responses	Okay, yes, right
	Evaluating responses	That's not what teacher said.
Organizing Devices	Regulates contact and conversation	Hi, bye, my turn, sorry
Performatives	Accomplishes event by speaking (protests, jokes, claims, teases, warnings)	Stop. Don't touch it.
		Josh is a baby.

Source: Dore (1978)

Development of Emotional Understanding

Appropriate use of communication in social interactions requires increasing awareness of one's own emotionality, the emotionality of others, and the social rules governing the appropriate display of emotions. Children's emotional understanding begins to develop early and follows a regular pattern of emergence (Harter, 1983; Michalson & Lewis, 1985; Pons, Harris, & de Rosnay, 2004).

Between ages three and four years, approximately 55% of children are able to recognize and name basic emotions (happy, sad, afraid, angry) on the basis of facial expression when presented with pictures. By age five years, 75% of children can do so. Moreover, by five years of age, a majority of children understand the relationship between emotions and memory—namely, they realize that the intensity of the emotion decreases with time and that some elements of a present situation can reactive past emotions. More than half of five-year-olds can also identify external causes of emotions and link a facial expression to a situation (e.g., one feels sad at the loss of a favorite toy or happy when receiving a desired gift).

By age seven years, the majority of children understand that a person's beliefs—whether true or false—will determine a person's emotional reaction to a situation. For example, if a child is afraid of snakes and thinks she sees a snake, she will be afraid, even if what she sees is a garden hose. Seven- to nine-year-olds develop an understanding of situations in which they should hide emotions. For example, if a neighbor gives them a piece of cake that tastes disgusting, they realize that they should smile and say, "Thank you," and not grimace and say, "This is really yukky."

By nine years of age, the majority of children understand that a person can have multiple, and even ambivalent or contradictory, emotions in a given situation. For example, the child might be both excited and fearful to go on a roller coaster. Furthermore, nine-year-olds understand that negative feelings are typically associated with morally inappropriate actions (lying, stealing) and positive feelings are associated with praiseworthy actions (making a sacrifice, resisting a temptation). By age 11 years, nearly all children understand that failure to confess a misdemeanor provokes sadness.

FACTORS AFFECTING SOCIAL–EMOTIONAL ASPECTS OF COMMUNICATION __

Social–emotional aspects of communication can be disrupted by both factors within the environment and factors within the child.

Factors in the Environment

Parents vary in the degree to which they respond sensitively to their infants' cues. In some instances, parents may be less able to read children's cues, may be less available to engage in interaction with children, or may misinterpret an infant's behavior (Field, 1987). Some parents may simply be poor matches with their infants. They may not be able to cope effectively with the temperamental style of their infants, or they may fail to attune to their infants affectively. *Affect attunement* refers to the ways in which internal emotional states are brought into communication within infant–caregiver interactions. Both the adult and the infant can be active in the attunement (Legerstee, 2005).

Alignment is one component of affect attunement in which an individual alters his or her state to approximate that of the other member in the dyad. For example, a parent might notice a child's smile and mirror back a smile; an infant may notice a parent's apprehensive or fearful look when watching the child crawl to some steps and mirror the parent's expression.

Alignment can be primarily a one-way process in which either the adult's or the infant's state changes to match and anticipate that of the other, or it can be a bilateral process, in which both the parent and infant modify their states.

When there are high levels of attunement between parents and children, they develop an emotional resonance that influences their sensitivity to other aspects of each other's minds. Some parents, however, do not easily attune to their infants. They may not be sensitive to their infant's states and hence may either overstimulate or understimulate their infants. Adults who overstimulate tend to engage in overcontrolling, intrusive behaviors with infants. Overstimulating adults may fail either to read or to respond to infants' efforts to control stimulation. What the baby does matters relatively little. Highly attuned or high-affect-monitoring parents spend more time than less attuned or low-affect-monitoring mothers focused on the objects their infants are focused on.

Attunement in secure parent–child interactions is related to later language development. Depressed, emotionally disturbed, or intellectually limited parents are more likely to be low-affect monitors and may understimulate their infants. Infants with understimulating or over-stimulating caregivers have fewer opportunities to participate in satisfying social interactions and to discover ways they can affect their environments through communication.

Children reared in abusive and/or emotionally neglectful circumstances may experience fewer instances of positive social interactions; even when such an interaction is available, the children may be in such a constant state of "fight or flight" that they cannot attend to the communication (Perry, 1997). Such children may suffer long-lasting social–behavioral–communicative deficits. The lack of appropriate affective experiences in early life can result in neurological differences and associated mal-organization of attachment capabilities. During development, abused/neglected children spend so much time in a low-level state of fear that they are constantly focusing on nonverbal cues. Such children feel no emotional attachment to other humans, and they fail to develop appropriate social-interactive relationships and communication skills (Alessandri & Lewis, 1996).

Factors Within the Child

Children with cognitive, syntactic, or semantic deficits are also likely to show delays and differences in social or pragmatic aspects of communication. Children who were born prematurely, and who have significant medical problems or cognitive impairments as a consequence, are less able to engage in the conversational dance during infancy. They are, therefore, at risk for pragmatic deficits beyond what would be expected based on their cognitive abilities alone.

Some conditions particularly affect the social–emotional or pragmatic aspects of communication development. A number of factors—many of which are profiled in this section—may result in the child being less able to be involved in communicative interactions or in the adult being less able to read the child's involvement.

Blindness

Early social interactions, gesturing, and the development of referencing are all dependent upon vision. Blind children are generally delayed in acquisition of first words and frequently exhibit pragmatic language impairments. They repeat words to themselves and fail to produce them to initiate interactions until well into their third year (Urwin, 1983). Later, they may ask many questions, sometimes inappropriately; they may use echolalia; and they may make 'off-the-wall' comments (Mills, 1993).

By six months of age, the sighted infant has developed a large repertoire of social interactions. Blind children, however, have no way of watching their mothers' facial expressions or of engaging in joint attention to visual events with her. Also, because blind babies stop looking at their mothers after the end of the reflex period, mothers do not pick them up as often. Consequently, infants miss out on these opportunities for communicating.

Lack of vision particularly affects the development of joint attention, which is essential for establishing referencing that is necessary for communicating. Blind children may have difficulty determining whether their intended listeners are attending to them, or even if the persons are present. Knowing that the person is present, however, is no guarantee that he or she is paying attention. Even if the person is present and has been listening, the child has no way of knowing if the person's attention has shifted to something else. The child must gain the listener's attention. Blind children do not have the option of establishing mutual gaze or gesturing. Instead, they must either touch the listener or vocalize. For sighted children, vocalizing to gain attention and establishing joint referencing are initially superimposed on earlier gestural strategies. Without vision, blind children develop few gestural communications. The blind child also may not be certain if the referent exists in the environment or if the listener is attending to it.

Many of the blind child's early referents are names of people rather than names of objects. Use of language for requesting purposes appears in sighted children by the end of the first year after birth, but emerges closer to the end of the second year in blind children. Because blind children's nonverbal behavior so often fails to provide topics for comment, parents frequently adopt a questioning mode of interaction. Although questioning may facilitate an early form of turn-taking between parent and child, because the initiative always remains with the adult, the practice inhibits the child's development of awareness of his own agency—that is, the ability to make things happen in the environment (McGurk, 1983).

Despite these early deficits, blind children who have no other handicapping conditions and who have adult caregivers who are alert to the interaction of blindness and language can develop normal communicative interaction patterns during the preschool years. Many, however, show patterns of delays and disorder in pragmatic communicative interactions (James & Stojanovik, 2006).

Deafness

Deafness causes not only a delay in language acquisition, but also a disruption in early parent–child interactions, particularly when the child is deaf and the parents are hearing. Deaf children of hearing parents and late-signing deaf children typically are also quite delayed in ToM associated with false belief (i.e., recognizing that what someone believes is untrue) and deception (i.e., recognizing that someone is intentionally trying to trick another) (Schick, de Villiers, de Villiers, & Hoffmeister, 2007). Deaf children of deaf parents typically pass formal ToM false-belief tasks at the same age as hearing children; however, the degree to which deaf children of deaf parents master higher levels of ToM or use ToM effectively is unknown. It is possible to pass ToM false-belief tasks yet not be able to comprehend all the nuances of perspective taking in naturalistic situations. Development of ToM requires not only an intact neurological system, but also experiences with persons who talk about the mind. The reduced communicative interactions experienced by deaf children limit their development of ToM (deVilliers, 2005).

A lack of development of higher-level ToM appears to influence deaf children's understanding of causes of emotions (Rieffe, Terwogt, & Smit, 2003). When identifying the emotion that would occur in a situation, deaf children tend to focus on the outcome of a situation in terms of whether a person's desires are fulfilled. As a consequence, they are likely to judge a person's emotional response to a situation in terms of being happy or sad, depending on whether the outcome was desired or not. In contrast, hearing children tend to consider both the controllability of a situation and the final outcome. Hence, if a child cannot go on a picnic because it is raining, they judge that the child will be sad; in contrast, if the child cannot go on a picnic because a parent insists that she clean her room instead, then they are likely to judge that the child will be angry. Deaf children are likely to judge to the child to be sad in both instances. Failure to distinguish the reasons behind an outcome will result in the latter children having fewer strategies to cope with social situations. These reduced strategies for coping with social situations may contribute to the frequently noted externalizing behavior problems of deaf children (Vostanis, Hayes, Du Feu, & Warren, 1997).

Specific Language Impairment

A strong correlation exists between language skills and social–emotional behavior (Baker & Cantwell, 1987; Brinton & Fujiki, 1993; Giddan, 1991). Although there is agreement that, in most instances, language and social impairments are causally linked, there is less agreement about the nature and direction of this relationship. Perhaps a biological or neurophysiological factor underlies both the social–emotional and linguistic difficulties. Deficits in one area might drive further deficits in the other area. Research is increasingly showing that children with specific language impairment (SLI) have more difficulties in social interactions than can be explained by their language impairment alone (Fujiki, Brinton, Isaacson, & Summers, 2001).

As a group, children with SLI are less competent in regulating their own emotions, and they experience fewer peer friendships and higher rates of bullying than their typical peers. Persons who accurately express and regulate their own emotions and understand the emotions of others are more successful socially than those who have difficulty with these behaviors (Denham, 1998). To participate effectively in social situations, children must be able to infer and interpret their partners' emotional reactions—a feat that requires an understanding of causal connections. Causal inferences may be based on physical events (e.g., inferring that wet clothes are caused by rain) or mental states (e.g., inferring that forgetting an umbrella might cause someone to be angry). Physical events are observable, but mental states are not; as a consequence, it may be more difficult for children to link events to mental states. Research indicates that children with SLI have difficulty making inferences based on both physical events and mental states (Botting & Adams, 2005; Ford & Milosky, 2003). Inability to make these inferences may contribute to the social difficulties children with SLI experience. Negative social consequences of SLI are manifested in the early preschool years when children as young as three years avoid conversing with language-impaired peers. By four years of age, children with SLI are chosen as least liked by their typically developing peers. This reduced popularity continues throughout the school years.

Some children with SLI may exhibit early appropriate social–emotional interactions, but later problems in word-finding, constructing requests or comments, repairing communication breakdowns, or comprehending what is said may adversely affect their social skills. Children with language impairments are less willing to engage in conversation, and they are more likely to be ignored or rejected when they do attempt to communicate (Fujiki, Brinton, & Todd, 1996; Rice, 1993). In addition, deficits in social and language skills frequently result in reduced opportunities for social interaction (Rice, 1993). Because social interactions are so critical in driving language and social development, the child with social and language impairments experiences further delays in development.

Autism Spectrum Disorders

Autism spectrum disorders (ASD) are probably the condition most commonly associated with deficits in social/emotional aspects of communication. Children with ASD exhibit a fundamental failure in socialization. The social dysfunction observed in children with autism is never observed in neurotypical children of any age and cannot be accounted for on the basis of cognitive impairments alone. Children with ASD show deficits in three areas related to social engagement: sociability and social communication, attachment, and understanding and express-ing emotions (Volkmar & Klin, 2005).

Deficits in socialization may be noted early. In fact, many children with ASD exhibit devi-ant patterns of gaze from early infancy. Young children with autism may avoid eye gaze, while some older children may stare fixedly and inappropriately. Deficits in joint attention and refer-ential pointing readily discriminate toddlers with and without ASD. Communication requires that one be able to conceive of another's sharing an interest about an object or topic. A key symptom of ASD is the child's inability to enter into joint attention and affective contact with other people.

The majority of children with autism eventually develop RJA and IBR, but they continue to exhibit deficits in IJA (Mundy, Sigman, & Kasari, 1994). Even though they may follow another's line of regard (RJA), they do not necessarily reference the emotional expression of the person they are observing; that is, they do not attempt to interpret the person's reason for looking or response to looking. Children who cannot engage in joint attention, or who avoid it, would have difficulty in grasping early language functions. Without RJA, IJA, and social–emotional referencing, children with ASD continue to exhibit poor skills in emotional sharing; without emotional sharing, they fail to develop higher levels of ToM essential for social under-standing and interpersonal relationships.

Children with autism exhibit a sparsity of intentional communicative behaviors. They use fewer communicative acts during interactions, and many of the communicative intentions they do use are not conventionalized. For example, some children with autism use echolalia (repeti-tions of words and phases they have heard spoken) to make a request. For example, they may say, *Do you want a drink?* instead of *I want water.* They use a high degree of nonreciprocal speech, fail to listen, make irrelevant comments, and fail to leave a topic of obsessive interest or to look for cues in the listener as to his or her interest or desire to take a turn (Dewey & Everard, 1974). They tend to be poor at initiating conversation, although they may not be un-responsive if another person initiates it (Loveland, Landry, Hughes, Hall, & McEvoy, 1988). When they do bring up a topic, it is often related to their own preoccupations, and their re-marks or questions are usually uttered without varied inflection (Rutter & Garmezy, 1983). Children with ASD are also likely to interrupt and respond inappropriately in conversations (Paccia-Cooper, Curcio, & Sacharko, 1981). Some engage in persistent and perseverative ques-tioning that does not serve the purpose of requesting information (Hurtig, Ensrud, & Tomblin, 1980). Although some basic intention to communicate exists, children with ASD have little skill in participating in communicative activities involving joint reference of shared topics, and particularly in supplying new information relevant to the listener's purposes (Tager-Flusberg, Paul, & Lord, 2005).

ASSESSING SOCIAL–EMOTIONAL BASES FOR COMMUNICATION _____

Caregiver–Child Interaction

Children's development of the social–emotional/intentional basis of communication is dependent on their interactions with those around them and on their own personality and abilities. Because communication in infancy is so related to caregiver–child interaction, when a young child is referred for communication evaluation, it is desirable to observe the nature of this interaction. Children require different types of interaction with caregivers at various stages of development.

Klein and Briggs (1987) developed a brief observation form to use in observing mothers and infants. They list 10 caregiver behaviors to observe:

1. Provides appropriate tactile and kinesthetic stimulation (e.g., gently strokes, pats, caresses, cuddles, rocks baby)
2. Displays pleasure while interacting
3. Responds to child's distress (changes verbalization, changes infant's position, provides positive physical stimuli)
4. Positions self and infant so eye-to-eye contact is possible (attempts to make eye contact, reciprocates eye gaze)
5. Smiles contingently at infant
6. Varies prosodic features (uses higher pitch, talks more slowly, exaggerates intonation)
7. Encourages conversation (uses rising intonation questions, waits after saying something, imitates child's sounds, answers when infant vocalizes)
8. Responds contingently to infant's behavior (vocalizes after infant movement or vocalization)
9. Modifies interaction in response to negative cues from infant (changes activity, reduces intensity of interaction, terminates interaction)
10. Uses communication to teach language concepts (interprets infant's behaviors appropriate—for example, *You're hungry, aren't you?*; comments on infant's attention to something in environment, matches infant's vocalization or word with slightly more elaborate language)

For each category, Klein and Briggs provide additional description of components of behavior. The observer is to rate the interaction on a scale of *rare, sometimes, often,* or *optimally.* This scale reflects ideas from mainstream literature on caregiver–child interactions and assumes that the mother is the primary caregiver. When using it with nondominant cultural groups, the assessor will want to observe the infants with other individuals who may be their caregivers and will want to observe other families from a similar cultural or socioeconomic level before interpreting the results of the observations.

Vigil and Westby (2004) have also proposed a parent–child interaction profile (**Table 5-3**). Their scheme differentiates behaviors according to whether they socialize children toward independence or toward interdependence.

TABLE 5-3   Patterns of Socialization Interaction

Behavior	Definition	Attentional Style	
		Independent (Attention Following)	Interdependent (Attention Directing)
Follow Lead	Caregiver attends to the object to which the child shows interest.		
Direct Attention	Caregiver uses vocalization, gesture, or object manipulation to engage the infant with an object or event that s/he wants the child to attend to.		
Alternate Attention	Caregiver alternates attention between competing events, focusing on one while momentarily stopping progress in another.		
Simultaneous Attention	Caregiver attends to several activities occurring at the same time. This does not necessarily involve simultaneous action, but rather simultaneous attention.		
Descriptives	An utterance in which information is given about an ongoing activity or behavior performed by either the caregiver or the child.		
Attentional Directives	Caregiver attempts to elicit the infant's attention to self or object through vocalization (i.e., "Look, look here").		
Behavioral Directives	Utterance that elicits or constrains the physical behavior of the infant by commanding, requesting and encouraging the child to do or desist from doing something (i.e., "Put your hand here").		
Holds Object	Caregiver holds object to support playing, but does not manipulate object or child's hands.		
Manipulates Object or Child	Caregiver manipulates an object to direct the child's play (i.e., shows child how to play with the toy).		

Assessment of Children's Communicative Behaviors

Assessment of children's communicative functions and intentions should consider the number of different communicative intentions they use, the proportion of each function, the rate of communicative intentions, and the child's developing theory of mind. The rate of communication may be a particularly useful measure of communicative development in language-impaired children who are using few or no words (Wetherby, Cain, Yonclas, & Walker, 1988). In particular, a lack of developing communicative functions may be a warning sign of broad-based communicative impairment. Assessment of children's communicative intentions can include standardized and norm-referenced questionnaires and tests, observation of caregiver–child/teacher–child interactions, interviews of family members and teachers regarding the child's communicative behavior, and observation of children's language use in naturalistic settings and in activities structured to trigger a variety of communicative intentions.

Formal/Standardized Assessments

An increasing number of formal tools, which often employ standardized methods for their administration, have been developed. Standardized, normed tests are useful when there is a need to compare an individual or group to some standard—for example, when screening children at risk for communication deficits. Formal, standardized questionnaires and tests may also be more time-efficient than observational approaches. The use of standardized tests for evaluating pragmatics is, however, controversial. Adults have control in test-like situations, and consequently children may not produce the same types and range of communicative intentions that they may produce in more natural situations. This outcome is particularly likely with children who are unfamiliar with test-like situations and unfamiliar with the examiner/examinee roles in testing (Westby, 2000).

Considering the important role of joint attention in the development of the social/emotional bases for communication, it is critical that joint attention be evaluated. Mundy and colleagues (2002) have provided a protocol, known as the *Early Social Communication Scales*, that can be used to evaluate the following types of joint attention in children between 8 and 30 months of age:

- Initiating joint attention to share an object or event
- Responding to joint attention (i.e., following the attention of a partner to an object or event)
- Initiating behavioral requests to obtain an action or object
- Responding to behavioral requests of partners to give an object or perform an action
- Initiating social interaction to elicit or maintain a turn-taking game or tease
- Responding to social interaction (turn-taking or teasing game) initiated by a partner

Although joint attention and its related behaviors of emotional sharing, referencing, and co-referencing develop in the first 12 to 18 months of life, they may not be well developed in older children, particularly those with autism spectrum disorders. Because joint attention is so essential for meaningful communication, it should be evaluated in individuals of all age levels who exhibit deficits is social communication.

Most formal developmental and language assessment tools that can be used with children younger than three years include items that evaluate early social–emotional and pragmatic communication development. These tools include the following assessments:

+ *Rossetti Infant–Toddler Language Scale* (Rossetti, 2006)
+ *Ages and Stages Questionnaires: A Parent-Completed Child Monitoring System* (Bricker & Squires, 1999) and *Ages and Stages Questionnaires: Social–Emotional* (Squires, Bricker, & Twombly, 2002)
+ *Communication and Symbolic Behavior Scales Developmental Profile* (Wetherby & Prizant, 2002)

Some standardized, normed assessments for older children also include assessment of pragmatic behaviors. For example, the *Clinical Evaluation of Language Fundamentals—Preschool* (for ages 3–6 years) (Semel, Wiig, & Secord, 2004) and the *Clinical Evaluation of Language Fundamentals—4* (CELF—4; for ages 5–21 years) (Semel, Wiig, & Secord, 2003) both include a pragmatics profile. The *Children's Communicative Checklist-2* (for children 4–16 years) (Bishop, 2006) rates speech, syntax, semantics, coherence, and several aspects of pragmatics. The availability of norming data enables differentiation of children with specific language impairment (deficits in syntax/semantics), pragmatics, or autism.

Standardized, non-normed assessments of pragmatics may use structured or scripted interactions or require judgments of what should be said in particular situations. For example, Creaghead (1984) provided a non-normed, scripted "Peanut Butter Protocol"(reproduced in Paul, 2007). With this tool, the adult attempts to elicit communication with the child while engaged in an activity with cookies, crackers, peanut butter, and jelly. During the evaluation, the adult notes the type and appropriateness of the child's pragmatic acts in response to the adult's comments.

Context	Expected Pragmatic Act
Child enters room.	Greeting
Crackers and cookies are in view but out of reach.	Requests object
Give child tightly closed jar with cookies in it.	Requests action
Ask, "How to you think we can open the jar?"	Hypothesizing
Say, "Do you want (mumble)?"	Requests clarification

Naturalistic Observations

The majority of studies on children's intentional communication have relied on naturalistic social contexts—that is, having children interact with familiar people, and allowing children to converse about topics of their choosing (Coggins, Olswang, & Guthrie, 1987). It has been assumed that nonobtrusive observation provides the best opportunity to obtain a representative sample of children's language use. This technique may, however, provide an incomplete picture of a child's capabilities. A combination of both natural, unstructured activities and structured activities designed to elicit particular communicative functions may be the best way of sampling children's capabilities. Children are more likely to use requests in structured conditions and comments during free-play situations (Coggins, Olswang, & Guthrie, 1987). In low-structured activities, toys are readily accessible and caregivers follow the child's leads; hence there is little need for children to request. In such situations, the child is in control and desires to share the experience with the adult. Consequently, the child is more likely to use comments to gain adult attention in nonstructured settings and less likely to use requests. Elicitation tasks are adult controlled in nature, with the adult manipulating the materials to direct the child's attention. The child does not need to gain the adult's attention, but to gain access to the materials the children has to make a request.

Young children will most readily communicate with familiar people in familiar settings. For infants and toddlers, it is best to carry out naturalistic observations of the child during daily routines at home—eating, bathing, or playing. When this is not possible, one can arrange naturalistic activities in a center and have the child's significant others (parents, grandparents, and siblings) carry out activities like they might do at home.

In practice, most clinicians use predetermined categories such as those outlined in Tables 5-1 and 5-2. A notation should be made each time a communicative behavior occurs. When using predetermined checklists, however, one should not feel compelled to make the child's responses fit the predetermined categories. The clinician should add new categories as necessary to explain the data.

In a completely naturalistic evaluation, children may not show the full range of intentionality of which they are capable. For this reason, one might want to structure the environment and interactions to trigger particular communicative functions. The activity may be loosely structured, in that the adult selects the materials and makes either leading comments or open-ended comments that could lead the child into using a particular communicative function. As adults play with the child, they may attempt to trigger requesting by not providing all the parts of a toy that are necessary; predicting by commenting, *I wonder what the fireman will do?*; projecting feelings by commenting, *I wonder how the baby feels?*; and so on.

The evaluator may want to use even greater structure and plan to present specific activities and interactions that might trigger specific communicative intentions. For young children or children who exhibit limited initiations, the evaluator can use activities that might tempt the child to communicate (Wetherby & Prizant, 1989). Some suggestions follow:

+ Eating a desired food in front of a child, without offering any to the child
+ Activating a toy, letting it wind down, and then handing it to the child
+ Opening a jar of bubbles, blowing some, and then closing the jar tightly and giving it to the child

Preschool and school-age children's communicative intentions can also be evaluated through the use of observational checklists. For example, the checklist in **Table 5-4** (based on Erickson, 1986) assesses both speech acts/communicative functions and discourse skills. Children in school should be observed in several contexts (i.e., reading class, math class, cafeteria, playground) and with both adults and peers.

The intent or function of a gesture or verbalization cannot be determined from the child's behavior alone. One must also take into account both the nonverbal and verbal aspects of the interactions and the linguistic and nonlinguistic contexts of the communication in determining communicative intentions and functions. What occurred prior to or following the behavior? How does the act relate to what came before and after? Does it repeat a prior behavior, respond to it, or provide further information? Did the child give clues that he was attempting to communicate, such as orienting his body to another person, looking toward another, or attempting to clarify a behavior? Following the child's behavior, did he wait as though expecting a response?

Interviews

A formal observational evaluation—whether it be nonstructured or structured—can be quite useful, but it does not demonstrate the variety and consistency of a child's behaviors in familiar environments. Although it may be possible to conduct an evaluation in the child's home or in the classroom, it is not possible to follow children in every aspect of their daily lives.

Interviewing significant others in children's lives can provide one with information regarding how children actually use their language. **Table 5-5** presents an interview format with cue questions and situations to explore five communicative functions that appear early in children's repertoires:

+ Requests for affection/interaction
+ Requests for adult actions
+ Requests for objects or food
+ Protests
+ Declaratives/comments (Schuler, Peck, Willard, & Theimer, 1989)

TABLE 5-4   Analysis of Communicative Competence

Discourse Skills	Speech Acts/Communicative Functions
☐ Starts a conversation	☐ Labels things/actions
☐ Shows listening behavior	☐ Asks for things/actions
☐ Passes turns	☐ Describes things/actions
☐ Receives turns/follows	☐ Asks for information
☐ Responds with appropriate content	☐ Gives information
☐ Interrupts legitimately	☐ Asks permission
☐ Stays on topic	☐ Promises
☐ Changes topic appropriately	☐ Agrees
☐ Appropriately ends conversation	☐ Threatens
☐ Recognizes listener's viewpoint	☐ Warns
☐ Demonstrates topic relevancy	☐ Apologizes
☐ Uses appropriate response length	☐ Protests/argues/disagrees
☐ Comments and examples of inappropriate conversational styles:	☐ Shows humor/teases
	☐ Gives greetings and leavings
	☐ Pleads
	☐ Commands/orders
	☐ Comments and examples of inappropriate language usage:

Source: Erickson (1986).

TABLE 5-5   Interview Questions for Communicative Functions

Requests for Affections/Interaction

What if child wants:

- ☐ Adult to sit near?
- ☐ Peer to sit near?
- ☐ Nonhandicapped peer to sit near?
- ☐ Adult to look at him?
- ☐ Adult to tickle him?
- ☐ To cuddle/embrace?
- ☐ To sit on adult's lap?
- ☐ Other:

Requests for Object, Food, or Things

What if child wants:

- ☐ An object out of reach?
- ☐ A door/container opened?
- ☐ A favorite food?
- ☐ Music/radio/tv?
- ☐ Keys/toys/book?
- ☐ Other:

Requests for Adult Action

What if child wants:

- ☐ Help with dressing?
- ☐ To read a book?
- ☐ To play ball/a game?
- ☐ To go outside?
- ☐ Other:

Protest

What if:

- ☐ Common routine is dropped?
- ☐ Favorite toy/food is taken away?
- ☐ Taken for ride with/without desire?
- ☐ Adult terminates interaction?
- ☐ Required to do something child doesn't want to?

Declaration/Comment

What if child wants:

- ☐ To show you something?
- ☐ You to look at something?
- ☐ Other:

Such intentional behaviors may include crying, pulling another's hand, touching/moving another's face, grabbing, walking away, vocalizing, pointing, facial expression, shaking the head yes or no, echoing something someone else said, a single word or single sign, or a phrase or sign combinations. Specific situations are presented and the adult is asked to describe what the child would do.

Assessing Theory of Mind and Emotion Understanding

The assessments discussed so far have focused on the nature of the parent–child interaction and the language functions (reasons for communicating) used by the child. Because intersubjectivity (the ability to appreciate the emotions, intentions, and beliefs of others) is so critical to the social basis of communication, it is useful to evaluate children's ToM and abilities to recognize and interpret the emotions and beliefs of others.

A number of strategies have been used to assess children's theory of mind—that is, their awareness and understanding of mental states in themselves and others. In the preschool years and early elementary years, children exhibit a predicable pattern of development of ToM and emotional understanding (Brinton, Spachman, Fujiki, & Ricks, 2007; Howlin, Baron-Cohen, Hadwin, & Swettenham, 1999; Pons, Harris, & deRosnay, 2004; Wellman & Liu, 2004). The following hierarchical list provides strategies for assessing some components of this line of development:

- *Recognition of emotion:* Name an emotion and ask the child to point to a photo of the person displaying this emotion
- *Identification of an external cause of emotion:* The child is shown a picture (without faces on the characters) and given a scenario (e.g., "This boy's dog ran away. He can't find his dog. How is the boy feeling?"). The child selects from photos showing happy, sad, scared, mad, and surprised and labels the emotion.
- *Diverse desires:* The child judges that two persons (the child versus someone else) have different desires about the same objects. Show the child a cartoon scenario with two boys, Mark and Jeff, on either side of a closed box with a moveable flap. Tell the child, "Mark hates carrots. Jeff likes carrots very much." Check to make certain the child remembers this "story," and then ask the child to open the flap to see the contents of the box. There are carrots in the box. Ask, "How is Mark feeling? Is he happy, sad, just alright, or scared? How is Jeff feeling? Is he happy, sad, just alright, or scared?"
- *Knowledge access:* The child sees what is in a box and judges (yes–no) the knowledge of another person who does not see what is in the box. The child is shown a small box and asked what is in it. The evaluator opens the box and shows the child a small plastic toy dog. He or she then produces a toy figure of girl and tells the child, "Polly has never seen what's inside this box. Here comes Polly. Does Polly know what's inside the box? Did Polly see inside the box?"

+ *Explicit false belief:* The child judges how a person will search, given the person's mistaken belief. The child is shown two dolls, Sally and Ann, and told, "While playing, Sally puts a marble into a basket and then goes outside. [The Sally doll disappears.] When Sally is gone, naughty Ann takes the marble out of the basket and puts it in a box. [Have the Ann doll move the marble from the basket to the box.] Sometime later, Sally comes back and wants to play with her marble. Where will Sally look for her marble?"

+ *Belief emotion:* The child judges how a person will feel, given a belief that is mistaken. The child is shown a book with a picture of a rabbit eating a carrot and told that the rabbit likes carrots very much. The child is then asked to lift a flap on the page, which reveals a hidden fox. Tell the child that the fox wants to eat the rabbit. Close the flap and ask the child if the rabbit knows the fox is there. If the child answers the false belief question correctly, say, "That's right—the rabbit doesn't know the fox is hiding behind the bushes." If the child answers incorrectly, say, "Well, actually the rabbit doesn't know the fox is hiding behind the bushes." Then ask, "How is the rabbit feeling? Is he happy, just alright, angry, or scared?"

+ *Regulation of emotion:* The child is shown a picture of Tom with tears in his eyes while looking at a photo of his rabbit. The child is told that Tom is very sad because his rabbit was eaten by the fox. Ask, "What is the best way for Tom to stop himself from being sad? Can Tom cover his eyes to stop himself from being sad? Can Tom go outside and do something else to stop himself being sad? Or is there nothing Tom can do to stop himself being sad?"

+ *Hiding emotions:* The child recognizes that there are situations where one should hide one's true emotions, such as showing pleasure rather than disappointment when receiving an undesirable birthday gift. The child is shown a picture of Chris and his grandmother and told, "This is Chris, and this is Chris's grandmother. Chris told his grandmother he wanted a really scary costume for Halloween. His grandmother makes him a Barney costume. [Show a picture of the grandmother with the Barney costume.] What does Chris say to his grandmother? What would Chris's parents want him to say?"

One should expect the majority of four-year-olds to be able to identify the expressions of happy, mad, sad, surprised, and afraid; by age four or five, children they should be able to match expressions to situations that would cause the expressions (Michaelson & Lewis, 1985; Pons, Harris, & deRosnay, 2004). Neurotypical four- to five-year-olds should also be able to pass tasks evaluating understanding of diverse beliefs, knowledge access, and false beliefs (Wellman & Liu, 2004). By the time they are in early elementary school, children should recognize how beliefs affect emotions, how to dissemble or hide emotions, and how to regulate emotions (Brinton, Spachman, Fujiki, & Ricks, 2007; Fujiki, Brinton, & Clarke, 2002). By nine to ten years of age, neurotypical children recognize that persons can have multiple emotions in response to situations (Harter, 1983).

One can also evaluate children's emotion understanding by asking them to identify emotions of characters in wordless picture books such *One Frog Too Many* (Mayer & Mayer, 1975) or *A Boy, a Dog, and a Frog* (Mayer, 1967), videos (such as *Max the Mouse*, 1989), or interactive computer story programs. One can also ask the child why the characters feel as they do and what they might do next. By age eight years, the majority of children should be able to explain the reasons for the feelings and predict what the characters will do in response to the emotion.

The DVD program *Mind Reading* (Baron-Cohen, Golan, Wheelwright, & Hill, 2004), which is intended to develop recognition of emotions in persons from age four years to adult, also provides assessment activities. Tasks include identifying emotional expressions, matching faces with similar emotions, and identifying emotions in voices. Videos and interactive computer programs provide additional movement and sound cues that signal emotions.

A word of caution about assessment of ToM and emotion understanding: Belief understanding does not guarantee emotion understanding; emotion understanding does not guarantee empathy; and empathy does not guarantee that the children will be kind to people they perceive as sad (Davis & Stone, 2003).

PHILOSOPHY OF INTERVENTION FOR SOCIAL–COMMUNICATIVE DEFICITS___

The social competence that underlies communication develops from the early emotional sharing relationships between caregivers and children. Because joint attention underlies the social interactive competence essential for true communication, interventions should address any deficits in the behaviors and interactions that underlie JA and that result from development of JA. Although IBR can be developed through use of clinician-directed behavioral approaches that use drill and practice, true RJA and IJA cannot. The social competence reflected in RJA and IJA cannot be trained outside of meaningful contexts. Instead, children must be motivated to engage with others in sharing experiences that will foster RJA and IJA. If children with social–emotional deficits are to share experiences with enthusiasm and enjoyment, parents and clinicians must provide them with real pleasures inherent in experience-sharing encounters.

Intervention approaches for social communicative deficits typically use a functional or naturalistic/ecological-based, child-centered framework rather than more directive, clinician-centered approaches. Three aspects of the social use of language are essential components of these language intervention programs: the social context in which intervention occurs, the embedding of communicative goals and objectives in daily activities, and the inclusion of caregivers (or children's significant others [SOs], such as parents, siblings, grandparents, and teachers) in the intervention. Some programs, such as *It Takes Two to Talk* (Pepper & Weitzman, 2004), *More Than Words* (Sussman, 1999), *Floortime* (Greenspan, 2006), and *Relationship Development Intervention* (Gutstein, 2002), focus on intervention with family members. Other approaches, such as the milieu approach and activity-based approach, are naturalistic intervention strategies that have been widely used in infant–toddler preschool programs. Milieu teaching uses everyday instances of social–communicative exchanges as opportunities to teach elaborated language and capitalizes on natural consequences as reinforcers (Hancock & Kaiser, 2006). Activity-based intervention is similar to milieu teaching, but is often directed to a group rather than an individual child and addresses all aspects of development, rather than just communication (Pretti-Frontczak & Bricker, 2004).

All ecologically based programs share some common assumptions:

+ The SOs are facilitators, not trainers.
+ The interactions should be contextualized and familiar.

As facilitators, SOs do not teach or control interactions with demands or questions. Instead, they follow the child's lead. For children who do not yet intentionally communicate, SOs imitate the infants' behavior. The facilitator looks for behaviors in the child and responds appropriately to the content and intent of the child's behavior. The child controls and initiates the conversational topics. The SO's job is to reinforce and maintain the communication naturally by responding in semantically and pragmatically contingent ways. Responses to children's behavior should be natural consequences. Thus a request for a cookie should be followed by giving the cookie and by words such as *Okay*, or *Just one*, or *What kind?*, but not by good talking.

The learning context should be meaningful to the child. Facilitory activities should occur in natural encounters throughout the day in the child's usual environments with familiar people and materials, not in contrived therapeutic settings. Highly routinized sequences of behavior have been shown to promote the development of intentional communication (Goetz, Gee, & Sailor, 1985). A strategy termed *interrupted behavior chain* can be used to trigger communicative behaviors. With this approach, the SO participates with the child in a familiar activity such as eating cereal, washing hands, or putting a doll to bed. The SO interrupts the behavior chain by delaying presentation of an item necessary for completion of the routine, placing a needed item just out of the child's reach or preventing the child from obtaining the desired object or person (e.g., by holding an object down, stepping back out of the child's reach, or preventing the child from going outside by putting hand on child). For example, the child may begin the hand washing activity by turning on the water, picking up the soap, and getting her hands wet and soapy. The adult may then turn off the water before the child rinses her hands. Because the routine is highly familiar, the child is likely to comment that she hasn't rinsed her hands, to complain that her hands are sticky, or to request that the water be turned back on. Adults must be conscious of a wide range of communicative functions and model them contingently in response to the child's behavior.

For young children with social–communicative deficits, ecologically based programs have the following goals:

+ *Establish interactional functions.* Turn-taking is essential for communication. SOs begin to establish turn-taking routines by attending to a child's behavior, responding to it, pausing and waiting for the behavior to recur, and then responding again. Turn-taking can occur in games in which the SO nuzzles the infant; stops; watches for the infant to smile, vocalize, or laugh; and then nuzzles the infant again. With older children, this may occur in play exchanges in which the SO and child roll a car back and forth, take turns stacking blocks, or take turns placing rings on a stand or dropping blocks in a bottle.

+ *Establish a clear intentional signaling system.* SOs treat an observed infant behavior as intentional (even when it isn't) and respond accordingly. If the infant looks toward a toy, the SO may say, *You want your teddy. Here it is,* as the SO brings the toy to the infant. If the infant moves its arms, the SO may say, *You want up;* raise the infant's arms; and then pick the infant up. By responding consistently to children's behavior, children discover that they have an effect on their environment. In time, their gestures and sounds acquire meaning because they elicit a predictable response.

+ *Develop socially appropriate and conventionalized signals.* Once the child is indicating intentions through gaze, vocalizations, or reaching, the adult begins to shape the behaviors by modeling appropriate gestures and words.

+ *Increase the variety and frequency of communicative intentions.* As the child becomes successful in indicating intentionality, SOs provide communicative temptations that will encourage active participation of the child.

These goals cannot be achieved unless children and SOs are engaging in activities in ways that promote *emotional sharing, social referencing,* and *coordination/coregulation* (i.e., ongoing mutual social referencing of the participants involved in social interactions). When playing with children, adults can provide surprising turns of events that promote heightened anticipation and excitement; adults can also amplify the shared emotion through facial expressions, gestures, and vocal tone. Development of social referencing can be promoted by creating simple decision points such as moving forward or stopping where the only way for the child to determine subsequent actions is to reference the partner's emotional reactions (i.e., Is the partner smiling and nodding, or frowning and shaking his or her head?).

Adults can encourage coordination/coregulation by setting up activities that require the child to continually check whether the partner is ready to participate or to continue interacting. For example, if playing ball, the child must check whether the partner is ready to catch the ball. Adults can also alter their own actions in relation to anticipated actions of their children. They can also gradually introduce activities where coordination begins to break down, and the child must notice this fact and repair the breakdown. For example, when playing catch, the adult may move so far away so that it is difficult for the child to catch the ball. The child must realize this fact and move closer. Or when walking, the adult can vary the pace so that the child must modify his pace to stay with the adult.

Emotional sharing, social referencing, and coordination/coregulation lay the foundation for the development of autobiographical memory, also known as *episodic memory*. Episodic memory links the emotional experience of an event with the what, when, and how of the event. This type of memory makes it possible for individuals to recollect happenings and events from their past and to use this information project anticipated events into one's future (Tulving, 1993). Episodic memory enables the individual to make predictions—and hence to make inferences in social interactions and in text comprehension. Episodic memory and ToM are interdependent. As children develop awareness of the relationship between their own feelings and experiences, they also begin to conceptualize the notion that others might have feelings about experiences. Beyond the early years, episodic memory and ToM form the cognitive underpinnings for social competence.

CONCLUSION

Parents, clinicians, and researchers are increasingly becoming aware of the social/pragmatic deficits exhibited by many children with a variety of language, learning, and behavioral difficulties. Age-level syntax, vocabulary, and semantic/procedural memory do not guarantee effective communication and academic success. Emergence of true communication and language depends on social–emotional competence and the motivation or goal to share emotional experiences. Then, developing language further promotes the development of social–emotional competence, which is essential for achieving friendships, working effectively with others, and comprehending narrative discourse.

The significance of the emergence of intentional communication in infants and toddlers has been recognized for some time. In recent years, research has provided insight into what underlies early social–emotional competence and what caregivers can do to promote this competence. Less attention has been given to the significance of social–emotional competence for older children. In fact, some school districts do not permit treatment of social–emotional/pragmatic deficits unless the clinician can show how these deficits affect academic performance. Nevertheless, such deficits in communicative competence have long-term consequences that affect all aspects of an individual's life.

KEY TERMS

Attachment

Attunement

Communicative competence

Coordination/coregulation

Emotions

Endogenous factors

Episodic memory

Exogenous factors

Horizontal development

Independent/individualist

Initiating joint attention (IJA)

Initiating behavior request (IBR)

Intentionality

Interdependent/collectivist

Joint attention (JA)

Pragmatics

Primary intersubjectivity

Referencing

Responding to joint attention (RJA)

Secondary intersubjectivity

Temperament

Theory of mind (ToM)

Vertical development

STUDY QUESTIONS

+ Describe the horizontal and vertical development of children's social communication from birth through the preschool years.

+ Explain how children's temperaments, attachment factors, and cultural differences in child-rearing practices may influence the development of children's language and social communicative competence.

+ Explain the significance of theory of mind in the development of children's language and social communication skills. In what ways can aspects of theory of mind be evaluated in infants, toddlers, and preschool children?

+ In what ways do different types of developmental disabilities affect children's social communicative competence?

+ How should a clinician approach intervention for a child's social communicative deficits?

REFERENCES

Ainsworth, M. D. S., Blehar, M. C., Waters, E., & Wall, S. (1978). *Patterns of attachment: A psychological study of the strange situation*. Hillsdale, NJ: Erlbaum.

Alessandri, S. M., & Lewis, M. (1996). Development of the self-conscious emotions in maltreated children. In M. Lewis & M. W. Sullivan (Eds.), *Emotional development in atypical children* (pp.185–202). Mahwah, NJ: Erlbaum.

Baker, L., & Cantwell, D. P. (1987). A prospective psychiatric follow-up of children with speech/language disorders. *Journal of the American Academy of Child and Adolescent Psychiatry, 26*, 546–553.

Baron-Cohen, S., Golan, O., Wheelright, S., & Hill, J. (2004). *Mindreading: The interactive guide to emotions*. London: Jessica Kingsley.

Bates, E. (1976). *Language in context*. New York: Academic Press.

Bates, E., Bretherton, I., Beeghly-Smith, M., & McNew, S. (1982). Social bases of language development: A reassessment. In H. W. Reese & L. P. Lipsett (Eds.), *Advances in child development and behavior* (Vol. 16, pp. 7–75). New York: Academic Press.

Bertenthal, B., & Longo, M. (2007). Is there evidence of a mirror system from birth? *Developmental Science, 10*, 526–529.

Bishop, D. V. M. (2006). *Children's Communication Checklist*, 2nd ed., U.S. ed. 2. San Antonio, TX: Harcourt Assessment.

Bloom, L. (1990). Developments in expression: Affect and speech. In N. L. Stein, B. Leventhal, & T. Trabasso (Eds.), *Psychological and biological approaches to emotion* (pp. 215–246). Hillsdale, NJ: Erlbaum.

Bloom, L. (1993). The transition form infancy to language: Acquiring the power of expression. New York: Cambridge University Press.

Botting, N., & Adams, C. (2005). Semantic and inferencing abilities in children with communication disorders. *Journal of Language & Communication Disorders, 40*, 49–66.

Bretherton, I. (1991). Intentional communication and the development of an understanding mind. In D. Frye & C. Moore (Eds.), *Children's theories of mind* (pp. 49–75). Hillsdale, NJ: Erlbaum.

Bretherton, I., & Beeghly, M. (1982). Talking about internal states: The acquisition of an explicit theory of mind. *Developmental Psychology, 18*, 906–921.

Bricker, D., & Squires, J. (1999). *Ages and Stages Questionnaire (ASQ): A parent-completed child monitoring system*, 2nd ed. Baltimore: Brookes.

Briggs, C. L. (1984). Learning how to ask: Native metacommunicative competence and the incompetence of fieldworkers. *Language in Society, 13*, 1–28.

Brinton, B., & Fujiki, M. (1993). Language, social skills, and socioemotional behavior. *Language, Speech, and Hearing Services in Schools, 24*, 194–198.

Brinton, B., Spachman, M. P., Fujiki, M., & Ricks, J. (2007). What should Chris say? The ability of children with specific language impairment to recognize the need to dissemble emotions in social situations. *Journal of Speech, Language, Hearing Research, 50*, 798–811.

Bruner, J. (1983). *Child's talk*. New York: W. W. Norton.

Bruner, J. (1986). *Actual minds, possible worlds*. Cambridge, MA: Harvard University Press.

Chapman, R. (1981). Exploring children's communicative intents. In J. F. Miller, *Assessing language production in children* (pp. 111–138). Austin, TX: Pro-Ed.

Coggins, T.E. & Carpenter, R.L. (1981). The communicative intention inventory: A system for observing and coding children's early intentional communication, *Applied Psycholinguistics 2*(3): 235–51.

Coggins, T. E., Oslwang, L. B., & Guthrie, J. (1987). Assessing communicative intents in young children: Low structured observation or elicitation tasks? *Journal of Speech and Hearing Disorders, 52*, 44–49.

Creaghead, N. (1984). Strategies for evaluating and targeting pragmatic behaviors in young children. *Seminars in Speech and Language, 5*, 241–252.

Davis, M., & Stone, T., (2003). Synthesis: Psychological understanding and social skills. In B. Repacholi & V. Slaugher (Eds.), *Individual differences in theory of mind: Implications for typical and atypical development* (pp. 306–352). New York: Psychology Press.

Denham, S. A. (1998). *Emotional development in young children*. New York: Guilford.

deVilliers, P. (2005). The role of language in theory-of-mind development: What deaf children tell us. In J. W. Astington & J. A. Baird (Eds.), *Why language matters for theory of mind* (pp. 266–297). New York: Oxford University Press.

Dewey, M., & Everard, M. (1974). The near normal autistic adolescent. *Journal of Autism and Childhood Schizophrenia, 4,* 348–356.

Dore, J. (1975). Holophrases, speech acts and language universals. *Journal of Child Language, 2,* 21–40.

Dore, J. (1978). Requestive systems in nursery school conversations: Analysis of talk in its social context. In R. Campbell & P. Smith (Eds.), *Recent advances in the psychology of language: Language development and mother–child interaction* (pp. 271–292). New York: Plenum Press.

Dunn, J., Bretherton, I., & Munn, P. (1987). Conversations about feeling states between mothers and their young children. *Developmental Psychology, 23,* 132–139.

Erickson, J. G. (1986). Analysis of communicative competence. In L. Cole & V. Deal (Eds.), *Communication disorders in multicultural populations.* Washington, DC: American Speech-Language-Hearing Association.

Ervin-Tripp, S. & Gordon, D. (1986). The development of requests. In. R. L.Schiefelbusch (Ed.), *Language competence: Assessment and intervention* (pp. 61–95). San Diego: College-Hill.

Field, T. (1987). Affective and interactive disturbances in infants. In J. D. Osofsky (Ed.), *Handbook of infant development* (pp. 972–1005). New York: Wiley.

Field, T., Sostek, A. M., Vietze, P., & Leiderman, P. H. (1981). *Culture and early interactions.* Hillsdale, NJ: Erlbaum.

Ford, J. A., & Milosky, L. M. (2003). Inferring emotional reactions in social situations: Differences in children with language impairment. *Journal of Speech, Language & Hearing Research, 46,* 21–30.

Fujiki, M., Brinton, B., & Clarke, D. (2002). Emotion regulation in children with specific language impairment. *Language, Speech, and Hearing Services in Schools, 33,* 102–111.

Fujiki, M., Brinton, B., Isaacson, T., & Summers, C. (2001). Social behaviors of children with language impairment on the playground: A pilot study. *Language, Speech, and Hearing Services in Schools, 32,* 101–113.

Fujiki, M., Brinton, B., & Todd, C.M. (1996). Social skills of children with specific language impairment. *Language, Speech, and Hearing Services in Schools, 27,* 195–202.

Giddan, J. J. (1991). School children with emotional problems and communication deficits: Implications for speech-language pathologists. *Language, Speech, and Hearing Services in Schools, 22,* 291–295.

Goetz, L., Gee, K., & Sailor, W. (1985). Using a behavior chain interruption strategy to teach communication skills to students with severe disabilities. *Journal of the Association of Persons with Severe Handicaps, 10,* 21–30.

Gordon, D., & Ervin-Tripp, S. (1984). Structure of children's requests. In R. L. Schiefelbusch &. J. Pickar (Eds.), *The acquisition of communicative competence* (pp. 295–322). Baltimore: University Park Press.

Greenfield, P. M., & Cocking, R. R. (1994). *Cross-cultural roots of minority child development.* Hillsdale, NJ: Erlbaum.

Greenspan, S. (2006). *Engaging children: Using the floortime approach to help children relate, communicate, and think.* Cambridge, MA: Da Capo Press.

Gutstein, S. E. (2002). *Autism Asperger's: Solving the relationship puzzle.* Arlington, TX: Future Horizons.

Halliday, M. A. K. (1975). *Learning how to mean: Explorations in the development of language.* London: Edward Arnold.

Hancock, T. B., & Kaiser, A. P. (2006). Enhanced milieu teaching. In R. McCauley & M. Fey (Eds.), *Treatment of language disorders in children* (pp. 175–202). Baltimore: Brookes.

Harter, S. (1983). Children's understanding of multiple emotions: A cognitive-developmental approach. In W. F. Overton (Ed.), *The relationship between social and cognitive development* (pp. 147–194). Hillsdale, NJ: Erlbaum.

Heath, S. B. (1983). *Ways with words.* Cambridge, MA: Cambridge University Press.

Hewitt, L.E. (1994). Narrative comprehension: The importance of subjectivity. In J. F. Duchan, L. E. Hewitt, & R. M. Sonnenmeier (Eds.), *Pragmatics: From theory to practice.* (pp. 88–104). Englewood Cliffs, NJ: Prentice-Hall.

Howlin, P., Baron-Cohen, S., Hadwin, J., & Swettenham, J. (1999). *Teaching children with autism to mind-read.* New York: Wiley.

Hurtig, R., Ensrud, S., & Tomblin, J. B. (1980). *Question production in children with autism: A linguistic pragmatic perspective.* Paper presented at the University of Wisconsin Symposium on Research in Child Language Disorders, Madison, WI.

James, D. M., & Stojanovik, V. (2006). Communication skills in blink children: A preliminary investigation. *Child Care, Health, and Development, 33,* 4–10.

Johnston, J. R., & Wong, M. Y. A. (2002). Cultural differences in beliefs and practices concerning talk to children. *Journal of Speech, Language, and Hearing Research, 45,* 916–926.

Klein, M. D., & Briggs, M. H. (1987). *Observation of communicative interaction.* Los Angeles: California State University–Los Angeles.

Laible, D. (2004). Mother–child discourse in two contexts: Links with child temperament, attachment security, and socioemotional competence. *Developmental Psychology, 40,* 979–992.

Legerstee, M. (2005). *Infants' sense of people: Precursors to a theory of mind.* New York: Cambridge University Press.

Loveland, K. A., Landry, S. H., Hughes, S. O., Hall, K. K. & McEvoy, R. E. (1988). Speech acts and the pragmatic deficits of autism. *Journal of Speech and Hearing Research, 31,* 593–604.

Lynch, E. W., & Hanson, M. J. (2004). *Developing cross-cultural competence.* Baltimore: Paul Brookes.

Main, M. (1996). Introduction to the special section on attachment and psychopathology: 2. Overview of the field of attachment. *Journal of Counseling and Clinical Psychology, 64,* 237–243.

Max in motion/adventuresome Max. (1989). SVE Videoplus.

Mayer, M. (1967). *A Boy, a dog, and a frog.* New York: Dial Press.

Mayer, M., & Mayer, M. (1975). *One frog too many.* New York: Dial Press.

McGurk, H. (1983). Effective motivation and the development of communicative competence in blind children. In A. E. Mills (Ed.), *Language acquisition in the blind child: Normal and deficient.* (pp. 114–132). San Diego: College-Hill.

Meltzoff, A., & Moore, W. (1977). Imitation of facial and manual gestures by human neonates. *Science, 198,* 75–78.

Michalson, L., & Lewis, M. (1985). What do children know about emotions and when do they know it. In M. Lewis & C. Saarni (Eds.), *The socialization of emotions* (pp. 117–139). New York: Plenum.

Mills, A. (1993). Visual handicap. In D. V. M. Bishop & K. Mogford (Eds.), *Language development in exceptional circumstances* (pp. 150–164). Hove, UK: Erlbaum.

Mundy, P., & Arca, F. (2006). Joint attention, social engagement, and the development of social competence. In P. Marshall & N. Fox (Eds.), *The development of social engagement neurobiological perspective* (pp. 81–117). New York: Oxford University Press.

Mundy, P., Delgado, C., Block, J., Venezia, M., Hogan, A., & Seibert, J. (2002). *Early Social Communication Scales.* Miami, FL: University of Miami.

Mundy, P., Sigman, M., & Kasari, C. (1994). Joint attention, developmental level, and symptom presentation in a young child with autism. *Developmental and Psychopathology, 6,* 389–401.

Mundy, P., & Thorp, D. (2006). The neural basis of early joint-attention behavior. In T. Charman & W. Stone (Eds.), *Social and communicative development in autism spectrum disorders* (pp. 296–336). New York: Guilford.

Nugent, J. K., Lester, B. M., & Brazelton, T. B. (1989). *The cultural context of infancy: Biology, culture, and infant development.* Norwood, NJ: Ablex.

Paccia-Cooper, J., Curcio, F., & Sacharko, G. (1981). *A comparison of discourse features in normal and autistic language.* Paper presented at the Boston University Child Language Conference, Boston.

Paul, R. (2007). *Language disorders from infancy through adolescence.* St. Louis, MO: Mosby.

Pepper, J., & Weitzman, E. (2004). *It takes two to talk: A practical guide for parents of children with language delays.* 3rd ed. Toronto: The Hanen Centre.

Perry, P. D. (1997). Incubated in terror: Neurodevelopmental factors in the "cycle of violence." In J. D. Osofsky (Ed.), *Children in a violent society.* (pp. 127–149). New York: Guilford.

Pons, R. Harris, P., & de Rosnay, M. (2004). Emotion comprehension between 3–11 years : Developmental periods and hierarchical organization. *European Journal of Developmental Psychology, 1,* 127–152.

Pretti-Frontczak, K., & Bricker, D. (2004). *An activity-based approach to early intervention.* Baltimore: Brookes.

Rice, M. L. (1993). "Don't talk to him; He's weird." A social consequences account of language and social interactions. In A. P. Kaiser & D. B. Gray (Eds.), *Enhancing children's communication: Research foundations for intervention* (pp. 139–158). Baltimore: Paul H. Brookes.

Rieffe, C., Terwogt, M. M., & Smit, C. (2003). Deaf children on the causes of emotions. *Educational Psychology, 23,* 159–168.

Rogoff, B. (2003). *The cultural nature of human development.* New York: Oxford University Press.

Rossetti, L. (2006). *The Rossetti infant–toddler language scale.* East Moline, IL: Linguisystems.

Rutter, M., & Garmezy, N. (1983). Developmental psychopathology. In E. J. Hetherington (Ed.), *Handbook of child psychology, Vol. IV: Socialization, personality, and social development.* (pp. 601–616). New York: Wiley.

Schaffer, H. R. (1984*). The child's entry into a social world.* New York: Academic Press.

Schick, B., de Villiers, P., de Villiers, J., & Hoffmeister, R. (2007). Language and theory of mind: A study of deaf children. *Child Development, 78,* 376–396.

Schieffelin, B. B., & Eisenberg, A. R. (1984). Cultural variation in children's conversation. In R. L. Schiefelbusch & J. Pickar (Eds.), *The acquisition of communicative competence* (pp. 378–420). Baltimore: University Park Press.

Schuler, A. L., Peck, C. A., Willard, C., & Theimer, K. (1989). Assessment of communicative means and functions through interview: Assessing the communicative capabilities of individuals with limited language. *Seminars in Speech and Language, 10,* 51–62.

Schulte-Ruther, M., Markowitsch, H. J., Fink, G. R., & Piefke, M. (2007). Mirror neuron and theory of mind mechanisms involved in face-to-face interactions: A functional magnetic resonance imaging approach to empathy. *Journal of Cognitive Neuroscience, 19,* 1354–1372.

Semel, E., Wiig, E., & Secord, W. (2003). *Clinical Evaluation of Language Fundamentals—4 (CELF—4).* San Antonio, TX: Harcourt Assessment.

Semel, E., Wiig., E., & Secord, W. (2004). *Clinical Evaluation of Language Fundamentals—Preschool 2. (CELF—P2).* San Antonio, TX: Harcourt Assessment.

Sheinkopf, S., Mundy, P., Claussen, A., & Willoughby, J. (2004). Infant joint attention skill and preschool behavioral outcomes in at-risk children. *Developmental Psychopathology, 16,* 273–291.

Snow, C. E., & Ferguson, C. A. (1977). *Talking to children: Language input and acquisition.* Cambridge, UK: Cambridge University Press.

Squires, J., Bricker, D., & Twombly, L. (2002). *Ages and stages questionnaires: Social–emotional.* Baltimore: Brookes.

Stern, D. (1977). *The first relationship: Infant and mother.* Cambridge, MA: Harvard University Press.

Sussman, F. (1999). *More than words: Helping parents promote communication and social skills in children with autism spectrum disorders.* Toronto: The Hanen Centre.

Thomas, A., & Chess, S. (1977). *Temperament and development.* New York: Brunner/Mazel.

Tomasello, M. (1995). Joint attention as social cognition. In C. Moore & P. Denham (Eds.), *Joint attention: Its origins and role in development* (pp. 103–130). Hillsdale, NJ: Erlbaum.

Tager-Flusberg, H., Paul, R., & Lord, C. (2005). Language and communication in autism. In F. Volkmar, R. Paul, A. Klin, & D. Cohen (Eds.), *Handbook of autism and pervasive developmental disorders: Vol. 1: Diagnosis, development, and neurobiology* (pp. 335–363). New York: Wiley.

Tulving, E. (1993). What is episodic memory? *Current Directions in Psychological Science, 2,* 67–70.

Urwin, C. (1983). Dialogue and cognitive functioning in the early development of three blind children. In A. E. Mills (Ed.), *Language acquisition in the blind child: Normal and deficient.* (pp. 18–41). San Diego: College-Hill.

Vigil, D. C. (2002). Cultural variations in attention regulation: A comparative analysis of British and Chinese-immigrant populations. *International Journal of Language & Communication Disorders, 37,* 433–458.

Vigil, D., & Westby, C. E. (2004). Caregiver interaction style. *Perspectives on Language Learning and Education, 11*(2), 10–14.

Volkmar, F., & Klin, A. (2005). Issues in classification of autism and related disorders. In F. Volkmar, R. Paul, A. Klin, & D. Cohen (Eds.), *Handbook of autism and pervasive developmental disorders: Vol. 1: Diagnosis, development, and neurobiology* (pp. 5–41). New York: Wiley.

Vostanis, P., Hayes, M., Du Feu, M., & Warren, J. (1997). Detection of behavioural and emotional problems in deaf children and adolescents: Comparison of two rating scales. *Child Care, Health, & Development, 23,* 233–246.

Wellman, H. M., & Liu, D. (2004). Scaling of theory-of-mind tasks. *Child Development, 75,* 523–541.

Westby, C. E. (2000). Multicultural issues in speech and language assessment. In J. B. Tomblin, H. L. Morris, & D. Spriesterbach (Eds.), *Diagnosis methods in speech-language pathology* (pp. 35–62). San Diego: Singular.

Wetherby, A. M., Cain, D. H., Yonclas, D. G., & Walker, V. G. (1988). Analysis of intentional communication in normal children from the prelinguistic to multiword stage. *Journal of Speech and Hearing Research, 31,* 242–252.

Wetherby, A. M., & Prizant, B. M. (1989). The expression of communicative intent: Assessment guidelines. *Seminars in Speech and Language, 10,* 77–91.

Wetherby, A. M., & Prizant, B. M. (2002). *Communication and Symbolic Behavior Scales Developmental Profile.* Baltimore: Brookes.

Whiting, B. B., & Edwards, C. P. (1988). *Children of different worlds.* Cambridge, MA: Harvard University Press.

CHAPTER 6

Gesture Development

Nina C. Capone, PhD

OBJECTIVES

- ◆ Define the term *gesture.*
- ◆ State the course of gesture development.
- ◆ Compare and contrast each category of gesture.
- ◆ State the relationship between gesture and other mental representations.

INTRODUCTION

The first chapter of this text introduced the clinical practice of speech-language pathology as being grounded in a strong developmental knowledge base. Chapter 2 reviewed early language development and the cognitive skills that underlie its development. This chapter continues this discussion by giving an overview of gesture development and its relationship with language. *Gestures* are manual, facial, or other bodily movements. These movements can communicate meaning or simply accompany the forward flow of speech.

The act of gesturing appears to be inherent to the act of speaking (e.g., Goldin-Meadow, Butcher, Mylander, & Dodge, 1994; Iverson & Goldin-Meadow, 2001). For example, children gesture regardless of their cultural background or the language that they speak. Further, blind speakers gesture to blind listeners, and deaf children create their own representational gestures to communicate even though their parents have not signed or modeled these gestures.

Gestures are not random movements. Indeed, many gestures convey meaning such that a child's gesture reflects what she knows (e.g., Capone, 2007; Evans, Alibali, & McNeil, 2001; Goldin-Meadow, 2003; Goldin-Meadow & Wagner, 2005). Gesturing becomes fully integrated with spoken language. School-age children are rarely observed to gesture in isolation, without speaking (e.g., Church & Goldin-Meadow, 1986).

When the child's gesture and spoken language are examined for the meaning each expresses, we see that the information conveyed by gesture may be the same or different from what she is saying. Thus gesture can express knowledge that the child has represented in memory but that information may or may not be expressed with spoken language. When the child conveys some information in gesture and different information in spoken language, it reflects how richly the child has knowledge represented in memory. As the child learns new information, she may not yet have consolidated or solidified it well enough in memory to formulate the language to talk about it. The child also pays attention to and uses the *adult's* gesturing to expand her own gesture repertoire and to learn spoken language. In this way, gesture is a rich source of information for the child as speaker and listener.

This chapter first defines types of gestures and delineates the developmental course of gesturing. The remainder of the chapter discusses the relationship between gesture and spoken language development.

DEFINING GESTURE TYPES

The first gestures to emerge in development are *deictic gestures*. Deictic gestures, which include *showing, giving, pointing* and *ritual request* gestures, are also referred to as prelinguistic gestures because they emerge before the child speaks her first word. Deictic gestures make reference to something in the environment and rely on that context to convey meaning. For example, a speaker may announce, "I can't find my book," while extending a hand toward the table. The gesture conveys the location that the book was last found, even though the speaker has not said this explicitly.

Deictic gestures have the pragmatic function (i.e., communicative intention) to gain or maintain adult interaction, or to request or draw attention to a referent. Infants may point to their cup before they have the word *cup* in their vocabulary. The infant's intention may be to draw attention to the cup or to request it, much like labeling it would. Other early communicative gestures are taught through social routines. These gestures include hand waving to signal greeting; shaking or nodding the head for *no* and *yes*, respectively; blowing kisses; shrugging to indicate an inability to answer the question *Where did it go?*; and placing a finger to the lips to indicate a *hush* (Fenson et al., 1993).

The second gesture type is the *representational gesture*. Representational gestures are iconic. They convey some aspect of the referent's meaning, so they can be understood even when they are produced without the referent in sight. The meaning conveyed by representational gestures might be the form of an object, the function of an object, the path or quality of an action, or the spatial relationship between two objects expressed by a preposition. For example, Goldin-Meadow and Butcher (2003) reported a child in their study to say the word *bear* while also producing scratching hand movements. From this clawing motion, we see that the child has some knowledge of what bears do as well as how we label them. As another example, the young child might extend his tongue in reference to a *frog* because this action is often characteristic of our idea of what frogs do. Similarly, the child may extend two fingers in a V to signal *bunny*. Here, the gesture represents the form of the bunny's ears. In another example, the child may extend an index finger upward toward a ceiling fan and use a quick circling motion. Here, he is commenting through gesture on the trajectory and quality of the fan's movement.

Representational gestures are also referred to as *iconic gestures* and *baby signs* (Acredolo & Goodwyn, 1996). Acredolo and Goodwyn (1996) published a popular-press book for parents about baby signs. It includes a glossary of representational gestures that were created by infants. The term *baby signs* should not be confused with sign language, such as *American Sign Language* (ASL). ASL signs are symbols, in the same way that spoken language is a symbol. That is, ASL signs convey meaning but many ASL signs are not iconic like representational gestures. They do not convey semantic content in the form they take (i.e., in the actual form of the sign itself). Signed languages are further differentiated from representational gesturing in that the child needs exposure to signed language to learn it, in the same way that spoken language must be taught. Another difference between gesturing and signing is that signed language encompasses more than single vocabulary items. Like spoken language, it adheres to a grammatical rule system.

Another symbolic gesture added later to the repertoire is the emblem gesture. *Emblems* are conventional symbols such as the *high-five* to convey camaraderie, *okay* or *thumbs up* gestures to signal agreement, and the *hand across the throat* to signal stop. These gestures are language-like in that they are abstract symbols. Like spoken language symbols, they do not change referents. Each gesture conveys a particular meaning consistently, and each gesture–referent pairing is agreed upon by the communication partners. This is also the case with representational gestures, although many times the representational gesture is dependent upon the spoken language or context that accompanies it. Also, the community that understands the child's representational gesture may be his immediate caregivers, whereas other early communicative and emblem gestures are shared by the larger community of the culture (Goldin-Meadow, 2003). Note that in some cases, an emblem gesture can be considered benign in one culture but offensive in another culture.

Another gesture to emerge in development is the *beat gesture*. These gestures follow the rhythm of speech, and may provide emphasis on a particular idea, but they do not convey semantic information. For example, you may notice that while your professor is lecturing her hands move up and down but then stop when she pauses. These movements are paced with the forward flow of speech.

The remainder of this chapter reviews the course of gesture development and the relationship between gesture and spoken language for the child as speaker and listener.

THE EMERGENCE OF GESTURE

Gesture development is predictable in terms of the sequence of gestures as they appear in the child's repertoire and the timeline of each gesture's emergence. This predictability provides the clinician with expectations regarding where the child falls along the continuum of communication development. The emergence of gestures predicts and parallels spoken language development.

Children first communicate intentionally during the illocutionary stage of communication development by using deictic gestures. At approximately 10 months of age, the infant begins to show objects to engage the adult partner in an interaction, though the infant will not hand over the object. Within weeks, however, the infant will give over the object to his partner to communicate. During the 10- to 12-month age range, infants also produce ritual request gestures. Ritual request gestures convey the infant's want or need for something by reaching with open hand or moving an adult's hand to the referent of interest. For example, an infant may take the adult's hand and move it to a bottle of bubbles indicating that she wants the mother to engage in this activity.

Once ritual request, showing, and then giving are in the infant's repertoire, and just before first words emerge, the infant begins pointing. Pointing is particularly important in communication development because it predicts the emergence of language symbols. This pre-naming behavior predicts the child's ability to use symbols. Specifically, the hearing child begins to point just before speaking his first word, and the hearing-impaired child points before his first signs (Folven & Bonvillian, 1991). Pointing seems to grow out of the child's use of his index finger to explore objects (Locke, Young, Service, & Chandler, 1990). The child will explore objects with the index finger while he is alone or while he is with others but he does not search for adult attention. Later, the index finger is extended and is not in contact with the object. This pointing gesture is coordinated with social interaction (e.g., eye contact with the caregiver). Other early communicative gestures are also being learned starting early in the second year (Fenson et al., 1993).

The emergence of representational gestures coincides with first words, at approximately 12 months of age. However, Goodwyn & Acredolo (1993) found infants had an advantage in expressing themselves via representational gestures when compared to spoken words. Their first gestured symbol was documented one month before their first word. This is the first piece of evidence that children will use gesture to express what they know before they have the spoken language to do so. Put another way, children know more than they say; if we pay attention to the child's gesture, we are also observing the knowledge she has represented in memory. This information could be missed if we attended to only spoken language.

On average, infants can have 3 to 5 representational gestures in their repertoire and as many as 17 gestures by toddlerhood (Acredolo & Goodwyn, 1988). Between 12 and approximately 16 months of age, infants communicate with gestures or words, used individually. Their gesture repertoires, although small, tend to complement or supplement their spoken vocabulary. That is, children in this age group do not have a word *and* a gesture for the same referent, but rather have a word *or* a gesture for a referent. When symbols (lexical and gestured) are combined, the sum is referred to as a conceptual vocabulary. Bilingual children (i.e., children learning two languages) also show a larger conceptual vocabulary than would be documented if the clinician only tallied lexical items from one language (Genesee, Paradis, & Crago, 2004).

As children's spoken vocabulary grows, they integrate gesturing with speech. The toddler starts to combine words between 18 and 24 months of age. Just before the emergence of two-word utterances, the child is putting gestures and words together into gesture–word combinations (Capirici, Iverson, Pizzuto, & Volterra, 1996; Goldin-Meadow & Butcher, 2003; Iverson & Goldin-Meadow, 2005; Morford & Goldin-Meadow, 1992; Özçalişkan & Goldin-Meadow, 2005). These gestures are predominately pointing gestures. The semantic relations expressed in spontaneous gesture–word combinations (e.g., *mommy* + POINT to chair) have been found in the first spoken word combinations (e.g., *mommy chair*) that toddlers produce (Iverson & Goldin-Meadow, 2005; Özçalişkan & Goldin-Meadow, 2005). Findings such as these provide a second piece of evidence that the child has more complex language represented than spoken language alone would indicate. It is, therefore, important for the clinician to observe gesture as a valid modality of expression.

Emblem gestures seem to appear in early toddlerhood and are most likely routine-based gestures at this point in children's development. For example, the *Rossetti Infant–Toddler Language Scale* (RITLS; Rossetti, 1990)— an assessment of children's language, social–emotional, play, and gesture development from birth to 36 months—first surveys children for emblem gesture (*give me five*) at the 24- to 27-month age interval. Beat gestures are the last type to emerge. Beat gestures have been reported for the child as she moves toward advancing morphological and syntactic domains of language development (Nicoladis, Mayberry, & Genesee, 1999). Nicoladis, Mayberry, & Genesee (1999) studied bilingual preschoolers who were learning French and English. These children varied in their proficiency with each language. More beat (and representational) gestures were produced for utterances in the child's more proficient language. As the child's vocabulary expands to include a variety of word classes, gesture will accompany not only nouns, but also verbs, adjectives, and adverbs (Nicoladis, Mayberry, & Genesee, 1999).

In summary, gesturing emerges as a natural course of development. Gestures include deictic gestures (ritual request, show, give, point), representational gestures, early communicative and emblem gestures, and beat gestures. Deictic gestures emerge during the prelinguistic period, before age 12 months, and pointing predicts first words. Representational and other early communicative gestures appear with first words and act to complement or supplement spoken vocabulary. Soon after, gesture–spoken language combinations predict two-word utterances. Beat gestures are observed once morpho-syntax begins developing.

Given the expectations of development, the clinician knows that the child who points is closer to first words than the child who is not yet pointing. If we examine the three case studies presented in Chapter 1 (typically developing 25-month-old Johnathon, late-bloomer 22-month-old Josephine, and late-talker 27-month-old Robert), we see that all three children are using prelinguistic gestures. This places each *at least* at the 12-month-old milestone for gesture development. Each child has the gestural precursor to the single-word stage of development.

Next, we have an expectation that the child who combines gestures and words is developmentally approaching the 18- to 24-month age range and is closer to two-word utterances than the child who is not yet producing cross-modal communications. All three children should be producing words in combination and gesture in combinations with words. Here, only Johnathon is combining gesture and words, and two words in utterances. This places Johnathon within normal limits for expressive language and gesture for his age. Josephine is not yet producing words, words in combinations, or words in combination with gestures. This represents a delay for Josephine in expressive language development. However, she demonstrates two strengths in gesture: (1) She combines gesture and vocalizations, and (2) she produces representational (iconic) gestures to communicate. These behaviors fall within the 12- to 18-month-old developmental range. Robert demonstrates the greatest delay. He is the oldest of the three children, yet he is using only prelinguistic gestures and some social gestures (e.g., shaking head *no*) for basic needs. He is not yet using words, representational gestures, or gesturing in combination with vocals. Therefore, he is delayed in expressive language as well as gesture development.

A strength for both Robert and Josephine is that, although their gesture repertoire differentiates their delays, they both used the gestures they had to communicate. Therefore, an initial intervention goal for Robert would be to expand his gesture repertoire to include representational gestures. This would provide him with more communication opportunities and establish semantic representations (meanings or concepts) of the words that he will eventually learn. The next section of this chapter discusses the relationship between spoken language and deictic and representational gestures.

GESTURE REFLECTS THE CHILD'S MENTAL REPRESENTATIONS

Gesture and spoken language tap the same mental representations in memory, particularly semantic representations. The term *mental representation* can be thought of as knowledge that is stored, or represented, in memory. For example, we have mental representations for the meaning of a word (i.e., semantic representation), for our understanding of how gears work, and for problem-solving procedures such as those for the Tower of Hanoi puzzle, conservation problems, or mathematical equivalence. We can on some level equate mental representation with knowledge, concept, or meaning. Something else we know is that mental representations evolve through experience (e.g., Barsalou, 1999). That is, learning is not an all-or-nothing phenomenon. Rather, learning is gradual and there is a process of trial and error to update our existing ideas, reorganize incorrect information, and establish accurate and rich mental representations of concepts. Gesture reflects not only the content of a mental representation (remember the *bear* example earlier in the chapter), but also the richness or stability of that mental representation (e.g., Capone, 2007; Church & Goldin-Meadow, 1986).

One underlying cognitive skill that gesture and spoken language share is the symbolic ability to decontextualize a mental representation. Decontextualization refers to the gradual distancing of a symbol from the original referent or learning context (Werner & Kaplan, 1963). It is a skill needed to use more complex and abstract spoken language, and later, written language. When children first learn words, their use tends to be contextualized, or tied to the original context of learning. For example, a child may use the word *cup* to label only his cup. The context of his cup (i.e., his red sipper cup) is the original context of learning the spoken symbol *cup*. Children gradually begin to decontextualize spoken language by using the word *cup* to refer to all cups that are similar in appearance (i.e., shape), and to request a cup without the object being present. Children extend known words to novel exemplars, even though no one has explicitly taught them each word–new referent pairing (e.g., *cup* refers to the mother's cup, too).

Before children do this with words, this ability to decontextualize, or distance the word from its referent or himself from a referent, is observed in the deictic gesture sequence. As the child progresses from showing an object to giving an object to pointing to an object, this evolution reflects the child's early ability to see objects as separate from him or herself, or to distance herself from an object when referring to it. As a second example, representational gestures can meet the same criteria of symbolic use that words satisfy (e.g., Goodwyn & Acredolo, 1993; McGregor & Capone, 2004). For example, in Goodwyn and Acredolo's work (1993), representational gestures met symbolic criteria that are applied to words as symbols. Specifically, the representational gestures that infant–toddlers produced (1) referred to multiple exemplars (e.g., objects and pictures), (2) were used in the absence of the referent, (3) were produced spontaneously, without models, and (4) were not part of a well-rehearsed routine (e.g., *eensy-weensy-spider*) (p. 695; see also McGregor & Capone, 2004).

An interesting parallel between the gesture lexicon and the spoken lexicon is found in their relationship to other developing language skills. Early in development, children tend to have many object words in their lexicon when compared to other word classes such as social words, verbs, and adjectives. Children with more objects in their spoken lexicons tend to have larger vocabularies overall and to meet semantic and early grammar milestones earlier than children who have fewer object labels in their spoken lexicons (Bates, Bretherton, & Snyder, 1988; Nelson, 1973). (This issue is also discussed in Chapter 7.) The early gesture lexicon parallels the infant's spoken vocabulary in this relationship. The early gesture lexicon also tends to have a high proportion of object gestures when compared to other word classes. Like children with a high proportion of spoken object labels in their vocabulary, children with more object gestures in their repertoire tend to have larger spoken vocabularies than do children with fewer object gestures in their repertoire.

A relationship between gesture and spoken language has also been observed in receptive language—specifically, in receptive vocabulary (O'Reilly, Painter, & Bornstein, 1997). O'Reilly, Painter, & Bornstein (1997) found that comprehension of representational gestures by four- and five-year-olds was positively correlated with their performance on a measure of receptive vocabulary but not related to their performance in morphological or syntactic comprehension. It appears, then, that representational gestures tap semantic representations specifically in the domain of language.

GESTURE REFLECTS THE CHILD'S READINESS TO LEARN

As gesture and spoken language become integrated and the child begins developing a variety of complex concepts, gesture continues to be a window into the child's developing mental representations. The relationship between what is expressed via gesture and via spoken language in an utterance becomes a marker of where the child is in acquiring a particular mental representation (e.g., Alibali & Goldin-Meadow, 1993; Capone, 2007; Church & Goldin-Meadow, 1986; Garber, Alibali, & Goldin-Meadow, 1998; Garber & Goldin-Meadow, 2002; Goldin-Meadow, 2000; Goldin-Meadow, Alibali, & Church, 1993; Kelly & Church, 1998; Perry, Church, & Goldin-Meadow, 1988; Pine, Lufkin, & Messer, 2004). To reiterate, we have mental representations of a word, understanding of how gears work, and solutions to conservation problems, mathematical equivalence problems, or the Tower of Hanoi puzzle, and many others. Because learning is gradual, children move from an inaccurate or incomplete understanding of a concept to an accurate and stable state of concept acquisition, over time. Gesture–spoken language combinations change and reflect where the child is in the process of acquiring concepts.

To understand the literature dealing with this issue, it is important to be clear on the methods used to document the phenomenon. Across many of these studies, participants are presented with a task that requires problem solving, and then the children are asked to explain its solution. Consider the concept of conservation of quantity as tested by Church and Goldin-Meadow (1986). In their study, five- to eight-year-old children were shown two equivalent glasses of liquid. The liquid from one glass was then poured into a dish. Children were first asked if the amount of liquid in the dish was equivalent to the liquid that was in the glass. This task tests whether children understand that liquid quantity is conserved (i.e., stays the same) even when the shape of the container holding it changes. The children's task solutions were analyzed for accuracy. Their accuracy in solving the problems served to classify them as having an inaccurate representation of the problem, a transitional representation of the problem, or a stable and accurate representation of the problem. The correct answer is that liquid quantity does not change simply because the shape of a container that holds it changes.

Second, children were asked to explain their response (e.g., "Why?", "How can you tell?"; p. 47). The children's explanations were analyzed for several variables, including the following:

- The modality of the child's response (spoken language, gesture–spoken language combination)
- The information expressed in gesture and the information expressed in their spoken language
- Whether gestured information was the same (matched) or different from (mismatched) the spoken information
- The accuracy of the information expressed in each modality

Three types of gesture–spoken language combinations were analyzed:

- Inaccurate match combination: gesture and spoken language match but express an inaccurate explanation (i.e., inaccurate or incomplete understanding)
- Mismatch combination: gesture and spoken language mismatch and may contain at least one piece of an accurate explanation (i.e., transitional understanding)
- Accurate match combination: gesture and spoken language match but express the accurate explanation (i.e., stable and acquired understanding)

For example, the child who understands that liquid quantity is conserved may explain that "The glass is tall and skinny" while producing a pouring motion from the *dish* to the *glass* (Church & Goldin-Meadow, 1986, p. 58). Here, the child expresses two beliefs about why liquid quantity conserves: the compensatory features of the container's shape in two dimensions (in spoken language) and the reversibility of the liquid's transformation (in gesture). Now that we understand the method, we can better understand the findings.

Research shows that as children transition from an incomplete understanding to a stable and accurate understanding of a concept, they transition from mismatch combinations to match combinations in their explanations over time with acquisition of the concept (e.g., Alibali & Goldin-Meadow, 1993; Church, 1999; Perry, Church, & Goldin-Meadow, 1988). Put another way, when children produce mismatch combinations in their explanations, it reflects a transitional knowledge state. During this stage of learning, the child is moving from an incomplete or inaccurate understanding of a concept toward a complete and accurate understanding of that concept. But why do these mismatches occur? It has been suggested that the child who is in transition is still considering multiple hypotheses—both accurate and inaccurate—about the solution to the problem. These hypotheses about the task's solution are simultaneously activated in memory as the child engages in thinking about the task. This simultaneous activation leads to some of those hypotheses being expressed via gesture and others with spoken language (Garber & Goldin-Meadow, 2002; Goldin-Meadow, Nusbaum, Garber, & Church, 1993).

When children's gesture–spoken language combinations are examined, children who produce many mismatch combinations during their explanations are more likely to benefit from instruction than children who produce few to no mismatch combinations (e.g., Alibali & Goldin-Meadow, 1993; Church & Goldin-Meadow, 1986; Perry, Church, & Goldin-Meadow, 1988). Take as an example a study by Alibali and Goldin-Meadow (1993). This study examined school-aged children's understanding of mathematical equivalence. In this study, children were asked to solve equivalence problems of addition and multiplication and then to explain their solutions. All children were provided with instruction on addition equivalence problems, but children who produced mismatch combinations in their explanations were more likely to advance to a correct understanding with this instruction. In addition, children who produced mismatch combinations generalized learning from trained items to untrained exemplars that also tested the concept. Children who did not produce mismatches were also provided with instruction but were less likely to generalize their knowledge to untrained exemplars. This result suggests that learning was richer for children who were already in a transitional phase of learning and that their mismatch combinations reflected their readiness to learn.

Gesture has access to the accurate ideas that the child has represented in memory even though it may not be heard in speech (Capone, 2007; Evans, Alibali, & McNeil, 2001; Garber, Alibali, & Goldin-Meadow, 1998; Goldin-Meadow, Alibali, & Church, 1993; Pine, Lufkin, & Messer, 2004). Goldin-Meadow, Alibali, and Church (1993) also found that children expressed more accurate explanations in gesture than in speech. That is, children had beliefs represented about the task's solution but this knowledge would have gone unnoticed had only speech been assessed. In the study carried out by Alibali and DiRusso (1999), undergraduates explained solutions to algebra word problems. In mismatch combinations, gesture was just as likely as speech to convey the strategy that the participant actually used to solve problems.

Capone (2007) examined gesturing in a developing language task reported on by Capone and McGregor (2005). This study extended the work of Goldin-Meadow and colleagues in two ways. First, a younger group of children (30-month-old toddlers) was the focus of study. Second, a new task—learning new words—was examined. Toddlers were placed in a transitional learning state by teaching them the names of new object words under three different conditions. In two learning conditions, semantic enrichment was provided by the adult. Semantic enrichment highlighted shape or function of the trained objects. The third learning condition was a control condition, so no semantic enrichment was provided beyond what experience with the object itself provided for the child. Learning was measured via naming of the objects at the end of the study. In this study, toddlers learned more names for objects taught in the semantic enrichment conditions than in the control condition (these results are discussed in more detail in Chapter 7).

Of importance to our discussion of gesture is an analysis of toddlers' gesture–spoken language combinations during this time of learning. Gesturing was analyzed at the beginning and end of instruction in a separate task that required children to state the functions of objects (*What do we do with this one?*). Several parallels were observed between these toddlers' gesturing and the older children's gesturing from previous studies. First, toddlers responded to these function probes with gestures and spoken language. Second, a transition from mismatched combinations at the beginning of training to accurate match combinations at the end of training was observed only under conditions where naming of the trained objects also occurred (i.e., stability in learning). Also consistent with other studies, accurate knowledge tended to be expressed in gesture before spoken language in mismatched combinations.

In summary, from the time that gesture and spoken language are becoming integrated, the relationship between gesture and spoken language serves as an index of the child's readiness to learn a variety of concepts, including new words.

GESTURE INPUT TO THE CHILD

Although gesture emerges as a natural course of development, the adult's gesture input to the child can be quite influential in shaping the child's gesture expression (Capone, 2007; Goodwyn, Acredolo, & Brown, 2000; Iverson, Capirici, Longobardi, & Caselli, 1999; Iverson, Capirici, Volterra, & Goldin-Meadow, in press). Iverson and colleagues (1999) found a gestural analogue to the motherese of speech directed to 16- and 20-month-old children. That is, mothers' gestures co-occurred with speech—approximately 15% of maternal utterances were supported by gesture. Gestures were conceptually simple, referred to the immediate context, and reinforced spoken messages (p. 70).

A cross-cultural study by Iverson, Capirici, Volterra, and Goldin-Meadow (in press) compared American toddlers to Italian youngsters. The Italian infants were part of a culture that is rich in its use of representational gesturing. This rich gesture input was reflected in Italian infants' repertoires of early symbols. When compared to their American counterparts, Italian infants had a larger repertoire of representational gestures and fewer spoken words. When gesture and spoken symbols were combined, Italian infants demonstrated total vocabulary sizes that were comparable to the size of the American infants' vocabularies.

Goodwyn, Acredolo, and Brown (2000) manipulated the representational gesture input to young toddlers and observed changes in their gesture repertoire. One group of parents was trained to use gestures and spoken words in combination while interacting with their children; two other groups of parents either were trained to increase spoken labeling or received no training. Children of parents who were trained to model gestures and words had larger gesture repertoires at the study's end than did the children in the other two groups. In addition, these children performed better than did the other groups on measures of spoken language development. Thus gesturing by adults produced a benefit not only on the children's own gesture communication but also on their language development more generally.

In the study described earlier, Capone and McGregor (2005) provided semantic enrichment during word learning via the experimenter's gesture cues to shape or function of the objects. These representational gestures took either the shape of the object being trained or the function of the object being trained. Capone (2007) observed that toddlers from Capone and McGregor's (2005) study produced more representational gestures in isolation when explaining object functions than is typically reported in studies of non-enriched environments. This outcome was partially attributed to the rich gesture environment that the children were provided during instruction by the experimenter.

Gesture input by adults to the child can also influence spoken language development. This type of input can serve as a visual cue or scaffold to the spoken language of the adult. For example, gesturing the function of an object while labeling it highlights important semantic information via the gesture and lexical information via the word model. Capone and McGregor (2005) found that gesture cues to salient object features (object shape or object function) enriched semantic knowledge of the objects and had an effect on word retrieval for naming the objects after instruction was provided (over a no gesture input condition). McNeil, Alibali, and Evans (2001) compared preschoolers' performance in following directions when provided gesture cues versus no gesture cues. Results showed that gesture cues were particularly helpful relative to no gesture cues when preschoolers were asked to follow complex directions versus simple directions.

Ellis Weismer and Hesketh (1993) examined the effect of gesture cues on learning words that conveyed spatial relations (e.g., *away from, on top of, beside*). They compared gesture and no-gesture conditions, but they also compared the effectiveness of this scaffold to other modalities of scaffolding, such as rate of speech in teaching the words and prosodic stress in saying the words (emphatic, neutral). These authors reported that children (with and without language delay) comprehended more words when they were taught with gesture cues than without gesture cues.

A recent study with adults showed that when a speaker uses gesture and spoken language in combination, the listener is sensitive to both (Wu & Coulson, 2007). Further, brain activation changes as a function of the speaker's use of gesture and spoken language together versus spoken language alone. In their work, Wu and Coulson (2007) measured evoked related potentials (ERP) while adults listened to and saw a speaker in discourse. Greater activation was observed for gesture–spoken language than for spoken language alone at the N400 mark. The N400 mark is a measure of semantic processing and integration in milliseconds after a stimulus is given. Wu and Coulson suggest that gesture activates visual–spatial representations that include shape, functions, and locations of entities.

In summary, gesture input to the child can influence both the child's own gesture repertoire and the child's performance on language tasks. Gesture appears to serve as a scaffold for the child's transition to more advanced language development.

If we, again, examine the three children from the case study, we see that Johnathon readily uses gesture cues by the adult to understand more complex directions and that Josephine readily imitates adults' gestures. These gesture cues are useful scaffolds for continued language development. In contrast, Robert does not consistently use gesture cues to scaffold his understanding of language, which puts him at a disadvantage in language learning. Improving Robert's attention to gesture cues by the adult, which will provide him with a scaffold for additional language learning, would be a prudent first goal of language intervention.

The next section reviews why gesturing may be useful for the child as both speaker and listener.

THE FUNCTION OF GESTURING

When linguistic or metalinguistic skills are immature, all that a child knows may be missed if only her spoken language is assessed. Infants, toddlers, and other children with limited spoken language abilities use gesture to compensate for limitations or immaturities in articulatory or language skills (Acredolo & Goodwyn, 1988; Iverson & Thelen, 1999). In addition, the retrieval and formulation of spoken language to convey what the child knows seems to rely on a rich mental representation, whereas gesture taps into the still evolving or weak mental representation (e.g., Alibali & Goldin-Meadow, 1993; Capone, 2007; Capone & McGregor, 2005; Church & Goldin-Meadow, 1986). Gesture allows the child to express ideas that are still forming (i.e., the immature, weak, and still evolving mental representation). This may be the case because gestures represent knowledge visually without the demand of formulating a verbal description (Goldin-Meadow, 2003). Speaking places greater demands on memory as compared to gesture, because speech is encoded sequentially, one piece of information at a time, over time, whereas gesture expresses information holistically, in a chunk.

Gesturing may also ease the child's thinking process. The brain has a limited set of processing resources (Baddeley, 2000). To use an analogy, we can think about neural processing resources as being akin to scholarship money. We have a limited set of resources, or scholarship money. The brain (university administration) can divide the processing resources among several aspects of a task (several students get a little bit of money toward tuition) or, alternatively, those resources can be redirected to one or fewer tasks (funding the entire tuition of one or two students). As with the supply of scholarship money, we cannot increase processing resources. Therefore, we must make the most efficient use of our resources to benefit learning or explaining the task at hand.

How might the child maximize this limited set of brain resources? When the child gestures, he externalizes a mental representation. Put another way, when the child gestures, the information that is gestured no longer needs to be remembered and kept track of in the mind because it is expressed externally, by the hands. Externalizing the thought process this way may free the brain's resources so that there are more resources for processing other aspects of a task (Alibali & DiRusso, 1999; Goldin-Meadow, Nusbaum, Kelly, & Wagner, 2001). In summary, gesturing may make the child's thought process more efficient for learning or performing.

The child's gesture can have an indirect effect on his learning as well, because adults can interpret the child's gestural communication. Researchers have shown that adults both with and without training in recognizing gesture communication can glean information from the child's gesture. These adults will subsequently tailor their instruction to the child according to what they understand the child to know (Goldin-Meadow & Singer, 2003; Kelly & Church, 1998; Kelly, Singer, Hicks, & Goldin-Meadow, 2002). In the same vein, the child's gesturing sets up opportunities for the adult to model the spoken language that labels what the child is gesturing. For example, a child may touch his lip with his index finger and round his lips in a blowing motion. This representational gesture conveys a request that the mother blow bubbles. The adult can then model the spoken language used to make this request—for example, "Mommy, blow more bubbles." The child now has an opportunity to imitate and learn the spoken language to request an activity.

The functions that gesturing serve for the child who is typically developing also can serve the child who has difficulty learning spoken language. For example, two of the three children in our case studies are delayed in spoken language. Their gesturing can serve as one focus of language modeling during the language intervention process. The next section of this chapter briefly gives examples of gesture development in children with language impairments.

CHILDREN WITH LANGUAGE LEARNING IMPAIRMENTS

The tight coupling of gesture and spoken language in development is illustrated by children with delays in learning language. Gesture development is a robust phenomenon. Even in the face of sensory, cognitive, and/or language impairments, gesturing emerges in children. Several characteristics of gesture development in typically developing children are also observed in children who are delayed in learning language. Children with language delays are limited in communication and verbal language (see Chapter 15 for full discussion of this issue).

Upon review of the developmental course and the functions of gesturing in typical development, we can see that gesture could serve the clinician in assessment and treatment of children with language delays. The speech-language pathologist encounters a variety of children with language delay, including those with early language delay (also referred to as late talkers), specific language impairment (SLI), Down syndrome, autism, and delays caused by multiple-birth pregnancy, to name a few. Gesture provides the speech-language clinician a modality of communication with which to better assess the child. Children with delays in learning language may show a delay in gesture development but, like younger, typically developing children, they also use gesture to compensate for limited spoken language in communication.

The robust relationship between the prelinguistic gesture sequence (showing, then giving, then pointing) and first words has been observed in children who demonstrate language delays due to multiple-birth risk factors. McGregor and Capone (2004) studied a set of quadruplets who were at risk for language delay as a result of biological (e.g., prematurity) and environmental (e.g., shared caregiver) factors. Although delayed in language development, the quadruplets were observed to progress from showing to giving to pointing before speaking their first words, albeit at a later age milestone.

Combinations of gesture and spoken language in an utterance were also observed in the set of at-risk quadruplets studied by McGregor and Capone (2004). As part of their study, these authors trained the quadruplets on a small vocabulary set by modeling words paired with representational gestures. These infants showed the developmental sequence of communicating these referents initially via gestures and then later with spoken words, just as observed in typical development. Further, the identical-twins pair of the four children showed a preference for combining gesture and spoken combinations as they transitioned to spoken naming.

Gesture serves a compensatory function for children who demonstrate a delay in language development (Evans, Alibali, & McNeil, 2001; Mainela-Arnold, Evans, & Alibali, 2006; Thal & Tobias, 1992). For example, Thal and Tobias (1992) reported that late talkers gestured more than language-mates but on par with age-mates, and Rescorla and Merrin (1998) found that late talkers relied more on several types of nonverbal communication, including gestures as well as gesture–spoken language combinations, to communicate when compared to their normally developing peers.

Evans, Alibali, and McNeil (2001) and Mainela and colleagues (2006) studied school-aged children with SLI and children who were matched for their ability to solve conservation problems like the ones discussed earlier in this chapter. Even though the younger children were just as accurate in solving the problems, the children with SLI conveyed more advanced explanations in their gestures in both studies. In particular, children with SLI expressed more information in gesture that was not heard in spoken language and expressed more advanced knowledge when gesture was combined with spoken language than when spoken language was used alone.

Gesture production is a strength for children with Down syndrome relative to their development in receptive and expressive language. When compared to typically developing children matched for vocabulary size, children with Down syndrome show greater gesture use (e.g., Caselli, Vicari, Longobardi, Lami, Pizzoli, & Stella, 1998; Singer Harris, Bellugi, Bates, Jones, & Rossen, 1997).

One group of children appear to show some deviation from typical development—children with autism spectrum disorder. Specifically, children with autism show impairments in pointing. They have been shown to use pointing to refer, as a prenaming activity while looking at a picture book. However, pointing in this kind of context is often accompanied by eye contact in the typically developing child. Children with autism do not point concurrent with eye contact with a communicative partner. Therefore, their atypical gesture development here appears to be related to their social–emotional development, rather than their referential development (Charman, 1998; Goodhart & Baron-Cohen, 1993).

Some very promising findings in this regard were reported by Capps, Kehres, and Signman (1998). These authors found that older children with autism use representational gestures in conversational contexts. Because children with autism tend to show great heterogeneity in their profiles, including behavioral, cognitive, and language profiles, greater attention needs to be paid to how gesture development relates to their development in other areas of language and cognition.

FINAL THOUGHTS FOR THE CLINICIAN

More research on gesture development in children with a variety of language impairments is still needed. Nevertheless, the clinician who is armed with the knowledge of the typical course of gesture development can begin to use this knowledge in the assessment and intervention of children. He or she can observe when children are not using gesture to communicate at expected age milestones and can identify this absence as indicative of a delay in development. At the same time, it is important to acknowledge the child who uses gesture to compensate for limited spoken language. It will be important for clinicians to also train parents and other caregivers to recognize gesture as a valid modality of communication.

As an intervention tool, the clinician can take the opportunity to observe what the child already has represented (and expressed via gesture) and provide language models for that knowledge. Modeling language, so that the child can hear and imitate it, is one useful scaffold that clinicians use to expand children's language learning. Gesture provides children with a means of expressing what they know and provides the clinician with a jumping-off point in language therapy. Finally, gesture cues can be useful as a visual scaffold for communication attempts as well as for enriching the mental representations of spoken language.

SUMMARY

The act of gesturing is a robust phenomenon. Children begin to gesture within the first 12 months of life. Gesturing never disappears—in fact, it becomes integrated with spoken language early on, by 24 months of age. Gesture development is predictable in its own developmental course and in relation to spoken language development. The clinician can use this predictability to his or her advantage in the clinical process.

Gesture serves many functions for children. Because it reflects what children know, it allows children to communicate before they have the spoken language to do so. Gesture reveals children's learning status through their use of gesture and spoken language in combination, as well as their readiness to learn. Some evidence indicates that gesturing eases children's thinking processes, both directly and indirectly (through adult interaction). In addition, when adults gesture, that behavior provides children with a rich source of information. Adults' gesturing positively influences children's gesturing and subsequently their spoken language.

Gesture development in children with language impairments proceeds in much the same way as it does in typically developing children. The exception is that the emergence of gesture may be delayed in children with language impairment, though such children may then use gesture longer to compensate for their difficulties related to spoken language. The clinician who is knowledgeable about gesture development can use this knowledge in the assessment and intervention process for children with language impairments.

KEY TERMS

American Sign Language

Baby signs

Beat gestures

Early communicative gestures

Emblems

Decontextualization

Deictic gestures

Gesture–spoken language match
 combination

Gesture–spoken language mismatch
 combination

Give gesture

Iconic gesture

Mental representation

Point gesture

Representational gestures

Ritual request

Show gesture

STUDY QUESTIONS

- ◆ List the types of gestures discussed in this chapter and create a timeline indicating when they emerge in development.

+ Compare and contrast the types of gestures. How does gesture differ from signed language such as ASL?
+ How does the clinician use the predictability of gesture development in clinical assessment of children?
+ What is one piece of information the adult can gain by paying attention to the child's gesture? More specifically, state the relationship between gesture and the child's mental representation.

REFERENCES

Acredolo, L., & Goodwyn, S. (1988). Symbolic gesturing in normal infants. *Child Development, 59,* 450–466.

Acredolo, L., & Goodwyn, S. (1996). *Baby signs: How to talk to your baby before your baby can talk.* Chicago: NTB/Contemporary.

Alibali, M. W., & DiRusso, A. A. (1999). The function of gesture in learning to count: More than keeping track. *Cognitive Development, 14,* 37–56.

Alibali, M. W., & Goldin-Meadow, S. (1993). Gesture–speech mismatch and mechanisms of learning: What the hands reveal about a child's state of mind. *Cognitive Psychology, 25,* 468–523.

Baddeley, A. (2000). The episodic buffer: a new component of working memory? *Trends in Cognitive Science, 4*(11), 417–423.

Barsalou, L. W. (1999). Perceptual symbol systems. *Behavioral and Brain Sciences, 22,* 577–660.

Bates, E., Bretherton, I., & Snyder, L. (1988). *From first words to grammar: Individual differences and dissociable mechanisms.* New York: Cambridge University Press.

Capirici, O., Iverson, J., Pizzuto, E., & Volterra, V. (1996). Gestures and words during the transition to two-word speech. *Journal of Child Language, 23,* 645–673.

Capone, N. C. (2007). Tapping toddlers' evolving semantic representation via gesture. *Journal of Speech, Language, and Hearing Research, 50*(3), 732–745.

Capone, N. C., & McGregor, K. K. (2005). The effect of semantic representation on toddlers' word retrieval. *Journal of Speech, Language, Hearing Research.,* 48(6), 1468–1480.

Capps, L., Kehres, J., & Sigman, M. (1998). Conversational abilities among children with autism and children with developmental delays. *Autism, 2*(4), 325–344.

Caselli, M. C., Vicari, S., Longobardi, E., Lami, L., Pizzoli, C., & Stella, G. (1998). Gestures and words in early development of children with Down Syndrome. *Journal of Speech-Language-Hearing Research, 41,* 1125–1135.

Charman, T. (1998). Specifying the nature and course of the joint attention impairment in autism in the preschool years: Implications for diagnosis and intervention. *Autism, 2*(1), 61–79.

Church, R. B. (1999). Using gesture and speech to capture transitions in learning. *Cognitive Development, 14,* 313–342.

Church, R. B., & Goldin-Meadow, S. (1986). The mismatch between gesture and speech as an index of transitional knowledge. *Cognition, 23,* 43–71.

Ellis Weismer, S. E., & Hesketh, L. J. (1993). The influence of prosodic and gestural cues on novel word acquisition by children with specific language impairment. *Journal of Speech* and Hearing Research, 36, 1013–1025.

Evans, J. A., Alibali, M. W., & McNeil, N. M. (2001). Divergence of verbal expression and embodied knowledge: Evidence from speech and gesture in children with specific language impairment. *Language and Cognitive Processes, 16*(2/3), 309–331.

Fenson, L., Dale, P., Reznick, J. S., et al. (1993). *MacArthur communicative development inventories*. San Diego, CA: Singular Publishing Group.

Folven, R., & Bonvillian, J. D. (1991). The transition from nonreferential to referential language in children acquiring American Sign Language. *Developmental Psychology, 27*(5), 806–816.

Garber, P., Alibali, M. W., & Goldin-Meadow, S. (1998). Knowledge conveyed in gesture is not tied to the hands. *Child Development, 69,* 75–84.

Garber, P., & Goldin-Meadow, S. (2002). Gesture offers insight into problem-solving in adults and children. *Cognitive Science, 26,* 817–831.

Genesee, F., Paradis, J., & Crago, M. B. (2004). *Dual language development and disorders: A handbook on bilingualism and second language learning*. Baltimore: Paul H. Brookes.

Goldin-Meadow, S. (2000). Beyond words: The importance of gesture to researchers and learners. *Child Development, 71*(1), 231–239.

Goldin-Meadow, S. (2003). *Hearing gesture: How our hands help us think*. Cambridge, MA: Harvard University Press.

Goldin-Meadow, S., Alibali, M. W., & Church, R. B. (1993). Transitions in concept acquisition: Using the hand to read the mind. *Psychological Review, 100*(2), 279–297.

Goldin-Meadow, S., & Butcher, C. (2003). Pointing toward two-word speech in young children. In S. Kita (Ed.), *Pointing: Where language, culture, and cognition meet* (pp. 85–107). Mahway, NJ: Lawrence Erlbaum Associates.

Goldin-Meadow, S., Butcher, C., Mylander, C., & Dodge, M. (1994). Nouns and verbs in a self-styled gesture system: What's in a name? *Cognitive Psychology, 27,* 259–319.

Goldin-Meadow, S., Nusbaum, H., Garber, P., & Church, R. B. (1993). Transitions in learning: Evidence for simultaneously activated strategies. *Journal of Experimental Psychology: Human Perception and Performance, 19*(1), 92–107.

Goldin-Meadow, S., Nusbaum, H., Kelly, S. D., & Wagner, S. (2001). Explaining math: Gesturing lightens the load. *Psychological Science, 12*(6), 516–522.

Goldin-Meadow, S., & Singer, M. A. (2003). From children's hands to adults' ears: Gesture's role in the learning process. *Developmental Psychology, 39*(3), 509–520.

Goldin-Meadow, S., & Wagner, S. M. (2005). How our hands help us learn. *Trends in Cognitive Sciences, 9*(5), 234–241.

Goodwyn, S., & Acredolo, L. (1993). Symbolic gesture versus word: Is there a modality advantage for onset of symbol use? *Child Development, 64,* 688–701.

Goodwyn, S. W., Acredolo, L. P., & Brown, C. A. (2000). Impact on symbolic gesturing on early language development. *Journal of Nonverbal Behavior, 24*(2), 81–103.

Goodhart, F., & Baron-Cohen, S. (1993). How many ways can the point be made? Evidence from children with and without autism. *First Language, 13,* 225–233.

Iverson, J. M., Capirici, O., Longobardi, E., & Caselli, M. C. (1999). Gesturing in mother–child interactions. *Cognitive Development, 14,* 57–75.

Iverson, J. M., Capirici, O., Volterra, V., & Goldin-Meadow S. G. (in press). Learning to talk in a gesture-rich world: Early communication in Italian vs. American children. *First Language.*

Iverson, J. M., & Goldin-Meadow, S. (2001). The resilience of gesture in talk: Gestures in blind speakers and listeners. *Developmental Science, 4*(4), 416–422.

Iverson, J. M., & Goldin-Meadow, S. (2005). Gesture paves the way for language development. *Psychological Science, 16*(5), 368–371.

Iverson, J. M., & Thelen, E. (1999). Hand, mouth, and brain: The dynamic emergence of speech and gesture. *Journal of Consciousness Studies, 6,* 19–40.

Kelly, S. D., & Church, R. B. (1998). A comparison between children's and adult's ability to detect conceptual information conveyed through representational gesture. *Child Development, 69*(1), 85–93.

Kelly, S. D., Singer, M., Hicks, J., & Goldin-Meadow, S. (2002). A helping hand in assessing children's knowledge: Instructing adults to attend to gesture. *Cognition and Instruction, 20*(1), 1–26.

Locke, A., Young, A., Service, B., & Chandler, P. (1990). Some observations on the origins of the pointing gesture. In V. Volterra and C. J. Erting (Eds.), *From gesture to language in hearing and deaf children* (pp. 42–55). New York: Springer-Verlag.

Mainela-Arnold, E., Evans, J. L., & Alibali, M. W. (2006). Understanding conservation delays in children with language impairment: Task representations revealed in speech and gesture. *Journal of Speech, Language, and Hearing Research, 49,* 1267–1279.

McGregor, K. K., & Capone, N. C. (2004). Genetic and environmental interactions in determining the early lexicon: Evidence from a set of tri-zygotic quadruplets. *Journal of Child Language, 31,* 311–337.

McNeil, N. M., Alibali, M. W., & Evans, J. (2001). The role of gesture in children's comprehension of spoken language: Now they need it, now they don't. *Journal of Nonverbal Behavior, 24*(2), 131–149.

Morford, M., & Goldin-Meadow, S. (1992). Comprehension and production of gesture in combination with speech in one-word speakers. *Journal of Child Language, 19,* 559–580.

Nelson, K. (1973). Structure and strategy in learning to talk. *Monographs of the Society for Research in Child Development, 143*(38).

Nicoladis, E., Mayberry, R., & Genesee, F. (1999). Gesture and early bilingual development. *Developmental Psychology, 35*(2), 514–526.

O'Reilly, A. W., Painter, K. M., & Bornstein, M. H. (1997). Relations between language and symbolic gesture development in early childhood. *Cognitive Development, 12,* 185–197.

Özçalişkan, S., & Goldin-Meadow, S. (2005). Gesture is at the cutting edge of early language development. *Cognition, 96,* B101–B113.

Perry, M., Church, R. B., & Goldin-Meadow, S. (1988). Transitional knowledge in the acquisition of concepts. *Cognitive Development, 3,* 359–400.

Pine, K. J., Lufkin, N., & Messer, D. (2004). More gestures than answers: Children learning about balance. *Developmental Psychology, 40*(6), 1059–1067.

Rescorla, L., & Merrin, L. (1998). Communicative intent in late-talking toddlers. *Applied Psycholinguistics, 19,* 393–414.

Rossetti, L. (1990). *The Rossetti Infant-Toddler Language Scale.* East Moline, IL: LinguiSystems, Inc.

Singer Harris, N. G., Bellugi, U., Bates, E., Jones, W., & Rossen, M. (1997). Contrasting profiles of language development in children with Williams and Down Syndromes. *Developmental Neuropsychology, 13*(3), 345–370.

Thal, D., & Tobias, S. (1992). Communicative gestures in children with delayed onset of oral expressive vocabulary. *Journal of Speech and Hearing Research, 35,* 1281–1289.

Werner, H., & Kaplan, B. (1963). *Symbol formation.* New York: John Wiley & Sons.

Wu, Y.C., & Coulson, S. (2007). How iconic gestures enhance communication: An ERP study. *Brain and Language, 101,* 234–245.

CHAPTER 7

Early Semantic Development: The Developing Lexicon

Nina C. Capone, PhD, William O. Haynes, PhD, and Kristy Grohne-Riley, MA

OBJECTIVES

+ To learn the milestones of early lexical–semantic development
+ To understand the course of word learning over time in development
+ To understand factors that influence word learning in children

INTRODUCTION

The child spends one year preparing for his first word with motor, pragmatic, cognitive, and phonological developments. For example, the child's ability to develop fine motor movements of the hand and mouth depends on the gross motor development of the body. Stability in the trunk muscles supports sitting at approximately six months of age. This development provides a stable base for mobility in the hands to explore objects and mobility for the muscles of the mouth for babbling and later word productions.

At the onset of first words, the child's utterances are one word in length until the child has accumulated an expressive vocabulary of approximately 50 words (Nelson, 1973). It is then, at the 50-word milestone, that these utterances are expanded into early word combinations of mostly two- and then some three-word utterances. It is also at this time that children begin to accrue new vocabulary at an exponential rate. This transition from word learning being a slow process to a rapid fire is termed the *word spurt* (Bates et al., 1994; Goldfield & Reznick, 1990). The single-word period typically extends from about 12 months of age until the child is nearly 2 years old.

Children, of course, have not read the developmental literature indicating exactly when they should enter and leave the single-word stage, so there is considerable variability among youngsters in traversing the single-word period. This chapter discusses the developmental course of early semantic milestones, the course of word learning, and factors that influence the child in learning a word.

PREPARING THE FIRST YEAR: PERLOCUTIONARY STAGE

Bates (1976) defined the development of communicative functions as consisting of three stages: *perlocutionary, illocutionary,* and *locutionary.* From birth to approximately 8 to 10 months of age, babies are in the perlocutionary stage of communication development. In this stage, the infant produces vegetative sounds (e.g., burping), sound play (e.g., coo-goo), and other behaviors (e.g., eye gaze) to which the adult infers a communicative intent. For instance, a child looks at a toy and the adult infers that the child wants it. Communication has taken place even though the child has not necessarily intended a specific message to the adult. Vegetative sounds such as cries and burps are also interpreted by the adult. The adult often responds to these with language (*Oh, you're hungry*), and so begins the child's journey onto a road of linking the intention (pragmatics), the meaning (semantics), and the form (phonology, morphology, and syntax) of language. Three important behaviors that are necessary for successful communication throughout the life span are already observed during the perlocutionary stage—namely, *eye contact, joint attention,* and *turn-taking.* These behaviors were discussed in Chapter 5.

Prelinguistic speech behaviors are also observed during this stage of development, including vocal play and babbling. These speech behaviors do not have meaning or intention to communicate. Nevertheless, a number of studies have shown that certain types of babbling appear to have some connection to later lexical development (e.g., de Boysson-Bardes & Vihman, 1991; Stoel-Gammon & Cooper, 1984; Vihman, 1996; Vihman, Macken, Miller, Simmons, & Miller, 1985). Chapter 8 discusses the relationship between babbling and first words.

INTENT TO COMMUNICATE: ILLOCUTIONARY STAGE

The second stage of communication is illocution. In this period the child displays the intention to communicate with gestures and nonlinguistic vocalizations. A major difference between the perlocutionary stage and the illocutionary stage is that the child has clear intention to communicate in the latter stage—it is not merely an adult inferring a communicative intent. The illocutionary stage is typically characterized by the child using gestural communication or using gestures accompanied by vocalizations (e.g., jargon, protowords) that are not words. Primarily, children attempt to communicate at this time for two purposes: (1) to regulate joint attention with the adult and (2) to regulate joint action with the adult (Bruner, 1975). For example, a child will repeatedly show an object to an adult to gain attention; when a child wants to have a wind-up toy activated, she will physically manipulate the adult by moving the adult's hand to the toy. The latter behavior is referred to as a *ritual request* gesture, as discussed in Chapter 6.

Children progress from a period of babbling to a point at which they begin to stabilize certain vocalizations around specific situations, events, and objects. These vocalizations have been called various names by researchers, including *protowords* (Halliday, 1975), *prelexical forms* (Bates, 1976), and *phonetically consistent forms* (PCF; Dore, Franklin, Miller, & Ramer, 1976). These vocalizations do not meet the criteria for classification as true words because they do not resemble adult productions. Prelexical transition utterances tend to be associated with a situation or event rather than with a particular physical referent. They are regarded by many as simply a part of an activity rather than language that is referential in nature. Dore and colleagues (1976) indicate that these forms have the following characteristics:

+ They are independent units bounded by pauses.
+ They are produced repeatedly, at different times.
+ They are correlated with recurring conditions.
+ They are phonetically more stable than babbling but not as stable as word productions.

These PCFs are not necessarily attempts at word approximations and are highly individual to specific children. One child might say /na na na/ every time he protests; another child may produce a different vocalization for protest. The key point is that the vocalization will be similar for each protest situation for an individual child.

One example of a PCF is an *affect expression*, in which a child stabilizes a vocalization around an emotional reaction such as anger, frustration, joy, protest, or some other affective situation.

A second PCF is an *instrumental expression*, in which a child vocalizes a consistent pattern whenever he is attempting to regulate adult behavior to obtain goods or joint activity. An example would be a child who vocalizes /uh/ whenever he is attempting to regulate an adult. Again, a child who says /uh/ to be lifted up is not necessarily saying *up* because the same vocalization is produced when the adult is enlisted to open a jar or wind a toy.

A final example of a PCF is an *indicating expression*. The indicating expression is produced in concert with pointing, where the goal is the direction of adult attention and not necessarily the regulation of action. The child may say /ba/ every time he points to an object to direct adult attention.

THE FIRST WORD: LOCUTIONARY STAGE

Most speech-language pathologists wish they had a dime for every parent who reported that their child spoke his first word at the age of six months. Parents typically scan the output of their infants with great interest early on for evidence of the first word, because this event marks the beginning of verbal communication. There is an important difference, however, between a six-month-old uttering /mama/ randomly and an adult using many words in specific, consistent, and appropriate contexts. The parent's criterion for the first word is probably phonological in nature, not semantic (Kamhi, 1988). Thus, if a word sounds like an adult word, the child is given credit for using it, even though it may have been void of semantic or pragmatic intent.

The notion of a true word should be separate from the mere uttering of a bisyllable by an infant. In babbling, infants often approximate an adult word such as /di/ and parents might say "Didn't she just say *dish?*", when actually it was just a phonetic accident that the child could never duplicate. A true word has to have "a phonetic relationship to some adult word" and the child must "use the word consistently to mark a particular situation or object" (Owens, 1988, p. 199). These criteria rule out babbling or jargon as true words.

The locutionary stage of communication begins at approximately 12 months, when the hearing child utters his first word. Twelve months is only the average age, however: Children typically vary in this milestone from 11 to 13 months. The child might say *ba* to indicate the bottle, say *up* and extend the arms toward the adult in an attempt to be picked up, or say *doggie* to direct the adult's attention to an oncoming canine. Nelson (1973) reported that the mean age of a 10-word vocabulary was 15 months, with a range of 13 to 19 months of age.

During the time that children are acquiring these first 10 words, their vocabulary is unstable. That is, they tend to have appearance and then disappearance of words. This phenomenon should not be confused with vocabulary regression, which is reported by parents of children with language impairments. In typical development, it is not uncommon for children to use a word for a few weeks and then stop using it. However, this disappearance is accompanied by new words being used. For children with language impairments, new words do not appear; rather, they experience a loss of using words more generally.

Nelson (1973) reported the mean age for acquisition of the 50-word lexicon was 19.75 months—though children vary widely around that milestone, with a range of 15 to 24 months. Word learning is fairly slow in the first half of the second year as compared to the second half of that same year and beyond. The 50-word lexicon milestone is important, however, because two key milestones follow it: Around the time the child accumulates 50 words, he enters a rapid period of word acquisition (i.e., the word spurt) and begins to combine words.

Between 18 and 24 months of age, most children will exhibit what has been variously referred to by researchers as *vocabulary spurt, naming insight, nominal insight,* or *naming explosion* (Bates et al., 1994; Bloom & Capatides, 1987; Goldfield & Reznick, 1990; Gopnik & Meltzoff, 1986). All of these terms refer to a discernable rapid increase in the number of words a child is learning and using. Various changes in development of related skills have been investigated to account for this sudden and rapid increase in word learning (e.g., object permanence; the ability to categorize objects—Gopnik & Meltzoff, 1986; temperament—Bloom & Capatides, 1987; connectionist learning algorithm—Plunkett, Sinha, Moller, & Strandsby, 1992). Findings are inconsistent in terms of whether these variables relate to the word spurt, however, and there remains no definitive explanation as to why or how these factors contribute to this rapid increase in the rate of new word learning.

Bloom (2004) has argued that the word spurt is a "myth" (p. 205) because other factors could account for the findings of an increase in rate of word learning. Two possible reasons Bloom suggests for the observed word spurt are the child's general talkativeness and the way in which the researcher of a study defines a word spurt (e.g., a child may be defined as having a word spurt when she acquires 12 new words in a 2-week period). On the first point, it is possible that the number of words children produce is simply a function of how much they talk, not how many new words they know. Put another way, the more one talks, the more words a researcher is likely to find (p. 213). On the second point, Bloom argues that researchers may define a child as having had a word spurt when 12 new words were acquired within a 2-week period but do not reference how many words were acquired the previous 2 weeks. The child may have learned 10 new words and then 12 new words in each respective time period, indicating a gradual increase in vocabulary rather than a sudden shift in word learning. These ideas are controversial, so it is wise to remember that children start out learning words slowly and then get better at it. It is unclear whether there needs to be a separate cognitive or social mechanism to explain this phenomenon.

The timely acquisition of early vocabulary milestones is important for continued language development. Marchman and Bates (1994) have suggested that the size of the lexicon must reach a necessary threshold if other language domains are to fully develop, particularly morpho-syntax. For example, the word spurt (if one exists) and two-word combination milestones tend to emerge after children have a threshold of at least 50 words in their lexicon. Nelson (1973) also found that vocabulary size at 2 years of age was related to mean length of utterance (MLU—a measure of syntactic development) at 30 months of age. Children who do not meet early vocabulary milestones in a timely manner are referred to as late talkers. While many late-talking toddlers outgrow their early delay and are reclassified as late bloomers, a proportion of these children persist in language impairments that transcend the domain of vocabulary to those of morphology, syntax, and written language (e.g., Rescorla, Dahlsgaard, & Roberts, 2000; Thal & Tobias, 1994; Thal, Tobias, & Morrison, 1991).

To see how this development is assessed, consider the early semantic milestones of the three case studies from Chapter 1. Johnathon was reported to speak his first word at 12 months, Josephine did not speak her first word until 15 months, and Robert's first word emerged at 18 months. Therefore, at the time of the evaluation, Josephine and Robert already had a history of delayed semantic development in expressive vocabulary. Josephine was

22 months at evaluation and had only 7 words in her vocabulary. Robert was 27 months at evaluation and had only 14 words in his vocabulary, some of which were sound effects. Only Johnathon was using new words and combining words. Josephine and Robert were both delayed for learning new words regularly and for combining words. Josephine and Robert have a history of delay that is persisting into toddlerhood. Their semantic delay could now be characterized as having (1) a small expressive vocabulary size for their age, (2) too few new words being added to their expressive vocabulary, and (3) a delay in combining words. Finally, while Johnathon relies on words to communicate, Josephine and Robert still rely on gestures and nonlinguistic vocalizations. Johnathon is evaluated as typical for his age, whereas Josephine and Robert show delays in vocabulary development that place them in a category of language impairment. During this time in development, we refer to them as late talkers.

A PREPONDERANCE OF NOUNS

Nelson (1973) analyzed the word classes present in the first 50-word lexicon using the classification system of *specific nominals*, *general nominals*, *action words*, *modifiers*, *personal–social words*, and *function words*. (See **Table 7-1** for definitions of these terms.) The proportion of total vocabulary that each word class (e.g., noun, action) represents in the early lexicon is remarkably

TABLE 7-1 Word Classifications	
Word Class	**Definition**
Specific Nominals	These words refer to a specific exemplar of a category whether or not it is a proper name (e.g., mommy, daddy, pet's name).
General Nominals	These words refer to all members of a category and include classes such as objects, substances, animals, people, letters, numbers, pronouns, and abstractions.
Action Words	These words are used to describe or demand an action.
Modifiers	These words refer to properties or qualities of things or events, such as attributes, states, locations, or possessives.
Personal–Social Words	These words express affective states and social relationships such as assertions (e.g., no, yes, want) and social expressive words (e.g., please, ouch).
Function Words	These words refer to items that serve a grammatical function in relating to other words (e.g., what, is, for, to).

Source: Nelson (1973).

similar across children. General nominals (i.e., common nouns) make up the largest proportion of the lexicon, accounting for 51% of vocabulary. Action words and specific nominals each account for 14% of the lexicon, and modifiers and personal–social words each represent 9% of the lexicon. Only 4% of the vocabulary is made up of function words. This same classification system is used today in clinical analyses of early language (e.g., Retherford, 2000).

Despite significant differences in language and culture, children learning Mandarin Chinese, Japanese, Kaluli, German, Italian, Hebrew, and Turkish are also observed to have more nouns than other word classes in their early lexicon (e.g., Caselli et al., 1995; Gentner, 1982; Goldfield, 1993). The universal nature of noun preference in early lexicons has garnered some attention by language researchers, and several hypotheses about the early predominance of nouns have been put forth.

For example, is there a frequency effect? That is, are nouns used more often than verbs? This is unlikely because even though adults use more nouns than other word classes, there is a larger variety of nouns. This means that individual nouns are used *less* frequently than the smaller lexicon of verbs in a language (Goldfield, 1993). With fewer verbs to use, adults will use each more often. Put another way, the pattern should be reversed (more verbs than nouns in the early lexicon) because children actually hear each of the smaller number of verbs more often than each of the larger number of nouns.

Another explanation might lie in the way parents teach language to their children. When speaking to their child, do adults organize their language around object naming? American parents largely focus heavily on object naming with their children (Nelson, Hampson, & Shaw, 1993). However, in Kaluli, parents are not particularly interested in teaching object names to their children, and Korean-speaking parents tend to focus their interactions around actions and activity (Kim, McGregor, & Thompson, 2000). With little difference in the early lexicons of children from these disparate cultures, it would appear that this is not a salient factor in noun acquisition.

Two factors that have received more attention for their part in this phenomenon are (1) the ordering of word classes in a sentence of a language and (2) conceptual differences between nouns and other word classes. We address each of these issues in turn.

The ordering of word classes in a sentence generally refers to the order of nouns, in subject (S) and object (O) position, and verbs (V). In English, we might say *The girl is reading a book,* where *The girl* is the noun phrase that occupies the subject position, *a book* is the noun phrase that occupies the object position, and *is reading* is the verb phrase that occupies the verb position. In English, nouns occupy the most salient positions in sentences. For example, the speech signal tends to change at the end of sentences and clauses (e.g., greater stress, elongated vowel, or fricative duration), making the words and morphemes that occur in this position more salient for the listener. It is possible that children acquire more nouns early on because they occur in salient sentence positions, and particularly in final sentence positions. In contrast, languages such as Korean, German, Kaluli, and Turkish have verbs in the final positions of sentence (S-O-V; O-S-V)—yet children learning these languages have lexicons that are predominantly made up of nominals as well.

Gentner (1982, 2006) proposes that concrete nouns promote more rapid learning than other word classes—particularly verbs—because they allow for greater transparency of the mapping between lexical and semantic information (natural partitions hypothesis; Gentner, 1982, p. 327). Nouns represent more perceptually stable entities than other word classes. Other word classes (verbs, prepositions, modifiers) are slower to be acquired because relationships among entities are less spatially cohesive and concrete than they are for objects. Predicates, for example, have more ambiguous relations to the perceptual world, and their meanings are harder to glean in a single exposure. Finally, because object concepts are concrete, they allow children to bootstrap into the language system. *Bootstrapping* is a term that refers to the child's use of known information to infer unknown information. In essence, knowing object concepts gives children a foothold in the speech stream, and it creates a scaffold from which to learn other word class–semantic relations. Simply put, learning nouns helps to you learn verbs, and so on.

It is likely that both language input and conceptual factors contribute to the universal pattern of noun learning. Kim, McGregor, & Thompson (2000) set out to compare early vocabularies of English- and Korean-speaking children to confirm or refute the claim that nouns dominate early vocabularies universally, and to explore why that might be. Specifically, their study followed eight English-speaking and eight Korean-speaking mother–child dyads to examine the influence of maternal language on the child's early vocabulary. Children were followed from 16 months of age to 21 months of age, just before or around their 50-word milestone. Kim and colleagues (2000) found that both Korean- and English-learning children acquired significantly more nouns than verbs, despite the differences the researchers observed between the two cultures in language input and parent activity. This dominance of nouns over verbs was found for Korean-speaking children even though their caregivers tended to emphasize verbs in their interactions with them. As expected, English-speaking caregivers tended to emphasize nouns in their talk to the children. These results suggest that all children come to the task of early word learning with a strong predisposition toward linking nouns to objects.

That being said, there was also an influence of the frequency and saliency of verbs in the Korean-speaking input. Specifically, even though Korean-speaking children had more nouns than verbs in their vocabulary, they had a greater proportion of verbs in their vocabulary as compared to the number of verbs in the English-speaking children's vocabulary. Therefore, while children appear to have some universal predisposition for noun learning, their environment also shapes the developing lexicon to some extent. In this case, the environment includes social activity and surface structure of the grammar that the child hears.

This pattern of noun learning over other word-class learning continues to be observed in the development of preschool and early school-age children, with and without language impairments. For example, two author teams—Rice, Buhr, and Nemeth (1990) and Oetting, Rice, and Swank (1995)—examined word learning after just a brief exposure to vocabulary items from a cartoon video. Both studies found that typically developing children and children with language impairments showed a preference for learning object terms over other word-class items, including action, attribute, and affective terms. Because non-object labels are difficult to map in a single exposure, more experience and contexts may be needed to map the meanings and linguistic specifications of these word classes (Oetting, Rice, & Swank, 1995; Waxman, 1994). We discuss the idea that richness of experience influences acquisition of words later in the chapter. First, however, we return to the early lexicon and the importance of noun learning.

EXPRESSIVE VERSUS REFERENTIAL WORD LEARNERS

When Nelson (1973) analyzed the first 50-word lexicon, she found that although the majority of children had a preponderance of general nominals, there was a group of children for which this was not the case. Nelson classified children as *referential* if general nominals accounted for more than 50% of their total vocabulary. Those children with general nominals accounting for less than 50% of their lexicon were referred to as *expressive*. The expressive children used many personal–social words, whereas the referential children used many nouns (see also Bates, Bretherton, & Snyder, 1988; Bloom, 1973; Goldfield, 1986, 1987; Snyder, Bates, & Bretherton, 1981). Snyder, Bates, & Bretherton (1981) found the expressive–referential distinction in children as young as 13 months, when the children had only 10 to 12 words in their lexicons. Note that expressive children and referential children should not be viewed dichotomously. Indeed, most authorities indicate that children who are categorized as expressive versus referential probably represent extreme points on a continuum, rather than separate classifications or typologies of language-developing children (Bates, Bretherton, & Snyder, 1988; Nelson, 1981; Nelson & Lucarielly, 1985).

As research began to focus on the differences between expressive and referential children, it was found that certain characteristics, in addition to lexical composition, were often observed in each group. For instance, referential children were reported to develop language earlier and more rapidly than expressive children did (Bates, Bretherton, & Snyder, 1988; Horgan, 1978, 1979; Nelson, 1973; Ramer, 1976).

Specifically, Bates and colleagues (1988) noted that referential children had larger vocabularies and reached morpho-syntactic milestones sooner than expressive children. Referential children had a word spurt, whereas expressive children tended to learn words at a slow and steady pace without a word spurt. Referential children showed greater growth of verb vocabulary at 20 months and more productive control over function words (e.g., determiners, prepositions) by 28 months. Initially, expressive children had more function words in their lexicon because they used phrases as holistic chunks. That is, they did not analyze the words of a phrase as individual words but rather as one lexical item. A U-shaped curve in function word development was observed: Once expressive children began analyzing individual words, these functional items dropped out and reappeared later as productive forms. Also, referential children tended to use words in context-flexible ways (e.g., saying *cup* to refer to many cups, not just their cup). They would *decontextualize* their word use by talking about absent objects. Decontextualization refers to the gradual distancing of a symbol from the original referent or learning context (Werner & Kaplan, 1963). The ability to decontextualize language is important for spoken and written language development as the child ages, particularly for social, emotional, and academic success.

The relationship between size of object vocabulary and vocabulary growth was also observed in the late talkers studied by Rescorla, Mirak, and Singh (2000). These authors found that even among children who were delayed in language development, if they had larger vocabularies (although smaller than is typical), the children tended to have greater growth in total vocabulary size over time than did the children who had the smallest vocabularies.

INNATE BIASES MAKE WORD LEARNING EFFICIENT

If children relied on explicit teaching (i.e., "this is a *cup*," "this is another *cup*") to learn each word of their language, language learning would be a laborious, effortful, and inefficient task. Luckily, children come to the task of word learning with some innate *biases* (also referred to as *constraints* or *principles* of word learning) that help them narrow down the many possible referents that could be paired with a word that they hear. For example, if mother says, "Oh, I see the *dax*," where *dax* is a novel word, the child must figure out which of the many objects, parts of objects, actions, and events going on in the room that *dax* is referencing.

Several biases can help the child achieve this feat. First, the child must differentiate between spoken language and other sounds as labels. The *principle of reference* states that words—but not other sounds—label objects, actions, and events (e.g., Hollich et al., 2000). When Balaban and Waxman (1997) presented nine-month-olds with objects paired with either a tone or a word, the infants showed a preference to link a word—but not a tone—with an object. This occurred even though both tones and words captured their attention in the learning phase.

Three related biases that help the child map a new word to the right referent are the *novel name–nameless category principle* (N3C; Golinkoff, Mervis, & Hirsh-Pasek, 1994), the *principle of mutual exclusivity*, and the *whole-object bias* (Markman, 1989). The principle of mutual exclusivity states that if the child already has a name for an object (*cup, comb*), it cannot receive another name. The flip side of this bias is the N3C principle, which states that a novel word will be taken as the name for a previously unnamed object. For example, in experiments examining how children map novel words to unfamiliar objects, an array of three objects may be presented to the child: a cup, a comb, and a novel object previously unseen or unnamed. When the experimenter states, "Give me the *dax*," the child will hand over the novel object because she already has names for the other objects. Children choose objects in this way even though they have never been explicitly taught, "This is a *dax*." Finally, the whole-object bias guides the child to infer that the word label refers to the entire object and not just a part, an attribute, or its motion. For example, the child knows that the word *car* refers to the whole entity, and not just the wheels, windows, or steering wheel of the vehicle.

Children also come to language learning armed with a *principle of conventionality* (Clark, 1993). That is, children know that there are culturally agreed-upon names for things and that these names do not change. Our use and understanding of language would be quite chaotic if the names given to things were ever changing. Children make this assumption early on.

Two additional biases that make word learning efficient for the child are the *principle of extendibility* (Hollich et al., 2000) and the *shape bias* (e.g., Clark, 1973; Landau, Smith, & Jones, 1988). These issues are addressed again later in the chapter, so they are mentioned only briefly here. Put simply, the principle of extendibility states that a word does not refer to only one object, but rather refers to a category of objects, events, or actions if they share similar properties. Therefore, a word will label all instances of an object if all of those instances have the same shape and/or function. The shape bias constrains word extension based on shared perceptual features of the original referent and the novel exemplar.

We can readily see the shape bias at work in some of children's naming errors. For example, a child may look at the moon and say *ball* because both moon and ball are round. The shape bias has been extensively studied in terms of its relationship with word learning (e.g., Booth & Waxman, 2002; Gershkoff-Stowe & Smith, 2004; Jones, 2003). Gershkoff-Stowe and Smith (2004) found a positive parallel relationship in toddlers' increasing use of the shape bias and an increase in their expressive noun vocabulary. Further, Jones (2003) found that late talkers—children defined by their small vocabulary size—do not demonstrate a shape bias. It would seem, then, that the shape bias is particularly important for vocabulary growth.

Even though a shared shape is one basis for word extension, a shared function between objects is also a salient feature that organizes a category of objects by one name (e.g., Booth & Waxman, 2002; Clark, 1973; Kemler Nelson, 1999). For example, Kemler Nelson (1999) assessed the role of shared function in word extensions made by 28-month-olds. These toddlers heard the names of objects and had opportunities to enact their functions. They were then tested on word extension to four types of objects: similar shape–similar function, similar shape–dissimilar function, dissimilar shape–similar function, and dissimilar shape–dissimilar function. In this study, toddlers were able to transcend shape similarities and extend words based on shared function. That is, they used the same name for two objects if the function was the same, even for objects that did not look alike.

Other object features, such as size of an object, have not been shown to influence extension decisions (e.g., Jones, Smith, & Landau, 1991). For example, children label a real car and a toy car both as *car* despite the obvious difference in size (and texture). Even though the size difference between their parent's car and their Fisher-Price miniature car is quite large, children call both *car* because the items share shape properties that include four wheels, doors, seats, windshield, steering wheel, and other salient features.

Toddlers are also quite smart about adjusting their shape bias. When Jones, Smith, and Landau, (1991) placed eyes on their objects, children accepted shape changes and extended a word label to another object that shared texture (e.g., fur). In this case, the presence of eyes signaled that the object was an animate entity, and animate entities tend to share material (e.g., bears have fur, humans have skin, birds have feathers) and change shape (i.e., we change shape as we move). Therefore, children appear to adapt to and integrate multiple perceptual cues to make inferences about what something is or is not.

THE EMERGENT COALITION MODEL OF WORD LEARNING

As stated earlier, little of language learning is accomplished by direct and explicit teaching. Instead, much of what the child learns is a result of what he infers about the language that he hears and what is going on around him. The previous section discussed the innate principles or biases that the child brings to the word learning task. Other cues in the environment also scaffold word learning for the child—for example, a parent's point or eye gaze, the grammatical structure of the language model, the perceptual salience of the object. The emergentist coalition model (ECM; Hollich et al., 2000) describes how children coalesce environmental cues and innate biases to learn new words. In addition to the interaction between cues and strategies, the ECM posits that children calculate their success and failure rate of mapping words to referents. This error signal feeds back into the learning system to improve the reliability of coalescing these cues and strategies as the child develops.

A full range of cues is always available to the child, though he weighs each cue differently over time. With development and experience, the child learns which cues are more reliable indicators of word–referent pairings. In turn, the child's accuracy in linking words to referents becomes more efficient. When a parent produces a word label, the child recruits attentional cues (e.g., perceptual salience of objects), social cues (e.g., eye gaze, pointing), and linguistic cues (e.g., regularities in syntax) in the environment to further constrain the possibilities of which referent that word is labeling. Infants aged 12 to 18 months initially consider perceptual salience (e.g., a moving object) to be a more important cue about what is being labeled than a social cue (e.g., eye gaze or pointing to it). Therefore, the child infers that the interesting moving object is what is being labeled, even though the parent may be looking at the boring object. By ages 18 to 24 months, children have learned that the social cue is a more reliable indicator of the word to referent mapping. Now when they hear a word, they pay attention to the adult's gesture and eye gaze to ensure a reliable word-to-referent mapping occurs. Put most simply, by toddlerhood children can accurately map the names of the boring objects as well as the interesting ones (Golinkoff & Hirsh-Pasek, 2006).

LEARNING A WORD

Learning a word is not an all-or-nothing phenomenon. Instead, as Carey (1978) described, word learning is a gradual and long-term process. Learning a word grossly encompasses learning the lexeme (word form or label), the semantic representation (word meaning), and grammatical specifications (e.g., word-class information), plus making connections between the various representations. As children encounter words in a variety of contexts, over time their knowledge of individual words is enriched.

Carey (1978) delineated two phases of word learning: *fast mapping* and *slow mapping*. A word is considered fast mapped if there is an initial association made between word and referent. A related phenomenon has been termed *quick incidental learning* (QUIL; Oetting, Rice, & Swank, 1995; Rice, Buhr, & Oetting, 1992). QUIL reflects more naturally occurring word learning situations—that is, situations that offer minimal environmental support with multiple cues in ongoing scenes.

In experimental studies, many new words may be presented as part of a cartoon program prior to the test of word learning. In contrast, the fast mapping phenomenon is often measured after a more explicit or structured task with fewer word–referent pairs needing to be inferred. The former scenario better matches the child's natural word learning experiences. What is important for the speech-language pathologist to keep in mind is that a child will not know much about a fast-mapped word–referent pair. Lexical and semantic information are weakly represented in memory after such a brief exposure. Therefore, the child needs several to many exposures to a word, depending on the word, to truly discern the subtleties of its meaning. This happens during the slow mapping phase of word learning.

Slow mapping is the process of enriching lexical–semantic representations after a word is fast mapped into memory. The child's representations are enriched through increased frequency of exposure and/or richer quality of exposure. This process has significant implications for the clinical practice of speech-language pathologists, because intervention provides the child with increased frequency of exposure to language and a richer quality of language learning. Quality of learning is enriched through the therapeutic scaffolds used by the clinician. Such therapeutic scaffolds could include the explicit use of verbal models of the word label being repeated with greater frequency for the child, or visual cues such as gesturing about the object while labeling it, or organizing objects by category to help the child build connections between related vocabulary items.

At any given time, words may vary in the richness of their lexical–semantic representations simply because some words are encountered more often than others. For example, as you are learning the vocabulary of speech-language pathology, you are mapping many new terms into memory. Your knowledge of these terms is still weak as compared to that of the master-level student who is about to enter the profession. The master-level student has had many more exposures through additional coursework and richer quality of each experience, and through advanced reading and clinical practicum. The richness of these professional terms in your own vocabulary will evolve over time as you move through undergraduate and graduate study. Conversely, if this is the last class you ever take in speech-language pathology, then your lexical–semantic knowledge of these terms will remain sparse and perhaps weaken as other words in your lexicon are continually updated and strengthened with repeated exposure.

AN ASSOCIATIONISTIC ACCOUNT OF LEXICAL–SEMANTIC REPRESENTATIONS

According to associationistic accounts, lexical and semantic information are stored and linked within a distributed neural network in the brain (e.g., Barsalou, 1999a, 1999b; Plunkett, Karmiloff-Smith, Bates, Elman, & Johnson, 1997). For example, the concept of *bone* comprises visual information (shape, color), thematic associates (dogs chew bones), actions (chewing), the proprioceptive–tactile experience of feeling its weight and rough texture, and its lexeme (/bon/). Lexemes are further divisible into phonemes (/b/, /o/, and /n/). Each of these is a node of information (semantic, phonological, lexical) in the network; connections within and between representations, in turn, allow for spreading of neural activation among semantic and lexical nodes. For example, when you see a bone, your shape node is activated. Through connections in the network, there is activation of the other nodes as well. This includes the lexeme /bon/.

The strength of those nodes and connections' activation weights influences whether nodes will be activated and information can be recalled from memory. When a semantic representation is stronger, it has many connected nodes of information, which leads to a greater number of connections to the lexeme. This richer quality and quantity of connections provides an activation strength that will reach the activation threshold of the lexeme such that it, too, will be activated (i.e., recalled).

Each node and connection pair carries an activation weight (excitatory or inhibitory). Fast-mapped words or infrequently encountered words tend to have few nodes with weak activation weights. These lexical–semantic representations are not distinct from other weakly represented words that share some, but not all, features. It is through the slow mapping phase that lexical–semantic representations are enriched. Richer lexical–semantic representations are distinct because a greater number of nodes and connections are present within and between lexical–semantic representations, and because their activation weights are stronger. When semantic activation weights and connections to the lexeme are strong, the likelihood of recalling the lexeme (i.e., activating it in memory) is quite good.

For example, upon seeing an image of a pig, the child may activate several lexical–semantic representations that are weak if he has little experience with farm animals. These representations perhaps all have two ears, four legs, and a tail. Several lexemes may exist to name this weak representation the child has of farm animals in memory (e.g., pig, horse, and cow). However, as the child enriches his knowledge of pigs, horses, and cows, only the relevant lexeme will be activated when he sees one of these, because the distinct semantic features are being activated for one of them. As part of this process, the unique feature nodes activate the correct lexeme for retrieval. At the same time, inhibitory signals are sent to the horse and cow lexeme nodes to forestall their activation.

Before the child develops a richer representation, she is more likely to fail to retrieve the name of an intended word (e.g., Capone & McGregor, 2005; McGregor & Appel, 2002; McGregor, Freidman, Reilly, & Newman, 2002; McGregor, Newman, Reilly, & Capone, 2002). For example, the child may say *doggie* instead of *cow*, where *cow* is the intended target word. The next sections of the chapter deal with the issue of naming errors in children.

NAMING ERRORS OF OVEREXTENSION AND UNDEREXTENSION

Parents and researchers have noted for years that children often misuse the words in their vocabularies. The early lexicon is in an almost continual state of flux and begins to stabilize only after the child's word spurt (Gershkoff-Stowe, 2001; Nelson, 1973). When a child calls a cow *doggie*, he is exhibiting the limitations of his vocabulary. Limitations can take the form of either weakness of knowledge or an immature retrieval process (Gershkoff-Stowe, 2002).

When a child uses a word too broadly to refer to referents that may be similar in perceptual feature or function, the error is referred to as an *overextension*. Some examples might be calling the moon a *ball* or calling a strange man *daddy*. Conversely, the child may also produce *underextensions*. Underextended words have too narrow a meaning. An example is the use of the word *dog* only when referring to the child's pet, and not when referring to other dogs. Clark (1973) has estimated that overextensions and underextensions occur frequently and can represent as much as one-third of a child's early vocabulary between the ages of one and two years. Two traditional theories attempt to explain extension errors.

First, the *semantic feature hypothesis* (Clark, 1973, 1975) states that children classify and organize referents in terms of perceptual features such as size, shape, animacy, and texture. This phenomenon could explain some overextensions in which a child generalizes a word based on perceptual similarity (e.g., *ball–moon*).

Second, the *functional core hypothesis* (Nelson, 1974) states that words are overextended because of the actions or functions performed on objects rather than the perceptual features of the referents. Thus a child may say the word *rake* when a person is sweeping because the actions are similar.

Aspects of each of these traditional theories are present in the current theories of word retrieval in children. While it is true that children organize categories around perceptual (e.g., shape) or functional features, several other factors also influence word learning and retrieval. These factors include the phonological make-up of the word (e.g., high versus low phonotactic probability; Storkel, 2001), the frequency with which the word is encountered and/or practiced (Dell, 1990; Gershkoff-Stowe, 2002), and the richness of the word's semantic representation (e.g., Capone & McGregor, 2005; McGregor, Friedman, Reilly, & Newman, 2002). For example, Storkel (2001) showed that preschoolers (ages three to six years) take advantage of how frequently phonological sequences is found in the language (phonotactic probability). When taught words made up of low-phonotactic-probability sequences and others consisting of high-phonotactic-probability sequences, preschoolers learned the high-phonotactic words faster.

The next section of the chapter delves into the nature of word retrieval/naming errors and explores how error and target are related in systematic ways.

NAMING ERRORS

The retrieval errors that children (and adults) make are often logically related to the word that was targeted for expression. Therefore, errors in word retrieval reflect a speaker's knowledge (Dell, 1990; Dell, Reed, Adams, & Meyer, 2000; McGregor, 1997).

For example, as the child's vocabulary grows in size, the semantic system begins to take on a hierarchical organization. Children acquire *basic-level* (or *ordinate terms*) lexical items first (e.g., *dog*) and later develop a hierarchy of *superordinate* (e.g., *animal*) and *subordinate* (e.g., *collie*) terms. If a target word is *dog*, the child's error is more likely to be *animal* than *spoon*, because *dog* and *animal* are more closely related (or connected) in the lexicon than are *dog* and *spoon*. These items are rarely, if ever, associated together in our experiences.

Word retrieval errors can actually relate to their targets in several ways:

+ Phonologically—for example, saying *chicken* instead of *kitchen* or *miracleride* for *merry-go-round*
+ Semantically—for example, saying *key* for *door* or *skating* for *skiing*
+ Phonologically and semantically—for example, saying *elevator* for *escalator*
+ An indeterminate response—for example, saying *thing* or *I don't know*
+ A perseverative response—that is, using the same word to label different objects within a set time interval
+ A visual misperception—for example, saying *lollipop* for *balloon*

McGregor (1997) found that the most prevalent type of word retrieval errors were semantic errors and indeterminate errors. These errors indicate that retrieval failure is likely
related to a weak or missing semantic representation of the target word or weak links between
semantic knowledge and lexical labels (Gershkoff-Stowe, 2001; Lahey & Edwards, 1999;
McGregor, 1997; McGregor, Newman, Reilly, & Capone, 2002; Plunkett, Karmiloff-Smith,
Bates, Elman, & Johnston, 1997). McGregor showed that preschoolers with and without language impairments make the same types of word retrieval errors (predominately semantic errors), but children with language impairments make more errors.

During the word spurt, the toddler begins mapping many new words into memory. Given
that the child has so many weak representations at this age, the word spurt is a good developmental time for examining the nature of word retrieval errors because the child makes so many
during this time (Gershkoff-Stowe, 2002; Gershkoff-Stowe & Smith, 1997). Gershkoff-Stowe
and Smith (1997) found that during this shift in rapidly learning new words, toddlers show a
parallel trend in increasing naming errors. As their word acquisition increases so rapidly, they
also have a sudden but temporary increase in retrieving words for the naming of known referents. Word retrieval errors during the word spurt period may occur related to words that toddlers had named accurately during the pre-spurt period. Consistent with the findings of other
studies, these naming errors are predominately semantically related to the target word, although
perseverative errors are also prevalent. Phonological errors were significantly less common.

Perseverative errors subsequently decline in the post-spurt period (Gershkoff-Stowe,
2002). Gershkoff-Stowe and Smith (1997) suggest that such errors reflect a general fragility in
the retrieval process and/or a weakness of word representations, reflecting the fact that children
of this age are new word learners. Semantic errors persist in the post-spurt period. This relationship is to be expected because the retrieval process itself has stabilized, yet new words are
continually fast mapped. As a consequence, the child will always have a continuum of weak to
richer representations. Weaker representations will be more prone to error in retrieving them
for naming purposes (Capone & McGregor, 2005). As the child practices saying words and
slow-mapping their semantics, the child may make increasingly fewer errors on those words
that are repeatedly encountered and enriched (Gershkoff-Stowe, 2002).

Recall the associationistic theory of the lexical–semantic system. We can think of lexical–
semantic representations as existing along a continuum of representations from weak to richer
forms, depending on the quantity and quality of experience with a particular word (Capone
& McGregor, 2005). Richer representations are distinct in that they have more unique nodes
of information and stronger activation weights. This summed excitatory activation at the target lexical node reduces the likelihood that the wrong lexeme (or no lexeme) will be retrieved.
Storkel (2001) found low phonotactic probability words are prone to error more than high
phonotactic probability words. She hypothesized that high phonotactic probability words are

learned faster, which most likely allows the child to map and integrate semantic information better for these words than for low phonotactic probability words. That is, high phonotactic probability words are less prone to error because they are more richly represented in memory than low phonotactic probability words.

In another study, Gershkoff-Stowe (2002) manipulated toddlers' frequency of experience in saying words via two conditions of naming practice. In one condition, toddlers had practice naming pictures from a picture book; in the second condition, toddlers had extra practice naming the same pictures (i.e., book, picture cards). Toddlers in the extra-practice condition produced fewer naming errors than the low-practice condition.

Richness of semantic representation also influences word retrieval (e.g., Capone & McGregor, 2005; McGregor, Friedman, Reilly, & Newman, 2002; McGregor, Newman, Reilly, & Capone, 2002). McGregor and colleagues have studied the richness of semantic representation associated with both accurate naming and naming errors by typically developing children and those with specific language impairment (SLI). Children with SLI are known for having difficulty with word retrieval (e.g., McGregor, 1997). In the studies conducted by McGregor, Friedman, Reilly, and Newman (2002) and McGregor, Newman, Reilly, and Capone (2002), children were asked to name a set of pictures to assess naming accuracy and then were subsequently asked to draw pictures of the target words and to define the target words. A group of adults rated pictures and definitions for quality and quantity of information, respectively. The results showed that for both groups of children, when they produced naming errors on target words, the corresponding drawings and definitions of those words were weak. Specifically, drawings were rated as poor in quality and definitions contained fewer pieces of semantic information than did drawings and definitions of accurately named targets. Drawings and definitions of accurately named targets contained more information in both drawings and definitions, indicating richer representations of these words. In summary, richer semantic knowledge was associated with accurate word retrieval for naming, while weaker semantic knowledge was associated with naming errors.

Experience with words is a key factor in creating a richer lexical–semantic network. Having more experience with certain words can lead to retrieval of them despite other factors that are often associated with expressive word use, such as older age and higher IQ (Bjorklund, 1987). Experience can be enriched via quantity (or frequency) of experience or via quality of each experience (e.g., through scaffolding). For example, in the Gershkoff-Stowe (2002) study discussed earlier, frequency of experience was manipulated by increasing practice in saying words; this extra practice had a positive effect on retrieving words for naming.

Capone and McGregor (2005) examined the influence of enriched quality of semantic learning for its effect on word retrieval. In their study, the frequency of word exposure was controlled but the semantic representation was enriched via representational gesture cues.

Frequency of word exposure was controlled by ensuring that the training objects and words were novel and the objects were labeled the same number of times in each condition. Semantic enrichment varied by three conditions: *shape*, *function*, and *control*. In the shape condition, toddlers heard the word label and also saw a gesture that highlighted the shape of the object. In the function condition, toddlers heard the word label and also saw a gesture that highlighted the function of the object. In the control condition, no gesture cues accompanied the word label. By the study's end, toddlers had learned the same number of words under all three learning conditions, but the quality of learning differed by condition. Toddlers retrieved more words for naming when semantic enrichment (shape, function) was provided than when words were learned without it (control). Indeed, when semantic learning was assessed, toddlers knew more about the objects in the shape and function conditions than in the control condition.

WORKING MEMORY

Our discussion thus far has largely referred to learning and retrieving words within the long-term memory system. Long-term memory is where information is stored after learning. Another memory system, known as working memory (Baddeley, 2000; Baddeley & Hitch, 1974), also plays a key role in word learning. The working memory system is involved in active, online processing of information; it allows for temporary storage of information while it is being manipulated or processed. Working memory has a limited capacity of resources to process information, so there is always a trade-off in terms of where those resources are being directed. For example, when the child sees an unknown referent and hears a novel word, she engages in a process of linking the word to the referent, but also fast-maps phonological and semantic information and integrates the entire picture with what she already knows (i.e., information from long-term memory). This kind of processing is termed *online processing*. Working memory is the system that allows us to process information online. It is the system used to make sense of new information and to integrate new information with known information stored in long-term memory.

Several distinct components constitute the working memory system. First, two workspaces process visual and verbal information. The workspace for verbal information, which is called the *phonological loop*, encodes, maintains, and manipulates speech-based input. The second workspace, called the *visuo-spatial sketchpad*, manipulates visual information for visual recognition and orientation of stimuli. These two subsystems compete for the limited processing resources available in the working memory system. The third component of the system, known as the *central executor*, acts as the overseer. It maximizes the processing of visuo-spatial and phonological information by allocating processing resources to one or the other of the two workspaces or by splitting the resources between the two. The central executor modulates attention to each type of information. A fourth component of the working memory system, the *episodic buffer*, provides a place for integration of information to occur after the initial processing. It allows temporary representations to be integrated (new and old information) prior to that final integrated representation being sent on for storage in long-term memory (Baddeley, 2000).

The integrity of the phonological loop is critical for vocabulary development (Gathercole & Baddeley, 1989, 1990; Gathercole, Willis, Emslie, & Baddeley, 1992; Jarrod & Baddeley, 1997). For example, Gathercole and Baddeley (1989) showed that the size of a child's receptive vocabulary was positively related to his ability to remember phonological information. Four- and five-year-olds were better at repeating nonwords when they had larger, rather than smaller, vocabularies. A child's performance accuracy in nonword repetition is a common measure of integrity of the phonological loop. Of course, all new words to the child are nonwords initially until they make a connection with their referents; therefore, nonword repetition is a good measure of the phonological loop's capacity for processing new words. Gathercole, Willis, Emslie, and Baddely (1992) identified the same relationship between the integrity of the phonological loop and vocabulary development in children four to eight years of age. Conversely, children with language learning impairments (e.g., SLI, Down syndrome) have been found to have poor nonword repetition and smaller vocabularies than typically developing children (Gathercole & Baddeley, 1990; Jarrod & Baddeley (1997). Therefore, the relationship is the same: Good nonword repeaters have larger vocabularies and poor nonword repeaters have smaller vocabularies.

To date, little research has focused on the integrity of the visuo-spatial sketchpad and vocabulary development. Jarrod and Baddeley (1997) found that children with Down syndrome showed a relative strength in tasks that required processing of visual information (visuo-spatial sketchpad measure) when compared to tasks requiring processing of verbal information (phonological loop).

LATER LEXICAL DEVELOPMENT

Word learning continues across the life span (Nippold, 2007). During the first half of the second year, the infant's vocabulary consists largely of nouns. As he passes into toddlerhood, the child's verb vocabulary expands. The size of other word classes grows as the child moves through the preschool years and beyond (e.g., spatial terms, temporal terms, pronouns, conjunctions). As the child enrolls in school, word learning opportunities shift from oral to written. The school-age child begins to learn many new vocabulary items via academic and social readings. Again, the child relies largely on inferences from the context that surrounds new words to glean their meanings. There is also some more direct teaching through instructors and text reading. For example, definitions are stated explicitly for some words.

One of the most significant accomplishments for the child from preschool to school age and into adolescence and adulthood is the ability to learn and use more abstract language. The child develops a flexibility in understanding that words can have multiple meanings and that sometimes these meanings are concrete (e.g., *cold* refers to temperature), and sometimes they are more abstract (e.g., *cold* refers to a person's temperament). More concrete meanings are learned first, in the preschool years; later, the psychological and abstract meanings are acquired. Also, the child expands the type of lexical items learned by including figurative language (e.g., metaphors, idioms, slang terms). Metaphors, idioms, and slang terms are extensions of lexical development. For example, idioms (e.g., *It's raining cats and dogs*) are believed to function as a single word. These constructs convey a single meaning that differs from the meaning that the words convey in isolation. Children's understanding of figurative language follows its own developmental course, with literal meanings being learned earlier (preschool and early school age) and figurative meanings being acquired later as the child moves through middle school, adolescence, and adulthood. Mastery of figurative language is essential for social and academic success. For example, humorous play on words is often a device used in advertising. Even in adulthood, however, performance on figurative language tasks does not reach a ceiling of 100% accuracy. Therefore, lexical acquisition and figurative language use are life-long in their development.

SUMMARY

Word learning is a lifelong, complex, and dynamic process. The child comes equipped with certain tools (i.e., biases) to help him jump into the word learning system; many scaffolds are also available for the child in the environment (e.g., gestures). The child readily takes advantage of these aids. The child spends a full year preparing for his first word. Although word learning is slow to start, by toddlerhood the child is a word-learning machine.

The early lexicon largely consists of nouns. As the child moves through toddlerhood and into the preschool years, however, vocabulary expands to include many other word classes, including verbs, prepositions, pronouns, conjunctions, and adjectives. The lexicon also expands to include words with multiple and figurative meanings, as well as larger language units that function as a single lexical item.

The process of learning a single word is an extended process that moves from an initial fast mapping to a longer period of slow mapping that enriches the lexical and semantic representation of the word. The richness of lexical–semantic representation is related to the likelihood of whether the child will retrieve that word from memory. Speech-language intervention provides the child with increased frequency and richer quality of word learning experiences, thereby narrowing the gap between a child with language impairments and his typically developing peers.

KEY TERMS

Action words

Basic-level terms

Central executor

Decontextualize

Emergentist coalition model

Expressive children

Distributed neural network

Episodic buffer

Fast mapping

Function words

Functional core hypothesis

General nominals

Hierarchical organization of the lexicon

Indeterminate errors/responses

Innate biases

Late bloomers

Late talkers

Lexeme

Lexical representation

Lexical–semantic network

Modifiers

Naming explosion

Naming insight

Natural partitions hypothesis

Nominal insight

Novel name–nameless category principle (N3C)

Ordering of word classes

Ordinate terms

Overextension

Perseverative errors

Personal–social words

Phonetically consistent form (PCF)

Phonological errors

Phonological loop

Prelexical forms

Principle of conventionality

Principle of extendibility

Principle of mutual exclusivity

Principles of word learning

Principle of reference

Protowords

Quick incidental learning (QUIL)

Referential children

Semantic errors

Semantic representation

Slow mapping

Semantic feature hypothesis

Sensorimotor morphemes

Shape bias

Specific nominals

Subordinate terms

Superordinate terms

Underextension

Visual misperception errors

Visuo-spatial sketchpad

Vocabulary spurt

Whole-object bias

Word learning constraints

Word retrieval errors

Word spurt

Working memory

STUDY QUESTIONS

- What are the precursor speech-language behaviors to first words observed in the infant?
- Describe lexical development from first words to two-word combinations, including the word class that predominates in this early lexicon.
- What is the word spurt? How does naming accuracy (word retrieval) change from pre- to post-word spurt?
- Define the principles of word learning, and explain how they aid the young child in learning words.
- Compare and contrast fast mapping and slow mapping of words.
- What is the effect of how richly a word is represented on retrieval of the lexeme?
- Describe the emergentist coalition model of word learning.
- Describe working memory, and explain how it relates to word learning.

REFERENCES

Baddeley, A. (2000). The episodic buffer: A new component of working memory? *Trends in Cognitive Sciences, 4*(11), 417–423.

Baddeley, A. D., & Hitch, G. J. (1974). *Working memory*. In G. Bower (Ed.), *The psychology of learning and motivation* (Vol. 8, pp. 47–90). New York: Academic Press.

Balaban, M. T., & Waxman, S. R. (1997). Do words facilitate object categorization in 9-month-old infants? *Journal of Experimental Child Psychology, 64*(1), 3–26.

Barsalou, L. W. (1999a). Perceptual symbol systems. *Behavioral and Brain Sciences, 22,* 577–660.

Barsalou, L. W. (1999b). Language comprehension: archival memory or preparation for situated action? *Discourse Processes, 28*(1), 61–80.

Bates, E. (1976). *Language in context: The acquisition of pragmatics*. New York: Academic Press.

Bates, E., Bretherton, I., & Snyder, L. (1988). *From first words to grammar: Individual differences and dissociable mechanisms*. New York: Cambridge University Press.

Bates, E., Marchman, V., Thal, D., et al. (1994). Developmental and stylistic variation in the coposition of early vocabulary. *Journal of Child Language, 21,* 85–123.

Bjorklund, D. F. (1987). How age changes in knowledge base contribute to the development of children's memory: An interpretive review. *Developmental Review, 7,* 93–130.

Bloom, L. (1973). *One word at a time*. The Hague: Mouton.

Bloom, L., & Capatides, B. (1987). Expression of affect and the emergence of language. *Child Development, 58,* 1513–1522.

Bloom, P. (2004). Myths of word learning. In G. Hall & S. Waxman (Eds.), *Weaving a lexicon* (pp. 205–224). Cambridge, MA: MIT Press.

Booth, A. E., & Waxman, S. R. (2002). Object names and object functions serve as cues to categories for infants. *Developmental Psychology, 38*(6), 948–957.

Bruner, J. (1975). The ontogenesis of speech acts. *Journal of Child Language, 2,* 1–19.

Capone, N. C., & McGregor, K. K. (2005). The effect of semantic representation on toddlers' word retrieval. *Journal of Speech, Language, and Hearing Research, 48*, 1468–1480.

Carey, S. (1978). The child as word learner. In M. Halle, J. Bresnan, & G. A. Miller (Eds.), *Linguistic theory and psychological reality* (pp. 264–293). Cambridge, MA: MIT Press.

Caselli, M. C., Bates, E., Casadio, P., et al. (1995). A cross-linguistic study of early lexical development. *Cognitive Development, 10*(2), 159–199.

Clark, E. (1973). What's in a word? On the child's acquisition of semantics in his first language. In T. Moore (Ed.), *Cognitive development and the acquisition of language* (pp. 65–110). New York: Academic Press.

Clark, E. (1975). Knowledge, context and strategy in the acquisition of meaning. In D. Dato (Ed.), *Developmental psycholinguistics: Theory and application*. Washington, DC: Georgetown University Press.

Clark, E. (1993). *The lexicon in acquisition*. Cambridge, England: Cambridge University Press.

de Boysson-Bardes, B., & Vihman, M. (1991). Adaptation to language: Evidence from babbling and first words in four languages. *Language, 67*, 297–319.

Dell, G. S. (1990). Effects of frequency and vocabulary type on phonological speech errors. *Language and Cognitive Processes, 5*, 313–349.

Dell, G. S., Reed, K. D., Adams, D. R., & Meyer, A. S. (2000). Speech errors, phonotactic constraints, and implicit learning: A study of the role of experience in language production. *Journal of Experimental Psychology, 26*(6), 1355–1367.

Dore, J., Franklin, M., Miller, R., & Ramer, A. (1976). Transitional phenomena in early language acquisition. *Journal of Child Language, 3*, 13–28.

Gathercole, S. E., & Baddeley, A. D. (1989). Evaluation of the role of phonological STM in the development of vocabulary in children: A longitudinal study. *Journal of Memory and Language, 28*, 200–213.

Gathercole, S. E., & Baddeley, A. D. (1990). Phonological memory deficits in language disordered children: Is there a causal connection. *Journal of Memory and Language, 29*, 336–360.

Gathercole, S. E., Willis, C. S., Emslie, H., & Baddeley, A. D. (1992). Phonological memory and vocabulary development during the early school years: A longitudinal study. *Developmental Psychology, 28*(5), 887–898.

Gentner, D. (1982). Why nouns are learned before verbs: Linguistic relativity versus natural partitioning. In S. Kuczaf (Ed.), *Language development: Volume 2: Language, thought and culture.* (pp. 301–334) Hillsdale, NJ: Lawrence Erlbaum.

Gentner, D. (2006). Why verbs are hard to learn. In K. Hirsh-Pasek & R. M. Golinkoff (Eds.), *Action meets word: How children learn verbs* (pp. 544–564). New York: Oxford University Press.

Gershkoff-Stowe, L. (2001). The course of children's naming errors in early word learning. *Journal of Cognition and Development, 2*(2), 131–155.

Gershkoff-Stowe, L. (2002). Object naming, vocabulary growth, and the development of word retrieval abilities. *Journal of Memory and Language, 46*, 665–687.

Gershkoff-Stowe, L., & Smith, L. B. (1997). A curvilinear trend in naming errors as a function of early vocabulary growth. *Cognitive Psychology, 34*, 37–71.

Gershkoff-Stowe, L., & Smith, L. B. (2004). Shape and the first hundred nouns. *Child Development, 75*(4), 1098–1174.

Goldfield, B. (1986). Referential and expressive language: A study of two mother–child dyads. *First Language, 6*, 119–131.

Goldfield, B. (1987). The contributions of child and caregiver to referential and expressive language. *Applied Psycholinguistics, 8*, 267–280.

Goldfield, B. (1993). Noun bias in maternal speech to one year olds. *Journal of Child Language, 20*, 85–99.

Goldfield, B. A., & Reznick, J. S. (1990). Early lexical acquisition: Rate, content and the vocabulary spurt. *Journal of Child Language, 17*, 171–283.

Golinkoff, R. M., & Hirsh-Pasek, K. (2006). Baby wordsmith: From associationist to social sophisticate. *Current Directions in Psychological Science, 15*(1), 30–33.

Golinkoff, R. M., Mervis, C. V., & Hirsh-Pasek, K. (1994). Early object labels: The case for a developmental lexical principles framework. *Journal of Child Language, 21*, 125–155.

Gopnik, A., & Meltzoff, A. (1986). Relations between semantic and cognitive development in the one word stage: The specificity hypothesis. *Child Development, 57*, 1040–1053.

Halliday, M. (1975). *Learning how to mean.* New York: Elsevier.

Hollich, G. J., Hirsh-Pasek, K., Golinkoff, R. M., et al. (2000). Breaking the language barrier: An emergentist coalition model for the origins of word learning. *Monographs of the Society for Research in Child Development, 65*(3).

Horgan, D. (1978). How to answer questions when you've got nothing to say. *Journal of Child Language, 5*, 159–165.

Horgan, D. (1979). *Nouns: Love 'em or leave 'em.* Address to the New York Academy of Sciences.

Jarrod, C., & Baddeley, A. D. (1997). Short-term memory for verbal and visuospatial information in Down's syndrome. *Cognitive Neuropsychiatry, 2*(2), 101–122.

Jones, S. S. (2003). Late talkers show no shape bias in a novel name extension task. *Developmental Science, 6*(5), 477–483.

Jones, S. S., Smith, L. B., & Landau, B. (1991). Object properties and knowledge in early lexical learning. *Child Development, 62*, 499–516.

Kamhi, A. (1988). Three popular myths about language development. *Child Language Teaching and Therapy, 4*(1), 1–12.

Kemler Nelson, D. G. (1999). Attention to functional properties in toddlers' naming and problem solving. *Cognitive Development, 14*, 77–100.

Kim, M., McGregor, K. K., & Thompson, C. K. (2000). Early lexical development in English- and Korean-speaking children: Language-general and language-specific patterns. *Journal of Child Language, 27*(2), 225–254.

Lahey, M., & Edwards, J. (1999). Naming errors of children with specific language impairment. *Journal of Speech, Language, and Hearing Research, 42*(1), 195–205.

Landau, B., Smith, L. B., & Jones, S. S. (1988). The importance of shape in early lexical learning. *Cognitive Development, 3*, 299–321.

Marchman, V. A., & Bates, E. (1994). Continuity in lexical and morphological development: A test of the critical mass hypothesis. *Journal of Child Language, 21*(2), 339–366.

Markman, E. M. (1989). *Categorization and naming in children: Problems in induction.* Cambridge, MA: MIT Press.

McGregor, K. K. (1997). The nature of word-finding errors of preschoolers with and without word-finding deficits. *Journal of Speech and Hearing Research, 40*(6), 1232–1244.

McGregor, K. K., & Appel, A. (2002). On the relation between mental representation and naming in a child with specific language impairment. *Clinical Linguistics and Phonetics, 16*(1), 1–20.

McGregor, K. K., Friedman, R. M., Reilly, R. M., & Newman, R. M. (2002) Semantic representation and naming in young children. *Journal of Speech, Language, and Hearing Research, 45*(2), 332–346.

McGregor, K. K., Newman, R. M., Reilly, R. M., & Capone, N. C. (2002) Semantic representation and naming in children with specific language impairment. *Journal of Speech, Language, and Hearing Research*, 45(5), 998–1014.

Nelson, K. (1973). Structure and strategy in learning to talk. *Monographs of the Society for Research in Child Development*, 143(38).

Nelson, K. (1974). Concept, word, and sentence: Interrelations in acquisition and development. *Psychological Review, 81*, 267–285.

Nelson, K. (1981). Individual differences in language development: Implications for development and language. *Developmental Psychology, 17*, 170–187.

Nelson, K., Hampson, J., & Shaw, L. K. (1993). Nouns in early lexicons: Evidence, explanations and implications: Erratum. *Journal of Child Language, 20*(2), 228.

Nelson, K., & Lucarielly, J. (1985). The development of meaning in first words. In M. Barrett (Ed.), *Children's single word speech* (p. 13). Chichester, UK: John Wiley and Sons.

Nippold, M. A. (2007). *Later language development: School-age children, adolescents, and young adults,* 3rd ed. Austin, TX: Pro-Ed.

Oetting, J., Rice, M., & Swank, L. (1995). Quick incidental learning (QUIL) of words by school-age children with and without SLI. *Journal of Speech and Hearing Research, 38*, 434–445.

Owens, R. (1988). *Language development: An introduction.* Boston: Allyn and Bacon.

Plunkett, K., Karmiloff-Smith, A., Bates, E., Elman, J. L., & Johnson, M. H. (1997). Connectionism and developmental psychology. *Journal of Child Psychological Psychiatry, 38*(1), 53–80.

Plunkett, K., Sinha, C., Moller, M. F., & Strandsby, O. (1992). Symbol grounding or the emergence of symbols? Vocabulary growth in children and a connectionist net. *Connection Science, Special Issue: Philosophical Issues in Connectionist Modeling,* 293–312.

Ramer, A. (1976). Syntactic styles in emerging language. *Journal of Child Language, 3*, 49–62.

Rescorla, L., Dahlsgaard, K., & Roberts, J. (2000). Late-talking toddlers: MLU and IPSyn outcomes at 3;0 and 4;0. *Journal of Child Language, 27*(3), 643–664.

Rescorla, L, Mirak, J., & Singh, L. (2000). Vocabulary growth in late talkers: Lexical development from 2;0 to 3;0. *Journal of Child Language, 27*(2), 293–311.

Retherford, K. (2000). *Guide to analysis of language transcripts,* 3rd ed. Eau Claire, WI: Thinking Publications.

Rice, M. L., Buhr, J. C., & Nemeth, M. (1990). Fast mapping word learning abilities of language-delayed preschoolers. *Journal of Speech and Hearing Disorders, 55*, 33–42.

Rice, M. L., Buhr, J. C., & Oetting, J. B. (1992). Specific-language-impaired children's quick incidental learning of words: The effect of a pause. *Journal of Speech and Hearing Research, 35*, 1040–1048.

Snyder, L., Bates, E., & Bretherton, I. (1981). Content and context in early lexical development. *Journal of Child Language, 8*, 565–582.

Stoel-Gammon, C., & Cooper, J. (1984). Patterns of early lexical and phonological development. *Journal of Child Language, 11*, 247–271.

Storkel, H. (2001) Learning new words: Phonotactic probability in language development. *Journal of Speech, Language, and Hearing Research, 44*(6), 1321–1337.

Thal, D., & Tobias, S. (1994). Relationships between language and gesture in normally developing and late-talking toddlers. *Journal of Speech and Hearing Research, 37*, 157–170.

Thal, D., Tobias, S., & Morrison, D. (1991). Language and gesture in late talkers: A one-year follow-up. *Journal of Speech and Hearing Research, 34*, 604–612.

Vihman, M. (1996). *Phonological development: The origins of language in the child.* Oxford, UK: Basil Blackwell.

Vihman, M., Macken, M., Miller, R., Simmmons, H., & Miller, J. (1985). From babbling to speech: A reassessment of the continuity issue. *Language, 61,* 397–445.

Waxman, S. R. (1994). The development of an appreciation of specific linkages between linguistic and conceptual organization. *Lingua, 92,* 229–257.

Werner, H., & Kaplan, B. (1963). *Symbol formation.* New York: John Wiley & Sons.

CHAPTER 8

Speech Sound Disorders: An Overview of Acquisition, Assessment, and Treatment

Lynn K. Flahive, MS, and Barbara W. Hodson, PhD

OBJECTIVES

- To demonstrate basic knowledge and skills in the area of speech sound disorders
- To differentiate the parts of the speech mechanism and describe their purposes
- To identify and categorize the phonemes, noting differences based on place, manner, and voicing as well as ages of acquisition
- To identify phonological deviations in children's speech productions
- To specify goals of an evaluation to assess a child for a possible speech sound disorder
- To write goals and procedures for a lesson plan for a child with highly unintelligible speech

INTRODUCTION

The term *speech sound disorders* refers to problems in producing the sounds of a language. The terms *articulation, phonology,* and *apraxia* are also used for these errors, but the American Speech-Language-Hearing Association (ASHA) has recommended using the term *speech sound disorders* to cover all of these disorders. As noted by Prezas and Hodson (2007), the term *articulation*, which refers to the process of producing speech sounds, is often used in conjunction with a child who has difficulty with only a few sounds. Children with a *phonological impairment* demonstrate problems with the sound system of language such that they have difficulties that involve more than one sound in a pattern. A child who omits an /s/ when it is part of cluster (e.g. *smoke* → /mok/) is said to have a phonological impairment. *Childhood apraxia of speech* (CAS) refers to problems with motor planning. Criteria for differentiating CAS from other speech sound disorders are generally lacking.

Although these terms are often used interchangeably, an articulation problem generally is mild to moderate in severity, and the child typically is understood most of the time. By comparison, children with disordered phonological systems and apraxia tend to have highly unintelligible speech and would be considered to have a severe to profound disorder. ASHA (2008) reports that 80% of children diagnosed with a speech sound disorder have a condition severe enough to warrant intervention.

Several different approaches to addressing speech sound disorders are possible. For example, one can examine the structures of the speech mechanism for muscle weakness, incoordination, or motor problems. One can also look for signs of CAS. Alternatively, one can address speech sound errors through the use of oral motor exercises.

Although all of these approaches are currently used, this chapter focuses on phonology—that is, the sound system of language. It includes the study of (1) syllable/word shapes/structures, (2) phonemes and allophones, and (3) prosody/suprasegmentals (Hodson, 2007). Phonological substitutions tend to show regularity in the language of children past the earliest stage of lexical acquisition (Bernthal & Bankson, 2004). The remediation process focuses on reorganizing the child's phonological system by helping the child learn to produce and acquire phonological patterns.

This chapter provides an overview of speech, including how it is produced. The sounds of English are explored, and general stages of development are reviewed. Regardless of which approach a speech-language pathologist (SLP) uses, this information is always needed for working with young children with speech sound disorders. Phonological patterns are described, and their importance in assessing and treating young children are explored. Although treatment for speech sound disorders may utilize a motor-based approach, a linguistic approach, or a combination of the two, this chapter focuses mostly on linguistic or phonologically based approaches.

THE SPEECH MECHANISM

Six major organs/subsystems are used in the production of speech. The respiratory system is where the air flow is generated. It includes the lungs, airways, ribcage, and diaphragm. The diaphragm is the chief muscle of inhalation. Speech begins here when the diaphragm pushes air through the respiratory system and into the airway. Air is then pushed through the thoracic cavity, past the trachea, to the larynx.

The larynx, often referred to as the 'voice box,' is composed of various cartilages and muscles. It is the chief structure for the production of sound. The vocal folds (or vocal cords) are found in the larynx. If the vocal folds vibrate as air flows through them, the sound is voiced. If the vocal folds remain open and do not vibrate, the sound produced is voiceless.

The air stream then enters the velopharyngeal area, which contains the velum, also known as the soft palate. This area separates the oral and nasal cavities. Thus air may go through the nasal cavity, through the oral cavity, or both. Nasal sounds are produced in the nasal cavity. The oral cavity contains the articulators. The tongue, which is the major articulator, is composed of muscles and can be divided into five parts: tip (apex), blade, back (dorsum), root, and body. After the air flows over the tongue, it crosses the jaws and lips. The lips are the most visible articulators. The jaws are bony structures that support the tissues of the tongue and lips.

PHONEMES

A *phoneme* is the smallest arbitrary unit of sound in a given language that can be recognized as being distinct from other sounds in the language (Nicolosi, Harryman, & Kresheck, 1996). Phonemes are the sounds of a language that combine to form words. American English has 44 symbols that are denoted in the International Phonetic Alphabet (IPA). English phonemes are divided into *consonants* and *vowels*. **Table 8-1** lists the phonemes with examples of each.

The position of the consonant in the word is described by the terms *initial, medial,* and *final.* When a consonant is described by its position in a word relative to the vowel, the terms *prevocalic, intervocalic,* and *postvocalic* are used. If the consonant is at the beginning of the word (e.g., *nose*), it is in the initial position. This can also be considered prevocalic because it precedes the vowel. Consonants that occur in the middle of a word are in the medial position. If the consonant is between two vowels (e.g., *bunny*), it is also referred to as intervocalic. Consonants that are the last sound in a word are said to be in the final position. If the consonant also follows a vowel in the word final position, it is postvocalic (e.g., *can*).

The 24 consonants of American English are typically described by their place, manner, and voicing. *Manner* refers to what happens to the air flow through the resonatory and articulatory systems (Scherz & Edwards, 2007). Consonants that involve some type of constriction of the air flow are *obstruents,* which include stops, fricatives, and affricates. *Sonorants,* which include nasals, glides, and liquids, are made with a relatively open vocal tract. When a complete closure of the vocal tract occurs at some point so that there is no air flow, thereby allowing for pressure to build and then be released, the sound is considered to be a *stop.* Stops /p, b, t, d, k, g/ are sometimes called plosives or stop-plosives. *Fricatives,* which include /f, v, s, z, ʃ, tʃ, θ, ð, h/, are noisy sounds caused by a turbulent air flow as the air stream goes through a narrow constriction. *Affricates* /tʃ, dʒ/ include two components: a stop and a fricative release. The sound begins with a stop and then ends with the air stream going through a narrow constriction.

The *nasals* /m, n, ŋ / are sounds in which the air flow goes through the nasal cavity. The *glides* /w, j/ are sometimes referred to as semivowels because of the relatively open vocal tract during production. *Liquids* /l, r/ are similar to glides, but have a bit more vocal tract obstruction than the glides or vowels. The only lateral sound in American English is /l/; the air flow goes over the sides of the tongue with an opening near the middle. The /r/ can be produced in

TABLE 8-1	Phonemes			
Phoneme	**Key Word**	**Place**	**Manner**	**Voicing**
/p/	*p*ie	bilabial	stop	voiceless
/b/	*b*ook	bilabial	stop	voiced
/t/	*t*ype	alveolar	stop	voiceless
/d/	*d*og	alveolar	stop	voiced
/k/	*c*ape	velar	stop	voiceless
/g/	*g*o	velar	stop	voiced
/f/	*f*ace	labiodental	fricative	voiceless
/v/	*v*ote	labiodental	fricative	voiced
/θ/	*th*umb	interdental	fricative	voiceless
/ð/	*th*em	interdental	fricative	voiced
/s/	*s*un	alveolar	fricative	voiceless
/z/	*z*oo	alveolar	fricative	voiced
/ʃ/	*sh*oe	palatal	fricative	voiceless
/ʒ/	trea*s*ure	palatal	fricative	voiced
/tʃ/	*ch*ip	palatal	affricative	voiceless
/dʒ/	*j*ump	palatal	affricative	voiced
/l/	*l*ip	alveolar	liquid	voiced
/r/	*r*un	palatal	liquid	voiced
/m/	*m*ap	bilabial	nasal	voiced
/n/	*n*ose	alveolar	nasal	voiced
/ŋ/	wi*ng*	velar	nasal	voiced
/w/	*w*in	bilabial	glide	voiced
/j/	*y*es	palatal	glide	voiced
/h/	*h*at	glottal	fricative	voiceless

many different ways (Secord, Boyce, Donohue, Fox, & Shine, 2007). A retroflex or rhoticized /r/ has the tongue tip curled back and up near the palate. The other major position involves bunching of the tongue near the palate.

When discussing manner, the terms *sibilants* and *stridents* also are useful. Sibilants, which include /s, z, ʃ, ʒ, tʃ, dʒ/, are consonants where the air stream going through the constriction produces a hissing sound. Strident sounds, which are created when the air stream hits the back of the teeth, include /f/ and /v/, as well as sibilants.

Consonants also may be described by noting which articulators are used to produce the sound. Typically, the place of articulation is the location along the vocal tract where the air stream constriction occurs. *Bilabials* /p, b, m, w/ are produced by the two lips coming together or by lip rounding. *Labiodentals* /f, v/ are created by the lower edge of the upper incisors coming into contact with the upper edge of the lower lip, thereby creating a slight constriction in the air flow. *Interdentals* are formed when a slight protrusion of the tongue tip touches the edges of the upper incisors, which creates a slight constriction over the tongue tip.

Alveolars /t, d, s, z, l, n/ involve constriction created by the tongue tip coming into contact with the alveolar ridge. Interestingly, alveolars are the sounds most frequently produced (50%) in American English, with /n/ being the most commonly occurring of the alveolars (Shriberg & Kwiatkowski, 1983). *Palatals* /ʃ, ʒ, tʃ, dʒ, r, j/ are formed when some part of the tongue comes into contact with the hard palate, typically with the contact occurring behind the alveolar ridge. The *velars* /k, g, ŋ/ are made by elevating the back of the tongue to the soft palate. The *glottal* /h/ is created by a partial opening of the vocal folds.

Besides describing the place and manner by which the sound is formed, consonants may also be designated as voiced or voiceless. This characteristic is based on the movement of vocal folds. If the vocal folds are vibrating during a sound production, it is *voiced*. Voiced sounds include /b, d, g, ð, z, v, ʒ, dʒ, m, n, ŋ, l, r, w, j/. When the vocal folds are not vibrating during production, the sound is said to be *voiceless* (i.e., /p, t, k, θ, s, f, ʃ, tʃ, h/). Sounds in the English language that vary only in terms of voicing are referred to as *cognates* (e.g., /p, b/).

Vowels are the other group of sounds in the English language. There are 12 vowels. During their production, the tongue typically does not come in contact with any of the other articulators. Vowels are always voiced and typically are not nasalized. Additionally, they are created with a relatively open vocal tract and have no point of constriction. Thus vowels are sonorants. Vowels can be described by identifying where the tongue is in relation to the palate using the terms *high, mid,* or *low.* They are also described by whether the tongue is near the front, middle (central), or back of the mouth. Finally, vowels may be distinguished as either lax or tense. *Lax* vowels are shorter in duration, indicating they are produced with less muscle effort. *Tense* (long) vowels have a longer duration and require more effort to produce.

Diphthongs are formed when two vowels are blended together, creating a change in the vocal tract (e.g., ɔɪ). Although a diphthong incorporates two vowels, it is only one phoneme.

All syllables must have a vowel, diphthong, or a vocalic/syllabic consonant to form the nucleus. Vowels are sometimes referred to as *syllabics* because they are necessary for syllable formation. Typically, a consonant combines with a vowel to make a syllable. When a syllable ends with a vowel (e.g., CV), it is an *open syllable*. If the syllable ends with a consonant (e.g., VC, CVC), it is a *closed syllable*.

SPEECH SOUND SYSTEM DEVELOPMENT

To determine the age of acquisition of the sounds of language, researchers use two different methodologies. In a *cross-sectional study*, which is the type of investigation often carried out by speech-language pathologists, children of different ages are tested on their abilities to produce speech sounds at a given point in time. *Longitudinal studies* involve testing children's productions over time. Comparing the results of the various studies can be difficult because various levels of mastery and means of eliciting responses have been used by different researchers. In some studies, a child needed to produce a sound correctly 100% of the time; in others, the criterion was 75%. Words were produced spontaneously in some studies, but were imitated in others. To further complicate the situation, different researchers required the mastery level to be met in all three positions, whereas others were concerned only with the initial and final positions.

Despite the variability in criteria, researchers have reached some general agreement about the progression in which individual sounds are acquired (see **Figure 8-1**). Nasals /m, n, ŋ/, stops /p, b, t, d, k, g/ and glides /w, j/ are acquired earliest, followed by the fricatives /f, v, θ, ð, s, z, ʃ, ʒ/, affricates / ʧ, ʤ/, and then the liquids /l, r/ (Sander, 1972). Sander's analysis of previous studies also noted that /θ, ð, ʒ/ were generally the latest phonemes to be acquired (Sander, 1972).

ACQUISITION

Prelinguistic Stages

The *prelinguistic stage* includes the time before the child's first true word. The early skills demonstrated in this stage—speech perception, infant speech production, and the transition from babbling to meaningful speech—lay the foundation for phonological development (Kelman, 2007).

Speech perception is the identification of phonemes—that is, the vowels and consonants of language—largely from acoustic cues, and the recognition of phonemes in combination as a word (Nicolosi, Harryman, & Kresheck, 1996). Being able to perceive the differences in speech sounds is critical to comprehending and developing language and is an essential precursor to speech production. Speech scientists have hypothesized that babies come 'prewired' to perceive minimal differences in speech sounds (Kelman, 2007). This ability occurs across languages. To acquire a given language, the child's brain must differentiate her language from the others. The

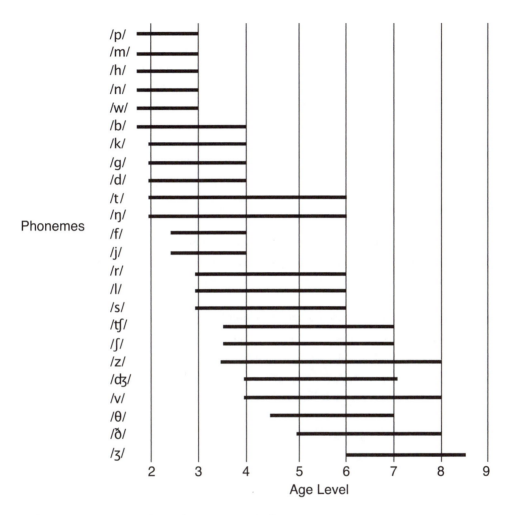

FIGURE 8-1   Ages at which phonemes typically occur.
Source: Sander, E. (1972).

sounds a child hears frequently become strengthened and are established as the basis for the individual's language (Cheour et al., 1998).

At birth, infants cry and soon make a variety of vocalizations that eventually become strings of consonant–vowel syllables. These vocalizations, which eventually resemble adult-like timing and intonation patterns, fall into two general categories: reflexive and nonreflexive vocalizations. *Reflexive vocalizations* include cries, coughs, and hiccups. *Nonreflexive vocalizations* are the sounds that eventually will be shaped into the adult form of words (Oller, 1980).

Oller's work serves as the basis for the establishment of the prelinguistic stages of vocalizations. He found that, regardless of the linguistic community in which they reside, all infants go through the same stages of vocal development. Although a certain time frame is identified for each stage in the following sections, it should be noted that these stages are not definitive; rather, they tend to be fluid and overlap.

Stage 1: Phonation Stage (birth to 1 month)

During the phonation stage, the infant exhibits reflexive vocalizations such as crying, fussing, coughing, burping, and sneezing. These sounds are similar to syllabic nasals and vowels.

Stage 2: Coo and Goo Stage (2–3 months)

In the coo and goo stage, the productions are acoustically similar to back vowels or to syllables consisting of back vowels and consonants. They are considered primitive because of the immature timing of the vocalizations, and they are the precursors to consonants.

Stage 3: Exploration and Expansion Stage (4–6 months)

The exploration and expansion stage is one of vocal play in which the child's productions range from repetitions of vowel-like elements to squeals, growls, yells, "raspberries," and friction noises. The infant begins to produce some sequences of CV syllables in which the vowels have better oral resonance, are more adult-like, and are considered marginal babbling.

Stage 4: Canonical Babbling Stage (7–9 months)

In *canonical babbling*, also known as *reduplicated babbling*, the child's vocalizations become longer and consist of CV syllables whose timing closely approximates adult speech. It is not uncommon during this stage to hear the infant say [mɑmɑ], although there is no sound-to-meaning relationship. At this time, the infant commonly uses stops, nasals, and glides, as well as lax vowels.

Stage 5: Variegated Babbling Stage (10–12 months)

Although the use of CV sequences continues in the variegated babbling stage, a greater variety of consonants and vowels is used (e.g., [dubaməa]). At this point, the child's utterances take on adult-like intonation patterns, especially as the child approaches the first birthday. The consonant and vowel inventories increase dramatically during this stage.

Later Stages

As children approach their first birthday, they begin the transition from babbling to meaningful speech, referred to as the *first word stage*. The first word appears around 12 months. By age 15 months, the child typically has a 15-word vocabulary. During this time, the child produces whole units rather than sequences of sounds. The first word stage continues until approximately 18 months. During this phase of development, the child has a rapidly increasing vocabulary and is developing a systematic relationship between the adult model and the child's pronunciation (Stoel-Gammon & Dunn, 1985).

It is also at this time that a child will use *protowords*, which are well-defined, meaningful sound patterns produced by young children that apparently are not modeled on any adult words (Nicolosi, Harryman, & Kresheck, 1996). Protowords are not considered to be the first "true" words, but rather tend to be simple CV shapes that are not phonetically related to the adult form. An example is the child who says [mi] for his favorite blanket. The child's production of [mi] is used consistently to indicate he wants his blanket. Yet [mi] does not have any phonemic characteristics of the adult word, *blanket*. Protowords are the link between babbling and adult-like speech.

During the next stage of phonemic development, from 18 months to 4 years, the child's vocabulary of true words increases rapidly from approximately 50 words around 18 months to approximately 1000 words by 36 months (Fenson et al., 1991). It is at this time that syllabic structures become more complex, with multisyllabic productions and consonant clusters beginning to appear.

Porter and Hodson (2001) noted various steps of phonological acquisition that serve as a guide during this time. During the first period, at approximately 12 months of age, the child does canonical babbling and uses vocables. By 18 months, the child has recognizable words, produces CV structures, and produces stops, nasals, and glides. By age 2, the child uses final consonants, communicates with words, and has "syllableness." The 3-year-old's speech will show an expansion of his phonemic repertoire, including /s/ clusters (although distortions are common) and anterior–posterior contrasts. By age 4, omissions are rare, most simplifications are suppressed, and the child's speech sounds adult-like. The child's phonemic inventory stabilizes between 5 and 6 years of age. Liquids become consistent, with /l/ appearing at age 5 years and /r/ at 6 years. The final step, at approximately 7 years of age, has the sibilants and "th" perfected, such that the child has "adult standard" speech (Creaghead, Newman, & Secord, 1989).

Of importance during the stabilization process, at approximately 6 years of age, the child is introduced to two important skills: reading and writing. Development of these skills helps to provide an extension of the understanding of the phonemic nature of the sound system and can add another modality for enhancing the child's phonemic repertoire.

PHONOLOGICAL DEVIATIONS

Speech sounds also can be discussed in terms of phonological patterns, which are accepted groupings of sounds within an oral language (Hodson, 2007). Speech pattern errors have been referred to as *phonological processes* (Ingram, 1976) or *deviations* (Hodson, 2004, 2007). According to Grunwell (1982), the concept of phonological "processes" in the clinical assessment of a child's speech is applied primarily as a descriptive device that identifies or analyzes systematic patterns in a child's pronunciations by comparing it with the targeted adult model. Phonological deviations can be viewed in terms of omissions, major substitutions, major assimilations, and syllable-structure/context-related changes (Hodson, 2007).

Omissions

Omissions at the syllable level include simplification of the word to one syllable (e.g., *rabbit* → [ræ]). With weak syllable deletion, an unstressed syllable is omitted (e.g., *banana* → [nænə]). "Multisyllabicity" problems involve difficulty producing all the syllables and sounds in a multisyllabic word (e.g., *ambulance* → [æmsən]).

Singleton consonant omissions can occur at the end of a word or postvocalic (e.g., *bat* → [bæ]), in the middle of a word or intervocalic (e.g., *happy* → [hæ i]), or at the beginning of a word or prevocalic (e.g., *pot* → [ɑt]). Prevocalic singleton omissions are not common in children who speak English. By contrast, final consonant omissions are common in children with disordered phonological systems.

Omissions are frequently observed in consonant clusters/sequences. A *consonant sequence* consists of all contiguous consonants in a word (e.g., [θbr] as in too*thbr*ush), whereas a *consonant cluster* comprises adjacent consonants in the same syllable (e.g., [gr] as in *green*). Consonant cluster reduction indicates one consonant is omitted (e.g., *spoon* → [pun]). Consonant cluster deletion would denote the omission of all consonants in the cluster, (e.g., *tree* → [i]). Consonant cluster reductions are common in the speech of highly unintelligible children and often influence children's morphologies.

Substitutions

In *fronting*, a sound made at the back of the mouth is substituted by a sound produced in the front. For example, the word *cup* would become [tʌp]. Anterior consonants include /p, b, m, w, t, d, s, z, n, l, f, v, θ, ð/, and posterior consonants are /k, g, ŋ, h/.

Backing is the reverse of fronting. In backing, a sound made in the front of the mouth is replaced by a back or posterior sound. Thus the word *tie* would become [kaɪ]. It should be noted that this not a common deviation.

Stopping refers to the use of a stop /p, b, t, d, k, g/ for a "nonstop" consonant, such as a glide, fricative, liquid, or nasal. An example is *sun* being said as [tʌn].

Gliding is another substitution pattern where the /w/ or /j/ is used for another consonant, typically a liquid. For example, *light* would become [jaɪt].

Vowelization, often referred to as *vocalization*, is the substitution of a pure vowel for a vocalic liquid. An example would be *paper* → [pepʊ].

In *palatalization* and *depalatiziation*, the palatal feature is added or omitted, respectively. This pattern typically occurs with sibilants. If the child says [sip] for the word *sheep*, the sibilant was depalatalized. If the child says [ʃi] for *see*, the sibilant is palatalized.

Affrication and *deaffrication* refer to addition or loss of the combination of a stop and fricative, respectively. If *chair* → [tɛɚ] or [ʃɛɚ], there was deaffrication. If *she* → [tʃi], affrication occurred.

Major Assimilations

Assimiliation involves a sound in a word taking on a characteristic of another sound in the same word. This change can occur even if a sound is omitted. Although labial assimilation is common in young children, children with expressive phonological impairments tend to use it excessively (Hodson, 2007). An example of labial assimilation would be *soap* → [pop]. Velar assimilation is also common; it occurs when a sound in a word containing a velar is replaced with a velar, such as *dog* → [gɔg]. Alveolar assimilation happens when an alveolar is used for a nonalveolar because of another alveolar in the word; for example, the word *fight* would become [taɪt].

Glottal Stop Replacement

Glottal stops are used by some children to 'mark' the final consonant in a word until the sounds are developed. Children with repaired cleft palates and other structural anomalies also often use glottal stops.

Syllable-Structure/Context-Related Changes

Metathesis occurs when two sounds or syllables in a word change places (e.g., *ask* → [æks]). In migration, only one sound moves within the word (e.g., *snake* → [neks]). *Coalescence* occurs when two sounds in a word are replaced by a single sound, which has the features of the two replaced sounds, but is neither of the original sounds. An example is *spoon* → [fun]: The /f/ has the stridency of /s/ and the labial component of /p/. *Reduplication* is the repetition of phonemes or syllables that young children demonstrate as a normal part of developing language (e.g., *bottle* → [baba]). *Epenthesis* is the insertion of a sound. The most common form of epenthesis is the addition of /ə/ between two consonants in a cluster, such as *black* → /[bəlæk]. *Diminutive* involves the addition of /i/ at the end of words (e.g., *pig* → [pɪgi]).

SUPPRESSION OF PHONOLOGICAL PROCESSES

Stoel-Gammon and Dunn's report (1985) now serves as a classic reference for suppression of phonological processes. As noted in **Table 8-2,** these processes are divided into those that typically disappear by the age of three years and those that commonly persist past three years of age.

Porter and Hodson (2001) evaluated phonological patterns and phonemes used by children ages three to six years. The study results in **Table 8-3** indicate the age of acquisition for phonological pattern/phonemes.

TABLE 8-2   Age of Suppression of Phonological Processes

Processes that Disappear by 3 Years of Age	Processes that Persist after 3 Years of Age
Unstressed Syllable Deletion	Cluster Reduction
Final Consonant Deletion	Epenthesis
Doubling	Gliding
Diminutization	Vocalization/Vowelization
Velar Fronting	Stopping
Consonant Assimiliation	Depalatalization
Prevocalic Voicing	Final Devoicing
Reduplication	

TABLE 8-3   Age of Acquisition of Phonological Patterns/Phonemes

Phonological Pattern	Age in Years
All phoneme classes except liquids; "syllableness" and singleton consonants (syllable/word structures)	3
Consonant clusters/sequences (two or more contigous consonants without omissions)	4
Liquid /l/	5
Liquid /r/	6

PHONOLOGICAL AWARENESS_____

Phonological awareness—a term that first began to appear in the literature in the late 1970s and early 1980s—refers to the child's knowledge that words are made up of smaller, discernable units (Gillon, 2004). The development of this skill indicates that a person has an awareness of the sound structure, or phonological structure, of spoken words independent of their meaning. Research has indicated that there is a strong link between literacy and phonological awareness (Gillon, 2004). The understanding of a word's sound structure enables a child to sound out, or decode, a word in print. Phonological awareness may also be referred to as *metaphonological awareness* because it is one aspect of the broader category of metalinguistics (Hodson, 2007). *Metalinguistic knowledge* refers to the child's ability to reflect on and discuss aspects of language separate from its meaning (Hodson, 2007).

Phonological awareness can be separated into syllable awareness, onset-rime awareness, and phoneme awareness. *Syllable awareness* requires knowledge that a word can be divided into large parts (i.e., syllables). Five tasks are included in this area:

- *Syllable segmentation* is the ability to tell how many syllables are in a word (e.g., *elephant* has three syllables/parts).
- *Syllable completion* is the ability to complete a word when given one or more syllables (e.g., Show the child a picture of a *computer* and ask child to finish the word when you say, "Finish this word, *compu_____*.")
- *Syllable matching* is the ability to discern which syllables are the same in two similar words. An example is asking the child to tell which part of *telephone* and *telegraph* are the same.
- *Syllable/word manipulation* includes (1) substitution—for example, substitute *foot* for *base* in *baseball* to yield *football*; (2) deletion—for example, *baseball* without *base* would be *ball*; and (3) transposition—for example, reversing the syllables in *ballbase* yields *baseball*.
- *Syllable/word blending* pertains to putting two or more syllables together to make a word. Words that yield compound words are generally easier than meaningless syllables (e.g., *base* plus *ball* yields *baseball*).

Another level of phonological awareness pertains to *onset-rime*. This level of phonological awareness is typically tested through rhyming tasks. This skill indicates the child knows that words share a common/same ending (rime) and understands that the beginning sound or sounds of the word are what differentiate them. The rime is the part of the word from the vowel to the end. The onset includes consonants before the vowel (e.g., *st* in *stun*). Alliteration involves only the beginning consonant (e.g., *s* in *stun*). Three tasks of onset-rime awareness follow:

+ *Judgment:* The ability to tell if two words rhyme (e.g., "Do *ball* and *call* rhyme?").
+ *Oddity:* The ability to tell which word does not rhyme, given a set of words (e.g., "Which word does not rhyme—*car, ball,* or *far?*").
+ *Rhyme generation/supply:* The ability to provide a word or a number of words that rhyme when given a word.

A third level is that of *phonemic awareness.* At this level, the child is able to break a word down into its smallest parts, the individual phonemes or sounds. Tasks at this level include these:

+ *Alliteration,* also referred to as phoneme detection, is tested by asking the child to tell which words have a different sound at the beginning (initial alliteration).
+ *Phoneme matching* asks the child to indicate which words have the same sound at the beginning when given a set of words. An example is "Which words begin with the same sound as *bat—ball, horn,* or *bone?*"
+ *Phoneme isolation* is being able to tell which sound is heard in a specific position within a word (e.g., "What sound do you hear at the beginning of *cat?*").
+ *Phoneme completion* is the ability to provide a missing sound (e.g., "Finish the word 'gla____.'").
+ *Phoneme blending* is a skill in which the child puts sounds given separately together to form a word (e.g., the child blends /k æ n/ to *can*).
+ *Phoneme deletion* is the ability to remove a specified sound from a word (e.g., "Say *boat.* Now say it without /t/.").
+ *Phoneme segmentation* is the ability to tell how many sounds are in a word (e.g., *neck* has three sounds: /n, ɛ, k/).
+ *Phoneme reversal* refers to changing positions of sounds in words (e.g., /ti/ becomes /it/).
+ *Phoneme substitution* implies changing a sound within a word (e.g., "Say *hop.* Now change the /ɑ/ to /ɪ/." [*hip*]).
+ *Spoonerisms* involve changing the first sound in two words (e.g., "*top man*" becomes "*mop tan*").

Phonological awareness skills are influenced by many factors, including vocabulary development, early language experiences, and the child's native language (Gillon, 2007). Research has shown that the size of a child's vocabulary is positively correlated with phonological awareness tasks, including onset-rime and phoneme-level skills. In addition, early language experiences appear to influence phonological awareness skills in children. Studies examining differences in these skills in children from different socioeconomic groups have found that children from middle-income families perform better on phonological awareness tasks than children from low-socioeconomic families (Lonigan, Burgess, Anthony, & Barker, 1998).

Researchers have also noted the importance of exposure to alphabetic knowledge and print referencing activities (Dodd & Carr, 2003). Both of these activities have been shown to help children understand the sound structure of words. Native languages that are alphabetic, such as English, Spanish, and French, support the progression of the skills outlined by Gillon (2004). Research on children whose first language is Cantonese or Japanese indicates phonological awareness skills are poorer in these children because they lack exposure to alphabetic scripts (Cheung, Chen, Lai, Wong, & Hills, 2001; Holm & Dodd, 1996). School-age children with moderate to severe expressive phonological impairment typically perform poorly on phonological awareness tasks (Hodson, 2004; Bird, Bishop, & Freeman, 1995; Webster & Plante, 1992). Justice and Schuele (2004) provided three tentative conclusions based on current studies, while noting that further study is needed in this area:

- Children with expressive phonological impairment are more likely to have difficulty with phonological awareness tasks and literacy skills.
- Children with expressive phonological impairment who also have receptive and/or expressive language difficulties are at greater risk than children with only phonological impairment.
- Some children with phonological impairment may have problems acquiring phonemic awareness, but they do not necessarily show obvious signs of difficulty in the early stages. As the academic demands placed on these children increase, however, their phonological awareness problems become apparent.

The American Speech-Language-Hearing Association issued a document outlining the roles and responsibilities of speech-language pathologists (SLPs) with respect to reading and writing. It noted that "as many as half of all poor readers have an early history of spoken-language disorders" (ASHA, 2001). Many of these children are part of the caseloads of SLPs who work in schools. Thus the SLP should make a focused effort to promote literacy skills in these children to help improve their future school success. Working on both expressive phonology and phonological awareness should improve both areas (Gillon, 2007).

EVALUATION OF CHILDREN WITH SPEECH SOUND DISORDERS

Major Etiological Factors

The acquisition of speech is affected by factors that relate to the structure and function of the speech mechanism as well as other variables. Effects on speech sound production may vary considerably. In addition, many variables may overlap.

Hearing

Adequate hearing is needed so that children are aware of the speech and language being used in their homes and surroundings. A hearing loss can affect the child's ability to hear, which in turn may affect the acquisition of speech. Additionally, hearing is needed so that the children can monitor their speech as it is developing. Of children with disabilities (ages 6–21) served in the schools, approximately 1.2% receive services for a hearing loss (ASHA, 2008).

The age of onset of a loss affects both speech and language acquisition. Children with severe/profound hearing losses since birth have a difficult time acquiring speech and language. If the hearing loss occurs after birth, the child may maintain some skills learned up to that point, but these skills typically deteriorate over time. Better language development is associated with early identification of hearing loss and early intervention (Yoshinaga-Itano, Sedey, Coulter, & Mehl, 1998).

Hearing loss and its effects on speech can be evaluated by noting the degree of loss. Individuals who are 'hard of hearing' have some residual hearing, which may assist them with speech and language acquisition. The less severe the loss, the less impact it typically has on speech and language.

Additionally, the type of loss will present with differing problems. A sensorineural loss involves a pathology in the inner ear or neural pathways. This type of loss may be helped by the use of a hearing aid; alternatively, the individual may be a candidate for a cochlear implant. A conductive loss, which occurs in the outer or middle ear, usually can be treated medically.

The prevalence of mild, moderate, or severe unilateral hearing loss (UHL) in the 'worse' ear and 'normal' hearing in the better ear was estimated at 4.9% and 5.7% in children 6–19 years of age in 1976 and 1994, respectively (NIDCD, 2006). Speech is audible for children with UHL, but it may not always be understandable, depending on the listening environment (Oyler & McKay, 2008).

A common cause of conductive loss is otitis media—that is, fluid in the middle ear. Studies indicate that among children who have had an episode of acute otitis media, as many as 45% have persistent fluid after 1 month (Thrasher & Gregory, 2005). Approximately 5% of children between the ages of 2 and 4 years have hearing loss due to middle ear effusion that lasts 3 months or longer. The prevalence of otitis media with effusion is highest in those age 2 years or younger, but sharply declines in children older than 6 years (Thrasher, 2007).

Oral Mechanism

Individuals can also have anomalies of the structures used for speech production such as the lips, teeth, tongue, and palate. These abnormalities can vary from slight to considerable; likewise, their impact on speech sound acquisition can range from negligible to severe. For this reason, it is important that the SLP examine the structure and function of the oral mechanism and evaluate the effects of any variation on speech production.

Personal Factors

Gender, age, intelligence, socioeconomic levels, and birth order may all have some effect on speech sound acquisition. Statistics indicate that males are at higher risk for speech and language difficulties than are females (Peña-Brookes & Hegde, 2007). Several studies have explored the age of acquisition of various phonemes. The ages identified vary across the studies, but all agree that by the age of 8 years, a child should have speech that is similar to an adult's. Therefore, as children age, they should have fewer speech sound errors.

Intelligence does not have a direct correlation to speech sound acquisition. That is, scores on articulation tests do not correlate with an individual's intelligence. When intelligence falls into the cognitively delayed range (e.g., intelligence quotient [IQ] < 70); however, there does tend to be a correlation: The lower the IQ, the higher the prevalence and frequency of speech sound errors (Peña-Brooks & Hegde, 2007).

Currently, there are no data to support the effect that birth order has on speech sound acquisition. The same is true in regard to socioeconomic status.

Ethnocultural Considerations

The 2000 U.S. Census indicated that 311 languages were spoken in the United States at that time (National Virtual Translation Center, 2007). Some of these languages are indigenous to the United States, whereas others are languages that immigrants used when they came to this country. Given this diversity, SLPs will most likely work with individuals whose English has been influenced by another language.

ASHA has published several technical reports and other documents that address cultural and linguistic diversity. Its social dialects position paper (ASHA, 1983) stated that "no dialectal variety of English is a disorder or a pathological form of speech or language."

The SLP needs to know about the child's background and consider cultural and linguistic issues when evaluating her. As noted by Peña-Brooke and Hegde (2007), children may speak (1) a language other than English, (2) English as a second language, (3) a dialectal variation of English (e.g., African American English), or (4) a different form of English (e.g., British English).

It is vital that the SLP recognize the use of standardized tests may not be appropriate for a given child, depending on the individuals on which the test was preformed. Likewise, it is important that individuals who speak English as a second language or a variation of English are not misdiagnosed simply because of that fact. The SLP needs to know (1) which language is used and what the phonological characteristics of the other/primary language are, (2) how the first language affects the learning of the second language, and (3) how to determine if there is a speech sound disorder in the primary language, the second language, or both (Peña-Brooks & Hegde, 2007).

Assessment

To fully assess the child's language in its cultural context, Bernthal and Bankson (2004) suggest that the SLP should take the following steps:

- Sample the adult speakers in the child's community.
- Obtain information from interpreters/support personnel.
- Become familiar with dialectal and language features of the child's linguistic community.

The monolingual SLP may need the assistance of a bilingual SLP in some cases. Given the diversity of the languages that can be encountered, however, it may be necessary to train an aide or interpreter. When that is not possible, the SLP will need to conduct the assessment using alternative strategies such as establishing an interdisciplinary team involving another professional (e.g., an educational diagnostician who is bilingual [ASHA, 1985]).

Evaluation is the process followed by the SLP to determine the presence or absence of a disorder. If a disorder is present, its characteristics are described and possible causes are explored. A screening can be done with a large number of children in a short period of time to determine if a more in-depth evaluation is necessary.

If a formal evaluation is needed, it will typically include a case history, an oral peripheral exam, administration of a standardized test, evaluation of stimulability in differing contexts, and a hearing screening. The case history can be obtained by written, oral, or both methods. The goal is to obtain information about the child as well as pertinent developmental, medical, familial, and social information that may affect the child's speech. Physical factors that should be considered include syndromes, sensory deficits, structural anomalies, and neurophysiological involvement (Hodson, 2007).

Tests

A standardized test of speech sounds should be administered as part of the evaluation. Most tests will assess the child's production of the various sounds in single-word productions. The test an SLP chooses should be based on several factors, including the amount of time it takes to administer the test, the stimulus materials, the difficulty of scoring, and the type of analysis. Testing results should aid the SLP in determining whether a disorder exists and, if so, in formulating treatment goals (Bernthal & Bankson, 2004). Norm-referenced tests allow for comparison of a child's score in terms of speech sound productions with scores of children who are the same age.

Many phoneme-oriented tests are used for this purpose (see **Table 8-4** for examples). These instruments are designed to evaluate how the child says a targeted sound in each position of a specified word. Typically, omissions, additions, substitutions, and distortions are noted on the form but not differentiated in the final score.

Other standardized tests focus more on phonological processes/deviations (see **Table 8-5**). These tests examine the child's sound system in terms of possible phonological deficiencies in an attempt to determine patterns that need to be targeted. Individual sounds are also assessed with these instruments.

In addition to assessment via a standardized test, the child's speech should be examined by collecting a continuous conversational speech sample. The speech of a child who is highly unintelligible, however, may be difficult or impossible to analyze. If analysis of the sample is possible, it allows the SLP to study the child's speech in a natural way. Note, however, that a continuous conversational sample may have a restricted range of phonemes (Stoel-Gammon & Dunn, 1985).

Stimulability should also be addressed when conducting a comprehensive speech evaluation. This measure indicates the degree to which a misarticulated sound can be produced correctly by imitation (Nicolosi, Harryman, & Kresheck, 2006). To test stimulability, the SLP gives the child simple instructions for where to place the articulators and says the targeted sound in the hope that the child will be able to imitate the target. This procedure provides valuable information when making a prognostic statement about the treatment process.

TABLE 8-4   Phoneme-Oriented Tests

Test	Author(s)	Publisher	Age Range
Arizona Articulation Proficiency Scale, Third Edition	Fudala (2000)	Western Psychological Services	1:5 to 18:0 years
Goldman–Fristoe Test of Articulation, Second Edition	Goldman & Fristoe (2000)	American Guidance Service	2–21 years
Photo Articulation Test, Third Edition	Lippke, Dickey, Selmar, & Soder (1997)	LinguiSystems	3–8 years

TABLE 8-5   Tests that Assess Phonological Processes/Deviations

Test	Author(s) & Publication Date	Publisher	Age Range
Bankson–Bernthal Test of Phonology (BBTOP)	Bankson & Bernthal (1990)	Harcourt Assessment, Inc.	3–9 years
Diagnostic Evaluation of Articulation and Phonology (DEAP)	Dodd, Hua, Crosbie, Holm, & Ozanne (2006)	Pearson Assessment	3–8:11
Hodson Assessment of Phonological Patterns, Third Edition (HAPP-3)	Hodson (2004)	Pro-Ed	Norms for 3:0–8:0
Khan–Lewis Phonological Analysis, Second Edition	Khan & Lewis (2002)	Pearson Assessment	2–21 years

Another part of the assessment should examine how intelligible the child is to the listener. When a child uses phonological deviations, speech intelligibility is usually reduced. Various studies have been done over the years to assess what level of intelligibility a child should have at various ages. Peña-Brooks and Hegde (2007) note that intelligibility will vary from child to child, but suggest that a 19- to 24-month-old child should be 25–50% intelligible, a child 2 to 3 years of age should be 50–75% intelligible, a 3- to 4-year-old should be 75–90% intelligible, and a child 5 years or older should be 90–100% intelligible. Of course, children older than age 5 years may still evidence some speech sound errors, but these typically do not affect the listener's ability to understand the child.

Hearing

Another area that is assessed is the hearing of the child. A SLP can, for example, screen the hearing of a child to determine if hearing is within normal limits or if the child needs to be referred to an audiologist for a complete hearing evaluation (ASHA, 2007).

Oral Mechanism

The various structures of the oral mechanism and their functions should be assessed. Typically, the SLP views the size and symmetry of the oral mechanism as well as the movements of the lips, tongue, and velum. "[O]nly gross abnormalities interfere with speech production" due to the flexibility and adaptability of the speech mechanism (Bleile, 2002).

Reporting

After all testing is completed, the SLP writes an evaluation report. Often the information contained in this report is explained orally to the client's parent(s) as well. This report becomes the official documentation of the evaluation results and recommendations. It should summarize pertinent case history information, hearing screening results, oral mechanism examination findings, test results, and recommendations.

TREATMENT

Phoneme-Oriented Approaches

Treatment of children with speech sound disorders can be approached in many different ways. Some approaches emphasize articulatory placement and motor or movement components, such as phonetic placement, moto-kinesthetic, sensory-motor, or oral-motor exercises. Perhaps the most commonly used approach in this area is Van Riper's stimulus approach, which is often referred to as the 'traditional approach.' Charles Van Riper (1939) brought together principles from various techniques and published his approach in 1939, with revisions following in later editions of his textbook, *Speech Correction: Principles and Methods* (Bernthal & Bankson, 2004; Van Riper, 1939). He advocated for an approach that used placement techniques combined with sensory-perceptual training. The stimulus approach proceeds through five stages: (1) auditory training, (2) elicitation of the sound, (3) stabilization of the sound, (4) carry-over, and (5) maintenance. As Bernthal and Bankson (2004) note, this approach has "withstood the test of time."

Contextual testing should be included as a part of the treatment process. Such an evaluation assesses the context, and its results may help the child produce the misarticulated sound. For example, certain vowels that come after the targeted sound make it easier for the child to produce the consonant; the vowels /i, ɪ, e/ after an /r/, for instance, may make it easier for the child to produce the consonant correctly. The information yielded from this kind of contextual analysis allows the SLP to make decisions about the consistency of errors and to decide which sounds should be targets. This information can be used as a starting point for treatment or in combination with other techniques (Secord, Boyce, Donohue, Fox, & Shine, 2007).

Linguistic-Based Approaches

Linguistic-based approaches recognize phonology as a component of the child's language system (Edwards, 2007; Hodson & Paden, 1983, 1991; Stoel-Gammon & Dunn, 1985). Although these methods improve the child's speech sounds, intelligibility is increased by helping reorganize the child's phonological system. At the same time, the processing of phonological information is enhanced (Grunwell, 1985; Strattman, 2007). Through these approaches, an awareness of patterns is developed.

The *cycles phonological remediation approach* was developed for use with children who have highly unintelligible speech. A *cycle* refers to the period of time required for the child to successfully focus on deficient patterns (Hodson & Paden, 1991). The length of the cycle depends on the number of patterns that need to be targeted and the number of phonemes that are stimulable within the pattern. Each phoneme or consonant cluster is targeted for approximately 60 minutes. Most patterns need to be recycled one or more times.

Hodson and Paden (1991) based this approach on seven principles, some of which reflect the natural acquisition of a child's sound system.

The first principle notes that phonological acquisition is a gradual process (Ingram, 1976). With the cycles approach, the child is given quick but limited exposure to a target, and the SLP typically returns to the pattern after a period of time. This approach allows for the child to internalize, sort, experiment with, and do self-rehearsal as a typically developing child does. Thus the concept of a cycle is used.

The second principle notes that children with normal hearing typically acquire the adult sound system primarily by listening (Van Riper, 1939). Most children with adequate hearing develop their speech sounds/patterns without any special assistance.

The third principle notes that as children gain new speech patterns, they associate kinesthetic with auditory sensations that help with later self-monitoring (Fairbanks, 1954). These two modalities—kinesthetic and auditory—need to be "synchronized" if the child is to develop self-monitoring.

The fourth cycles approach principle states that phonetic environment can facilitate correct sound production (Buteau & Hodson, 1989; Kent, 1982). In other words, it is easier to produce some sounds in certain words than in others. As a part of the clinical process, words initially are chosen with facilitative phonetic environments.

Children need to be actively involved in their phonological acquisition, as indicated in the fifth principle. Children with disordered phonological systems need to be active (rather than passive) participants in their treatment.

The sixth principle states that children tend to generalize new speech production skills to other targets (McReynolds & Bennett, 1972). This principle implies that not all sounds in a pattern need to be targeted; rather, a few sounds can be taught, with time then allowed for their generalization.

The last principle explains the need for an optimal match to facilitate the child's learning (Hunt, 1961). With this approach, the SLP finds the child's current functioning level and then begins work one step above that level. Complexity is increased gradually so that the child is challenged, yet experiences success and gains satisfaction (Hunt, 1961).

Using these principles, the SLP can work on the speech of highly unintelligible children using the cycles approach. Through this process, the child's sound system is reorganized. The child learns new rules to use in producing the sounds of the words of his language.

The primary strength of the cycles approach is its efficiency (Hodson, 1982, 1997, 2004, 2007; Hodson & Paden, 1991). Indeed, many preschoolers require less than a year of this type of phonological intervention to become intelligible. Typically, three to four cycles (30–40 hours of SLP contact time) are required for the child to become intelligible when this treatment approach is used (Hodson, 2007).

To decide which patterns should be targeted, the *Hodson Assessment of Phonological Patterns, Third Edition* (HAPP-3; Hodson, 2004), is administered. Patterns identified as deficient through this tool's results then become possible targets. Early-developing patterns that would be first targets include syllableness, singleton consonants (for omissions), /s/ clusters, posterior–anterior contrasts, and liquids (Hodson, Scherz, & Strattman, 2002).

Syllableness is a first target when deficient, as most young children are readily able to sequence at least two syllables. When this area is targeted, the emphasis is on the appropriate number of syllables rather than on the specific consonants. This pattern is important for language because it has a direct reflection on increasing length of utterances. If a child can use syllableness, the child can put words together.

Improved production of /s/ clusters can have a beneficial impact on morphology. Examples include plurals (e.g., *hats*), third person present verb tense (e.g., *She eats*), and possessives (e.g., the *cat's mat*).

A treatment session using the cycles approach uses an easy-to-follow structure. Each session begins with a period of auditory stimulation using slight amplification, in which the SLP reads a list of words that contain the day's target. Next, approximately five picture cards are provided with the child's target. With this therapy, words (rather than nonsense syllables) are always used. During the first cycles, monosyllabic words with facilitative phonetic environments are selected (Hodson, 2007). Semantic considerations during this stage may also include the use of verbs, such as *spin* for /s/ clusters. Actual objects are also used with preschoolers. In the final cycles, minimal pairs are often incorporated to ensure the child understands the semantic differences between the error and the target productions (Hodson, 2007).

Experiential-play and production-practice activities follow the listening activities, with these exercises incorporating the child's picture cards into the session's activity. This part of the session allows the child to practice the targeted pattern during a play-based task. The next step is to check stimulability for the next session's target patterns/phonemes. This testing is followed by a brief metaphonological activity (e.g., rhyme). The session ends with a repeat of the listening activity.

Daily home practice is also a component of the cycles approach. Both the reading list and the picture cards used that day are sent home for practice (approximately two minutes per day).

The metaphonological activity is incorporated because research has shown that children with disordered expressive phonological systems have greater difficulty completing phonological awareness tasks than do their typically developing peers; as a consequence, the former's literacy acquisition may be hindered.

Focused Auditory Input/Stimulation

For children who are functioning below the age of three years, *focused stimulation* serves to lay the foundation for acquiring language aspects. According to Weismer and Robertson (2006), through this intervention, "the child is provided with concentrated exposures of specific linguistic forms/functions/uses within naturalistic communicative contexts" (p. 175). Focused stimulation differs from general stimulation in that specific patterns are targeted during each session.

For example, a common goal is helping a child become aware of and eventually produce word endings. During the first session for this goal, the final /p/ is often targeted, with the room being filled with objects and activities for final /p/ (e.g., *up, hop, top, jump, mop, cup*). The SLP demonstrates /p/ and models the words (with slight emphasis on the /p/) during parallel play, but does not at this time ask the child to imitate. After a few months of focused auditory stimulation, the child typically is ready for production-practice activities for target patterns (Hodson, 2007).

CASE STUDIES

When assessing the speech sound system of young children, needed information includes the phonemic inventory, including both consonants and vowels, syllable shapes, and intelligibility. An attempt should be made to examine phonological patterns.

One of the best ways to assess these parameters is to have the parent and the child play together. This natural interaction typically will elicit speech from the child. During the play time, the parent can gloss the child's utterances; that is, the parent can restate what the child said to aid identification of words.

The case study of Johnathon, 25 months of age, indicates that he is at least 60% intelligible; has a solid phonemic inventory, including stops, nasals, and glides; and shows varied syllable shapes. Although some phonological deviations are being used, they are developmentally appropriate. The recommendation for the mother to return to the clinic if she has further concerns is appropriate.

The second case study, involving 22-month-old Josephine, indicates that she has a restricted consonant and vowel inventory. Josephine does use a good variety of syllable shapes with limited reduplicated babbling. Her intelligibility was judged to be 50%, which falls within acceptable limits, according to Peña-Brooks and Hegde (2007). If possible, another area that might be assessed is Josephine's use of phonological patterns. The screening portion of the HAPP-3 could be administered to do so. If Josephine does not respond to the items spontaneously, modeling could be used, preferably incorporating delayed imitation. The screening portion of the HAPP-3 would assess early-developing patterns. The recommendation for the mother to enroll her child in an early intervention program is appropriate. Josephine's speech skills should be reevaluated in approximately 6 months to assess her progress.

Robert presents some interesting challenges. At 27 months of age, he appears to have global developmental delays. Notably, he appears to have a unilateral hearing loss. When evaluating a child for speech sound disorders, this type of deficiency may be a contributing factor. Robert's intelligibility level, which is less than 25%, is cause for concern. Moreover, he has a restricted consonant inventory. His syllable shapes are also limited.

It would be helpful to screen Robert for potential phonological patterns using the HAPP-3 preschool screening instrument. Modeling could be used, if needed, during the assessment. This screening information could provide a temporary baseline for deficient phonological patterns and assist in the selection of initial treatment goals. Enrolling Robert in speech and language intervention is recommended. Treatment should focus on developing both his speech and language, as this approach would allow for work to be done in both language and phonology. The use of a play-based approach incorporating words with patterns that are deficient and need to be targeted (e.g., syllableness, final consonants, /s/ clusters, velars, liquids) would be appropriate. Robert's parents should be included in the treatment process and be given home assignments.

SUMMARY

Phonology, which is one of the five components of language, is important for morphology, syntax, and semantics. The process of acquiring speech sounds begins at birth, when the child expresses wants and needs through reflexive vocalizations, such as crying, burping, and coughing. From birth, the speech sounds are formed and improved. The sounds are acquired at different ages, with all sounds becoming a part of the child's phonemic inventory by 8 years of age. The sounds of our language can be differentiated by noting their place, manner, and voicing. Phonological patterns can also be used for classification.

A variety of factors may affect speech sound acquisition. In particular, hearing—including hearing loss—influences speech acquisition. Ethnocultural considerations must also be taken into account.

The assessment of children with possible speech sound disorders should include a standardized test that examines the sounds and phonological patterns. A connected speech sample should also be obtained and analyzed, if possible, to determine the percentage of intelligibility and to note the consistency with which errors occur. The oral mechanism should be evaluated, as should hearing. This information is then analyzed, and the results are summarized in a written report.

Treatment for children with speech sound disorders can take either a motor-based approach or a linguistic-based approach, or it may involve a combination of these strategies. Children whose speech is highly unintelligible are best treated with a linguistic approach. The cycles approach is an effective means of working with children with disordered phonological systems.

KEY TERMS

Articulation

Consonants

Cycles phonological approach

Phonemes

Phonological awareness

Phonological deviations

Phonological intervention

Phonological patterns

Phonology

Sound system development

Speech mechanism

Speech sound disorders

Vowels

STUDY QUESTIONS

+ What are the six principal organs/subsystems of speech production? Discuss each part as well as the progression and flow of speech through it.
+ Discuss the prelinguistic stages of speech development. Name the stage, define the age range at which it is expected to occur, and describe the expected characteristics of speech at each stage.
+ Identify the different phonemic awareness tasks, giving an example of each skill addressed by the task.
+ Phonemes are described by their place, manner, and voicing. List the 24 phonemes, and note the place, manner, and voicing for each.
+ Phonological deviations can be designated by omissions, assimilations, and syllable structure. Note patterns that would be classified by each of these descriptors.
+ Discuss how hearing loss relates to speech sound acquisition.
+ What is the purpose of an evaluation? Which steps are taken during an evaluation?
+ Which factors would an SLP consider in selecting a test for evaluating speech sound production?
+ Briefly outline the structure of a session using the cycles approach for phonological remediation.

REFERENCES

American Speech-Language-Hearing Association (ASHA). (1983). Social dialects and implications of the position on social dialects. *ASHA, 25*, 23–27.

American Speech-Language-Hearing Association (ASHA). (1985). *Clinical management of communicatively handicapped minority language populations* [position statement]. www.asha.org/policy.

American Speech-Language-Hearing Association. (2001). *Roles and responsibilities of speech-language pathologists with respect to reading and writing in children and adolescents* (position statement, executive summary of guidelines, technical report). ASHA *Supplement, 21*, 17–27. Rockville, MD.

American Speech-Language-Hearing Association (ASHA). (2007). *Scope of practice in speech-language pathology. www.asha.org/policy.*

American Speech-Language-Hearing Association (ASHA). (2008). Incidence and prevalence of communication disorders and hearing loss in children. http://www.asha.org/members/research/reports/children.htm.

Bankson, N. W., & Bernthal, J. E. (1990). *Bankson-Bernthal test of phonology.* San Antonio: Harcourt Assessment, Inc.

Bernthal, J. E., & Bankston, N. W. (2004). *Articulation and phonological disorders,* 5th ed. Boston: Allyn & Bacon.

Bird, J., Bishop, D., & Freeman, N. (1995). Phonological awareness and literacy development in children with expressive phonological impairments. *Journal of Speech and Hearing Research, 38,* 446–462.

Bleile, K. (2002). Evaluating articulation and phonological disorders when the clock is running. *American Journal of Speech-Language Pathology, 11,* 243–249.

Buteau, C., & Hodson, B. (1989). *Phonological remediation targets: Words and primary pictures for highly unintelligible children.* Austin, TX: Pro-Ed.

Cheor, M., Ceponiene, R., Lehtokoski, A., et al. (1998). Development of language-specific phoneme representations in the human brain. *Nature Neuroscience, 1,* 351–353.

Cheung, H., Chen, H. C., Lai, C. Y., Wong, O. C., & Hills, M. (2001). The development of phonological awareness: Effects of spoken language experience and orthography. *Cognition, 81*(3), 227–241.

Creaghead, N., Newman, P., & Secord, W. (1989). *Assessment and remediation of articulatory and phonological disorders,* 2nd ed. New York: Macmillan.

Dodd, B. W., & Carr, A. (2003). Young children's letter-sound knowledge. *Language, Speech, and Hearing Services in Schools, 34,* 128–137.

Dodd, B., Hua, Z., Crosbie, S., Holm, A., & Ozanne, A. (2006). *Diagnostic evaluation of articulation and phonology.* Bloomington, MN: Pearson Assessment.

Edwards, M.L. (2006). Phonological theories. In B.W. Hodson (Ed). *Evaluating and enhancing children's phonological systems* (pp. 145–170). Greenville, SC: Thinking Publications University.

Fairbanks, G. (1954). Systematic research in experimental phonetics: A theory of the speech mechanisms as a servosytem. *Journal of Speech and Hearing Disorders, 19,* 133–139.

Fenson, L., Dale, P., Reznick, J. S., et al. (1991). *Technical manual for MacArthur communicative development inventories.* San Diego: San Diego State University Department of Psychology.

Fudala, J. B. (2000). *Arizona Articulation Proficiency Scale,* 3rd. ed. Los Angeles: Western Psychological Services.

Gillon, G. (2004). *Phonological awareness: From research to practice.* New York: Guilford Press.

Gillon, G. (2007). Effective practice in phonological awareness intervention for children with speech sound disorder. *Perspectives on Language Learning and Education, 14,* 18–23.

Goldman, R., & Fristoe, M. (2000). *Goldman-Frisoe Test of Articulation,* 2nd ed. Circle Pines, MN: American Guidance Service.

Grunwell, P. (1982). *Clinical phonology.* Rockville, MD: Aspen.

Grunwell, P. (1985). *Phonological assessment of child speech.* Windsor, UK: NFER-Nelson.

Hodson, B. (1982). Remediation of speech patterns associated with low levels of phonological performance. In M. Crary (Ed.), *Phonological intervention: Concepts and procedures* (pp. 91–115). San Diego: College-Hill.

Hodson, B. (1997). Disordered phonologies: What have we learned about assessment and treatment? In B. Hodson & M. Edwards (Eds.), *Perspectives in applied phonology* (pp. 197–224). Gaithersburg, MD: Aspen.

Hodson, B. (2004). *Hodson Assessment of Phonological Patterns*, 3rd. ed. Austin, TX: Pro-Ed.

Hodson, B. (2007). *Evaluating and enhancing children's phonological systems*. Greenville, SC: Thinking Publications University.

Hodson, B., & Paden, E. (1983). *Targeting intelligible speech: A phonological approach to remediation*. Austin, TX: Pro-Ed.

Hodson, B., & Paden, E. (1991). *Targeting intelligible speech: A phonological approach to remediation*, 2nd ed. Austin, TX: Pro-Ed.

Hodson, B., Scherz, J., & Strattman, K. (2002). Evaluating communicative abilities of a highly unintelligible preschooler. *American Journal of Speech-Language Pathology, 11*, 236–242.

Holm, A., & Dodd, B. (1996). The effect of first written language on the acquisition of literacy. *Cognition, 59*, 119–147.

Hunt, J. (1961). *Intelligence and experience*. New York: Ronald Press.

Ingram, D. (1976). *Phonological disability in children*. New York: Elsevier.

Justice, L. M., & Schuele, C. M. (2004). Phonological awareness: Description, assessment, and intervention. In J. Bernthal & N. Bankson (Eds.), *Articulation and phonological disorders*, 5th ed. (pp. 376–403). Boston: Allyn & Bacon.

Kelman, M. (2007). Acquisition of speech sounds and phonological patterns. In B. W. Hodson (Ed.), *Evaluating and enhancing children's phonological systems* (pp. 23–41). Greenville, SC: Thinking Publications.

Kent, R. D. (1982). Contextual facilitation of correct sound production. *Language, Speech, and Hearing Services in Schools, 13*, 66–76.

Khan, L. M. & Lewis, N. P. (2002). *Khan-Lewis Phonological Analysis*, 2nd ed. Bloomington, MN: Pearson Assessment.

Lippke, B. A., Dickey, S.E., Selmar, J.W., & Soder, A.L. (1997). *Photo Articulation Test*, 3rd. ed. Moline, IL: LinguiSystems.

Lonigan, C., Burgess, S., Anthony, J. L., & Barker, T. A. (1998). Development of phonological sensitivity in 2- to 5-year old children. *Journal of Educational Psychology, 90*(2), 294–311.

McReynolds, L.V., & Bennett, S. (1972). Distinctive feature generalization in articulation training. *Journal of Speech and Hearing Disorders, 37*, 462–470.

National Virtual Translation Center. (2007). http://www.nvtc.gov/lotw/months/november/USlanguages.html.

National Institute on Deafness and Other Communication Disorders. (December 2006). *NIDCD outcomes research in children with hearing loss*. http://www.nidcd.nih.gov/funding/programs/nb/outcomes/report.htm.

Nicolosi, L., Harryman, E., & Kresheck, J. (2006). *Terminology of communication disorders*, 4th ed. Baltimore: Williams & Wilkins.

Oller, D. K. (1980). The emergence of the sounds of speech in infancy. In G. Yeni-Komshian, J. Kavanagh, & C.A. Ferguson (Eds.), *Child phonology: Vol.1. production* (pp. 93–112). New York: Academic Press.

Oyler, R., & McKay, S. (22 January 2008). Unilateral hearing loss in children: Challenges and opportunities. ASHA Leader, 13(1), 12–15.

Peña-Brooks, A., & Hegde, M. N. (2007). *Assessment and treatment of articulation and phonological disorders in children*. Austin, TX: Pro-Ed.

Porter, J. H., & Hodson, B. W. (2001). Collaborating to obtain phonological acquisition data for local schools. *Language, Speech, and Hearing Services in Schools, 32*(3), 165–171.

Prezas, R., & Hodson, B. (2007). Diagnostic evaluation of children with speech sound disorders. In S. Rvachew (Ed.), *Encyclopedia of language and literacy development* (p. 107). London, Ontario: Canadian Language and Literacy Research Network [http://ww.literacyencyclopedia.ca/].

Sander, E. (1972). When are speech sounds learned? *Journal of Speech and Hearing Disorders, 37*, 55–63.

Scherz, J., & Edwards, H. (2007). Review of phonetics. In B. W. Hodson (Ed.), *Evaluating and enhancing children's phonological systems* (pp. 9–22). Greenville, SC: Thinking Publications.

Secord, W., Boyce, S., Donohue, J., Fox, R., & Shine, R. (2007). *Eliciting sounds: Techniques and strategies for clinicians.* Clinton Park, NY: Thomson Delmar Learning.

Shriberg, L., & Kwiatkowski, J. (1983). Computer-assisted natural process analysis: Recent issues and data. In J. Locke (Ed.), *Assessing and treating phonological disorders: Current approaches. Seminars in speech and language* (Vol. 4, p. 397). New York: Thieme.

Stoel-Gammon, C., & Dunn, C. (1985). *Normal and disordered phonology in children.* Austin, TX: Pro-Ed.

Strattman, K. (2007). Overview of intervention approaches, methods, and targets. In B. W. Hodson (Ed.), *Evaluating and enhancing children's phonological systems* (pp. 23–41). Greenville, SC: Thinking Publications.

Thrasher, R. D. (19 April 2007). Middle ear, otitis media with effusion. *EMedicine.* American Academy of Otolaryngology—Head and Neck Surgery. Retrieved February 19, 2008, from http://www.emedicine.com/ent/topic209.htm.

Thrasher, R. D., & Gregory, C. A. (October 2005). Middle ear, otitis media with effusion. *EMedicine.* American Academy of Otolaryngology—Head and Neck Surgery, University of Colorado School of Medicine, and Ehrling Berquist Hospital. Retrieved October 20, 2007, from http://www.emedicine.com/ent/topic209.htm.

Van Riper, C. (1939). *Speech correction: Principles and methods.* Englewood Cliffs, NJ: Prentice-Hall.

Webster, P., & Plante, A. (1992). Effects of phonological impairment on word, syllable, and phoneme segmentation and reading. *Language, Speech, and Hearing Services in Schools, 23*, 176–182.

Weismer, S. E., & Robertson, S. (2006). Focused stimulation approach to language intervention. In R. McCauley & M. Fey (Eds.), *Treatment of language disorders in children* (pp. 175–202). Baltimore: Paul H. Brookes.

Yoshinaga-Itano, C., Sedey, A., Coulter, D., & Mehl, A. (1998). Language of early- and later-identified children with hearing loss. *Pediatrics, 102*(5), 1161–1171.

CHAPTER 9

Morphology

Theresa E. Bartolotta, PhD, and Brian B. Shulman, PhD

OBJECTIVES

+ Define morphemes.
+ Describe the stages of morphological development as part of the larger language development process.
+ Review assessment of morphological development and mean length of utterance (MLU) calculation.
+ Describe clinical applications of morphological acquisition.

INTRODUCTION

When a child asks, "Can I have two of the biggest cookies?", while looking at a plate full of treats, the adult is given a great deal of information about the child's intent based on the form of the utterance the child has produced. We know that the child wants more than one cookie—two, to be precise. That information is provided by two key elements of the utterance: the word *two* and the *s* at the end of the word *cookie*. We also know that the child has an expectation for the size of his cookies, as signaled by the use of the word *biggest*. These key elements that add critical information and specificity to this utterance are called morphemes, which are part of the form, or syntax, of an utterance. Consider what the utterance would sound like without those three key components: "Can I have the cookie?" The meaning is greatly changed, and the child's intent of the utterance is altered.

This example serves to illustrate the critical role that morphemes play in expressing meaning in our language. In this chapter, we'll review the types of morphemes, see how morphemes develop, and explore the key role they play in adding length and complexity to children's expressive language.

DEFINITION

A *morpheme* is the smallest unit of language that carries meaning. For example, the word *shoe* is a morpheme whose meaning is "an item worn on the foot by people." The word *shoe* is a single morpheme that cannot be broken down further into smaller meaningful components. You have learned that words are composed of individual phonemes, and the word *shoe* is composed of two phonemes: /ʃ/ and /u/. On their own, these individual phonemes do not carry any meaning. Instead, each must be combined with other phonemes to create meaningful syllables. In our example, *shoe* fulfills the definition of being a small unit of language that carries meaning. It cannot be further subdivided into any meaningful parts. Thus the word *shoe* is composed of one morpheme.

When we combine *shoe* with the /s/ phoneme, we create the word *shoes*, which refers to more than one shoe, thereby changing the meaning of the original word. The word *shoes* is composed of two morphemes, as the /s/ ending adds meaning by referring to plurality or "more than one." More generally, we change the meanings of words by adding or modifying morphemes. As children progress through the stages of language acquisition, they add length and complexity to their language by gradually using more morphemes and combining morphemes in new ways. The study of morphology refers to words and parts of words, and the ways in which those segments of language are combined to create meanings.

Two types of morphemes are distinguished: *free* and *bound*. Free morphemes are those morphemes that can stand alone and carry meaning. In our example, *shoe* is a free morpheme. By contrast, bound morphemes must be combined with free morphemes to be meaningful. You have undoubtedly guessed by now that the -*s* in *shoes* is a bound morpheme. Bound morphemes are often referred to as grammatical markers that cannot function independently.

Bound morphemes may be either derivational morphemes or inflectional morphemes. Derivational morphemes are added to words as prefixes (e.g., *un-, in-, pre-, trans-*) or suffixes (e.g., *-ly, -est, -er, -ness*). These types of morphemes are used to change one word into another word, resulting in the emergence of a different part of speech. For example, when the derivational morpheme -*ness* is added to the adjective *happy*, the adverb *happiness* is created. Inflectional morphemes don't change the overall meaning or word class of words, but rather are used to modify or add meaning to the free morphemes with which they are combined. The plural -*s* marker is an inflectional morpheme, as are the -*s* added for possession (e.g., John's coat) and the -*ing* and -*ed* endings added to change tense (e.g., jump*ing*, jump*ed*). See **Table 9-1** for examples of the different types of bound morphemes.

MORPHOLOGICAL DEVELOPMENT

The development of morphology is a lengthy process, which begins when the child first begins to combine words and typically ends at approximately age five, when a child has learned to

TABLE 9-1   Types of Bound Morphemes

	Derivational		Inflectional
Prefixes		**Suffixes**	shoes
*un*usual		eas*ily*	Lisa'*s* movie
*in*sufficient		larg*est*	runn*ing*
*pre*term		bold*er*	crash*ed*
*trans*continental		warm*ness*	sit*s*

use most of the major types of English sentences, suffixes, and phonological patterns. Under the *form–content–use* model of linguistic development (Bloom & Lahey, 1978), morphology is considered as part of the *form* or *syntax* of language, but is greatly influenced by related "developments" in phonology (also part of *form*) and semantics (as part of *content*). Although a great deal of variation is observed across children as they move through the stages of linguistic development, it has been helpful to study the work of Roger Brown (1973) when learning about the process of morphological development.

Brown conducted a longitudinal study based on three children, through which he identified certain critical stages of syntactic development. These stages were characterized by changes in the child's utterance length and, in turn, syntactic complexity. Brown termed the key parameter *mean length of utterance* (MLU), and he used changes in MLU to delineate each stage of linguistic development. MLU is a measure of utterance length based on the average number of free and bound morphemes contained in a designated set of spontaneously produced utterances. Length of an utterance is determined by the number of morphemes rather than by the number of words. To calculate a child's MLU, one first determines the total number of free and bound morphemes in the language sample and then divides the morpheme total by the number of utterances analyzed. The number obtained is the MLU for that specific sample, which can then be compared to the data on MLU stages (**Table 9-2**) to determine which stage of *morphosyntactic development* a child has achieved.

These stages should be used with caution. Research conducted since Brown's early work has demonstrated that substantial individual differences occur among children with similar MLU levels (Leonard & Finneran, 2003). Additionally, Brown's (1973) position was that if no evidence of the use of a morpheme by a child was found, then the child did not have productive knowledge of that structure. That theory has been the subject of much debate over the years.

At this point, it is helpful to introduce certain terminology that is relevant to the description of morphemes. The time when a child first begins to use a morpheme correctly is called

TABLE 9-2   MLU Stages

Stage	MLU	Approximate Chronological Age (months)
Early I	1.01–1.49	19–22
Late I/early II	1.50–1.99	23–26
II	2.00–2.49	27–30
III	2.50–2.99	31–34
Early IV	3.00–3.49	35–38
Late IV/early V	3.50–3.99	39–42
Late V	4.00–4.99	43–46
V+	4.50–4.99	47–50
V++	5.00–5.99	51–67

Sources: Data from Brown (1973), Owens (2008), and Retherford (2000).

emergence, and the time when a morpheme is fully acquired is called *mastery.* The section of an utterance where morpheme use is required for the utterance to be meaningful and syntactically accurate is termed the *obligatory context.* A morpheme is considered mastered, or fully acquired, when it is used 90% of the time in obligatory contexts (Brown, 1973). The assessment of mastery—that is, "knowledge" of a morpheme—and the way a child learns to use each morpheme has been and continues to be studied carefully, as discussed later in this chapter.

MLU is considered to be a *moderate* predictor of the complexity of a child's language, although this measure is considered only fairly reliable until MLU reaches 4.0. Beyond 4.0, internal complexity and variability increase without necessarily adding length to an utterance. That is, children demonstrate linguistic complexity based on the types of words used, rather than by stringing more words together (Owens, 2008). There is a demonstrated relationship between age and MLU in the first few years of life that does not continue past age four or five years. From age 18 months, when MLU is somewhere between 1.0 and 2.0, MLU increases by approximately 1.2 morphemes per year until age five years. This progression roughly correlates with one-year-old children having a predicted MLU of approximately 1.0, two-year-olds having an MLU of approximately 2.0, and so on (Scarborough, Wyckoff, & Davidson, 1986).

Computing MLU

As we have discussed, MLU can be a fairly useful tool in helping to describe a child's level of linguistic complexity. It may also be used as a clinical tool by speech-language pathologists to identify areas of concern. The clinician should begin by collecting a spontaneous conversational language sample of 50 to 100 utterances (100 is ideal) in a naturalistic setting. Each utterance is analyzed to determine the number of morphemes using rules for counting morphemes originally developed by Brown (1973). **Table 9-3** summarizes rules for assigning morphemes to utterances.

TABLE 9-3   Rules for Assigning Morphemes to Utterances

1. Select a portion of the language sample transcript that appears to be representative of the child's abilities. Number 50–100 consecutive utterances that are completely intelligible, as selecting individual utterances for calculation can inflate the MLU. Do not assign numbers to repeated, incomplete, or interrupted utterances.

2. Count as one morpheme: single words, compound words (e.g., *pocketbook, birthday*), proper names, ritualized reduplications (e.g., *night-night*), irregular past tense verbs (e.g., *ate, threw*), diminutives (e.g., *doggie*), auxiliary verbs and catenatives (e.g., *is, have, do, gonna, hafta*), irregular plurals (e.g., *men, feet*). These words, although they consist of two or more free morphemes, are believed to be learned as complete units by children and therefore are treated like single words. An incorrect use of an inflection added to an irregular past tense or past participle form (e.g., *runned*) should not be counted as a separate morpheme. Assign these unique productions one morpheme.

3. Count as two morphemes (inflected verbs and nouns): possessive nouns, plural nouns, third person singular verbs in the present tense (e.g., *walks*), regular past-tense verbs (e.g., *walked, talked*), present progressive verbs (e.g., *running, eating*)

4. Do not assign morphemes to repetitions of words that occur as a result of stuttering or false starts unless the word is added for emphasis (e.g., *my dad is big big*).

5. Do not assign morphemes to fillers (e.g., *um, yeah, like*).

6. Assign morphemes to short words such as *hi, yeah,* and *no*.

7. Inflections on gerunds and predicate adjectives are not counted as individual morphemes (e.g., I like jogg*ing*, I am bor*ed*). Assign only one morpheme to the entire word.

8. Assign two morphemes to negative contractions (e.g., *can't, don't*) only if there is evidence in the language sample that the child uses each part of the contraction independently. The reason for this is similar to the example cited in number 2. Without confirmation that the child created this contraction and has independent knowledge of each component, we assume that the word is learned as a whole and represents one morpheme.

9. Assign two morphemes to all non-negative contractions (e.g., *I'm, he'll, you'll, she'd, they're*).

10. Common derivational prefixes and suffixes should be assigned their own morpheme (e.g., *re-, un-, pre-, -ly, -ful, -en*).

Sources: Data from Brown (1973), Owens (2008), and Retherford (2000).

Using the guidelines from Table 9-3, we would analyze the following utterances as such:

leave _it_ _in_ _the_ _water_	5 morphemes
that _'s_ _dirty_	3 morphemes
happy _birthday_ _mommy_	3 morphemes
_I_ _hafta_ _clean_ _my_ _shoe_ _s_	6 morphemes
play _ing_ _with_ _my_ _toy_ _s_	6 morphemes
_go_ _night-night_	2 morphemes
_he_ _fell_ _down_	3 morphemes

When calculating MLU for an entire sample, the clinician continues analyzing each utterance until the target number has been analyzed. The total number of morphemes is added and then divided by the total number of utterances analyzed to yield the MLU value. This number, which represents the _average_ length of a child's utterances, can then be used to assign a stage of linguistic development. Although the preceding sample of seven utterances is far smaller than the number of utterances that would provide a truly representative sample of a child's language, we can compute the MLU for it as an exercise. By adding the total number of morphemes in the sample, we obtain a sum of 28 morphemes. That is divided by the number of utterances, which is 7, and results in an MLU for this brief sample of 4.0.

Stages of Morphological Development

Brown (1973) determined a set of stages that were characteristic of certain changes in grammatical (or morphosyntactic) development. In Stage I, the child's language is primarily comprised of single-word utterances. Additionally, we can observe the child beginning to combine two words such that the two words are meaningfully related to each other. For example, in "Mommy eat," the child orders the words to signify that Mommy is the person performing the action of eating. Thus the child is beginning to make word associations that convey meaningful information about the world around him.

Brown and Fraser (1963) described these early words as _telegraphic_. These utterances contain content words (also called open-class words) such as nouns, adjectives, and verbs, but lack functor words (also called closed-class words) so that they resemble telegrams. These utterances would be typical of telegraphic speech in Stage I: "no more"; "Daddy book"; "all wet"; "more cookie"; "bye-bye Papa."

Early word combinations are extended in Stage II and further characterized by the appearance of grammatical morphemes that serve to add _syntactic specificity_ to the child's language. In contrast to Stage I, the child in Stage II will typically produce utterances such as "Mommy eat*ing*" or "*in* car" to mark the syntactic relations implied by the word order. In Stage II, we see the appearance of grammatical morphemes that allow the child to mark these relations. The emergence of these grammatical inflections, known as Brown's 14 morphemes, is covered later in this chapter.

In Stage III, we see the emergence of simple sentences, along with the child's use of yes/ no and *wh*-question forms, imperative statements, and negatives. Stage IV is characterized by refinements in sentence complexity. Namely, the child begins *clausal* and *phrasal embedding*. Here, for example, the child places a clause such as "who smiled" within another sentence to create a sentence such as "The boy, *who smiled*, spilled the milk." As the child enters Stage V, syntactic modifications are exhibited in the form of compound sentences (e.g., "Mom dusted and I swept.").

Table 9-4 provides a summary of the acquisition of grammatical morphemes as a function of Brown's stages.

The application of the information in Table 9-4 to clinical use can be illustrated by referring to our brief language sample, in which we calculated a child's MLU at 4.0 based on the morphemes used in seven utterances. With an MLU of 4.0, this child is expected to be in late Stage V and to be approximately 43–46 months of age.

The next step is to study the sample and identify the morphemes that are expected to be used at this stage, and those that are, indeed, present in the utterances analyzed. In this sample, we have evidence of the preposition *in*, the plural *-s*, the present progressive *-ing*, the irregular past tense verb *fell*, and the definite article *the*. Our next task it to search the entire transcript (remember—the transcript should be approximately 100 utterances long) for evidence of use of the remaining morphemes expected to be used in *obligatory contexts* by Stage V. These include the preposition *on*, possessive *-s*, regular past tense of verbs, regular third person singular present tense *-s*, indefinite article *a*, and the contractible copula.

If there is no evidence of use of these morphemes in obligatory contexts, then the speech-language pathologist will likely design scenarios in which these morphemes will be elicited. For example, to elicit the possessive *-s*, the clinician may present a child with items belonging to a classmate, and then ask the child, "Whose gloves are these?" Ideally, multiple opportunities for the child to use the possessive marker will be offered. If the child fails to use the *-s* when required, the clinician may decide to target this morpheme as a goal in therapy. If the morpheme is used inconsistently, the clinician may decide that the morpheme is emerging, and instruct adults in the child's environment to provide opportunities to hear and practice use of the possessive *-s*. The clinician may also decide to reassess the child's use of this morpheme (and any others that are not yet mastered, but expected) at a later date.

TABLE 9-4   Grammatical Morpheme Production Organized by Brown's Stages

Stage	MLU	Approximate Age (months)	Grammatical Morphemes	Examples
Early I	1.01–1.49	19–22	Occasional use	
Late I/early II	1.50–1.99	23–26	Occasional use	
II	2.00–2.49	27–30	1. Present progressive tense of verb -ing	1. Mommy *driving*.
			2. Regular plural -s	2. My *shoes* hurt.
			3. Preposition *in*	3. Ball *in* cup.
III	2.50–2.99	31–34	4. Preposition *on*	4. Cup *on* table.
			5. Possessive -s	5. *Daddy's* car blue.
Early IV	3.00–3.49	35–38	No others mastered	
Late IV/early V	3.50–3.99	39–42	No others mastered	
Late V	4.00–4.49	43–46	6. Regular past tense of verb -ed	6. I *pulled* my bike.
			7. Irregular past tense of verb	7. I *ate* my ice cream.
			8. Regular third person singular present tense -s	8. Chris *hits*.
			9. Definite and indefinite articles	9. *a* doggie; *the* car
			10. Contractible copula	10. *Boy's* big.
V+	4.50–4.99	47–50	11. Contractible auxiliary	11. Steven's eating cake.
			12. Uncontractible copula	12. She *is*. (in response to the question "Who is home?").
			13. Uncontractible auxiliary	13. He *is*. (in response to the question "Who is drinking your juice?").
			14. Irregular third person singular	14. He *does* it.
V++	5.00–5.99	51–67	No data	

Sources: Data from Brown (1973) and Retherford (2000).

Brown's Fourteen Grammatical Morphemes

In his research, Brown (1973) isolated 14 obligatory morphemes that appeared early in the sample of the children he studied. He termed these morphemes as "obligatory," meaning that they are required to mark inflection in English language. These morphemes (which are listed in **Table 9-5**) share the following characteristics (adapted from Owens, 2008):

+ *They are phonetically minimal.* They are not composed of complex syllables, and they typically include simple changes in phonemic production, such as the addition of the *-s* phoneme.
+ *They receive light vocal emphasis.* They are not stressed in utterances.
+ *They belong to a small class of constructions.* They are few in number.
+ *Their phonological form can vary* based on the grammatical and phonetic properties of the free morpheme they are linked with. For example, in the word *trees,* the *-s* morpheme is pronounced as /z/, yet in the word *hats* the *-s* is pronounced as /s/. This rule

TABLE 9-5   Brown's Fourteen Grammatical Morphemes

Morpheme	Age of Mastery* (months)
present progressive *-ing*	19–28
in	27–30
on	27–30
regular plural *-s*	27–33
irregular past	25–46
possessive *-s*	26–40
uncontractible copula (verb *to be* as main verb)	27–39
articles *-a, the*	28–46
regular past *-ed*	26–48
regular third person *-s*	26–46
irregular third person	28–50
uncontractible auxiliary	29–48
contractible copula	29–49
contractible auxiliary	30–50

* Mastery defined as correct use in 90% of obligatory contexts

Source: Data from Brown (1973), Miller (1981), and Owens (2008).

is based on the type of phoneme that precedes the morpheme. If a plural morpheme is added to a free morpheme that ends in a voiced phoneme, such as a vowel, then the -s is pronounced as its voiced cognate, /z/.

+ *They develop gradually and there is much individual variation.* Although we can use Brown's stages as a guide to the order of acquisition of grammatical structures and the expected age of acquisition, the order of emergence and mastery will vary considerably across children.

Brown believed that absence of a particular morpheme in a child's language indicated that the child had not yet learned to use the structure. Hence, speech-language pathologists use the list of Brown's morphemes as a clinical tool to assess morphologicalal development as *an aspect* of syntactic development. The morphemes emerge in Stage II, and most develop in the order that they are listed in Table 9-5. However, it is not unusual for the order to vary for individual children. For example, the regular plural -s may emerge before the irregular past verb tense for some children, and vice versa for others. Most of the morphemes are not fully mastered (used correctly 90% of the time when required or obligated) until later in development (Owens, 2008). The order in which morphemes are listed in Table 9-5 indicates when morphemes are mastered, *not* when they are first used by children.

Young children develop additional morphemes within Brown's stages. However, these morphemes were not studied by Brown and, consequently, do not appear in Table 9-5. In turn, less is known about their acquisition. Such morphemes include pronouns (e.g., *I, it, one, some, other, him, her*), other auxiliary verbs (e.g., "have + -en," "will"/"can"/"may" + verb), and noun and adjective suffixes (e.g., the adjectival comparative and superlatives -er and -est, respectively (as in "cold*er*" and "cold*est*").

The process of acquiring these major grammatical morphemes is both gradual and lengthy (Tager-Flusberg, 1989). While these morphemes are initially observed in the child's linguistic repertoire upon reaching an MLU of 2.0, all are not *consistently* used until after the child enters school. As grammatical morphemes continue to develop into Stage III, the child also begins to develop different types of sentences in the form of negatives (e.g., "*no* eat cookie") and questions (e.g., "*Where* Mommy go?"). Retherford (2000) provides additional data relative to production of negative sentences, yes/no questions, *wh*-questions, noun/verb phrase elaboration, and the development of complex sentences across Brown's (1973) stages. These developmental markers are covered in greater depth elsewhere in this text.

Researchers are not entirely certain how children acquire morphemes. In fact, multiple theories have been proposed to explain how children acquire grammar/syntax, including some that consider the role of imitation to be quite strong. Other theories suggest that a child plays an active role in analyzing words and assigning them to particular syntactic categories based on her knowledge of language and a particular stage of linguistic development. In a classic study,

Berko (1958) assessed preschool and first-grade children's productive control of English morphology using a set of "creatures" performing certain actions. Termed the *Wug Test*, a sentence completion task (or *structured elicited production task*) was employed to facilitate the child's use of invented (or nonsense) words containing grammatical morphemes in the form of plurals, possessives, the third-person present tense, the past tense, and the present progressive tense. The children in the study performed well, and the findings led Berko (1958) to state that young children internalize knowledge about the English morphological system such that they can add correct morphemes to novel words. In turn, this study further demonstrated that children do not simply learn grammatical morphemes through imitation, but rather through a *rule-governed morphological system*.

Tomasello (2000) suggested that when children first begin to combine words, they have a strong verb orientation. Their early sentences contain inflections paired with verbs only if they have heard the verb used in that exact way. In this way, the child does not generalize morphemes across verbs (and other word types) in the early Stages (I–III) but uses only those structures that have been modeled by adults. By age three years, most children have learned to use enough verb structures that they can begin to generalize and use new verbs in a variety of syntactic contexts. In a study that examined how typically developing children and children with specific language impairment learn grammatical morphemes, Miller and Deevy (2003) found that memorization did not account for the learning of morphemes for the majority of their subjects. Instead, these researchers noted a tendency for typically developing children to rely on memorization only in the early stages of language acquisition. They suggested that learning by rote plays a role in early morphosyntactic development, as children have to practice these new forms before generalizing this learning to new structures. Children then play a more active role in learning to use morphemes accurately. Children make multiple errors as they attempt to master these complex grammatical structures. It is this process that we do not fully understand.

In a study that examined the acquisition of three inflected morphemes (the copula *be*, the auxiliary *be*, and the third person present tense -*s*) in a sample of transcripts from five children, Wilson (2003) found that learning to use inflection was much more dependent on use with particular words rather than on application of a certain linguistic rule. This suggests that at the start of morphological production, at approximately Brown's Stage II, children's use of morphemes is related to accurate use of a *word* in an obligatory context. After a morpheme has been used correctly with a number of words (the specific number is not yet known), a child is then able to apply the "rule" more abstractly across new words and multiple sentence types.

Clearly, we still have much to learn about the process of morpheme acquisition. Miller and Deevy (2003) recommend that combining descriptive measures (such as eliciting spontaneous productions and examining language samples) with elicited tasks, such as the "Wug" task, may be an ideal research strategy for studying morphological productivity in young children.

CLINICAL APPLICATIONS: EXAMINATION OF THE CASE STUDIES_____

The case studies you have been reviewing provide us with some real-life examples of using Brown's stages to examine the morphosyntactic aspect of children's language development.

JOHNATHON (TD)

Johnathon, the TD case, was evaluated at age 25 months. That age would place him in late Stage I/early Stage II with an expected MLU of 1.50–1.99 (see Table 9-2). Recall that MLU is a calculation of the *average* length of utterance, so we would expect a child in this stage to use a combination of one- and two-word utterances. Review of Johnathon's assessment data indicates that his expressive language performance on the *Rossetti Infant Toddler Language Scale* (RITLS; Rossetti, 1990) was measured at the 21- to 24-month level, with scattered skills up to the 24- to 27-month level. Johnathon was reported to use new words, combine words, and use many action words. He was not described as using sentences, but his ability to combine words suggests that he is moving toward producing sentences in a typical fashion.

At this stage of development, we would not expect that any morphemes would yet be "mastered," or used 90% of the time in obligatory contexts. The morphemes that we might expect to emerge at this time are the present progressive -*ing*, the regular plural -*s*, and the prepositions *in* and *on*.

Recall from the case study that Jonathon's mother was concerned that his language development may have been delayed. As part of the assessment process, the speech-language pathologist counseled Johnathon's mother regarding typical language behaviors that Johnathon would be exhibiting. Part of this counseling might include some suggestions on developmental milestones that she would look for to make sure Jonathon was continuing to progress at a good rate. The clinician might also suggest ways to model the morphemes that will be emerging in the upcoming developmental period (e.g., *in, on, -s, -ing*) and provide Jonathon's mother with suggestions on how to elicit imitations of her models of these targeted structures. For example, to facilitate the emergence of the -*ing* morpheme, the adult can provide lots of opportunities for Johnathon to engage in actions (e.g., run*ning*, jump*ing*, clapp*ing*) and, while these actions are occurring, provide models for the target word (e.g., "Oh, you're jumping"; "Wow! Great jumping"; "Do you want to do more jumping?") and suggest that Johnathon use the word to label the activity. These types of focused language modeling sessions can provide a young language learner, such as Johnathon, with rich opportunities to experience the targeted morpheme in a variety of naturalistic contexts to enrich understanding and production.

JOSEPHINE (LB)

Josephine, the LB case, was evaluated at age 22 months. At that time, she was described as communicating through gesture and use of phoneme sequences that marked two syllables. She did not readily imitate words and had produced only a small number of true words. This child's performance on the RITLS for expressive language was measured at the 9- to 12-month level, which was a significant delay compared to her receptive language skills, which were within age expectations. Josephine communicated through gesture, babbling, jargon, and spontaneous vocalizations. She was reported to use only 7 words in her expressive vocabulary, which is typical of a 12-month-old child.

Referring to Table 9-2, we see that Josephine should be at the end of early Stage I, based on her chronological age of 22 months. Children in this stage have an expected MLU of 1.01–1.49 and demonstrate only very occasional use of grammatical morphemes. This expected MLU (remember—it is an *average* value) would suggest that the child is primarily using one-word utterances with occasional use of two-word utterances. Josephine, however, uses fewer than 10 words consistently, and we know that children typically begin to combine words when their productive vocabularies approach 50 words. This suggests that Josephine has a great deal of "developmental ground" to cover before she can begin to combine words to make new utterances.

The evaluating speech-language pathologist recommended that Josephine enroll in speech-language therapy where goals would focus on parent education and training of language facilitation techniques. Early efforts should focus on expanding Josephine's core vocabulary so that she can build a repertoire of words to meet her daily communication needs. The clinician can work with the family to identify words that will help Josephine to convey a range of meanings (i.e., using nouns and verbs) in functional activities throughout the day. These words will give her a strong foundation on which to build morphology.

ROBERT (LT)

Robert, the LT case, was evaluated at age 27 months. His first words did not emerge until age 18 months (age adjusted for premature birth) and, at the time of the evaluation, he was not yet combining words. On the RITLS, Robert's expressive language skills were measured at the 9- to 12-month level with scattered skills up to the 15- to 18-month level. His mother reported an expressive vocabulary of 14 words. He did not yet use any morphemes, nor did he combine words.

At age 27 months, Robert would be expected to be developmentally in Brown's Stage II (see Table 9-2), with an MLU of 2.00–2.49. The grammatical morphemes that should be emerging in Robert's expressive language at this time include present progressive -*ing*, prepositions *in* and *on*, regular plural -*s*, irregular past tense, possessive -*s*, and the uncontractible copula -*is*.

As with Josephine, the speech-language pathologist who conducted the evaluation recommended that Robert be enrolled in therapy to address speech as well as receptive and expressive language development. A play-based approach to intervention was recommended to capitalize on the use of naturalistic contexts to facilitate linguistic development. One of the goals for expressive language development was to establish Robert's ability to produce early developing morphemes that mark present progressive tense (-*ing*) and spatial relations (*in*, *on*). For Robert and other children with language development concerns, clinicians can use the information from Brown's stages (Table 9-2) and Brown's grammatical morphemes (Tables 9-4 and 9-5) to plan the sequence of intervention targets and also track progress. Once the target morphemes are noted to emerge in Robert's productive language, the clinician can subsequently target new morphemes that are next expected to emerge (an example would be regular plural -*s*) while using the tables to track mastery of morphemes as that occurs.

SUMMARY _____

In this chapter, we defined and described the types of morphemes found in the English language and examined the role these morphemes play in building the complexity of children's language. It is important for speech-language pathologists to understand the developmental process of morphological acquisition, including the way in which morphemes develop, as well as other aspects of grammatical (phonology and syntax) and semantic development. After reading this chapter, you should have a good understanding of how to assess an individual child's level of morphological development, identify aspects of deficiency, and plan targets for intervention. At each step of this process, speech-language pathologists use data from language sampling to guide their clinical decision making. Calculation of the mean length of utterance (MLU) is a key tool used to identify where a child is positioned developmentally along the process of language acquisition, and whether the child and his family need assistance in facilitating continued linguistic growth.

Although we are not certain exactly how children learn to use morphemes and apply them to novel utterances, current research suggests that children rely on a combination of strategies. These include imitating morphemes used by caregivers as well as actively testing and applying rules for morpheme use based on linguistic context. Most of the research findings in this area of inquiry have been based on small groups of children, so this area of study is an excellent venue for collaboration between researchers and clinicians. Speech-language pathologists in clinical practice and researchers should work collaboratively to further build the literature base by collecting language samples produced by young children and studying the process of morphological acquisition. It is an exciting area of study to pursue, and we look forward to new developments in this critically important area of communication development.

KEY TERMS

Bound morpheme   Morpheme
Free morpheme   Obligatory contexts
Mastery

STUDY QUESTIONS

- Demonstrate your understanding of the different kinds of morphemes by defining *free* and *bound* morphemes and providing examples of each.
- Review Table 9-4 and provide multiple examples of each of Brown's 14 grammatical morphemes.
- Tape-record a young child telling a story and, after transcribing the child's utterances, compute the MLU of the sample using the guidelines in Table 9-3. Compare your findings with the guidelines listed in Table 9-4, and identify the stage of development and which expected morphemes are present in the sample.
- Choose three of Brown's morphemes and design contexts to elicit the use of each morpheme with a young child.

REFERENCES

Berko, J. (1958). The child's learning of English morphology. *Word, 14,* 150–177.

Bloom, L., & Lahey, M. (1978). *Language development and language disorders.* New York: Wiley.

Brown, R. (1973). *A first language.* Cambridge, MA: Harvard University Press.

Brown, R., & Fraser, C. (1963). The acquisition of syntax. In C. N. Cofer & B. Musgrave (Eds.), *Verbal behavior and learning: Problems and processes* (pp. 158–209). New York: McGraw-Hill.

Leonard, L. B., & Finneran, D. (2003). Grammatical morpheme effects on MLU: "The same can be less" revisited. *Journal of Speech, Language and Hearing Research, 46,* 878–888.

Miller, C. A., & Deevy, P. (2003). A method for examining productivity of grammatical morphology in children with and without specific language impairment. *Journal of Speech, Language and Hearing Research, 46,* 1154–1165.

Miller, J. (1981). *Assessing language production in children.* Baltimore: University Park Press.

Owens, R. E. (2008). *Language development: An introduction.* 7th ed. Boston: Pearson Education.

Retherford, K. S. (2000). *Guide to analysis of language transcripts.* 3rd ed. Eau Claire, WI: Thinking Publications.

Rossetti, L. (1990). *The Rossetti Infant–Toddler Language Scale.* East Moline, IL: LinguiSystems.

Scarborough, H., Wyckoff, J., & Davidson, R. (1986). A reconsideration of the relationship between age and mean utterance length. *Journal of Speech and Hearing Research, 29,* 394–399.

Tager-Flusberg, H. (1989). Atypical children. In J. Berko-Gleason (Ed.), *The development of language* (pp. 311–348). Columbus, OH: Merrill.

Tomasello, M. (2000). Acquiring syntax is not what you think. In D. V. M. Bishop & L. B. Leonard (Eds.), *Speech and language impairments in children: Causes, characteristics, intervention, and outcome* (pp. 1–15). Hove, East Sussex, UK: Psychology Press.

Wilson, S. (2003). Lexically specific constructions in the acquisition of inflection in English. *Journal of Child Language, 30,* 75–115.

CHAPTER 10

The Development of Grammar

Patricia J. Brooks, PhD, and Liat Seiger-Gardner, PhD

OBJECTIVES

- Provide an overview of syntactic development under typical circumstances.
- Identify difficulties in grammar learning in late talkers and children with specific language impairment (SLI).
- Familiarize students with theoretical accounts of syntactic difficulties associated with language impairments.

INTRODUCTION

During their third year of life, children begin in earnest to combine words into phrases of increasing length and complexity. Grammatical development unfolds gradually and extends throughout childhood as children master constructions such as passives (e.g., *The cat was chased by the dog*), relative clauses (e.g., *The cat chased by the dog climbed up a tree*), and sentential complements (e.g., *Max saw the dog chase the cat up the tree*). Starting with their first word combinations, children acquire grammatical patterns that they then extend to new vocabulary, even occasionally using words in unconventional ways—for example, by saying *goed* instead of *went*, or *He falled it* instead of *He made it fall* or *He dropped it*. At each stage of development, children show highly variable rates of learning, ranging from precocious toddlers who produce considerable numbers of multiword utterances prior to their second birthdays to late talkers who produce very few, if any, intelligible words at the same age. Persistent difficulties in producing and understanding grammatical constructions are a hallmark symptom of specific language impairment (SLI) and may remain unresolved.

This chapter describes how grammatical abilities emerge in early childhood and change over time. It compares learning trajectories of children with typical development, late talkers, and children with SLI, and explores various theoretical approaches to understanding the grammatical difficulties of children with SLI.

THE DEVELOPMENT OF GRAMMAR
IN TYPICALLY DEVELOPING CHILDREN

The development of grammar involves the child's acquisition of a structured inventory of *linguistic constructions* that convey "who did what to whom" (Goldberg, 2006; Tomasello, 2003). Linguistic constructions are often associated with specific speech acts, such as asking a question or making a promise. Constructions vary with respect to their complexity, ranging from single-word constructions to more complex constructions involving multiple verbs. Under some circumstances, a single word can convey an entire communicate intention—for example, when a person commands his dog with the utterance *sit* or a child requests some juice with the utterance *more*. At the other extreme are constructions that include complex features such as embedded sentences, relative clauses, and long-distance dependencies (as in subject-verb agreement or co-reference between nouns and pronouns). For example, the assertion *I hope to spend the holidays visiting my brother who lives in the Midwest* contains a main verb *hope*, followed by an embedded sentence containing the verb *spend*, with its three arguments comprising an omitted subject (*I*), the direct object *the holidays*, and the gerund *visiting*, followed by its direct object *my brother*, which is modified by the relative clause *who lives in the Midwest*.

The building blocks of a language are the content words that refer to objects and other entities, and that convey the properties and relationships of those entities. These content words are combined with function words and inflections, the so-called grammatical morphemes, to create templates for possible sentences. One can conceive of a language's constructions as a set of mental instructions for how to build a sentence; in effect, they explain how to arrange nouns, verbs, prepositions, adjectives, adverbs, function words, and other grammatical morphemes to convey one's communicative intention in a way that is consistent with the conventions of a language community. These instructions can be applied recursively (e.g., *This is the cow with the crumpled horn, that tossed the dog, that worried the cat, that killed the rat, that lay in the house that Jack built*) or conjoined (e.g., *She got out of bed and got dressed and brushed her teeth and ate her breakfast and headed off to school*) to yield an infinite variety of possible utterances.

A language's inventory of linguistic constructions is structured in the sense that there is regularity in the instantiated patterns (often described as syntactic rules). It is systematic in the sense that verbs that convey similar meanings (e.g., *wash* and *scrub*) tend to be used in a similar range of construction types (e.g., *I washed the dishes; I scrubbed the dishes; The dishes are being washed; The dishes are being scrubbed*) (Levin, 1993). The acquisition of verbs is crucial to the child's acquisition of grammar, because verb meanings dictate the number of nouns that are required for sentences to be complete. Sentences are built around verbs, with the verb projecting its "argument structure," which comprises its verb-specific expectations about the number of noun phrases, sentential complements, or prepositional phrases required. Intransitive verbs, such as *sleep*, have only one argument (e.g., the one sleeping); transitive verbs, such as *throw*, have two arguments (e.g., the one throwing the object and the object being thrown); and ditransitive verbs, such as *give*, have three arguments (e.g., the giver, the recipient, and the object being given to the recipient). English verbs have a variety of argument structures. For example, *think* takes a sentential complement, as in *I think Bob will join us for dinner*, and *put* requires both a prepositional phrase and a noun phrase, as in *She put the milk in the refrigerator*.

The semantic roles of the nouns in a sentence are determined by the verbs involved as well as the constructions in which they occur. This is most obvious in verb pairs, such as *chase* and *flee* or *buy* and *sell*, which are distinguished by which role is associated with the noun in subject position (for example, *Marcia bought a TV from the store* versus *The store sold a TV to Marcia*). In English, there is a strong tendency to associate the agent role (i.e., the one performing the action) with the noun in the pre-verbal subject position and the patient role (i.e., the entity acted upon or affected by the action) with the noun in the post-verbal direct object position. This tendency is not absolute, however, owing to the great variety of semantic roles associated with the subject position of English verbs. For example, contrast the role of the subject *Max* in the following sentences containing the transitive verbs *smash, break, receive*, and *weigh*:

Max smashed the pumpkin.

Max broke his arm.

Max received a letter.

Max weighs 50 pounds.

Only in the first sentence is *Max* a prototypical agent directly acting on an object, leading to a visible change of state in that object.

Despite this variability in the semantic roles associated with the sentence subject, English speakers rapidly come to expect the first noun in the subject–verb–object construction to refer to the one performing the action. This bias makes both children and adults susceptible to comprehension errors in processing grammatical structures with atypical word orders, such as reversible passive sentences (e.g., *The boy was chased by the dog*) and object cleft sentences (e.g., *It was the boy the dog chased*) (Sudhalter & Braine, 1985; Ferreira, 2003).

Statistical Learning

Children discover syntactic regularities through a process of *statistical learning*, by which they accumulate information about the frequency of occurrence of different types of linguistic elements (e.g., speech sounds, words, phrases) and their quasi-regular co-occurrence patterns in speech (Chang, Dell, & Bock, 2006; Gomez & Gerken, 2000; Saffran, 2003; Seidenberg & MacDonald, 1999). Statistical learning is supported by domain-general associative learning mechanisms, and begins in utero, as demonstrated by fetal sensitivity to the prosodic or rhythmic qualities of maternal speech prior to birth (DeCasper, Lacanuet, Busnel, Granier-Deferre, & Maugeals, 1994; Kisilevsky et al., 2003; Krueger, Holditch-David, Quint, & DeCasper, 2004). Infants in the first months of life readily distinguish the language spoken by their mother from other languages (Mehler, Jusczyk, Lambertz, Halsted, Bertoncini, & Amiel-Tison, 1988), and they are able to do so solely on the basis of prosodic information (Dehaene-Lambertz & Houston, 1998; Mehler et al., 1988). By 7 months of age, infants can generalize recurrent patterns among syllables (e.g., the ABA pattern of *ko-ga-ko*) to new vocabulary (e.g., *ba-po-ba*) (Marcus, Vijayan, Bandi Rao, & Vishton, 1999); by 12 months, they can generalize their knowledge of a finite-state grammar, generating four- to six-syllable phrases, to novel vocabulary (Gomez & Gerkin, 1999). At 18 months, infants are able to track nonadjacent dependencies among first and last syllables in three-syllable phrases (Gomez, 2002). This type of dependency is prominent in natural languages in contexts requiring "agreement" in number, gender, or case between nouns and verbs, adjectives, or pronouns, as in *Tom wants his mother to drive him to the store*, where *Tom* requires number agreement on the verb *want* and gender agreement on the pronouns *his* and *him*.

Statistical learning plays a major role in the acquisition of word classes such as nouns, verbs, and adjectives as children discover how members of these word classes combine with function words and other grammatical morphemes (Maratsos, 1990; Mintz, Newport, & Bever, 2002; Redington, Chater, & Finch, 1998). For example, in English, determiners such as *a, one*, and *the* collocate with nouns, whereas auxiliaries such as *is, can*, and *do* and inflections such as *-ed* and *-ing* collocate with verbs.

In addition to conducting distributional analyses of the semantic and syntactic contexts of word use, children track statistics pertaining to the phonological features of words, which are correlated with grammatical word classes (Cassidy & Kelly, 2001; Saffran, 2003). With respect to the distinction between function words (e.g., determiners and auxiliaries) and content words (e.g., nouns and verbs), content words tend to have more phonemes and more complex consonant clusters and syllables than do function words. Function words, in contrast, are more likely than content words to have phonologically reduced vowels (i.e., schwa) (Monaghan, Chater, & Christiansen, 2005). Phonological features also provide useful cues for distinguishing nouns and verbs: Nouns tend to have more syllables than verbs, whereas verbs tend to have more syllabic complexity and fewer reduced syllables than nouns, and are more likely to end in *-ed* (Kelly, 1992; Monaghan, Chater, & Christiansen, 2005). In languages with complex morphological systems (e.g., Spanish, Russian or Lithuanian), children use statistical learning of phonological and distributional information to acquire noun gender and declension subclasses (Gerken, Wilson, & Lewis, 2005).

Acquiring Word-Specific Formulae

Although word meanings map systematically onto construction types with verbs playing a pre-dominant role, children must nonetheless master the specific combinatorial properties of each and every word in their language to fully master their language's grammatical system. For example, verbs with highly similar meanings often combine with different sets of prepositions (e.g., *We came to the party at 8:00* versus *We arrived at the party at 8:00*). Many verbs alternate between intransitive (one argument) and transitive (two arguments) construction types; these alternation patterns are quasi-regular, with verbs occurring in an alternation pattern tending to have similar meanings, although numerous exceptions to the pattern may exist. For example, the verb *trip* occurs in both intransitive and transitive constructions (e.g., *I tripped on the broken sidewalk; The broken sidewalk tripped me*), whereas the verb *stumble* is grammatical only in the intransitive construction (e.g., *I stumbled over the broken sidewalk*, but not *The broken sidewalk stumbled me*). In general, the most frequent words in a language tend to be the most irregular in their patterns of usage. This irregularity is easiest to observe in the context of inflectional mor-phology, where the verbs with irregular past tense forms (e.g., *go–went, do–did, fall–fell, come–came*), as opposed to regular past tense forms (e.g., *walk–walked, drop–dropped, kiss–kissed*), tend to be among the earliest verbs acquired. Similarly, the most frequent English verbs (e.g., *be, get, go, have*) occur in the widest range of grammatical constructions, with highly idiosyn-cratic patterns of usage.

Children learn linguistic constructions by attending to how others use words to convey their communicative intentions. From their first single-word utterances at about 10 to 12 months of age, children use language both imperatively to ask things of others and declaratively to point out things to others (Bates, Benigni, Bretherton, Camaioni, & Volterra, 1979). Over their second year of life, toddlers show a variety of paths in making the transition to multi-word language—sometimes learning to connect words into phrases, and sometimes learning to isolate individual words out of connected phrases (Nelson, 1981; Pine & Lieven, 1993; Pine, Lieven, & Rowland, 1997). Some children start out producing many utterances consisting of single words spoken in isolation, whereas other children construct longer utterances with many unintelligible segments, but with a recognizable prosodic contour.

Children's first word combinations often involve a verb, preposition, or other relational term (e.g., *all-gone*) used in combination with a noun (e.g., *all-gone juice*). Two-year-old chil-dren's two-word utterances convey a wide range of semantic relationships and cannot be reli-ably categorized in terms of semantic categories such as "agent–action," "object–location," and so on (Howe, 1976; Ninio, 2006). Many toddlers master a variety of simple syntactic patterns, typically consisting of a specific word preceded or followed by a slot for a noun or a pronoun (Braine, 1976). These *word-specific formulae* (e.g., *all-gone* _____) are the child's first construc-tions and are sufficient to allow the child to creatively construct novel utterances, such as saying *all-gone sticky* following a hand washing (Braine, 1971). Basic processes of inserting different nouns into the slots of word-specific formulae and concatenating single words onto the beginnings of ends of word-specific formulae account for much of the early creativity in toddlers' multiword speech (Lieven, Behrens, Speares, & Tomasello, 2003).

Verb Acquisition and Its Influence on Grammatical Structures

Because verbs serve as the key to organizing elements in sentence construction (Pinker, 1989), much attention has been paid to the child's first word combinations containing actual verbs, as opposed to other relational words, such as prepositions, adjectives, and adverbs. Learning of both verbs and constructions is gradual and continuous, and most likely involves the same learning mechanisms (Bates & Goodman, 1997). As noted by Tomasello (1992), the best predictor of how a toddler will use a particular verb in his language is the toddler's prior history of usage of that particular verb. Thus each verb follows its own learning trajectory, and much of what the toddler is discovering about syntactic structure is tied to specific lexical items.

At the same time, the toddler is acquiring the most basic constructions of her language, and each construction has its own learning curve (Ninio, 2006). In English, the most basic constructions are the simple transitive subject–verb–object and intransitive subject–verb structures (Tomasello & Brooks, 1998). English-speaking two-year-olds very often omit the subject–noun phrase in their utterances (Valian, 1991; Valian & Aubry, 2005), thereby producing early transitive utterances with verb–object structure (e.g., *Want juice*). The likelihood that a child will produce a verb–object construction with a new verb increases as a function of the number of other verbs the child has previously used in verb–object combinations (Ninio, 1999). That is, the more verbs a child already knows how to use in a particular construction, the faster he will learn to use new verbs in that construction.

The order of acquisition of specific verbs in specific constructions largely reflects the patterns of verb usage in the input (Theakston, Lieven, Pine, & Rowland, 2004). That is, the first verbs used in the basic construction types are not semantically restricted (i.e., they have a diversity of associated meanings), but rather reflect the distribution of highly frequent verbs in caretaker language (Ninio, 2006). Furthermore, children learn verbs in a diversity of constructions, including the passive voice (as in *The baby was born last night*), with the specific verb–construction pairings reflecting the patterns of verb usage in child-directed speech.

Because children acquire words and their combinatorial properties at the same time, throughout childhood a very tight link is observed between vocabulary and grammar acquisition (Bates & Goodman, 1997). It has been argued that grammar acquisition requires children to have a critical mass of vocabulary to identify recurrent combinatory patterns (Marchman &

Bates, 1994) that can be applied productively in language production. In this process, which is referred to as *lexical bootstrapping*, as the child acquires a sufficient number of lexical exemplars, she constructs the abstract grammatical patterns required for *syntactic productivity*. In other words, grammar emerges from an accumulation of word-specific combinatorial formulae. According to this view, the same learning mechanisms support the acquisition of words and the extraction of grammatical regularities based on similarities among stored items (Thordardottir, Weismer, & Evans, 2002).

Syntactic Overgeneralizations

During the preschool years, children demonstrate syntactic productivity in their usage of basic sentence constructions by producing *overgeneralization errors* such as *Don't giggle me* or *Stay it there*. These errors involve the child's use of a verb in a construction that is not conventional in his language community (Bowerman, 1988; Pinker, 1989). Many of these utterances involve usage of transitive subject–verb–object or verb–object constructions with intransitive verbs (Bowerman & Croft, 2007; Loeb, Pye, Richardson, & Redmond, 1998). Nevertheless, errors with other syntactic patterns are also common, as in *Explain me your answer* or *I spilled it of orange juice*. Children at this age also creatively devise *lexical innovations* such as *Let me broom the floor* (meaning "sweep the floor"), *I'm softing you right here* (meaning "stroke softly"), or *I'm gonna higher you up* (meaning "lift you higher"), in which the child uses a noun or an adjective as if it were a verb (Clark, 1993).

To explore the onset of syntactic productivity, a large number of experimental studies have tested whether toddlers will use a newly introduced non-verb in a construction other than the one(s) in which the verb is introduced by an adult. For example, if the made-up verb *tam* (with a meaning similar to the English verb *swing*), is introduced in the sentence *The apple is being tammed by Big Bird*, the experiment tests whether children will answer the question *What is Big Bird doing?* using the subject–verb–object construction, as in *Big Bird is tamming the apple*. These studies (e.g., Akhtar & Tomasello, 1997; Brooks & Tomasello, 1999b; Childers & Tomasello, 2001; Tomasello & Brooks, 1998) demonstrate a very strong preference among two-year-olds to use a newly introduced verb in exactly the same constructions as they have heard it used by others. However, by age three to four, the majority of children with typical development will flexibly use a novel verb in a variety of construction types.

Although toddlers tend to be conservative learners who avoid using novel verbs in unattested constructions, they generally show good comprehension of novel verbs in transitive and intransitive constructions (Fernandes, Marcus, Di Nubila, & Vouloumanos, 2006; Fisher, 2002; Naigles, 1990, 1996). That is, two-year-olds will select different actions as the referent for a novel verb as a function of the construction in which they have heard the novel verb used. More specifically, the results of the comprehension studies demonstrate that toddlers have a preference to associate a novel verb occurring in a subject–verb–object construction with an event in which someone is directly acting on something or someone, and they are *not* likely to associate a novel verb occurring in a subject–verb construction with an action directed toward an object. This ability to use the construction in which a novel verb is used to make inferences about the possible meaning of the verb is called *syntactic bootstrapping* and typically develops in the third year of life (Gleitman, 1990; Gleitman, Cassidy, Nappa, Papafragou, & Trueswell, 2005).

Once syntactic productivity with the basic construction types has been established, virtually all children will make overgeneralization errors by using verbs in constructions that sound ungrammatical to adult native speakers. These errors seem to be especially common in three- to six-year-olds, but gradually become less frequent as children mature. Nevertheless, even among preschoolers, in the majority of their utterances they follow the conventions of their language community and use verbs in the same constructions as they have heard others use the verbs. That is, overgeneralization errors occur, but they are relatively rare, and likely reflect on-the-spot pressures to produce fluent speech as opposed to systematic discrepancies in the child's grammar (Braine & Brooks, 1995; MacWhinney, 2004). Of course, even adults occasionally produce such errors (Pinker, 1989), which may be a consequence of fatigue or distraction.

In accounting for the gradual decrease in the frequency of overgeneralization errors during childhood, several factors have been implicated. First, children gradually learn that verbs with similar meanings tend to occur in the same sets of constructions (Levin, 1993). English-speaking children are more willing to extend an intransitive verb denoting a manner of motion (e.g., verbs such as *roll, swing, bounce, jiggle*) to the transitive subject–verb–object construction than an intransitive verb referring to a motion in a specific direction (e.g., verbs such as *fall, come, descend, rise*) (Brooks & Tomasello, 1999a) or an intransitive verb referring to an internally caused action (e.g., verbs such as *cough, laugh, blush, squeal*) (Ambridge, Pine, Rowland, & Young, 2008). Although correlations between verb meanings and syntactic patterns are less than perfect, children are sensitive to these regularities, as are adults when they learn new verbs (e.g., *e-mail*) and use them in appropriate constructions (e.g., *E-mail me your answer*), even if they have never heard the verb used in that construction.

A second factor is *entrenchment*—in effect, the frequency of usage of specific verbs in specific constructions. From infancy, children are highly sensitive to the co-occurrence patterns of speech sounds, words, and phrases. Patterns that are repeated often come to sound natural and are preferred over patterns that are rarely, if ever, heard. Thus, if a child repeatedly hears sentences of the form *The magician made the rabbit disappear* but not *The magician disappeared the rabbit*, the former construction will come to be preferred over the latter (Braine & Brooks, 1995; Brooks & Tomasello, 1999a; Brooks & Zizak, 2002). Children have more certainty about how to use the most common verbs in their language, owing to their higher frequency of usage, and they are more likely to make errors with newly introduced verbs for which they lack the relevant experience (Brooks, Tomasello, Dodson, & Lewis, 1999; Theakston, 2004).

Erroneous Syntactic Operations

Typically developing children make occasional errors in executing syntactic operations throughout childhood. A great deal of research has explored the difficulties English-speaking children experience in mastering the subject–auxiliary inversion operation crucial for question formation. Children make errors in producing questions by omitting auxiliaries (e.g., *What he doing?*), failing to invert the subject and auxiliary (e.g., *Who she is hitting?*), generating double auxiliaries (e.g., *What does she does like?*), or double tensing (e.g., *What does he likes?*) (Ambridge, Rowland, Theakston, & Tomasello, 2006; Rowland, 2007; Santelmann, Berk, Austin, Somashekar, & Lust, 2002). The frequency of these errors varies as a function of the specific *wh*-word + auxiliary combination, with highly entrenched combinations (i.e., those that arise most frequently in caretaker speech) seemingly protected from errors in children's language (Ambridge et al., 2006; Rowland, 2007).

On the side of sentence processing, children make numerous errors in comprehending sentences containing reduced relative clauses, such as *Put the frog on the napkin in the box* (Hurewitz, Brown-Schmidt, Thorpe, Gleitman, & Trueswell, 2000; Trueswell, Sekerina, Hill, & Logrip, 1999), by interpreting *on the napkin* as a destination for the frog's movement as opposed to a modifier of the frog, as in *Put the frog who is on the napkin in the box*. Children also make errors in their comprehension of sentences containing universal quantifiers, such as *Every boy is riding a donkey*, in which the child must determine which noun phrase is modified by the quantifier *every* (Brooks & Braine, 1996; Brooks & Sekerina, 2005/2006). That is, when shown a picture of three boys, each of whom is riding a donkey, along with an extra donkey with no rider, children will argue that not every boy is riding a donkey, due to the extra donkey. It has been argued that young children often generate shallow, or incomplete, interpretations of sentences with complex grammatical structures or atypical word order (e.g., passive-voice sentences such as *The boy was chased by the dog*), and they generally fail to revise their initial interpretations of sentences, even in the face of information (e.g., additional words in the sentence) that conflicts with their initial interpretation (Trueswell et al., 1999).

THE DEVELOPMENT OF GRAMMAR IN LATE TALKERS

Toddlers with delays in receptive and expressive language development show deficits in both vocabulary and grammar acquisition. Two of the most common metrics for evaluating syntactic development in children from spontaneous language samples are *mean length of utterance*

(*MLU*; Brown, 1973) and *index of productive syntax* (*IPSyn*; Scarborough, 1990), with the latter providing a more sensitive assessment in older preschoolers.

On both of these measures, late talkers, identified at ages 2;0 to 2;7 using the Language Development Survey (Rescorla, 1989), continued to show deficits in grammatical complexity at 3;0 and 4;0 relative to their typically developing peers (Rescorla, Dahlsgaard, & Roberts, 2000). Late talkers appeared to recover more rapidly in the area of lexical development than in areas of syntactic and morphological development (Rescorla, Roberts, & Dahlsgaard, 1997). However, in long-term follow-ups of these late talkers at ages 9 and 13 (Rescorla, 2002, 2005), although scoring within the normal range, these children showed significant deficits on most language measures relative to a control group matched on socioeconomic status and nonverbal intelligence. Scores on the Language Development Survey taken at ages 2;0 to 2;7 significantly predicted outcome measures in vocabulary, grammar, verbal memory, and reading comprehension through age 13. Other longitudinal studies (e.g., Bishop & Edmundson, 1987; Moyle, Weismer, Evans, & Lindstrom, 2007; Stothard, Snowling, Bishop, Chipchase, & Kaplan, 1998) have yielded similar findings of persistent subclinical weaknesses across language domains in many children identified as late talkers in comparison to their typically developing peers.

Confirmation of the tight relationship between vocabulary and grammatical development in late talkers as well as in children with typical development is provided by a recent longitudinal study carried out by Moyle, Weismer, Evans, and Lindstrom (2007). These researchers followed 30 late talkers and 30 typically developing children from ages 2;0 to 5;6, using both standardized tests and spontaneous language sampling to measure vocabulary and grammar growth at 6-month intervals. In both groups, vocabulary and grammar measures showed strong concurrent correlations (i.e., vocabulary measures at time 1 related significantly to grammar measures at time 1, vocabulary measures at time 2 related significantly to grammar measures at time 2, and so on). However, when using cross-lagged statistics (i.e., correlating vocabulary measures at time 1 with grammar at time 2, grammar measures at time 1 with vocabulary at time 2, and so on), grammatical abilities were less predictive of future vocabulary growth in the late talkers in comparison to the children with typical development. This pattern suggests that the late talkers were less able to use grammatical information to constrain word meaning than the control group; in effect, they were less capable of utilizing syntactic bootstrapping as a mechanism for vocabulary acquisition. In contrast, in both groups, vocabulary size was predictive of future grammatical abilities, although the significant cross-lagged statistics were observed at younger ages in the children with typical development in comparison to the late talkers. This pattern is consistent with the lexical bootstrapping hypothesis that the abstract grammatical constructions supporting syntactic productivity emerge from accumulated word-specific formulae.

THE DEVELOPMENT OF GRAMMAR IN CHILDREN
WITH SPECIFIC LANGUAGE IMPAIRMENT

Specific language impairment (SLI) is characterized by dramatic and profound difficulties in the acquisition and processing of syntax and grammatical morphology (Bishop, 1992; Bishop, Bright, James, Bishop, & van der Lely, 2000), which are coupled with difficulties in acquiring vocabulary, especially verbs (Windfuhr, Faraghter, & Conti-Ramsden, 2002). Children with SLI are less accurate in labeling events than their language-matched younger peers (Loeb, Pye, Redmond, & Richardson, 1996; Loeb, Pye, Richardson, & Redmond, 1998); they are inefficient word learners with less diverse vocabularies (Oetting, Rice, & Swank, 1995; Stokes & Fletcher, 2000), more rapid forgetting of newly acquired words (Riches, Tomasello, & Conti-Ramsden, 2005), and greater dependence on high frequency of occurrence in the input for learning to be successful (Windfuhr, Faraghter, & Conti-Ramsden, 2002). Children with SLI appear to have difficulties working out the precise functions of grammatical elements. In particular, they show a prolonged period of item-by-item learning and are subsequently delayed in generalizing syntactic knowledge across items (Fletcher, Stokes, & Wong, 2005).

Syntactic Bootstrapping and Knowledge of Constructions

One factor contributing to the verb-learning difficulties observed in children with SLI is their inability to use syntactic bootstrapping as a word learning strategy (Shulman & Guberman, 2007; van der Lely, 1994). Children with SLI are less capable of using syntactic cues in sentences to make inferences about the possible meanings of novel verbs. For example, when shown two scenes—one depicting a causative action and the other depicting a repetitive motion—preschool children with typical development are strongly biased to associate a novel verb in a transitive construction (e.g., *Look the rabbit is gorping the duck*) with the causative action, and a novel verb introduced in an intransitive construction (e.g., *Look the rabbit and duck are gorping*) with the repetitive motion (Naigles, 1990; Shulman & Guberman, 2007). In contrast, language-matched five-year-old children with SLI perform at chance levels of responding (Shulman & Guberman, 2007). Similarly, six-year-old children with SLI are much less successful in acting out the meaning of a novel verb on the basis of the syntactic construction in which it is introduced than their typically developing peers (van der Lely, 1994).

A growing body of literature indicates that children with SLI show considerable delays in acquiring their language's inventory of grammatical constructions. English-speaking five-year-olds with SLI show very limited syntactic productivity, even with the most basic transitive and intransitive constructions, and they are reluctant to use a verb in a construction with which they have not heard it used in the input (Conti-Ramsden & Windfuhr, 2002; Riches, Faraghter, & Conti-Ramsden, 2006). To examine rates of overgeneralization errors in children with SLI,

Loeb and colleagues (1998) used agent-focused questions (e.g., *What did I do to the baby?*) to elicit transitive sentences with intransitive verbs (e.g., *You slept the baby*) and patient-focused questions (e.g., *What did the ball do?*) to elicit intransitive sentences with transitive verbs (e.g., *It threw*). Although overgeneralization errors were rare, Loeb and colleagues (1998) observed that five- and six-year-old children with SLI were less likely than language-matched younger children to use the periphrastic causative construction (e.g., *You made the baby sleep*) to answer the agent-focused question and were less likely to use the passive construction (e.g., *It was thrown*) to answer the patient-focused question. Thus the children with SLI were less flexible in varying the constructions in which they used English verbs in response to the discourse pressures of the elicitation questions.

Evans and MacWhinney (1999) reported that English-speaking children with expressive–receptive SLI are much less likely to use word order as a cue to sentence interpretation than their typically developing peers or children with expressive SLI. That is, when presented with sentences such as *Chair chases horse*, seven-year-old children with expressive–receptive SLI tend to base their responses on noun animacy, selecting the horse as the one doing the chasing, rather than utilizing knowledge that the first noun in the subject–verb–object construction refers to the entity performing the action. In contrast to the children with expressive–receptive SLI, children with expressive SLI tend to rely exclusively on a first noun as agent strategy. This preference persists even for sentences such as *Horse camel chases*, for which the second noun is the preferred agent (i.e., the one doing the chasing) for children with typical development. In Evans and MacWhinney's study, reliance on word order as a cue to sentence interpretation was strongly correlated with receptive language abilities.

Representational Deficits and Grammatical SLI

Perhaps the most important debate in the field relates to the source of grammatical difficulties in children with SLI—in particular, whether there is a representational deficit in a specialized grammar module (e.g., Rice & Wexler, 1996; van der Lely, 1994, 1998, 2005) or whether more general processing mechanisms can account for grammatical difficulties (e.g., Joanisse & Seidenberg, 2003; Leonard, Weismer, Miller, Francis, Tomblin, & Kail, 2007; Ullman & Pierpont, 2005). According to the Representational Deficit for Dependent Relations (RDDR) account, the deficit lies in the computational syntactic system as opposed to general processing mechanisms (van der Lely, 1994; van der Lely & Stollwerck, 1997). Central to the RDDR account is the identification of a subgroup of children with *grammatical SLI (G-SLI)* who are characterized by persistent receptive and expressive language impairments that are restricted to core grammatical operations. The grammatical representations of these children have been viewed as "underspecified" (van der Lely, 1996; van der Lely & Stollwerck, 1997) owing to their incomplete syntactic analysis. In addition to their deficits in the domains of morphology and syntax, children with G-SLI often have difficulties processing phonology, especially with more complex linguistic stimuli (van der Lely, 2005). The auditory processing of speech is impaired in the majority of children with G-SLI, whereas auditory processing of nonspeech sounds does not distinguish children with G-SLI from their typically developing peers (van der Lely, Rosen, & Adlard, 2004).

A more recent formulation of the RRDR account, called the Computational Grammatical Complexity (CGC) hypothesis, proposes that children with SLI are impaired in the computations underlying hierarchical, structurally complex forms across one or more components of grammar (van der Lely, 1998, 2005). According to the CGC hypothesis, the underlying deficit in the linguistic system markedly affects syntactic dependencies such as "movement" operations or intrasentential co-reference. For example, in the question *What book did Jack read?*, the *wh*-phrase *what book* is said to move from its position as the direct object of the verb *read* to its sentence initial position. Maranis and van der Lely (2007) observed that children with G-SLI show an atypical pattern in processing *wh*-questions, and they rely on lexical and thematic information in question interpretation. Similarly, sentences involving anaphoric or pronominal co-reference require a detailed syntactic analysis to constrain co-reference relationships within a sentence. For example, in the sentence *Elmo says Oscar was tickling himself*, the anaphor *himself* must refer to Oscar; in contrast, in *Elmo says Oscar is tickling him*, the pronoun *him* must refer either to Elmo or to some other entity not mentioned in the sentence. Children with G-SLI perform at chance levels of responding when sentence interpretation depends on syntactic information to rule out inappropriate co-reference relationships, but they are adept at utilizing semantic or contextual cues (e.g., gender of the pronoun, herself = female) in sentence interpretation (van der Lely & Stollwerck, 1997).

Because of their heavy reliance on lexical, semantic, and contextual cues in sentence interpretation, children with G-SLI have difficulties with "reversible" active-voice sentences involving the transitive construction (e.g., *The girl carries the baby*) or the ditransitive construction (e.g., *The boy gives the girl the baby*) (van der Lely & Harris, 1990). In reversible transitive sentences, either noun in the sentence could be assigned to either thematic role on semantic grounds. For example, the sentence *The boy pushed the girl* is reversible because both nouns can be assigned the thematic role of the agent as in *The girl pushed the boy*; in contrast, in the sentence *The boy pushed the chair*, only *the boy* is animate and is likely, on semantic grounds, to be the one doing the pushing. Reversible sentences are difficult for children with G-SLI to process because the children must use grammatical information (i.e., word order) to construct a correct sentence interpretation.

Tomblin and Pandich (1999) have argued against the account put forth by van der Lely and her colleagues that grammatical abilities can be selectively impaired in SLI, leaving vocabulary acquisition unimpaired. Tomblin and Pandich (1999) observed a statistically significant, moderately sized correlation between vocabulary and grammar acquisition in a large sample of children with SLI. In their study, children's performance on language and nonlanguage tasks was subjected to factor analysis to identify principal components of variation in task performance. The results indicated that measures of grammar and semantics loaded onto the same underlying factor, whereas phonology and speech sound-production loaded onto a separate factor. These findings, in turn, suggest that grammatical abilities were not selectively impaired relative to semantics in these children.

The Extended Optional Infinitive Hypothesis

Another domain-specific account, the *Extended Optional Infinitive (EOI) hypothesis* (Rice & Wexler, 1996; Rice, Wexler, & Cleave, 1995), argues that the deficits seen in children with SLI affect many language components but that the central deficit occurs in the part of morphosyntax responsible for tense marking. According to this account, children with SLI treat tense marking as optional, although, in English, it is obligatory. Rice and Wexler have proposed that typically developing children go through an optional infinitive stage as well; however, in children with SLI, this stage extends over a longer period of time. Whereas the RDDR and CGC accounts assume difficulties with the application of grammatical rules and the construction of hierarchical linguistic representations, respectively, the EOI hypothesis suggests that children with SLI know the rules for tense marking but lack the knowledge that tense marking is obligatory in certain linguistic contexts.

In children with SLI, support for the EOI hypothesis comes from four sources:

- Their inconsistent use of finite verb morphology in speech production (Miller & Leonard, 1998)
- The rarity of errors suggesting use of incorrect grammatical rules (e.g., *The dogs bark<u>s</u> at the girl* or *They <u>is</u> swimming*) (Rice, Wexler, & Cleave, 1995)
- Morphological overgeneralization errors (*e.g., He eated the apple*) (Leonard, Eyer, Bedore, & Grela, 1997)
- The finding that their production of auxiliaries (e.g., *is, are*) is influenced by the presence or absence of an auxiliary in their preceding utterance (Leonard, Miller, Deevy, Rauf, Gerber, & Charest, 2002)

That is, children with SLI are more likely to produce an auxiliary in an obligatory context when their previous utterance contained an auxiliary than when it did not. Taken together, these observations suggest that children with SLI have some awareness of morphological rules, but lack knowledge of the specific contexts in which those rules' application is required.

Performance Accounts of Grammatical Difficulties

Leonard (1989) has proposed the *Surface Account,* which focuses on children's difficulties in acquiring low-saliency morphemes such as tense-marking inflections (e.g., past tense -*ed,* third person singular -*s*). According to this model, children with SLI have a general processing capacity limitation, which profoundly affects both their perception of grammatical morphemes that are brief in duration and their ability to infer their grammatical functions. Using a computational model of the language-processing system, Joanisse and Seidenberg (2003) have argued in similar fashion that the grammatical difficulties observed in SLI may occur secondary to an underlying deficit in speech perception.

In support of the Surface Account, Montgomery and Leonard (1998) observed that children with SLI have greater difficulty in a on-line (reaction time) word-recognition task as well as an off-line grammaticality judgment task when the task involved a low-phonetic-substance inflection, such as the third person singular -*s* or the past tense -*ed,* in comparison to a high-phonetic-substance inflection, such as the present progressive -*ing.* Children with SLI also perform worse than their age-matched peers in a speech perception task involving discrimination of the consonant vowel pair /ba/ and /da/, which requires attention to brief-duration acoustic cues. Children with SLI perform comparably to younger children matched on receptive syntax on the grammaticality judgment task, but show a different profile in the on-line reaction time task, which suggests that real-time language processing is especially difficult for these children.

Leonard (1995) examined the production of a wide range of functional morphemes (determiners, inflections, complementizers) in the spontaneous speech of children with SLI. In this work, children with SLI were found to utilize the full range of function word types in their speech, albeit with lesser frequency and consistency than their typically developing peers matched on MLU. These results indicate a broader difficulty with grammar than that suggested by the EOI hypothesis and Surface Account, and they encourage further exploration of performance factors that might predict whether children with SLI will successfully provide grammatical morphemes in obligatory contexts.

Recognizing that children with SLI exhibit errors in marking verbs for tense, Owen and Leonard (2006) compared the proficiency of children with SLI in producing finite and nonfinite complement clauses (e.g., *Big Bird knew that Elmo fed the dog* versus *Big Bird knew to feed the dog*). They found that children with SLI have difficulties using complement clauses, relative to their typically developing peers matched on language abilities or age, regardless of the type of complement clause being considered (i.e., finite or nonfinite). These authors suggest that nonfinite complement clauses are the first to emerge and are somewhat easier to acquire than finite complement clauses for two reasons: (1) Nonfinite complement clauses do not involve finite verb morphology (i.e., they involve a bare verb) and (2) they involve one fewer noun argument than the corresponding finite complement clause.

Generalized Slowing and Limited Verbal Working Memory Capacity

By focusing on grammatical morphology, the Surface Account and the EOI hypothesis provide too narrow of a characterization of the grammatical difficulties of children with SLI, and neither theory adequately accounts for children's difficulties with complex syntactic constructions such as passives (Leonard, Wong, Deevy, Stokes, & Fletcher, 2006; van der Lely, 1996), *wh*-questions (Deevy & Leonard, 2004; Maranis & van der Lely, 2007; van der Lely & Battell, 2003), and complement clauses (Owen & Leonard, 2006). In contrast to the perspective taken by the Surface Account, more recent proposals attribute grammatical difficulties to deficits in higher-order linguistic processing, as opposed to basic acoustic-phonetic processing (Montgomery, 2006).

It is widely accepted that children with SLI are slower to process spoken language than their typically developing peers (Miller, Kail, Leonard, & Tomblin, 2001; Leonard et al., 2007). Given that sentence processing requires the ability to hold verbal information long enough in memory to process it fully and integrate it with previously heard information, Montgomery (2002, 2005, 2006) has argued that limited *verbal working memory capacity* may underlie the reduced *information-processing speed* of children with SLI. In children as well as in adults, language learning and sentence processing have been consistently linked to individual differences in verbal working memory capacity (Baddeley, Gathercole, & Papagno, 1998; Carpenter, Miyake, & Just, 1995). Children with SLI have lesser verbal working memory capacity and, consequently, are less efficient in allocating attention to multiple sources of information. As a result, they are less capable of executing the multiple operations required for retrieving, evaluating, and integrating the semantic–syntactic properties of incoming words to construct sentence interpretations (Montgomery, 2002, 2005, 2006).

Support for this information-processing account comes from observations that children with SLI have considerable difficulties during sentence processing in assigning syntactic structures to sentences, both in off-line tasks and in real-time processing of connected speech (Montgomery, 1995, 2000a, 2000b, 2002, 2005, 2006). Children with SLI show a limited ability to comprehend sentences containing double relative embedded clauses (e.g., *The girl who is crying is pointing to the boy who is laughing*), sentences with a single relative embedded clause (e.g., *The boy who is sitting behind the girl is very big*), and sentences with extra verbiage (e.g., *The little old blue car is going to hit the great big fast speeding train*). In processing complex and lengthy constructions, children have to allocate considerable working memory resources to storing the initial sentence information while processing the semantic–syntactic information of the final clause(s) and integrating all of the information to construct a detailed syntactic analysis. In processing *wh*-questions, children with SLI are highly sensitive to a manipulation of question length, which drastically increases the processing demands of the task (Deevy & Leonard, 2004). Similarly, children with SLI produce more errors in supplying auxiliaries in obligatory contexts as sentences increase in length and argument structure complexity (Grela & Leonard, 2000). Thus the detrimental effects of a limited working memory capacity and a slower speed of information processing are more pronounced when the amount of linguistic information to be processed is increased (Deevy & Leonard, 2004; Grela & Leonard, 2000).

Additional support for the information-processing capacity model comes from a study that simulated SLI in typically developing children by introducing cognitive stress factors into a grammaticality judgment task (Hayiou-Thomas, Bishop, & Plunkett, 2004). In one condition, the speech rate of spoken sentences was compressed to 50% of its original rate; in another condition, the memory load was increased by adding redundant verbiage to sentence stimuli. Under both circumstances, children with SLI showed a linguistic profile similar to that of typically developing children, with reduced accuracy in making grammaticality judgments of sentences containing past tense -ed and third person singular -s verb inflections.

Impaired Statistical Learning

Recently, Ullman and Pierpont (2005) have advanced a novel perspective on how the grammatical difficulties observed in SLI might be explained in terms of a general-purpose learning mechanism. Specifically, they propose that children with SLI are characterized by abnormal development in the *procedural memory system*. This system supports statistical learning of sequences of linguistic elements; thus children with SLI are expected to show deficits in the learning of *probabilistic patterns* and *sequential dependencies*. By this account, children with SLI have deficient associate learning mechanisms and are slow to accumulate information about the frequency of occurrence of different types of linguistic elements and their co-occurrence patterns (see the earlier discussion of the role of statistical learning in language development in typically developing children). To date, only two studies have been conducted to test this hypothesis (Plante, Gomez, & Gerken, 2002; Tomblin, Mainela-Arnold, & Zhang, 2007); both yielded evidence of difficulties in sequence learning in individuals with disordered language development.

Plante, Gomez, and Gerken (2002) used a finite-state grammar to generate sentences in an artificial language consisting of CVC nonce words (an example sentence is *fim sag tup dak sag tup*), and then determined whether young adults with a learning disability or dyslexia would show impaired learning of the word-order rules of the artificial grammar. Consistent with the proposed deficit in procedural learning, after exposure to a representative set of sentences, the adults with language/learning disability showed impaired performance in judging new sentences as obeying or violating the rules of the artificial grammar, relative to a non–learning-disabled group.

Tomblin, Mainela-Arnold, and Zhang (2007) tested teenagers with SLI on a serial reaction time (SRT) task in which they had to press a button corresponding to the spatial location of a visual stimulus (i.e., a creature in a box), which varied in its location over trials. In the "random" blocks, the spatial location of the creature varied pseudo-randomly across trials. In the "patterned" blocks, the order of the varying spatial locations was generated by a 10-element sequence, which was repeated 10 times to produce 100 trials. In support of the hypothesized deficit in procedural learning, teenagers with SLI showed a slower learning rate during the patterned blocks in comparison to their peers but did not differ on the random blocks. This difference in learning rate for the patterned blocks was observed when groups were defined by grammatical abilities, but not when they were defined by vocabulary size. This result suggests that performance on the SRT task is specifically predictive of grammar learning.

Remediation of Syntactic Difficulties

Despite the substantial evidence for the grammatical deficits of children with SLI, research that explores remediation of these difficulties in children with SLI is sparse, particularly in school-aged children (Bishop, Adams, & Rosen, 2006). In an efficacy study that examined grammatical comprehension with and without speech modification in children with SLI, resistance of syntactic difficulties to remediation was apparent (Bishop, Adams, & Rosen, 2006). In this treatment study, two types of training regimes were used: (1) speech was introduced to the child with pauses appearing before salient words to give the child more processing time, and (2) the speech was both introduced with pauses and modified to accommodate a slower rate of speech processing. Constructions included in the grammar comprehension task were those involving spatial concepts (e.g., over/under, above/below), active/passive sentences, comparative sentences (e.g., *The wall is smaller than the boy*) and double comparative sentences (e.g., *The tree is smaller than the girl and bigger than the boy*). Children were trained for at least 20 sessions, each lasting 15 minutes. Results revealed only modest gains that could be explained by practice with the task rather than the efficacy of the specific training programs. There was no evidence that the modified speech led to any improvement in children's grammatical understanding.

More recently, Ebbels, van der Lely, and Dockrell (2007) tested the efficacy of a grammar intervention in 11- to 16-year-olds with SLI. As noted by van der Lely (2005); Bishop, Adams, & Rosen, (2006); and others, syntactic difficulties are extremely persistent in children with SLI of ages 9 years and older, and are generally resistant to treatment. Ebbels and colleagues (2007) targeted children's acquisition of verb argument structures in nine weekly half-hour therapy sessions. One group received "syntactic–semantic" therapy utilizing a combination of shapes, colors, and arrows to code phrases, parts of speech, and morphology (Ebbels, 2007). A second group received "semantic" therapy that provided detailed information about the definitions of verbs. A third (control) group learned to use "clues" from words in sentences to draw inferences from text (Yuill & Oakhill, 1998). To assess their use of verb argument structures in speech production, children viewed a series of video-depicted actions and were asked to describe what was happening in each scene. To ensure that children recognized the actions, for each scene the target verb was introduced as a gerund (e.g., *This is telling, This is walking, This is spilling*) prior to the elicitation question. In this study, relative to the control group, children receiving "syntactic–semantic" or "semantic" therapy improved in providing syntactically complete and accurate descriptions of the scenes, and children receiving the "syntactic–semantic" therapy produced utterances containing a greater number of syntactically optional verb arguments.

As these results demonstrate, therapies aimed at improving knowledge of verb meanings and their associated syntactic requirements have great potential to improve grammatical functioning, even in older children with SLI. Nevertheless, more efficacy studies are needed to elucidate the underlying source of the grammatical deficits of children with SLI, as well as to facilitate treatment of these difficulties in this population.

SUMMARY

Statistical learning of probabilistic grammatical patterns and sequential dependencies begins in the first year of life and contributes to children's discovery of the grammatical constructions of their language. Grammatical development in typically developing children is closely tied to vocabulary acquisition, and especially to the acquisition of verbs. Typically developing children make occasional errors in production and comprehension of complex syntactic constructions throughout childhood.

Late talkers exhibit subclinical weakness in grammatical skills that are identified during the preschool years and persist through childhood. Although these children may fall within the normal range on standardized tests, their difficulties are apparent when they are compared to their typically developing peers matched for age and socioeconomic status (maternal education). Children with SLI show profound deficits in grammatical development that may be unresolved. Much research is needed to develop remedial programs that will address the grammatical deficits exhibited by children with language impairments.

KEY TERMS

Extended Optional Infinitive (EOI) hypothesis

grammatical SLI (G-SLI)

index of productive syntax (IPSyn)

information-processing speed

linguistic constructions

mean length of utterance (MLU)

overgeneralization errors

probabilistic patterns

procedural memory system

sequential dependencies

statistical learning

Surface Account

syntactic bootstrapping

syntactic productivity

verbal working memory capacity

word-specific formulae

STUDY QUESTIONS

+ What are the processes by which children discover syntactic regularities in the adult language?
+ Describe the role of verb acquisition in grammatical development.
+ Describe the characteristics of grammatical development in late talkers.
+ Describe the various accounts of pervasive difficulties in grammatical abilities in children with SLI.

REFERENCES

Akhtar, N., & Tomasello, M. (1997). Young children's productivity with word order and verb morphology. *Developmental Psychology, 33*, 952–965.

Ambridge, B., Pine, J. M., Rowland, C. F., & Young, C. R. (2008). The effect of verb semantic class and verb frequency (entrenchment) on children's and adults' graded judgments of argument structure. *Cognition, 106*, 87–129.

Ambridge, B., Rowland, C. F., Theakston, A. L., & Tomasello, M. (2006). Comparing different accounts of inversion errors in children's non-subject *wh*-questions: What experiment data can tell us. *Journal of Child Language, 33*, 519–557.

Baddeley, A., Gathercole, S., & Papagno, C. (1998). The phonological loop as a language learning device. *Psychological Review, 105*, 158–173.

Bates, E., Benigni, L., Bretherton, I., Camaioni, L., & Volterra, V. (1979). *The emergence of symbols: Cognition and communication in infancy.* New York: Cambridge University Press.

Bates, E., & Goodman, J. (1997). On the inseparability of grammar and the lexicon: Evidence from acquisition, aphasia, and real-time processing. *Language and Cognitive Processes, 12*, 507–584.

Biship, D.V.M. (1992). The underlying nature of specific language impairment. *Journal of Child Psychology and Psychiatry, 33*(1), 3–66.

Bishop, D. V. M., Adams, C. V., & Rosen, S. (2006). Resistance of grammatical impairment to computerized comprehension training in children with specific and non-specific language impairments. *International Journal of Language and Communication Disorders, 41*, 19–40.

Bishop, D. V. M., Bright, P., James, C., Bishop, S. J., & van der Lely, H. K. J. (2000). Grammatical SLI: A distinct subtype of developmental language impairment? *Applied Psycholinguistics, 21*, 159–181.

Bishop, D. V. M., & Edmundson, A. (1987). Language impaired 4-year-olds: Distinguishing transient from persistent impairment. *Journal of Speech and Hearing Disorders, 52*, 156–173.

Bowerman, M. (1988). The "no-negative evidence" problem: How do children avoid constructing an overly general grammar? In J. Hawkins (Ed.), *Explaining language universals* (pp. 73–101). Oxford, UK: Blackwell.

Bowerman, M., & Croft, W. (2007). The acquisition of the English causative alternation. In M. Bowerman & P. Brown (Eds.), *Crosslinguistic perspectives on argument structure: Implications for learnability* (pp. 279–308). Hillsdale, NJ: Lawrence Erlbaum.

Braine, M. D. S. (1971). On two types of models of the internalization of grammars. In D. I. Slobin (Ed.), *The ontogenesis of grammar* (pp. 153–186). New York: Academic Press.

Braine, M. D. S. (1976). Children's first word combinations. *Monographs of the Society for Research in Child Development, Serial No. 164, 41*(1).

Braine, M. D. S., & Brooks, P. J. (1995). Verb argument structure and the problem of avoiding an overgeneral grammar. In M. Tomasello & W. E. Merriman (Eds.), *Beyond names for things: Young children's acquisition of verbs* (pp. 352–376). Hillsdale, NJ: Lawrence Erlbaum.

Brooks, P. J., & Braine, M. D. S. (1996). What do children know about the universal quantifiers *all* and *each*? *Cognition, 60,* 235–268.

Brooks, P. J., & Sekerina, I. A. (2005/2006). Shortcuts to quantifier interpretation in children and adults. *Language Acquisition, 13,* 177–206.

Brooks, P. J., & Tomasello, M. (1999a). How children constrain their argument structure constructions. *Language, 75,* 720–738.

Brooks, P. J., & Tomasello, M. (1999b). Young children learn to produce passives with novel verbs. *Developmental Psychology, 35,* 29–44.

Brooks, P. J., Tomasello, M., Dodson, K., & Lewis, L. (1999). Young children's overgeneralizations with fixed transitivity verbs. *Child Development, 70,* 1325–1337.

Brooks, P. J., & Zizak, O. (2002). Does preemption help children learn verb transitivity? *Journal of Child Language, 29,* 759–781.

Brown, R. (1973). *A first language: The early stages.* Cambridge, MA: Harvard University Press.

Carpenter, P. A., Miyake, A., & Just, M. A. (1995). Language comprehension: Sentence and discourse processing. *Annual Review of Psychology, 46,* 91–100.

Cassidy, K. W., & Kelly, M. H. (2001). Children's use of phonology to infer grammatical class in vocabulary learning. *Psychonomic Bulletin and Review, 8,* 519–523.

Chang, F., Dell, G. S., & Bock, K. (2006). Becoming syntactic. *Psychological Review, 113,* 234–272.

Childers, J. B., & Tomasello, M. (2001). The role of pronouns in young children's acquisition of the English transitive construction. *Developmental Psychology, 37,* 739–748.

Clark, E. (1993). *The lexicon in acquisition.* Cambridge, UK: Cambridge University Press.

Conti-Ramsden, G., & Windfuhr, K. (2002). Productivity with word-order and morphology: A comparative look at children with SLI and children with normal language abilities. *International Journal of Language and Communication Disorders, 37,* 17–30.

DeCasper, A. J., Lacanuet, J. P., Busnel, M. C., Granier-Deferre, C., & Maugeals, R. (1994). Fetal reactions to recurrent maternal speech. *Infant Behavior and Development, 2,* 159–164.

Deevy, P., & Leonard, L. B. (2004). The comprehension of *wh*-questions in children with specific language impairment. *Journal of Speech, Language, and Hearing Research, 47,* 802–815.

Dehaene-Lambertz, G., & Houston, D. (1998). Faster orientation latency toward native language in two-month-old infants. *Language and Speech, 41,* 21–43.

Ebbels, S. H. (2007). Teaching grammar to school-aged children with specific language impairment using shape coding. *Child Language Teaching and Therapy, 23,* 67–93.

Ebbels, S. H., van der Lely, H. K. J., & Dockrell, J. E. (2007). Intervention for verb argument structure in children with persistent SLI: A randomized control trial. *Journal of Speech, Language, and Hearing Research, 50,* 1330–1349.

Evans, J. L., & MacWhinney, B. (1999). Sentence processing strategies in children with expressive and expressive–receptive specific language impairments. *International Journal of Language and Communication Disorders, 34,* 117–134.

Fernandes, K. J., Marcus, G. F., Di Nubila, J. A., & Vouloumanos, A. (2006). From semantics to syntax and back again: Argument structure in the third year of life. *Cognition, 100,* B10–B20.

Ferreira, F. (2003). The misinterpretation of noncanonical sentences. *Cognitive Psychology, 47*, 164–203.

Fisher, C. (2002). Structural limits on verb mapping: The role of abstract structure in 2.5-year-olds' interpretations of novel verbs. *Developmental Science, 5*, 55–64.

Fletcher, P., Stokes, S., & Wong, A. (2005). Constructions and language development: Implications for language impairment. In P. Fletcher & J. F. Miller (Eds.), *Developmental theory and language disorders* (pp. 35–51). Amsterdam: John Benjamins.

Gerken, L., Wilson, R., & Lewis, W. (2005). Infants can use distributional cues to form syntactic categories. *Journal of Child Language, 32*, 249–268.

Gleitman, L. R. (1990). The structural sources of verb meanings. *Language Acquisition, 1*, 3–55.

Gleitman, L. R., Cassidy, K., Nappa, R., Papafragou, A., & Trueswell, J. C. (2005). Hard words. *Language Learning and Development, 1*, 23–64.

Goldberg, A. E. (2006). *Constructions at work: The nature of generalization in language.* Oxford, UK: Oxford University Press.

Gomez, R. L. (2002). Variability and the detection of invariant structure. *Psychological Science, 13*, 431–436.

Gomez, R. L., & Gerken, L. A. (1999). Artificial language learning by one-year-olds leads to specific and abstract knowledge. *Cognition, 70*, 109–135.

Gomez, R. L., & Gerken, L. A. (2000). Infant artificial language learning and language acquisition. *Trends in Cognitive Sciences, 4*, 178–186.

Grela, B. G., & Leonard, L. B. (2000). The influence of argument-structure complexity on the use of auxiliary verbs by children with SLI. *Journal of Speech, Language, and Hearing Research, 43*, 1115–1125.

Hayiou-Thomas, M. E., Bishop, D. V. M., & Plunkett, K. (2004). Simulating SLI: General cognitive processing stressors can produce a specific linguistic profile. *Journal of Speech, Language, and Hearing Research, 47*, 1347–1362.

Howe, C. (1976). The meaning of two-word utterances I the speech of young children. *Journal of Child Language, 3*, 29–48.

Hurewitz, F., Brown-Schmidt, S., Thorpe, K., Gleitman, L. R., & Trueswell, J. C. (2000). One frog, two frog, red frog, blue frog: Factors affecting children's syntactic choices in production and comprehension. *Journal of Psycholinguistic Research, 29*, 597–626.

Joanisse, M. F., & Seidenberg, M. S. (2003). Phonology and syntax in specific language impairment: Evidence from a connectionist model. *Brain and Language, 86*, 40–56.

Kelly, M. H. (1992). Using sound to solve syntactic problems: The role of phonology in grammatical category assignments. *Psychological Review, 99*, 349–364.

Kisilevsky, B. S., Hains, S. M. J., Lee, K., et al. (2003). Effects of experience on fetal voice recognition. *Psychological Science, 14*, 220–224.

Krueger, C., Holditch-David, D., Quint, S., & DeCasper, A. (2004). Recurring auditory experience in the 28- to 34-week-old fetus. *Infant Behavior and Development, 27*, 537–543.

Leonard, L. B. (1989). Language learnability and specific language impairment in children. *Applied Psycholinguistics, 10*, 179–202.

Leonard, L. B. (1995). Functional categories in the grammars of children with specific language impairment. *Journal of Speech and Hearing Research, 38*, 1270–1283.

Leonard, L.B., Ellis Weismer, S., Miller, C.A., Fracis, D.J., Tomblin, J.B., & Kail, R.V. (2007). Speech of processing, working memory, and language impairment in children. *Journal of Speech, Language, and Hearing Research, 50*(2), 408–428.

Leonard, L. B., Eyer , J. A., Bedore, L. M., & Grela, B. G. (1997). Three accounts of the grammatical morpheme difficulties of English-speaking children with specific language impairment. *Journal of Speech, Language, and Hearing Research, 40,* 741–753.

Leonard, L. B., Miller, C. A., Deevy, P., Rauf, L., Gerber, E., & Charest, M. (2002). Production operations and the use of nonfinite verbs by children with specific language impairment. *Journal of Speech, Language, and Hearing Research, 45,* 744–758.

Leonard, L. B., Wong, A. M. Y., Deevy, P., Stokes, S. F., & Fletcher, P. (2006). The production of passives by children with specific language impairment: Acquiring English or Cantonese. *Applied Psycholinguistics, 27,* 267–299.

Levin, B. (1993). *English verb classes and alternations.* Chicago: Chicago University Press.

Lieven, E., Behrens, H., Speares, J., & Tomasello, M. (2003). Early syntactic creativity: A usage-based approach. *Journal of Child Language, 30,* 333–367.

Loeb, D. F., Pye, C., Redmond, S., & Richardson, L. Z. (1996). Eliciting verbs from children with specific language impairment. *American Journal of Speech-Language Pathology, 5,* 17–30.

Loeb, D. F., Pye, C., Richardson, L. Z., & Redmond, S. (1998). Causative alternations of children with specific language impairment. *Journal of Speech, Language, and Hearing Research, 41,* 1103–1114.

MacWhinney, B. (2004). A multiple process solution to the logical problem of language acquisition. *Journal of Child Language, 31,* 883–914.

Maranis, T., & van der Lely, H. K. J. (2007). On-line processing of *wh*-questions in children with G-SLI and typically developing children. *International Journal of Language and Communication Disorders, 42,* 557–582.

Maratsos, M. (1990). Are actions to verbs as objects are to nouns? On the differential semantic bases of form, class, category. *Linguistics, 28,* 1351–1379.

Marchman, V., & Bates, E. (1994). Continuity in lexical and morphological development: A test of the critical mass hypothesis. *Journal of Child Language, 21,* 339–366.

Marcus, G., Vijayan, S., Bandi Rao, S., & Vishton, P. M. (1999). Rule learning by seven-month-old infants. *Science, 283,* 77–80.

Mehler, J., Jusczyk, P. W., Lambertz, G., Halsted, G., Bertoncini, J., & Amiel-Tison, C. (1988). A precursor of language acquisition in young infants. *Cognition, 29,* 143–178.

Miller, C. A., Kail, R., Leonard, L. B., & Tomblin, J. B. (2001). Speed of processing in children with specific language impairment. *Journal of Speech, Language, and Hearing Research, 44,* 416–433.

Miller, C. A., & Leonard, L. B. (1998). Deficits in finite verb morphology: Some assumptions in recent accounts of specific language impairment. *Journal of Speech, Language, and Hearing Research, 41,* 701–707.

Mintz, T. H., Newport, E. L., & Bever, T. G. (2002). The distributional structure of grammatical categories in speech to young children. *Cognitive Science, 26,* 393–424.

Monaghan, P., Chater, N., & Christiansen, M. H. (2005). The differential role of phonological and distributional cues in grammatical categorisation. *Cognition, 96,* 143–182.

Montgomery, J. W. (1995). Sentence comprehension in children with specific language impairment: The role of phonological working memory. *Journal of Speech and Hearing Research, 38,* 187–199.

Montgomery, J. W. (2000a). Relation of working memory to off-line and real-time sentence processing in children with specific language impairment. *Applied Psycholinguistics, 21,* 117–148.

Montgomery, J. W. (2000b). Verbal working memory and sentence comprehension in children with specific language impairment. *Journal of Speech, Language, and Hearing Research, 43,* 293–308.

Montgomery, J. W. (2002). Understanding the language difficulties of children with specific language impairments: Does verbal working memory matter? *American Journal of Speech-Language Pathology, 11,* 77–91.

Montgomery, J. W. (2005). Effects of input rate and age on the real-time language processing of children with specific language impairment. *International Journal of Language and Communication Disorders, 40,* 171–188.

Montgomery, J. W. (2006). Real-time language processing in school-age children with specific language impairment. *International Journal of Language and Communication Disorders, 41,* 275–291.

Montgomery, J. W., & Leonard, L. B. (1998). Real-time inflectional processing by children with specific language impairment: Effects of phonetic substance. *Journal of Speech, Language, and Hearing Research, 41,* 1432–1443.

Moyle, M. J., Weismer, S. E., Evans, J. L., & Lindstrom, M. J. (2007). Longitudinal relationships between lexical and grammatical development in typical and late-talking children. *Journal of Speech, Language, and Hearing Research, 50,* 508–528.

Naigles, L. R. (1990). Children use syntax to learn verb meanings. *Journal of Child Language, 17,* 357–374.

Naigles, L. R. (1996). The use of multiple frames in verb learning via syntactic bootstrapping. *Cognition, 58,* 221–251.

Nelson, K. (1981). Individual differences in language development: Implications for development and language. *Developmental Psychology, 17,* 170–187.

Ninio, A. (1999). Pathbreaking verbs in syntactic development and the question of prototypical transitivity. *Journal of Child Language, 26,* 619–653.

Ninio, A. (2006). *Language and the learning curve: A new theory of syntactic development.* Oxford, UK: Oxford University Press.

Oetting, J. B., Rice, M. L., & Swank, L. K. (1995). Quick incidental learning (QUIL) of words by school-age children with and without SLI. *Journal of Speech and Hearing Research, 38,* 434–445.

Owen, A. J., & Leonard, L. B. (2006). The production of finite and nonfinite complement clauses by children with specific language impairment and their typically developing peers. *Journal of Speech, Language, and Hearing Research, 29,* 548–571.

Pine, J. M., & Lieven, E. V. M. (1993). Reanalysing rote-learned phrases: Individual differences in the transition to multi-word speech. *Journal of Child Language, 20,* 551–571.

Pine, J. M., Lieven, E. V. M., & Rowland, C. F. (1997). Stylistic variation at the "single-word" stage: Relations between maternal speech characteristics and children's vocabulary composition and usage. *Child Development, 68,* 807–819.

Pinker, S. (1989). *Learnability and cognition: The acquisition of argument structure.* Cambridge, MA: MIT Press.

Plante, E., Gomez, R. L., & Gerken, L. A. (2002). Sensitivity to word order cues by normal and language/learning disabled adults. *Journal of Communication Disorders, 35,* 453–462.

Redington, M., Chater, N., & Finch, S. (1998). Distributional information: A powerful cue for acquiring syntactic categories. *Cognitive Science, 22,* 425–469.

Rescorla, L. (1989). The language development survey: A screening tool for delayed language in toddlers. *Journal of Speech and Hearing Disorders, 54,* 587–599.

Rescorla, L. (2002). Language and reading outcomes to age 9 in late-talking toddlers. *Journal of Speech, Language, and Hearing Research, 45,* 360–371.

Rescorla, L. (2005). Age 13 language and reading outcomes in late-talking toddlers. *Journal of Speech, Language, and Hearing Research, 48,* 459–472.

Rescorla, L., Dahlsgaard, K., & Roberts, J. (2000). Late-talking toddlers: MLU and IPSyn outcomes at 3;0 and 4;0. *Journal of Child Language, 27*, 643–664.

Rescorla, L., Roberts, J., & Dahlsgaard, K. (1997). Late talkers at 2: Outcome at age 3. *Journal of Speech and Hearing Research, 40*, 556–566.

Rice, M. L., & Wexler, K. (1996). Toward tense as a clinical marker of specific language impairment in English-speaking children. *Journal of Speech and Hearing Research, 39*, 1239–1257.

Rice, M. L., Wexler, K., & Cleave, P. L. (1995). Specific language impairment as a period of extended optional infinitive. *Journal of Speech and Hearing Research, 38*, 850–863.

Riches, N. G., Faraghter, B., & Conti-Ramsden, G. (2006). Verb schema use and input dependence in 5-year-old children with specific language impairment (SLI). *International Journal of Language and Communication Disorders, 41*, 117–135.

Riches, N. G., Tomasello, M., & Conti-Ramsden, G. (2005). Verb learning in children with SLI: Frequency and spacing effects. *Journal of Speech, Language, and Hearing Research, 48*, 1397–1411.

Rowland, C. F. (2007). Explaining errors in children's questions. *Cognition, 104*, 106–134.

Saffran, J. R. (2003). Statistical language learning: Mechanisms and constraints. *Current Directions in Psychological Science, 12*, 110–114.

Santelmann, L., Berk, S., Austin, J., Somashekar, S., & Lust, B. (2002). Continuity and development in the acquisition of inversion in yes/no questions: Dissociating movement and inflection. *Journal of Child Language, 29*, 813–842.

Scarborough, H. S. (1990). Index of productive syntax. *Applied Psycholinguistics, 11*, 1–12.

Seidenberg, M. S., & MacDonald, M. C. (1999). A probabilistic constraints approach to language acquisition and processing. *Cognitive Science, 23*, 569–588.

Shulman, C., & Guberman, A. (2007). Acquisition of verb meaning through syntactic cues: A comparison of children with autism, children with specific language impairment (SLI) and children with typical language development (TLD). *Journal of Child Language, 34*, 411–423.

Stokes, S. F., & Fletcher, P. (2000). Lexical diversity and productivity in Cantonese-speaking children with specific language impairment. *International Journal of Language and Communication Disorders, 35*, 527–541.

Stothard, S. E., Snowling, M. J., Bishop, D. V. M., Chipchase, B. B., & Kaplan, C. A. (1998). Language impaired preschoolers: A follow-up into adolescence. *Journal of Speech, Language, and Hearing Research, 41*, 407–418.

Sudhalter, V., & Braine, M. D. S. (1985). How does comprehension of passives develop? A comparison of actional and experiential verbs. *Journal of Child Language, 12*, 455–470.

Theakston, A. L. (2004). A role of entrenchment in children's and adults' performance on grammaticality judgment tasks. *Cognitive Development, 19*, 15–34.

Theakston, A. L., Lieven, E. V. M., Pine, J. M., & Rowland, C. F. (2004). Semantic generality, input frequency, and the acquisition of syntax. *Journal of Child Language, 31*, 61–99.

Thordardottir, E. T., Weismer, S. E., & Evans, J. L. (2002). Continuity in lexical and morphological development in Icelandic and English-speaking 2-year-olds. *First Language, 22*, 3–28.

Tomasello, M. (1992). *First verbs: A case study of early syntactic development.* New York: Cambridge University Press.

Tomasello, M. (2003). *Constructing a language: A usage-based theory of language acquisition.* Cambridge, MA: Harvard University Press.

Tomasello, M., & Brooks, P. J. (1998). Young children's earliest transitive and intransitive constructions. *Cognitive Linguistics, 9,* 379–395.

Tomblin, J. B., Mainela-Arnold, E., & Zhang, X. (2007). Procedural learning in adolescents with and without specific language impairment. *Language Learning and Development, 3,* 269–293.

Tomblin, J. B., & Pandich, J. (1999). Lessons from children with specific language impairment. *Trends in Cognitive Sciences, 3,* 283–285.

Trueswell, J. C., Sekerina, I. A., Hill, N. M., & Logrip, M. L. (1999). The kindergarten-path effect: Studying on-line sentence processing in young children. *Cognition, 73,* 89–134.

Ullman, M. T., & Pierpont, E. I. (2005). Specific language impairment is not specific to language. *Cortex, 41,* 399–433.

Valian, V. (1991). Syntactic subjects in the early speech of American and Italian children. *Cognition, 40,* 21–81.

Valian, V., & Aubry, S. (2005). When opportunity knocks twice: Two-year-olds' repetition of sentence subjects. *Journal of Child Language, 32,* 617–641.

van der Lely, H. K. J. (1994). Canonical linking rules: Forward vs. reverse linking in normally developing and specifically language impaired children. *Cognition, 51,* 29–72.

van der Lely, H. K. J. (1996). Specifically language impaired and normally developing children: Verbal passive vs. adjectival passive sentence interpretation. *Lingua, 98,* 243–272.

van der Lely, H. K. J. (1998). SLI in children: Movement, economy, and deficits in the computational–syntactic system. *Language Acquisition, 7,* 161–192.

van der Lely, H. K. J. (2005). Domain-specific cognitive systems: Insight from grammatical SLI. *Trends in Cognitive Sciences, 9,* 53–57.

van der Lely, H. K. J., & Battell, J. (2003). *Wh*-movement in children with grammatical SLI: A test of the RDDR hypothesis. *Language, 79,* 153–181.

van der Lely, H. K. J., & Harris, M. (1990). Comprehension of reversible sentences in specifically language-impaired children. *Journal of Speech and Hearing Disorders, 55,* 101–117.

van der Lely, H. K. J., Rosen, S., & Adlard, A. (2004). Grammatical language impairment and the specificity of cognitive domains: Relations between auditory and language abilities. *Cognition, 94,* 167–183.

van der Lely, H. K. J., & Stollwerck, L. (1997). Binding theory and specifically language impaired children. *Cognition, 62,* 245–290.

Windfuhr, K., Faraghter, B., & Conti-Ramsden, G. (2002). Lexical learning skills in young children with specific language impairment (SLI). *International Journal of Language and Communication Disorders, 37,* 415–432.

Yuill, N., & Oakhill, J. (1988). Effects of inference awareness training on poor reading: Comprehension. *Applied Cognitive Psychology, 2,* 33–45.

CHAPTER 11

Comprehension of Language

Amy L. Weiss, PhD

OBJECTIVES

+ Identify developmental principles of children's language comprehension and list several developmental milestones.
+ Explain why the comprehension competencies of young children are more difficult to measure than their expressive language competencies, and provide several solutions for this problem.
+ Become familiar with several techniques for standardized assessment of language comprehension.

INTRODUCTION

A careful perusal of the available textbooks focusing on the scope of children's language development yields relatively little information about language comprehension. This omission is surprising because language comprehension represents one of the two major processes of language acquisition (along with language production, of course) that young children are learning (Miller & Paul, 1995). The dearth of information in this area may stem from the inherent difficulty of studying language comprehension, rather than because the topic is viewed as a trivial matter.

This chapter explores several principles that appear to hold true for children's development of language comprehension, describes what we know about the specific developmental milestones achieved by children during the preschool years, and introduces several different methods for evaluating that development. Several suggestions about how to best incorporate this information into clinical work are also provided.

STUDYING LANGUAGE COMPREHENSION IN YOUNG CHILDREN _____

What Is the Challenge?

There are at least two compelling reasons for clinicians and researchers to carefully study and consider the development of young children's language comprehension. The first has to do with the important role that language comprehension plays in young children's understanding of their world, including how it works and how to participate in its workings. The second has to do with the difficulties inherent in accurately evaluating language comprehension. Unlike the study of expressive syntax, phonology, or morphology, comprehension is not right "out there," but rather has to be inferred from the context (both linguistic and nonlinguistic) as well as the linguistic units provided. Therein lies the daily challenge for both clinicians and family members with young children who are developing language.

Because the evaluation of comprehension is largely inferred from children's nonverbal responses to tasks, it is relatively easy to overestimate their language comprehension competencies instead of accurately determining what young children understand. Language comprehension competencies are also easy to overestimate because young children who are developing language tend to make guesses about the language they hear around them that they cannot quite understand. Sometimes those guesses are correct or appear correct; as a consequence, we sometimes give credit for a correct response based on what was actually the result of a child's incorrect or incomplete decoding process. For speech-language pathologists, these errors can be useful, because the way we derive the most insight about language learning is often by analyzing the mistakes that young children make in their attempts to understand.

An Example

To illustrate how mistakes can yield important information, consider this example of a five-year-old with age-appropriate language abilities who revealed where the limits of her language understanding were. Notice how important nonverbal context is in this case for interpreting what is going on comprehension-wise. Careful consideration of nonverbal or nonlinguistic context is one crucial clinical tool that we should routinely apply.

> The setting was a preschool classroom with multiple centers of activity. One of these centers was designated for painting, and the child in question was busily painting on a piece of paper secured to a large easel. Adorned in an over-sized apron, she had a juice can filled with bright orange paint at her disposal, situated on the ledge of the easel in front of her. With great care, the child would dip her paintbrush into the can and, without much dripping, stroke the brush across the paper. She appeared to be more engrossed in the brush and paint process than in creating anything recognizable. Absorbed in her work, the child did not even look up when one

of the undergraduate students who volunteered in the classroom walked by the easel. Seeing the child's painting efforts, the student said, "Modern art, huh?" To this comment (and without making eye content with the speaker), the child replied, "Yeah. Orange."

I frequently use this example with my students to gauge their insights into language learning and especially comprehension. This vignette provides a nice illustration of a preschool-age child who understands her role in a conversation, although she does not understand the specific allusion the speaker has made to modern art. In a pragmatic sense, the child has recognized that a door was opened for her to respond (i.e., a tag question, "huh?," includes a request for a response, thus relating both syntax and semantics as well as pragmatic competencies), and the response she provided had something to do with her painting (i.e., she provided the color of her paint). Clearly, though, this five-year-old was not able to relate to the more abstract meaning of the student's comment. When evaluating the child's response, you should give her credit for understanding that she has been asked to comment on the statement made by the older, more competent speaker (pragmatics), but acknowledge that her conceptual development has not yet extended to understanding different genres of art (lexical/semantics) or to recognizing that the student was probably being just a little bit sarcastic and has actually made a rhetorical comment that needs no response (pragmatics).

Rather than view the older participant's comment as a disingenuous attempt at communication, I look at it as fortuitous. It provided an opportunity to achieve some insight into the young child's ability to understand the words spoken, the world around her, and her role in the communication process. We do not expect a five-year-old to understand the abstract term "modern art" or to recognize a rhetorical comment when she hears one; thus her response does not raise any developmental concerns about the young artist's comprehension competencies based on this particular interaction. Nevertheless, analysis of the vignette does provide us with some insight into how context—in this case, the use of orange paint and painting—influenced how the child revealed her level of comprehension for the language used in this adult–child conversation.

One additional point is also brought to light through analysis of this brief interaction. Note how different components of language work together in the child's attempt to make sense of the language input: The child's pragmatics, semantics, and syntax knowledge are all being called upon to resolve the matter of language comprehension. This is a commonly observed phenomenon. That is, demonstration of language comprehension involves much more than simply knowing what individual words mean. Language comprehension is much more than receptive vocabulary. Everything the child understands about language in its broadest sense, including pragmatics, semantics, syntax, morphology, and especially phonology, must become part of the processing of language input for an accurate response to result. Just as it is quite artificial to say that we can study the development of syntax without considering semantics and phonology, so we cannot fully evaluate a child's language comprehension without considering the rest of the child's breadth of language knowledge.

WHAT IS LANGUAGE COMPREHENSION?

Speech-language pathologists (SLPs), developmental psychologists, linguists, and others involved in studying language development use a number of different terms to refer to the acquisition of language comprehension. Most often, in addition to language comprehension, the terms "receptive language (learning)" or "the understanding of language" may be used. In all cases, the terminology refers to decoding the language input present in the child's environment as opposed to the production of language. Bishop (1997) refers to language comprehension as "a process whereby information is successfully transformed from one kind of representation to another" (p. 2). That is, language comprehension relates to the process of turning a highly complicated set of acoustic signals into a meaningful message.

In this chapter, understanding of spoken language will be considered. To be sure, much can be gained by studying the development of comprehension when the input is visual rather than spoken, as in American Sign Language, or written, as when we study reading comprehension. Those topics are beyond the scope of this chapter and are addressed elsewhere.

Understanding the Role of Context

Language comprehension refers to an individual's ability to understand the linguistic information contained in a message, which is almost always augmented by the message's specific nonlinguistic context (e.g., what is going on at the same time, who is speaking, what was previously said, what visual information is available) and by the listener's world knowledge (i.e., how the course of typical events as they occur in the world affects the interpretation of this linguistic message). Milosky (1992) provides a comprehensive discussion of the role of world knowledge in comprehension.

The balance enforced among these information sources is not always predictable. When children are in the process of acquiring language comprehension, the relative contributions of these information sources are determined by where the child is in development. That is, if complete linguistic knowledge is unavailable, more reliance will probably be placed on the nonlinguistic information available and context becomes more critical for understanding. Miller and Paul (1995) list a number of areas of knowledge that are crucial to successful language comprehension, including but not limited to social knowledge and the understanding of intentionality, inferencing, and scriptal knowledge. These authors note, as does Bishop (1997), that the necessity for such a holistic approach to understanding the process of language comprehension likely explains the difficulties computer programs have in making translations between languages. Put simply, translation is more than a word-by-word transformation from one language to another.

The following example demonstrates the interplay between linguistic and nonlinguistic information. Note the role played by nonlinguistic information (context).

Setting: A mother is busy getting ready for work. Her young child, age 18 months, is watching her mother quickly move around the bedroom, lifting up papers and the bed linens, obviously searching for something. The mother repeatedly mutters to herself but loud enough for the child to hear, "My shoes. Where are my shoes?" The child glances down at her own shoes, reaches forward to touch her right shoe, and chortles, "Mine," as she grasps the shoe. The child then looks up to her mother for approval.

Interpretation: The child probably just understands the word "shoes" (although probably not the plural morpheme). A veteran of many turn-taking exchanges that are prompted by being asked, "Where is your X?", this child provides a response relative to herself and not to her mother. Thus the child has incorporated world knowledge into an attempt to understand the situation unfolding around her in the bedroom. The usual course of events from the child's perspective is that "My mother often asks me where my body parts are and where different items of my clothing are, so that is probably what is happening now." Although she is not specifically being asked a question requiring a response, the child has personalized the exchange by referencing her own shoe.

Does this child have complete understanding of her mother's comment and question? No, it is highly unlikely that she could understand all of the nuances of this communication. In the same situation, an adult might respond with the question, "Which pair of shoes are you looking for?" Another possible adult rejoinder could be, "Where did you last see them?" In both instances, an adult would know that to understand the intended message, one would have to recognize that the mother's shoes are at issue, not her own. Additional world knowledge would reveal that when we are in a hurry, we often cannot find the things we need most, and that comments of encouragement, clarification, and assistance are what are needed. In the example, the child demonstrated incomplete knowledge, both linguistic and nonlinguistic, but still provided a turn in the form of a response to the hypothesized "Where?" question. In the absence of complete information, just as in the example of our five-year-old artist, this young child attempted to use the information that was at her disposal to participate in the communication exchange.

Interactions Between Context and Comprehension of Meaning

Given the close association between linguistic and nonlinguistic information, a confound may potentially arise from the latter information if we believe we are exclusively looking at linguistic comprehension competencies without making special provisions. Clinicians and researchers who are concerned with the confounding of linguistic and nonlinguistic comprehension make sure to eliminate as much nonlinguistic information as possible when testing young children, for example. Asking questions or making requests in a manner where all gestures are eliminated reduces the possibility that nonlinguistic cues have been relied on for comprehension. Similarly, objects that might serve to cue the child are placed out of sight. Another strategy used by some has been to make requests that run counter to real-world expectations. More information about the elimination of nonlinguistic cues will be provided later in this chapter when we address the measurement of children's language comprehension.

Why do clinicians and caregivers disagree about young children's language comprehension?

The use of, and perhaps reliance on, nonlinguistic information by young children may lead many caregivers to state with certainty that their toddlers understand everything that is said to them. This expression has been a common occurrence in my clinical experience. What leads to caregivers' very strong beliefs that their children, at approximately two years of age, understand everything said to them? This is an especially important question because comprehension data collected with tasks that carefully control for extraneous cuing have shown that young children younger than age two understand a corpus of single words, some two-word combinations, and possibly an occasional three-word combination—but they certainly do not understand everything said to them (Miller, Chapman, Branston, & Reichle, 1980).

Given that we empirically know that toddlers cannot understand everything said to them, Chapman, Klee, and Miller (1980) sought to determine why caregivers so often report that their two-year-olds understand everything said to them. They reported the findings of a preliminary investigation focused on this clinical quandary: Why do researchers and caregivers disagree in their perception of young children's comprehension abilities? These researchers looked at half-hour videotaped samples collected from young children, ranging in age from approximately 8 months to 21 months who were engaged in play with their mothers. The investigators carefully analyzed all of the instances where the mothers had made either requests for objects (e.g., *Give me the block*) or requests for action (e.g., *Come over here*) and all of the children's responses. The investigators catalogued use of gestures made on the part of the mothers that may have cued the children to the mothers' linguistic message as well as the use of the children's names to get their attention. In addition, Chapman and her colleagues considered the timing of the requests relative to the children's responses.

A summary of the study's findings demonstrated that not only did the mothers frequently use gesture to gain and direct their children's attention, but they also timed their requests to match the production of their children's responses. This timing sequence had the effect of making the children's responses appear to be correct. Because these responses were actually under way before the request was made, Chapman, Klee, and Miller (1980) called these events "pseudo-successes." This term derives from the decision by the researchers that credit for a successful response could not be given, although the caregivers may have concluded that their children understood them.

Here is an example of how such an interaction might look. A mother might say, "Give me the cup," when the child is, in fact, already in the act of handing the mother the cup. In another example, the child might turn his gaze to the mother, and the mother says, "Look at me." In both instances, the mother's requests are made after the child begins the requested action. In Western culture, middle-class mothers have been observed to shape their utterances to create turn-taking conversation frameworks with their young, language-immature children; the mothers in the Chapman, Klee, and Miller (1980) study may have had the same goal. The effect of their timing, however, was to render the children's participation as looking like comprehension.

Chapman and colleagues (1980) concluded that many mothers who have observed this enhanced connection between requests for action and requests for objects and their children's apparent compliance over many instances have assumed this relationship was evidence of their children's genuine language comprehension. We cannot discount the perspective that parents enjoy seeing their young children's compliant behavior and may not question whether the compliance can be attributed to genuine comprehension.

My own anecdotal observation has been that parents of children with bona fide expressive language deficits appear to be even more likely to comment on the strength of their children's language understanding. Part of this perception may derive from the *relative* strength of language understanding when compared with language expression for these children. Also, in lieu of age-appropriate language production skills, anything these parents perceive their children to have mastered—in this case, language comprehension—is viewed with great relief! Experience shows that caregivers who are pleased with their children's apparent skill at language comprehension are less than pleased when told that their perspective is not shared by the SLP.

How do we incorporate this information into our clinical work?

The findings of the Chapman, Klee, and Miller (1980) study, although preliminary, raise two important issues. First, SLPs need to do more than just take parents' opinion of their children's language comprehension as the final word in language comprehension assessment. This need for further action reflects the difficulty we all experience in getting a pure sample of language comprehension behavior and accurately interpreting what we have. This point is not meant to be dismissive of the important role caregivers play in evaluating their children's language. Second, SLPs have to be sure that, when assessing language comprehension skills in young children, they provide tasks that are not confounded by nonlinguistic cues that provide children with the opportunity to look savvier in terms of their linguistic language comprehension than they actually are.

What do we know about the development of language comprehension?

A child setting out to understand his first language faces an extraordinary task. If you have attempted to learn a second language (or third or fourth) later in life, you probably remember how difficult it was at first to even parse the stream of language that assaulted your ears to determine where one sentence ended and another began. Even more difficult was to determine where one word ended and another began. Infants and toddlers encounter many of the same challenges in making sense of language input and learning language: They have to determine where to segment the stream of sounds they hear. Once segmented, the job of making sense of the phonological information is left to accomplish.

Which types of competencies are being developed to cope with the acoustic information of speech?

For children to effectively use phonological information from the speech stream they hear, children must be able to detect, discriminate, and classify sounds. First, at the most rudimentary level, children must detect the sounds in the speech stream. That is, can they be heard? Second, children must be able to discriminate between sounds in their input so that they recognize when a /b/ versus a /p/ is produced, although the relevance of that discrimination for first-language learning is not yet understood. Third, and much more central to specific language-learning, is the ability to classify sounds into meaningful categories such as the phonemes in a given language (i.e., /b/ and /p/ are phonemes in English because when used as the initial sound in words formed with _____at, a meaningful lexical difference results).

Bishop (1997, p. 51) refers to a fourth competency, known as "phonological constancy," as being critical to the ability to utilize the speech signal. This last consideration is related to classification—children have to develop a set of boundaries within which sound productions reflect the same intended sound. In essence, because not every /b/ will sound identical to every other /b/ heard, the child has to set parameters that are forgiving enough so that it will be rare that sounds are confused for others or ignored in terms of their meaningfulness.

Assistance from the Environment

Most of word learning probably is associative in nature. Thus children who are developing language normally look to nonlinguistic information to help them map meaning to the consistent sound strings they hear. The strategy of relying on nonlinguistic context to map meaning to sound strings is similar to what adults experience when trying to learn a second language. You may have had the experience of being in a situation where you can understand very little of the language spoken by the people around you. I remember grabbing hold of one word I could understand—like a life saver—in a stream of words that I largely could not understand and attempting to figure out the rest of the message from that one word.

Not long ago the following experience happened to me when I was in a Spanish-speaking country. It was lunchtime, so the fact that I had understood the word for "lunch" made sense. Yes, of course, I would like to join a group of acquaintances who were local to the area for lunch. As it turned out, I had actually been asked if I knew which dining room was serving lunch that day; I had not received an invitation from the group to join them. I was embarrassed to be sure, but the experience was a helpful one because it reflected a problem not all that dissimilar from that of language-learning children. The more we can appreciate the disadvantages faced by young children learning language in their attempts to understand the language around them, and the immense resourcefulness they demonstrate in this situation, the better our perspective for accurately evaluating their comprehension efforts.

Quality of Input and Context: Helping Children "Map" Language

The study of caregivers' speech and language to young children has provided us with evidence that the input young children receive—at least in Western, middle-class households—is not identical in quantity or quality to the input produced in adult–adult conversation. Specifically, adult–infant/toddler speech and language typically includes more repetition, especially of content words (e.g., *apple*, *hungry*); longer pauses at grammatical junctures; emphasis of content words; more dramatic shifts of prosody and intonation contours; and longer turn-taking transitions than would be found in adult–adult conversation in the same cultural milieu (Fernald & Kuhl, 1987). It has been speculated that these differences serve to focus a young child's attention on the stream of speech, specifically on those parts that are most relevant to understanding the message communicated by the adult (Fernald, Taeschner, Dunn, Papousek, deBoysson-Bardies, & Fukui, 1989).

Many adults also utilize specific gestures to facilitate communication with young children (Bruner, 1978). For example, it is not unusual for a caregiver to accompany use of the word *here* with a gesture that makes obvious to the young child where *here* is intended to be, as in "Put your cup *here*." The use of the same strategy with another adult could be viewed as insulting by the adult on the receiving end. The implied message in the latter case would be, "I do not believe you can understand me with my words alone."

We assume that the goal of any child learning language is to determine how to connect or map language input to the context or event that is occurring. Consider the following example of an infant's incorporation into a farewell routine. When the grandmother has put on her coat and headed for the door after giving daddy and infant a very substantial hug and kiss, and then daddy says to the infant, "Grandma is going home now," the infant has been provided with an opportunity to more easily connect the language to the event than if the language occurred without the context. The more assistance that an adult (or more sophisticated language user) provides to draw the infant's attention to the symmetry between language and context, the easier the mapping task will be for the language-learning child. We can call this symmetry *mapping*, meaning the connecting of language to event or person or object.

Consider this example of facilitation of mapping that occurred when a friend's son was approximately eight months old. The infant's six-year-old sister held out his pacifier (referred to in the family as a "passy") so that it was right in front of him within easy grasp as she slowly intoned, "Want passy? Want passy, Joe?" It is not clear whether the child's subsequent grab for his "passy" was prompted by the linguistic information or by the presence of the very attractive pacifier in close proximity to his person. The important information may be that the nonlinguistic context—the presence of the pacifier held by his sister within his reach—was coupled with the production of a linguistic message that fit the scenario. Joe was incorporated into a turn-taking set because his sister asked a question and paused, waiting for her brother to reach for the accessible pacifier. Down the road, multiple instances of this or similar linguistic messages paired with symmetrical nonlinguistic contexts may serve to assist a young child in mapping the likely meaning of "passy" and other words.

Can we credit Joe with understanding the words "want" and "passy," either singly or in combination? The evidence we have would not allow us to conclusively assume we can or cannot. Our indecision rests on the remarkable use of comprehension strategies by young children that make the most of nonlinguistic information and/or partial linguistic information in the absence of complete linguistic knowledge.

Development and Use of Comprehension Strategies

Chapman (1978; see also Miller & Paul, 1995; Paul, 1990) has written extensively about the existence of language comprehension strategies in the normal development of children's understanding of spoken language. Her conceptualization is a helpful one because it incorporates what young children are doing in terms of cognitive development with their use of what Chapman refers to as formulas for getting around a lack of complete information. Young children learning language will be much more reliant on nonlinguistic or context information than the more linguistically sophisticated, older child.

For the unsophisticated language user, gesture, proximity to the speaker, attention to what the speaker is attending to, and previous situation experience or world knowledge take on extraordinary importance in decoding language input. Young children are focused on the here and now. Whatever is physically present will significantly figure into the child's attempts to understand any linguistic message.

Examples of "Comprehension" When Little Linguistic Knowledge Has Been Acquired

The example of Joe and his pacifier presented earlier could illustrate one of the comprehension strategies described by Chapman (1978): "Act on objects at hand." That is, when an attractive object is placed in front of Joe, he will try to grasp it. It probably does not matter what his sister said. It does not matter that her utterances are an attempt to help him map language onto context. If Joe is physically able and the pacifier is something he wants, in the absence of linguistic knowledge you probably could say, "Want hedge trimmer?" and Joe would reach for the pacifier anyway. At eight months of age, asking Joe if he wants anything that is not physically present would probably be less successful. Given his eight-month-old motor skills, reaching for something he wants is his response to seeing the pacifier, because he can.

An example of another early-developing comprehension strategy described by Chapman (1978) has likely been observed by most readers of this text. A nine-month-old child is held in her parents' arms and incorporated into a leave-taking routine by the caregiver. The caregiver starts to wave good by to a visitor and tells the baby, "Wave bye-bye." Soon after, the baby begins to wave at the departing visitor. The caregiver is convinced that this movement is occurring in response to the request for action, specifically to wave. According to Chapman's taxonomy, however, the baby is much more likely following a comprehension strategy called "Imitate ongoing actions." That is, the caregiver is waving and, regardless of what has actually been said, the child begins to wave, too. This situation could be considered a case of actions speaking louder than words.

Why does this response occur? The imitation occurs because at the baby's age, imitation of what caregivers do constitutes a frequent activity on the part of many normally developing children. According to Tomasello (1995), young children learn early on that there is a benefit to attending to what the speaker attends to for mapping clues. The adult waves and so the baby waves. If you want your baby to look really smart at this age, just keep saying, "Do what I do;" perform actions your toddler can do; and let cognition take its course! The key is to remember that the ensuing activity is not necessarily the result of linguistic comprehension, but rather a response likely to have occurred regardless of what was said.

Here is yet another example that meshes well with clinical attempts to estimate young children's language comprehension abilities. Two prepositions that emerge and are mastered quite early in children's expressive and receptive repertoires are the morphemes "in" and "on." Both are part of Brown's (1973) 14 grammatical morphemes used to chart the development of morphology in preschool-age children. SLPs often attempt to determine whether two-year-olds can understand these prepositions, but the nonlinguistic context for assessment must be carefully controlled for test results to have any validity. For example, if children are presented with a cup and asked to "Put the blocks in the bucket," it is very likely that young children, whether or not they understand the linguistic request, will place the blocks into the bucket. Buckets are receptacles: In "doing what you usually do with objects at hand" (Chapman, 1978), you place smaller things inside something with a natural inside. Similarly, if the SLP tells a child to "put the book on the box" (and supplies the child with a closed cardboard box), it is very likely that the child will place the book on top of the box, not underneath it or next to it. The box has a natural top, so even a child who does not understand more than the words *book* and *box* (and may know quite a bit less) will do what is usually done—that is, place one object on top of another where the top is clearly demarcated.

Comprehension Strategy Use Continues into the Linguistic Period

Chapman (1978) follows the use of comprehension strategies through the young child's early vocabulary acquisition and semantic/syntactic development. The process of making best guesses given knowledge of only part of the linguistic message is related to a phenomenon called *bootstrapping*. That is, children learning language tend to use what they already know to extend their understanding into realms of language where their knowledge is sketchy (Owens, 2008).

For example, children quickly become familiar with the high-frequency occurrence of subject–verb–object (S-V-O) sentence productions. But what happens when they are presented with a less familiar sentence type, such as a passive construction where the subject and object have exchanged locations in the sentence? Consider the following two sentences, the first in the active voice and the second expressed in the passive voice: (1) The *dog* chased the *cat* and (2) The *cat* was chased by the *dog*. If you provide preschool-age children with a toy dog and cat, and ask them to act out these two sentences one at a time, they are likely to indicate that the first noun is the actor and the second noun is the recipient of the action in both sentences. Mature English-language users know that in both cases the actor and the recipient are the same; it is only the grammatical structure that varies between the two sentences.

In this scenario, the child has used a strategy that can be likened to "playing the percentages." If you are a devoted baseball aficionado, you will more easily understand the reference. Given the high frequency of S-V-O sentences, the child will impose that template on new, unknown grammatical structures such as the passive construction. Thus, in the first sentence, the child correctly understands that the dog (S) chases (V) the cat (O); in the second sentence, the child erroneously assumes that the cat (S) chases (V) the dog (O). A child who relies on application of the S-V-O rule to unknown sentence constructions may be following a *word-order strategy*. Recall that because the child had mastered the template in which the first noun is always the subject and the second noun is the object/patient, passive-voice sentences will be misinterpreted if the word-order strategy is applied.

Another more sophisticated example of a comprehension strategy is application of the *order of mention strategy*, which may occur when children are asked to comprehend sentences with multiple clauses. An example of a situation where this comprehension dilemma could occur is when the adverbs *before* and *after* are used. If the child does not understand the adverbs, a mistake may result. Look at the four sentences that follow and determine which action would occur first and which action would occur second when children are asked to order two pictures according to the information provided by each sentence:

1. "Show me: 'Before he took a bath, he worked on his homework.'"
2. "Show me: 'He took a bath after he worked on his homework.'"
3. "Show me: 'After he took a bath, he worked on his homework.'"
4. "Show me: 'He took a bath before he worked on his homework.'"

Relying on linguistic knowledge only, you would understand that in the first two sentences, homework was worked on before taking a bath. In the final two sentences, the bath was taken before homework was worked on. For the child applying the order of mention strategy, each of the four sentences would be acted out in the same way. Specifically, the bath occurred first and the homework was worked on second because the first clause includes the word *bath* and the second includes *homework*. The adverbs *before* and *after* are inconsequential to the child who has no knowledge of their role in lending meaning to sequenced actions. Therefore, if a child is presented with only statements such as those in examples 3 and 4, "correct" responses would not necessarily mean that the child understood the adverbs.

SLPs must carefully develop probe test items that will determine whether comprehension strategies are being used and if the child has true linguistic comprehension of the structure in question. More information about the development of nonstandardized probe items is provided later in this chapter.

One final example of comprehension strategies warrants mention because it represents a very crucial portion of the information that children bring to the table in attempting to decipher language input. This piece is referred to as *world knowledge*, and the strategy is referred to as the *probable relation of events strategy* by Chapman (1978; see also Miller & Paul, 1995). Using the example sentences given earlier for *before* and *after* comprehension, consider the case of young children who use world knowledge to figure out sentences that are beyond their competence level. When they are less sophisticated in a linguistic sense, younger children use a "do what you usually do" strategy—for example, when given a brush, they brush hair. When they become more sophisticated in the ways of the world, they interpret what they do not know by thinking about what would make the most sense in that situation based on past experience or how the world typically operates for them. For example, if a child lives in a household where the bedtime routine always includes homework first and then a bath, the use of adverbs the child cannot understand will not hinder him from attempting to understand those four sentences. The answer to the question of which activity occurred first would also be "first homework, then a bath" when a probable relation of events strategy was used.

Guessing May Be a Good Strategy for Learning

Children can facilitate adults' miscalculations of their language comprehension because they often make a guess at what is being said when they have understood only a portion of the input. This kind of guessing can be a good thing. Unlike on some of the standardized tests we have taken as adults (or nearly adults) where the directions specify that we are not to guess if we do not feel sure of an answer, children's use of partial information, as in the examples of children who have used comprehension strategies to attempt to answer a question, is not without its benefits.

In language-learning contexts, an incorrect response often prompts feedback from a more language-competent person (Demetras, Post, & Snow, 1986; Farrar, 1990). To see how this works, suppose a child makes what could be called a "best guess" using the information she does have available, but the response is wrong. That response may prompt a correction, a model, or a clarification by a caregiver, for example. If she is paying attention, the child can use this feedback to determine why the answer was wrong and then generalize this information to another, similar situation in the future. If the response is accepted by the caregiver and the conversation continues, this is also feedback for the child. In this second case, the response produced was probably correct or at least acceptable.

Here is an example of this type of exchange between a caregiver and a 22-month-old child. Notice how the conversation framework plays a vital role.

> Adult: You found the brush for the dolly's hair.
> Child: (Vigorously shakes her head in affirmation and begins to style the doll's hair with the brush.)
> Adult: Well, okay, if you want to brush the dolly's hair, that's fine. Brush the doll's hair. (Child continues to brush the child's hair.)

In this example, the child identified the brush as belonging to the doll or being appropriate for the brushing of the doll's hair: brush–doll–hair. These three words, or some combination thereof, were likely understood by the child. The intention of the adult, which was probably just to comment on the child's finding of the brush, was incorrectly taken to mean that a request for action had been made. Note how the caregiver has shaped her response to the child's action to fit the conversation flow despite the child's misunderstanding of the adult's original intent. By adding the imperative form, "Brush the doll's hair," the adult has modeled for the child what she would have likely said if the response she had been looking for was the action produced by the child.

Comprehension of Single Words

A number of studies have demonstrated that the vocabularies of young children who are developing normally appear to be somewhat similar in several respects. One feature that appears common to most children is that their *receptive vocabularies*—that is, the single words they understand but do not necessarily produce—begin their development prior to the emergence of their *expressive vocabularies*; early on, the former vocabularies are typically larger than the child's corresponding expressive vocabulary. Both Nelson (1973) and Benedict (1979) found that children often have receptive vocabularies of approximately 50 different words by the time they have acquired their first 10 expressive vocabulary words. The size differential between receptive and expressive vocabulary appears to diminish as the child moves through the preschool years. Fenson and colleagues (1994) have demonstrated that by 10 months of age, children may have as many as 10 words in their receptive vocabularies. In fact, thanks to advances in computer technology, investigators such as Tincoff and Jusczyk (1999) have demonstrated that 6-month-old infants will reliably attend to video images of their own mothers when the word *mommy* is presented. Reznick (1990) and others have also demonstrated that infants as young as 6 months can reliably demonstrate visual preference for words they comprehend.

Clinicians should note that a child's early comprehension (or production) of a word does not necessarily mean that we can expect the child to have the same sophisticated conceptual understanding for a word that an adult or a much older child might have. To a young child who has just learned to reliably pick out the picture of *"apple"* from a set of four pictures, each depicting something to eat, the actual prototypicality of the apple picture matters. That is, to the child, an apple may have a specific set of features (e.g., is red, can be rolled, has a stem) that describes a very narrowly defined apple by adult standards. Adults know that any trip to a grocery store will likely provide the opportunity to see fruits that do not share these three characteristics yet are considered apples nonetheless.

Over time, and with repeated exposures, we can expect the child's own boundaries of the word to gradually take shape where the adult semantic boundaries lie until, for both child and adult, an apple is an apple. If the boundaries are too narrow, underextension occurs (e.g., *doggy* refers only to my dog); if they are too broadly spaced, overextension occurs (e.g., *doggy* refers to any four-legged animal) (MacWhinney, 1989; Thomson & Chapman, 1977). For young children, overextensions and underextensions appear in both their receptive and expressive vocabularies. Caregiver feedback is often useful in assisting children to revise their word meaning boundaries (Chapman, Leonard, & Mervis, 1986).

Another aspect of vocabulary learning is the development of word category hierarchies from general terms, such as *"vehicle,"* to more specific terms, such as *"car"* or *"Toyota."* When children develop their first vocabularies, words characterizing mid-level generalities (Owens, 2008), such as "car," predominate. The internalized organization of these hierarchies likely facilitates word recall and the eventual ability to associate words across abstract domains like opposites or synonyms. The ability to develop a complex system of semantic linkages is related to both general cognitive development and an increased vocabulary size. The strategy of creating semantic maps helps students to consider related words and concepts prior to writing a story, for example. The ability to utilize semantic mapping relies on a foundation of semantic linkages.

Word Learning Mechanisms: Links Between Phonology and Semantics

Vocabulary learning is an activity that extends over one's lifetime but is particularly prodigious during the infant/toddler period. In the last 30 years, researchers have adopted an information-processing paradigm to study vocabulary acquisition. For example, researchers have realized for some time that for children to learn words, they must be able to recognize repeated strings of phonological information and somehow accurately determine what that phonological string references. At the same time, children are increasing their understanding of the world and the things, people, and events in it. They parlay what they have learned about things, people, and events when they were in the preverbal stage into conceptual units, adding information as they go about experiencing their world.

To be successful word learners, children must develop robust phonological representations for words in short-term memory (Gathercole & Baddeley, 1989). This ability provides them with the opportunity to connect specific phonological strings with specific conceptual constructs. It is hypothesized that not only do children have to create phonological representations for short-term memory store, but they also have to be able to retain those representations long enough for the connections to be made. Investigators have also shown that strong nonword repetition skills are related to successful vocabulary learning. That is, children who have formed templates of potential phonological combinations are more likely to draw upon these templates for task repetition purposes than children who lack this type of internalized phonological knowledge.

Bishop's (1997) model of language comprehension focuses on the bridge between phonological representation and meaning. She takes the perspective that determining meaning is a function of all that the young child understands about how language works from the components of the language input message code itself, as well as its relationship to the context in which the message has occurred. As Bishop (1997) notes, "[T]he segmentation of a speech stream cannot be a simple bottom-up process, driven solely by perceptual input; the listener uses prior knowledge, context, and expectations, to achieve this task, and to select a meaning from a range of possibilities" (p. 13). Instead, she argues, comprehension probably involves both bottom-up (e.g., phonological representation) and top-down (e.g., world knowledge) processes. Top-down influences on word learning also include what the child knows about the semantic and syntactic neighborhood in which a novel word appears.

Fast Mapping

Fast mapping refers to the degree of word learning that can occur the first few times a child is exposed to a novel word but not provided with any explicit information about the word (Carey & Bartlett, 1978). To accurately understand a word presented only once or twice, a child must rely heavily on context to provide salient cues to the word's meaning. Children who are successful "fast mappers" have an advantage in vocabulary learning because fewer exposures to a word are needed before they begin to use the new word. It is likely that some of the context information inferred by the child to be related to the new word is not needed or is incorrectly linked to the new word. This differentiation between what is essential to the new word's meaning and what can be discarded will be refined over multiple exposures to the word (Harris, Barrett, Jones, & Brookes, 1988).

Comprehension of Semantic Relationships and Syntax

Usually after young children have acquired 50 different words in their expressive vocabularies, they begin to produce two-word combinations. For most children, this language production milestone occurs between 18 and 24 months of age. In fact, many children experience a substantive vocabulary growth spurt once their productive vocabulary includes approximately 100 words (Bates & Carnevale, 1993). This vocabulary spurt may be related to greater ease in the combining of phonological representations and mapped meanings.

For most children, the understanding of two-word combinations begins somewhat before the time those combinations appear in production (Miller, Chapman, Branston, & Reichle, 1980). Combining two words together requires that children understand more about the meaning of individual words than the characteristics that define them. In addition, children must learn something about the roles that words serve.

To see how this process works, we will return to learning about the word *"apple"* as already discussed. Not only are children learning the characteristics that define the group of items that can be called *"apple"* and not *"peach,"* for example, but they are also learning how *"apple"* can be linked with other words such as *"eat," "throw,"* and *"pick."* With each of these three action words, *"apple"* can be the recipient of the specified action. Thus we can talk about *"eat apple," "throw apple,"* and *"pick apple."* Children probably hear these combinations as parts of larger, more complex sentences or in sentence fragments directed at their less mature receptive language competencies. As a result, they add to their internal database the information that *"apple"* not only has distinguishable perceptual characteristics but also plays a definite part when linked with certain other words.

"Apple" can also be described as *"red apple"* or *"wormy apple."* Here the initial word in the two-word utterance is not an action but a descriptor. The descriptor and what it describes can be linked together to achieve more clarity when indicating which apple is referenced.

As emphasized later in this chapter, when assessing semantic relationships, clinicians must take into consideration how routine the two-word combinations are. If the clinician's goal is to determine when comprehension strategies are being used, it will be important to select combinations of words that are not transparent or rote learned, but require true linguistic comprehension.

Generally, between one and two years of age, children begin to demonstrate comprehension when actions are paired with expected, familiar words in three-word commands such as *"eat the apple," "throw the ball,"* and *"kiss the dolly."* If we insert unexpected or unfamiliar nouns into those action + object pairs, such as *"kiss the apple," "throw the dolly,"* or *"eat the ball,"* we are more likely to elicit confusion than compliance. When confused, children often rely on either context cues or world knowledge to determine how to respond. This brings us full circle back to a consideration of comprehension strategies.

When children master syntactic development in comprehension, where different types of sentences are understood (e.g., declaratives, interrogatives, imperatives), and when they begin to understand how to decode combined clauses and phrases when they have created lengthier and more complicated grammatical structures (e.g., conjoining and embedding), the use of nonlinguistic cues becomes increasingly less necessary. The use of comprehension strategies diminishes as the child begins to rely on linguistic information more often. Once syntactic information is available, young children have the foundation for making predictions about the meanings of novel words from this more sophisticated type of context cue. That is, it becomes possible for children to recognize when the new word is likely to be a noun versus a verb. As noted by Bishop (1997), "syntactic relationships between an unknown word and the other sentence elements can also give critical cues to meaning" (p. 106). This process is also considered to be a top-down method of word learning.

During their third year, children typically add some prepositions (e.g., *in, on, over*), opposites (e.g., *big* and *little, stop* and *go, big* and *small*), and descriptors (e.g., *happy, yellow, beautiful*) to their productive vocabularies and presumably understand the relationships expressed by these elements. With the addition of these concepts to their receptive lexicon, children will be better equipped to understand (and perhaps comply with) one- and two-stage commands such as *"Give me the yellow pen"* or *"Pull the blanket over the pillow and bring me the dolly."* Although preschool-age children use conjunctions to combine clauses and phrases (e.g., *and, because*) into the same sentences, it is not until the early school years—ages seven to nine years, according to Owens (2008)—that children understand and are able to incorporate more sophisticated and subtle adverbial "connectors, such as *before, after, during,* and *while*" (p. 156).

Does Language Comprehension Always Exceed Production?

Generally speaking, although there are anecdotal examples to the contrary (Paul, 2007), children's receptive language competencies exceed their production capabilities. That is, when children are reliably demonstrating understanding of three- and four-word utterances, they may be consistently producing somewhat less lengthy and less sophisticated expressions. Examples where children appear to be producing language in the absence of comprehension generally occur when they have rote-learned a phrase but have not parsed it into its component parts (e.g., "forever and ever"). There is additional evidence from work by Chapman and Miller (1975) and Paul (2000) that some children have shown production of word-order constraints that cannot be demonstrated in their comprehension. Thus it is crucial for SLPs not to presume that language comprehension always surpasses production abilities for a given child and to be sure to have ample clinical evidence to back up any statements made about relative language abilities.

There are at least two reasons why differential competencies in language comprehension and production must be considered. First, when making recommendations for intervention-targeted structures that are neither comprehended nor produced by a young child, it is probably a good idea to include both comprehension and production training. This is not to say that comprehension teaching must inevitably precede all production training. Lahey (1988) has argued for simultaneous teaching of targets in comprehension and production targets to reflect the way she believes normal language learners acquire language structure. When addressing a child's language disorder in the clinic, for example, the SLP will focus somewhat differently on the problem of inconsistent correct plural use depending on whether the child has demonstrated understanding of the plural concept ("Show me: '*The cat chases the mice.*'"; "Show me: '*The cat chases the mouse.*'").

The second reason for carefully considering whether comprehension deficits exist has to do with the following research findings. The results of studies conducted by Thal, Reilly, Seibert, Jeffries, and Fenson (2004) and Whitehurst and Fischel (1994) with children diagnosed with specific language impairment have demonstrated that children with bona fide language disorders who present with deficiencies in only language production have a better prognosis for catching up with their peers than do children with deficiencies in both language comprehension and production. This may sound intuitive to the reader: Having problems in two language modalities is a more significant therapeutic challenge to overcome than a problem in one modality—specifically, language production.

Question Comprehension: Accurate, Appropriate, or Both?

Question comprehension is an important topic because questions are frequently used by adults and others to invite children into conversations (requests for participation are implicitly made), which is where language learning often takes place. Accurate comprehension of questions versus non-questions may rely not only on children's ability to detect a rising intonation at the ends of utterances, but also on the grammatical structure that signals a question. Comprehension of question types has been shown to follow a fairly specific order (Parnell, Patterson, & Harding, 1984; Tyack & Ingram, 1977). At a relatively early age, toddlers have been shown to indicate comprehension of yes/no questions by attending to them versus ignoring of *wh*-questions that are beyond their comprehension. Chapman (1978) has noted that young children will use a strategy called "Supply missing information" in response to *wh*-questions they do not fully understand.

Parnell and colleagues (1984) found that their subjects, ages three through six, responded to *wh*-questions in the following order of difficulty from easiest to most challenging: Where?, Which?, What + be?, Who?, What + do?, When?, Whose?, Why?, and What happened? Specifically, between ages three and four, most children are able to answer "who," "what," and "where" questions as long as they are well supported by context. It is not surprising that the three question types whose answers require the cognitive underpinnings of time ("when"), manner ("how"), and causality ("why") concepts were among the last four question types acquired.

For children to be credited with question comprehension, they must demonstrate their ability to answer questions appropriately, though not necessarily accurately. Parnell and colleagues (1984) made this distinction when categorizing their results, as illustrated in the following example:

> Adult: When do you go to bed?
> Child: At 10 o'clock.
> Adult: *When?*
> Child: At 8 o'clock.
> Adult: That's better!

In both of the child's responses to the adult's "When?" question, the child supplied a mandatory time segment, indicating understanding the constraint of answering a "When?" question. Regardless of the adult's indication that the first response given by the child was incorrect (i.e., the child's bedtime is not at 10 P.M.), the answer was appropriate from a comprehension point of view. Leach (1972) provides a comprehensive taxonomy of the constraints on responses inherent in different question types. Question comprehension will be revisited later in this chapter as the basis of a nonstandardized comprehension probe.

MEASURING CHILDREN'S LANGUAGE COMPREHENSION

This chapter has made a compelling argument concerning why SLPs must actually assess children's language comprehension and not simply make assumptions of normalcy. The comment in a diagnostic report to the effect that "The child's comprehension appears to be within normal limits" is one that has been known to elicit a reflexive "How do you know that?" from me either as a clinical instructor or as a clinician reading a report completed by a colleague.

A number of standardized tests are available with which to assess aspects of the language comprehension of preschool-age children. On many occasions, however, it is necessary for SLPs to design nonstandardized probes to look more carefully at what preschool-age children actually understand when they need to evaluate the range of a comprehension deficit of a particular grammatical type.

Whether employing standardized or nonstandardized testing, the tasks SLPs use to evaluate comprehension typically fall into one of three categories: identification, acting-out, or judgment tasks (Weiss, Tomblin, & Robin, 1999). These tasks will require pointing to a picture that best fits the word(s) or answers the question asked. Acting-out tasks are less frequently used than identification tasks and involve having three-dimensional materials available to the child to demonstrate the action reflected in a sentence (e.g., "Give me the bottle," "Show me the baby drives the Jeep.") Judgment tasks typically tap the child's ability to make grammaticality judgments. They may involve asking a child to indicate which sentence sounds "silly" or "okay" to avoid the terms *grammatical* and *ungrammatical*. Regardless of the task type, comprehension tasks tend to be limited in the amount of verbal output needed from the examinee; for this reason, comprehension testing may be the preferred place to start when evaluating reticent children.

A Summary of Caveats

As mentioned previously, young children learning to understand the spoken language in their environment may depend heavily on the nonlinguistic context in which that language is produced to fill in any gaps that may exist in their linguistic understanding. Therefore, *if* the clinician's goal is to determine a child's competence to understand the linguistic portion of a message, he or she must carefully construct tasks that eliminate the nonlinguistic component as much as possible. To do so in a valid manner, SLPs should eliminate unintended gestures that provide clues to understanding. They should also select examples for testing that do not represent routines. For example, handing a child a dolly and saying, "Hug the dolly," is a task more likely to bypass comprehension processing than asking the same child to "Hug the apple." For the clinician, a clear understanding of how comprehension strategies are likely to function in the comprehension development of the young child will save the SLP from many instances of misinterpretation, and possibly misdiagnosis or *missed* diagnosis.

When designing comprehension tasks to provide children with multiple examples of a comprehension task type, it is also important to carefully take into account the vocabulary included in the task, and to watch the timing of any requests to the child so that you do not create the "pseudo-successes" that Chapman and her colleagues (1980) found to be so prevalent in the interactions between caregivers and their children. Using multiple examples will reduce the likelihood that the child's response was the result of some extraneous variable connected to that one item. When clinicians use vocabulary in test items that is unfamiliar to the child, they may find that they are testing vocabulary and not comprehension of sentences, for example.

Perhaps the *most* important advice that can be given to clinicians who question the language abilities of young children, whether or not language comprehension is the primary focus of concern, is to be absolutely certain of the child's hearing status prior to formalized language testing. Fortunately, many states have mandated newborn screenings and follow-up for children suspected of hearing loss. Nevertheless, these measures are not a panacea for catching all losses that might lead to negative academic and social ramifications. Given the propensity of middle ear disease in childhood, including repeated episodes of serous otitis media, often with accompanying hearing loss, it is critical to monitor children's hearing levels and determine whether the language input is in unaltered condition and available for their consumption (Roberts, Sanyal, Burchini, Collier, Ramey, & Henderson, 1986).

Standardized Assessment

Standardized assessment involves two aspects of test giving. The first aspect is that there is a set procedure for the administration and interpretation of the test as well as a standard set of stimuli provided for the examiner's use. These stimuli could consist of specific tasks using specific materials, or they might comprise a prescribed list of questions that are posed to a caregiver familiar with the child's development. The second aspect of standardization involves the substantiation of the psychometric rigor of the test. In addition to evidence of validity and reliability, normative data gleaned from use of a standardized sample of subjects to whom the test has been administered are typically available. The norms can be applied to the performance of a child (i.e., if appropriate for the test, given the criteria delineated in the test manual), thereby enabling the examiner to determine whether the child falls within the range of age-expected ability. For the purposes of this chapter, this section profiles tests that meet either one or both of these criteria for standardized tests.

Assessing Infants and Toddlers

For the clinical assessment of language comprehension in young children, two standardized tools are frequently employed and appear in the case studies found in this text: the *Rossetti Infant-*

Toddler Language Scale (Rossetti, 1990) and the *MacArthur–Bates Communicative Development Inventories* (Fenson et al., 1993). Although a number of other assessment tools have been published for use with this young population (see Paul, 2007, for a more complete list), these two tests will serve as examples for the types of tasks used for comprehension assessment.

Rossetti Infant-Toddler Language Scale. Rossetti's assessment tool, the *Rossetti Infant-Toddler Language Scale* (RITLS; Rossetti, 1990), is appropriate for children from birth through age three and yields an overall developmental age, individual developmental ages for language comprehension or language production, or developmental age equivalents for each of six language-learning areas. Of course, given the age range specified for its use, prelinguistic behaviors are also evaluated in terms of whether they have emerged at an accepted age.

The RITLS can be used as the basis of a caregiver interview about language development. The SLP can supplement the caregiver's responses to queries about the specific language competencies listed on the test (e.g., report) with observation or elicitation of behaviors.

The specific developmental achievements listed in each age group have been gleaned from other developmental resources; there are no normative data accompanying this test. According to Rossetti, the validity of the test derives from the excellence of the developmental sources used for item selection. The author refers to this test as a criterion-referenced measure, noting that it is useful for following a particular child's progress over time with reference to norms from the general population at large.

The items have been gleaned from other developmental assessment tools and the author's own experiences evaluating infants, toddlers, and young preschoolers. Examples of items from the language comprehension portion of the test are as follows for infants from birth to three months of age:

+ Shows awareness of a speaker
+ Attends to a speaker's mouth
+ Moves in response to a voice

For a child to receive credit for reaching a specific language comprehension age, *all* items at that age level must be achieved. That is, all of the items are viewed to be equally representative of the age level in question.

MacArthur–Bates Communicative Development Inventories. The *MacArthur–Bates Communicative Development Inventories* developed by Fenson et al. (1993) consists of two different test protocols: the Infant form (Words and Gestures), which is appropriate for children ranging in age from 8 to 16 months of age, and the Toddler form (Words and Sentences), which is appropriate for children ranging in age from 16 to 30 months of age. These inventories are identical to the *MacArthur Communicative Development Inventory*—the name has recently been altered by the authors to honor the contributions of the late Dr. Elizabeth Bates, one of the test's co-authors.

In terms of language comprehension testing, this test provides a standardized format for collecting information about a young child's early single-word and phrase vocabulary. By providing caregivers with closed sets of options for selecting words and phrases that their children comprehend (and produce), the authors generally find that parents are easily able to complete the checklist in a brief period of time with minimal, if any, assistance from professional examiners. The normative data provided by the authors are extensive (Dale & Fenson, 1996), but comprehension data are available for the Infant form only. This limitation likely reflects the fact that as children's vocabularies grow substantially into their second year, it becomes more difficult to determine in the absence of production which words the toddler actually understands and which words are perceived as understood due to context confounds. The normative data are also divided between males and females.

A look at the vocabulary comprehension data provided by Fenson and colleagues (1993) demonstrates the rapid acquisition of single-word vocabulary. For example, girls ranking at the 50th percentile comprehend 14 different words at 8 months of age and 191 at 16 months of age. Vocabulary "stars" functioning at the 99th percentile have 142 words at 8 months of age and 392 words by 16 months! When we consider these same "stars" in terms of their vocabulary production, they have an average of 7 words at 8 months of age and 281 words at 16 months of age, demonstrating a substantive difference between the size of their comprehension and production vocabularies.

Standardized Testing Procedures for Older Preschool-Age Children

Most often, standardized assessment of children in the two- through five-year age range involves having children identify pictures that are the best referents for the words, phrases, or sentences produced by the examiner. Typically several foil items appear on the page in addition to the correct answer. Children are encouraged to look at all of the options before selecting the picture that answers the query, and the test administrator should use any sample items to be sure that they understand the task. Examiners should be alert to children who appear to persevere in pointing to one location for all pictures, because this behavior may mean that they are not considering all of the picture options. Examiners also need to be careful not to accidentally point to the correct picture choice.

Paul (2007) lists 33 language assessment tools that are appropriate for use with children at the developing language level. Of these, only 14 are identified as focusing on the assessment of comprehension competencies of preschool-age children. Some of these tests provide SLPs with the opportunity to evaluate both comprehension and production. A smaller number evaluate language comprehension only.

Two of the most commonly used tests in this age group are the *Peabody Picture Vocabulary Test-4* (PPVT-4; Dunn & Dunn, 2007), a test of hearing vocabulary only, and the *Test for Auditory Comprehension of Language-3* (TACL-3; Carrow-Woolfolk, 1999), an assessment tool that consists of three parts—vocabulary, grammatical morphemes, and elaborated phrases and sentences. Both of these tests use identification tasks to elicit responses from test takers and utilize a basal/ceiling scoring regimen. The pictures that make up the PPVT-4 items are displayed four on a page; the TACL-3 items consist of three pictures located side-by-side. Because examiners are asked to determine basal and ceiling scores, they are provided with suggestions for where to start in the test given the child's chronological age.

Examiners can derive the following scores from the PPVT-4: standard scores, percentiles, normal curve equivalents, stanine scores, age equivalents, grade equivalents, and growth scale value scores. The TACL-3 provides the SLP with the opportunity to compare the child's performance with normative data so as to derive percentile ranks, standard scores, and age equivalents.

As psychometrically sound as these standardized tests are, their usefulness—especially when deciding where to begin therapy—can be limited. For that reason, the use of nonstandardized probes to fine-tune the results from diagnostic tests is often recommended (Weiss, Tomblin, & Robin, 1999).

Nonstandardized Comprehension Probes

Sometimes the standardized tests do not provide SLPs with the opportunity to fully evaluate specific areas of language comprehension. To perform a more complete assessment of a child's comprehension competencies, SLPs may have to devise their own tasks to collect the information we need for clinical decision making. That is, SLPs may need to develop their own nonstandardized probes.

Here is one example of a nonstandardized comprehension probe that may prove very useful—it was designed to fill a gap in available testing. This tool is meant to account for the fact that standardized tests do not do a particularly good job in providing clinicians with the means to assess children's comprehension of different question forms. For example, the TACL-3 (Carrow-Woolfolk, 1999) contains very few items that directly address *wh*-question comprehension. Specifically, these questions are framed as follows: "When do you sleep?" and "What do you eat?" Children are told to point to the one of three pictures that best represents an answer to the question. Actually, the task is a little less specific than that: Examiners tell children to show the examiner the picture that best represents the utterance produced by the examiner. Note how decontextualized the use of the question is in this test-taking situation. Typically a question turns the speaking floor over to another conversation partner. During test taking, however, no verbal response is called for. It is no wonder that many children will answer the question when it is produced by the examiner!

Given that question comprehension plays a vital role in children's ability to function in academic and social settings, determining the adequacy of a child's question comprehension is not a trivial matter. Relying on the TACL-3 will not achieve this goal. Thus a nonstandardized assessment tool can be developed to provide more and different examples of questions.

Table 11-1 shows one such nonstandardized probe. Note that several examples per question type are used. The question types selected reflect the results of a study that demonstrated

TABLE 11-1   A Nonstandardized Probe for *Wh*-Questions

Question Type and Examples	Functionally Appropriate
What + be: e.g., "What is this?"	
What is a banana?, etc.	
What is your name?, etc.	
Which: e.g., "Which puppy is cuter?"	
Which ball is orange?, etc.	
Which boat is a sailboat?, etc.	
Where: e.g., "Where do you live?"	
Where are your toys?, etc.	
Where do you sleep?, etc.	
Who: e.g., "Who takes you to school?"	
Who do you play with?, etc.	
Who is your best friend?, etc.	
Whose: e.g., "Whose hat is that?"	
Whose toy is that?, etc.	
Whose hair is curliest?, etc.	
What do: e.g., "What are you doing?"	
Why: e.g., "Why did he fall down?"	
When: e.g., "When is your bedtime?"	
What happened: e.g., "What happened yesterday?"	

the question forms typically understood by children ages three through six (Parnell, Patterson, & Harding, 1984). This article serves as the only normative referent. Completion of this non-standardized test will provide a clinician with the data needed to determine whether question comprehension is progressing within normal limits or if it represents an appropriate goal for therapy for a particular child.

One advantage of developing nonstandardized assessment probes is that you can design the tool to fit the specific children whom you are evaluating. Not only can you be sure to focus attention on the area of language comprehension you may be curious about, but you can also select the type of task that you believe will work best (e.g., identification, acting out, judgment, response to question) for the child. In addition, you can control for the vocabulary used so that the performance of the child is not confounded by use of unfamiliar words in the tasks (Weiss, 2001).

CASE STUDIES

Given our discussions about language comprehension in this chapter, how can we relate that information to the three case studies?

JOHNATHON, a typically developing child at age 25 months

The speech-language evaluation report provided for the typically developing two-year-old, Johnathon, includes some information in the history paragraph about the child's receptive language abilities. As noted in the report, Johnathon was able to follow age-appropriate directions provided without contextual support. Although there might be a problem with the example used (i.e., "Bring me your bottle" is fairly stereotypical of what one would be asked to do with a bottle), at least the clinician viewed comprehension as important enough to inquire about it on the front end of the evaluation. The section chronicling Johnathon's receptive language could have been supplemented with nonstandardized tasks that would determine the extent to which the child used comprehension strategies in response to requests for actions or objects.

The comment that Johnathon understands new words rapidly should be clarified. An example or two would be helpful here. Does this comment refer to Johnathon's penchant for fast mapping? That is, is he likely to use a word correctly after being exposed to it only one or two times? We know that children who are considered good at fast mapping typically show accelerated word learning. These children are risk takers in terms of language learning. Their ability to observe how a word is used is keen, meaning that they can pick out the salient features of the verbal and nonverbal context to generalize the word to future circumstances. Also, they do not seem to be shy about trying out their new words.

A comparison between the child's receptive and expressive language abilities demonstrated that Johnathon's skills were closely aligned; that is, there was no discrepancy between receptive and expressive competencies as indicated by the RITLS (Rossetti, 1990). We have already discussed the importance of not making assumptions about expressive language skills based on receptive skills, and vice versa.

JOSEPHINE, a late talker at age 22 months

Josephine's significant history included the observation that her receptive language was a relative strength. Although Josephine did not produce her first word until the age of 15 months, and her mother's perception was that her daughter had a smaller expressive vocabulary than would be expected for her age, the child was reported to be following two-step commands. Note that the example given by the mother could be reflective of an overestimate of Josephine's language comprehension: "Go to the family room and get your diaper." If Josephine recognizes the word "diaper" and, as most children do, knows where they are kept, the first portion of the command is unnecessary. That is, when retrieving a diaper, Josephine will go to the family room whether told to or not. Thus Josephine's response to this particular two-step command may mean as little as comprehension of the word *diaper* and "locate the objects mentioned," one of Chapman's comprehension strategies.

According to her performance on the RITLS, Josephine's receptive language abilities slightly exceeded those expected for her chronological age. This estimate included successful completion of tasks requiring responses to two-step commands. When comparing Josephine's expressive and receptive test results, it is clear that her language comprehension abilities significantly exceed her language production abilities. This is a child whose caregivers may believe "she understands everything" partly because of the discrepancy between receptive and expressive language and partly because of the facility with which her comprehension strategies are used. Clinicians should take care to explain to the parents that certainly Josephine's strength is her understanding of language and that this strength will be used in therapy to help increase her expressive language abilities. Under no circumstances, however, should the parents be encouraged to believe that their child understands everything that is said to her: No two-year-old does.

Research has demonstrated that children whose problems are confined to expressive language tend to make swifter language development gains than those with both receptive and expressive language needs (Thal, Reilly, Seibert, Jeffries, & Fenson, 2004). Because Josephine's receptive language or language comprehension is a relative strength for her, this child's ability to catch up to her same-age peers in terms of her language development is more likely than that of another child who demonstrated both comprehension and expressive language deficits.

ROBERT, a child with a bona fide language impairment at age 27 months

Robert has presented with a number of developmental concerns, only one of which is language learning. Diagnosed with developmental delay by a physician, Robert's language comprehension development was not addressed in his history other than the mention of his ability to follow simple directions. Of some concern is the lack of definitive information provided regarding Robert's hearing levels. Accurate/adequate hearing will supply Robert with not only the verbal information necessary to understand language, but also the context information necessary for understanding the more subtle nuances of communicated messages.

Standardized testing on the MCDI: Words and Gestures form (normally used for children somewhat younger than Robert) revealed that Robert's receptive vocabulary was typical of a 1;6- to 2;0-year-old child. Results from the RITLS revealed a less mature picture, with his receptive language developmental age being closer to one year, although the report did note a scattering of skills up to the 21- to 24-month-old level. Because both receptive and expressive language competencies appear to be slow to develop, and given the pervasive delays observed in Robert's other developmental areas, the prognosis for Robert to make significant gains without continued provision of dedicated, intensive speech-language therapy is not very positive.

SUMMARY

Language comprehension, though an important aspect of language development, does not always receive the attention it deserves. Whether our interest is in normally developing or clinical populations, focusing on language comprehension competencies allows us to forge a more holistic picture of a child's language competencies, provide some hypotheses about how the child learns best, or, in the case of children with language deficits, give some insight into how to approach their language problems in the clinic. Further, the study of language comprehension provides a wealth of evidence indicating that children's learning of language necessitates the interweaving of knowledge not only about specific linguistic parameters, but also about how their world operates.

KEY TERMS

Assessment   Development
Comprehension   Language

STUDY QUESTIONS

+ You have received a catalogue from a publisher of speech and language tests. While perusing its pages, you notice that one of the products highlighted is a brand-new comprehension test advertised as appropriate for children ages three to six years of age. Before purchasing this test for your use in your work setting, you think about your practice. Which specific information about language comprehension in children will assist you in evaluating the benefit of owning this new test instrument?

+ Using a university library's research engine, find an issue of a journal that publishes information about language learning in either normal or atypical children (e.g., *First Language; Journal of Child Language; Journal of Speech, Language, and Hearing Research*), including an article chronicling some aspect of children's developing language comprehension. Determine which types of tasks were used to assess comprehension. Were the procedures used for data collection valid? That is, did the tasks account for the possibility of an overestimation of children's comprehension abilities?

+ Link to the http://www.youtube.com Web site and find a video clip called "Baby Alison." Its URL is as follows: http://www.youtube.com/watch?v=yz_czUxd2w0. The video stars a toddler who is being held by her dad, who asks her to wave "bye-bye." Watch the segment carefully. Given what you know about children's early language comprehension and the appearance of early language, would you or would you not give this child credit for understanding the command "Wave bye-bye"? If this particular video clip is not available, find another using the key words "baby" and "waving." Be sure that there is a caregiver involved in the clip as well.

REFERENCES

Bates, E., & Carnevale, G. (1993). New directions in research on language development. *Developmental Review, 13,* 436–470.

Benedict, H. (1979). Early lexical development: Comprehension and production. *Journal of Child Language, 6,* 183–200.

Bishop, D. (1997). *Uncommon understanding: Development and disorders of language comprehension in children.* East Essex, UK: Psychology Press.

Brown, R. (1973). *A first language: The early stages.* Cambridge, MA: Harvard University Press.

Bruner, J. (1978). The role of dialogue in language acquisition. In A. Sinclair, R. Jarvella, & W. Levelt (Eds.), *The child's conception of language* (pp. 241–256). New York: Springer-Verlag.

Carey, S., & Bartlett, E. (1978). Acquiring a single new word. *Papers and Reports on Child Language Development, 15,* 17–29.

Carrow-Woolfolk, E. (1999). *Test for Auditory Comprehension of Language.* 3rd ed. Austin, TX: Pro-Ed.

Chapman, K., Leonard, L., & Mervis, C. (1986). The effect of feedback on children's inappropriate word use. *Journal of Child Language, 13,* 101–117.

Chapman, R. (1978). Comprehension strategies in children. In J. Kavanaugh & W. Strange (Eds.), *Speech and language in the laboratory, school and clinic* (pp. 308–327). Cambridge, MA: MIT Press.

Chapman, R., Klee, T., & Miller, J. (November 1980). *Pragmatic comprehension skills: How mothers get some action.* Presented at the annual meeting of the American Speech and Hearing Association (Detroit, MI).

Chapman, R., & Miller, J. (1975). Word order in early two- and three-word utterances: Does production precede comprehension? *Journal of Speech and Hearing Research, 18,* 355–371.

Dale, P. S., & Fenson, L. (1996). Lexical development norms for young children. *Behavior Research Methods, Instruments, & Computers, 28,* 125–127.

Demetras, M., Post, K., & Snow, C. (1986). Feedback to first language learners: The role of repetitions and clarification questions. *Journal of Child Language, 13,* 275–292.

Dunn, L., & Dunn, L. (2007). *Peabody Picture Vocabulary Test—IV.* 4th ed. Circle Pines, MN: American Guidance Service.

Farrar, M. (1990). Discourse and the acquisition of grammatical morphemes. *Journal of Child Language, 17,* 607–624.

Fenson, L., Dale, P., Reznick, S., et al. (1993). *The MacArthur Communicative Development Inventories.* San Diego: Singular Publishing.

Fenson, L., Dale, P., Reznick, S., Bates, E., Thal, D., & Pethick, S. (1994). Variability in early communicative development. *Monographs of the Society for Research in Child Development, 59* (Serial No. 242).

Fernald, A., & Kuhl, P. (1987). Acoustic determinants of infant preference for motherese speech. *Infant Behavior and Development, 10,* 279–293.

Fernald, A., Taeschner, T., Dunn, J., Papousek, M., deBoysson-Bardies, B., & Fukui, I. (1989). A cross-language study of prosody modifications in mothers' and fathers' speech to preverbal infants. *Journal of Child Language, 16,* 477–501.

Gathercole, S., & Baddeley, A. (1989). Evaluation of the role of phonological STM in the development of vocabulary in children: A longitudinal study. *Journal of Memory and Language, 28,* 200–213.

Harris, M., Barrett, M., Jones, D., & Brookes, S. (1988). Linguistic input and early word meanings. *Journal of Child Language, 15,* 77–94.

Lahey, M. (1988). *Language development and language disorders.* New York: MacMillan.

Leach, E. (1972). Interrogation: A model and some implications. *Journal of Speech and Hearing Disorders, 37*, 33–46.

MacWhinney, B. (1989). Competition and lexical categorization. In R. Corrigan, F. Eckman, & M. Noonan (Eds.), *Linguistic categorization* (pp. 195–242). New York: John Benjamins.

Miller, J., Chapman, R., Branston, M., & Reichle, J. (1980). Language comprehension in sensory motor stages 5 and 6. *Journal of Speech and Hearing Research, 23*, 1–12.

Miller, J., & Paul, R. (1995). *The Clinical Assessment of Language Comprehension*. Baltimore: Paul H. Brookes.

Milosky, L. (1992). Children listening: The role of world knowledge in comprehension. In R. Chapman (Ed.), *Processes in language acquisition and disorders* (pp. 20–44). St. Louis: Mosby Year Book.

Nelson, K. (1973). Structure and strategy in learning to talk. *Monographs of the Society for Research in Child Development, 38*.

Owens, R. (2008). *Language development: An introduction*. 7th ed. Boston: Pearson/Allyn & Bacon.

Parnell, M., Patterson, S., & Harding, M. (1984). Answers to *wh*-questions: A developmental study. *Journal of Speech and Hearing Research, 27*, 297–305.

Paul, R. (1990). Comprehension strategies: interactions between world knowledge and the development of sentence comprehension. *Topics in Language Disorders, 10*(3), 63–75.

Paul, R. (2000). *Understanding the "whole" of it: Comprehension assessment*. Seminars in Speech and Language, 21(3), 10–17.

Paul, R. (2007). *Language disorders from infancy through adolescence: Assessment and intervention*. 3rd ed. St. Louis: Mosby Elsevier.

Reznick, J. (1990). Visual preference as a test of infant word comprehension. *Applied Psycholinguistics, 11*, 145–166.

Roberts, J., Sanyal, M., Burchini, M., Collier, A., Ramey, C., & Henderson, F. (1986). Otitis media in early childhood and its relationship to later verbal and academic performance. *Pediatrics, 78*, 423–430.

Rossetti, L. (1990). *The Rossetti Infant–Toddler Language Scale: A measure of communication and interaction*. East Moline, IL: Linguisystems.

Thal, D., Reilly, J., Seibert, L., Jeffries, R., & Fenson, J. (2004). Language development in children at risk for language impairment: Cross-population comparisons. *Brain & Language, 88*(2), 167–179.

Thomson, J., & Chapman, R. (1977). Who is "Daddy" revisited: The status of two year olds' over-extended words in use and comprehension. *Journal of Child Language, 4*, 359–375.

Tincoff, R., & Jusczyk, P. (1999). Some beginning of word comprehension in 6 month olds. *Psychological Science, 10*, 172–175.

Tomasello, M. (1995). Pragmatic contexts for early verb learning. In M. Tomasello & W. Merriman (Eds.), *Beyond names for things: Young children's acquisition of verbs* (pp. 115–146). Hillsdale, NJ: Erlbaum.

Tyack, D., & Ingram, D. (1977). Children's production and comprehension of questions. *Journal of Child Language, 4*, 211–224.

Weiss, A. (2001). *Preschool language disorders: Resource guide*. San Diego: Singular Publishing/Thomson Learning.

Weiss, A., Tomblin, J., & Robin, D. (1999). Language disorders. In J. Tomblin, H. Morris, & D. Spriestersbach (Eds.), *Diagnosis in speech-language pathology*, 2nd ed. (pp. 129–173). San Diego: Singular Publishing.

Whitehurst, G., & Fischel, J. (1994). Early developmental delay: What, if anything, should the clinician do about it? *Journal of Child Psychology and Psychiatry, 35*, 613–648.

CHAPTER 12

The Transition to the School-Age Years: Literacy Development

SallyAnn Giess, PhD

OBJECTIVES

+ Understand the complexity of the term literacy.
+ State the key components of the emergent literacy period according to van Kleeck and Schuele.
+ Describe the role of phonological awareness in reading development.
+ Understand the relationship between spoken and written language.
+ Be familiar with normal literacy development.

INTRODUCTION

There are many definitions of literacy, and being literate has different connotations in different cultures. *Literacy* may best be thought of as both a foundational skill of lifelong learning and a lifelong learning process (United Nations Educational, Scientific, and Cultural Organization [UNESCO], 2004). UNESCO (2004) has drafted the following definition:

> Literacy is the ability to identify, understand, interpret, create, communicate, and compute, using printed and written materials associated with varying contexts. Literacy involves a continuum of learning in enabling individuals to achieve their goals, to develop their knowledge and potential, and to participate fully in their community and wider society. (p. 13)

Within that definition is the fundamental necessity of creating meaning from print.

When one thinks of "being literate," perhaps the first connotation that comes to mind is "being able to read." At a foundational level, reading involves the process of associating a letter sound with a written, orthographic symbol. At a more skilled level, reading involves a complex interaction between the reader and the text as the reader creates meaning from the printed material (Catts & Kamhi, 2005). As the definition put forth by UNESCO illustrates, literacy is a multidimensional, multifaceted construct, and one that takes route early in a child's life. How do children come to arrive at this ability? How do they transition from a world where the focus is on language as a spoken event to a world where the focus is on language as a written event? Clearly, children have a great deal to learn as they make this transition.

This chapter considers literacy development along a continuum from the emergent literacy period, typically occurring during the preschool years, through the early literacy period, which consists of the first years of formal schooling. Long before a child enters formal schooling, the foundations of literacy must already be in place; thus the foundational skills of literacy that develop during the preschool years will be discussed first. The next section will focus on the initial years of a child's formal education, the early literacy years, and the necessary components of effective literacy education. Finally, the three case studies are discussed in line with longitudinal research that has predicted later literacy skills from early speech and language development.

THE FOUNDATIONS OF LITERACY: THE EMERGENT LITERACY PERIOD _____

During the period of a child's life from birth through kindergarten, the foundations of literacy development are being laid. Teale and Sulzby (1986) introduced the term *emergent literacy* to describe the reading and writing behaviors that precede and develop into conventional literacy. This period occurs before a child learns the formal mechanics of print and can actually decode (i.e., read) a printed word (van Kleeck & Schuele, 1987). Whitehurst and Lonigan (1998) define emergent literacy as "the skills, knowledge, and attitudes that are presumed to be developmental precursors to conventional forms of reading and writing and the environments that support these developments" (p. 849).

Although they were first described more than two decades ago, the conclusions Teale and Sulzby (1986) make regarding the underpinnings of emergent literacy are just as relevant today to understanding the foundations of literacy:

  + Listening, speaking, reading, and writing abilities develop concurrently and interrelatedly.
  + Literacy develops in real-life settings for real-life activities; in other words, it is a functional activity.
  + Children acquire written language skills through active engagement with their world—both in independent activities and through interactions with adults.

van Kleeck and Schuele (1987) describe two key domains that characterize the emergent literacy period: literacy socialization and language awareness. *Literacy socialization* reflects the social and cultural aspects of reading that a child acquires by being a member of a literate society, whereas *language awareness* focuses on the specific knowledge about the linguistic code that a child needs to master to become literate. The literacy socialization period can be further characterized according to literacy artifacts, literacy events and functions, and literacy knowledge acquired before learning to read (van Kleeck & Schuele, 1987).

Literacy artifacts are those representations of print that enrich a child's environment. Common examples of literacy artifacts include pictures of characters from nursery rhymes and *Sesame Street* that decorate a child's room, clothing, and picture books, alphabet blocks, stickers, and even character toothbrushes (van Kleeck & Schuele, 1987). Literacy artifacts also show up in less obvious places. For example, logos on a cereal box, store labels on a grocery bag, and an address on an envelope all expose a child to the importance of print in both his world and the world of his parents.

Although literacy artifacts are certainly important for exposing a child to print, it is the *literacy events and functions* that surround these artifacts that serve as real teaching opportunities during the emergent literacy period. One literacy event that has become part of mainstream American talk about literacy is shared or joint book reading. While joint book reading may not be "the single most important activity for . . . eventual success in reading" (Commission on Reading, 1985, p. 23), it serves as a rich source of information and opportunity to learn (Whitehurst & Lonigan, 2001). As children engage in joint book reading with a caregiver, they are exposed to a "book-language" way of talking (Mason, 1992) and to routines involving book reading.

In summarizing earlier work, van Kleeck and Schuele (1987) relate the rising expectations parents have for children in shared book reading to the rising expectations teachers have for students' reading curriculum in school. These expectations are reflected in the following developmental progression in questioning and commenting:

- Item labels: What's that? Who is that?
- Item elaborations (labels for subclasses, type, number): What kind of animal is that? How many fish do you see?
- Event: What happened?
- Event elaborations: (talk about already-introduced events by elaborating on location or consequences)
- Motive or cause: Why? How come?
- Evaluation/reaction: What a silly little boy!
- Relation to the real world: That looks just like the fish you caught with Grandpa!

These question/answer interactions provide opportunities for children to hear new words in meaningful contexts and to build a vocabulary that will be instrumental in the early school years (Mason, 1992). Given the exposure and emphasis placed on shared book reading, one could easily be swayed to agree that it is the single most important event for literacy success. Nevertheless, not all researchers support such a belief.

Scarborough and Dobrich (1990) concluded from their review of the literature that, while parent–preschooler shared reading experiences do influence language and literacy development, the strength of the influence is variable and may only be modest at best. Factors such as demographics, attitude, and skill level must also be considered as important and strong influences on early reading success. Children from lower-socioeconomic backgrounds and low-print homes may experience less benefit from shared book reading but may benefit from other activities that serve a similar function, such as those associated with daily living (e.g., paying bills) and entertainment (e.g., reading a tabloid or television guide). Similarly, a negative attitude about reading may lead to what Scarborough and Dobrich consider a "broccoli effect" (1990, p. 295). Not all young children are interested in books, and forcing an uninterested child to interact in a shared book activity may have the opposite of the desired effect. Catts and Kamhi (2005) stress that a negative attitude and a preference to not read are not the same as an inability to read; thus negative attitudes may not have long-term effects on literacy achievement.

The third aspect of literacy socialization is the print knowledge children gain from literacy experiences, referred to as *literacy knowledge*. In fact, literacy artifacts and literacy events may be most valuable for providing a context for this learning. By watching, doing, and handling, children learn the spatial orientation of books—that they have covers and backs, that pages turn from left to right, and that there is a right-side up position. More importantly, children are exposed to fundamental concepts of print—that sentences are read from left to right, that words have boundaries, that there is a spoken counterpart to the orthographic symbol, and that words tell stories. A caregiver sharing an alphabet book with a child is a prime example of how a literacy artifact can be used in a literacy event to teach knowledge of the alphabet principle. As the caregiver says the name of the letter and then the sound that the letter makes while simultaneously pointing to the letter and corresponding picture that represents the sound, the child learns that letters represent sounds in a predictable system, and words comprise patterns of letters and corresponding patterns of sounds.

This discussion of print knowledge alludes to the concept of phonological awareness. While phonological awareness is a skill that develops predominately during the early literacy period (kindergarten and first grade), it also has a place in discussion of emergent literacy skills. *Phonological awareness* is a broad term that refers to an individual's knowledge or sensitivity to the sound structure of words (Pullen & Justice, 2003) and at the emergent literacy level is reflected in activities such as rhyming, word play, and phonological corrections (van Kleeck & Schuele, 1987). For young children who are at risk for developing a reading disability or who come from homes where there is limited opportunity for language play, phonological awareness is a skill whose development may require explicitly engaging the child in meaningful and enjoyable activities that focus on the internal structure of words.

To this point in the chapter, the focus has been on the written precursors to literacy development. In fact, oral language skills have also been associated with later reading achievement, especially reading comprehension (Pullen & Justice, 2003). Although children are able to understand and use language long before they begin to read, their early experiences and successes with spoken language serve as the foundation for later reading development (Whitehurst & Lonigan, 1998). Indeed, preschool children's knowledge of vocabulary and grammar accounts for significant variance in later literacy skills. The ability to comprehend and produce increasingly complex syntactic structures influences literacy development. In her investigation of early language deficits of children who later develop dyslexia, Scarborough (1990) identified oral language skills that predicted later reading disability. In a sample of children, she found that syntactic deficits among two-year-olds and vocabulary deficits among older preschool children corresponded most closely with children's later literacy outcomes.

Linguistic awareness, which is a metalinguistic skill, also plays a role in emergent literacy and later reading success (Whitehurst & Lonigan, 1998). *Linguistic awareness* is the ability to understand language as a cognitive construct and to possess information about the manner in which language is constructed and used. Whitehurst and Lonigan (1998) describe it as awareness that *cat* and *sat* are units of language called words, that words are constructed from units of sound, and that these words differ in one letter but share two other letters. Such sensitivity to phonemes is critical to learning to read, but learning to read also increases one's phonemic sensitivity. Higher levels of linguistic awareness are essential for later reading skills when a child transitions to reading to learn (Whitehurst & Lonigan, 1998).

Van Kleeck and Schuele's (1987) presentation of the literacy socialization period explains some key events that occur during the preschool years and foster later literacy development. However, it does not explain how children become proficient in decoding words, a skill that is at the root of proficient reading. The ability to accurately and effortlessly recognize words is a key—perhaps *the* key—component to proficient reading. Stage theories of reading development are useful in understanding the development changes children go through as they become proficient readers.

STAGE THEORIES OF READING DEVELOPMENT

In 1983, Chall introduced her influential *stages of reading development* model based on a theory that reading development resembles cognitive and language development (other influential stage theorists include Ehri and Frith). Chall based her theory of reading development on several hypotheses that reflect Piaget's cognitive theories of development. Several of Chall's theories are mentioned below:

- Reading stages have a definite structure and differ from one another in qualitative ways, following a hierarchical progression.
- Reading is a problem-solving activity in which readers adapt to their environment.
- Individuals pass through the stages through interactions in their home, school, and community.
- Successive stages are characterized by growth in ability to read language that is more complex and more abstract.
- As readers advance through the stages, they are required to bring more sophisticated knowledge of the world and of the topic to the reading event.
- Readers may get stuck on techniques of an earlier stage, such as the decoding stage, and struggle with the demands of a more difficult stage (Chall, 1996, pp. 11–12).

Catts and Kamhi (2005) summarize the key components of the stage, models as follows: logographic stage, alphabetic stage, and orthographic stage, and automatic word recognition. The *logographic stage* may best be regarded as a prereading stage where children focus on the salient visual features of words. In this stage, children associate unanalyzed spoken words with salient graphic features of printing words and their surrounding context; they do not use letter names or sound–letter relationships to recognize words (Catts & Kamhi, 2005). As such, the logographic stage is not considered a prerequisite to reading. Indeed, this stage may be bypassed in children from low-print homes who go on to become proficient readers.

In contrast to the logographic stage, the *alphabetic stage* is essential. This stage is characterized by the onset of reading words by processing letter–sound correspondences and may be considered the first step to automatic word recognition. The key event in the alphabetic stage is the development of the *alphabetic principle*—the insight or awareness that letters correspond to sounds and that those same sounds make up our spoken language (Adams, 1994). At this stage, children spend a considerable amount of time phonologically decoding words.

Considering the arbitrariness of the English language, learning letter–sound correspondences is a difficult task for children. Put simply, phonological decoding is an inefficient strategy to word reading for the young child. Orthographic knowledge is necessary to the development of automatic, effortless word recognition, a knowledge that will eventually allow the reader to become "unglued" from the print (Chall, 1996). When a child reaches the *orthographic stage* of reading, she is able to use letter sequences and spelling patterns to recognize words visually without engaging in the cumbersome task of phonologically decoding each word (Catts & Kamhi, 2005).

A direct visual route to access semantic memory and word meaning, free of phonological mediation, is necessary to develop *automatic word recognition*. To develop this direct route, children must develop sufficient knowledge of spelling patterns. Such knowledge comes about with repeated encounters with similar letter sequences that are stored in semantic memory.

This is a place where spoken language knowledge will influence acquisition of written language. To develop automatic word recognition, a child must recognize and understand morphological endings such as *-ing*, *-ed*, and *-able* and function words such as *the*, *a*, and *an*. Understanding the importance and obligatory function of these words in spoken language will facilitate the recognition of these words in written language.

Stage theories of reading development are useful as a framework to explain the knowledge and skills children must have to become accomplished readers, but they fail to explain the actual processes that are used to acquire these skills (Catts & Kamhi, 2005). As an alternative to the stage-based theories, Share (1995) and Share and Stanovich (1995) have proposed a self-teaching hypothesis to explain how children learn to read.

THE SELF-TEACHING HYPOTHESIS

In considering direct instruction, contextual guessing, and phonological recoding as possible options for developing a literate lexicon, Share (1995) proposed that only *phonological recoding* (print-to-sound translation, also commonly referred to as *decoding*) offers the most viable means for developing fast, efficient, visual word recognition. The problem with direct instruction as a means to word recognition is that children encounter far too many words in printed text to possibly memorize them. Similarly, the use of semantic, syntactic, and pragmatic cues in written text is far too unreliable to facilitate fast and efficient word recognition (Share, 1995). Thus Share sees phonological recoding as the only viable means of efficient word recognition and the central component to the *self-teaching hypothesis*. According to the self-teaching hypothesis:

> . . . each successful decoding encounter with an unfamiliar word provides an opportunity to acquire the word-specific orthographic information that is the foundation of skilled word recognition. A relatively small number of (successful) exposures appear to be sufficient for acquiring orthographic representations . . . [in] this way, phonological recoding acts as a self-teaching mechanism or built-in teacher enabling a child to independently develop both (word)-specific and general orthographic knowledge. (p. 155)

The self-teaching hypothesis relies on an item-based role of decoding in development. The process of word recognition depends on the frequency with which a child has been exposed to a word and on successful identification of that word. Because children rapidly acquire orthographic information of a word, they are likely to visually recognize high-frequency words with little effort paid to phonological processing. Words that are encountered less frequently, and thus are less orthographically salient, will be more dependent on phonological processing (Share, 1995). Share describes this as a "phonology by familiarity account" (p. 155).

A second key feature of the self-teaching hypothesis is the lexicalization of phonological recoding (Share, 1995). Young readers initially begin the word recognition process with a basic knowledge of simple letter–sound correspondences that become associated with particular words (i.e., they are "lexicalized"). Children modify these simple one-to-one grapheme–morpheme correspondences by using constraints such as context, word position, and morphological endings (a grapheme is a written symbol [letter] that represents a phoneme [sound]). Share recognized that these initial decoding successes are much different than the decoding of the complex words that skilled readers eventually encounter. Nevertheless, according to Share, these early, manageable encounters are enough to kick-start the self-teaching mechanism, which in turn refines itself in light of orthographic knowledge. *Orthography* refers to the way a language is represented in print. *Orthographic representation* of a word refers to the way the word is stored visually in one's memory (Torgesen, 2004). The early lexicalization of sound–letter correspondences may best be considered a bootstrap or scaffold for developing the "complex, lexically constrained knowledge of spelling–sound relationships that characterize the expert reader" (Share, 1995, p. 165).

A third key feature of the self-teaching hypothesis relates to the contributions of the phonological and orthographical processes to fluent word recognition. While both processes make independent contributions to fluent word recognition, the phonological component is considered primary, accounting for the majority of individual differences in reading ability (Share, 1995). The ability to store and retrieve word-specific visual/orthographic information depends heavily on the ability to use spelling–sound relationships to identify unfamiliar words.

EARLY LITERACY: THE TRANSITION TO SCHOOL

The early literacy years reflect the events surrounding literacy that take place during the first few years of a child's formal education—typically kindergarten through second grade. During this period, children tackle the formidable task of learning how to read. Children arrive at their formal schooling years with different literacy experiences during the emergent literacy period. Some may already know how to spell their names and are creatively spelling words; others may be experiencing literacy artifacts (e.g., paper, crayons) for the first time (van Kleeck & Schuele, 1987). Both sets of children face the daunting task of becoming skilled at the same components of early literacy. The ultimate goal in the early literacy period is for a child to develop sufficient orthographic knowledge to allow for automatic, effortless word recognition that eventually leads to the end goal of reading comprehension. The National Reading Panel (NRP) identified five areas of reading instruction that are necessary to teaching children to read: phonemic awareness, phonics, fluency, vocabulary, and text comprehension (National Institute of Child Health and Human Development [NICHHD], 2000). Skill in each of these areas has a basis in oral language.

Phonemic awareness is the ability to notice, think about, and work with the individual sounds in spoken words (NICHHD, 2000). It is the understanding that sounds of spoken language work together to make words (NICHHD, 2000). Phonemes are the building blocks of spoken words, whereas letters are the building blocks of written words (Ehri & Roberts, 2006). As Ehri and Roberts (2006) state, phonemic awareness is conceptually separate from print; its function is to enable beginning readers to connect speech to print. Without this connection, children will likely struggle with early literacy.

As one type of phonological awareness skill, phonemic awareness is considered necessary, but not sufficient, for the development of word reading accuracy (Phillips & Torgesen, 2006). An example of a phonemic awareness activity is instructing a child to say the word *bat* and then to say the word again, replacing the /b/ with the /k/ sound (*cat*). As children develop oral language, they learn about the sounds of English through sound games such as singing the alphabet song and engaging in word play with their caregivers. Eventually, they come to experience these same sounds with their written (i.e., orthographic) counterparts. Repeated exposure to the sounds in words in both their spoken and written forms leads a child to discover the consistency and regularity in words. Knowledge and awareness of this consistency then allow a child to read words that he encounters for the first time in print (Phillips & Torgesen, 2006). Without such awareness, a child would see each printed word as a new experience and would not experience reading as a fluent process. Without the ability to read fluently, reading comprehension will suffer.

Phonics is a second building block of early literacy (NICHHD, 2000). As defined by Adams (1994), "phonics refers to a system of teaching reading that builds on the alphabetic principle, a system of which a central component is the teaching of correspondences between letters or groups of letters and their pronunciations" (p. 50). The connection between spoken and written language is central to phonics. To learn to read, children must understand the linguistic importance of sounds (phonemes) and must know the letters of the alphabet (Adams, 2001). This knowledge, in turn, facilitates reading words both in isolation and in connected text. Perhaps the emphasis on phonemic awareness instructions in early literacy programs can be tied to Juel's (2006) statement that, "without phonemic awareness, phonics instruction is meaningless" (p. 410). Although some children come to school already equipped with this knowledge, explicit instruction in phonics has been shown to be useful for all children (Torgesen, 2004).

A third component of early literacy is *fluency*. Various definitions of fluency exist (Phillips & Torgesen, 2006). Some definitions include the components of reading text accurately, quickly, and without effort (NICHHD, 2000; Meyer & Felton, 1999). The ability to group words into meaningful phrases, to read with prosody, or to read with intonation and stress may also be included in a definition of fluency. Phillips and Torgesen (2006) base their understanding of fluency in curriculum-based assessment, defining fluency as rate and accuracy in oral read-ing. The authors of the NRP report (NICHHD, 2000) differentiate automaticity from flu-ency. *Automaticity* is the fast, effortless word recognition that is a product of consistent reading practice. Fluent readers, by contrast, read aloud effortlessly and with expression. Automaticity is necessary, but not sufficient, for fluency (NICHHD, 2000).

One skill that facilitates reading fluency is the ability to detect orthographic patterns (Catts & Kamhi, 2005). Young readers learn early on to detect common morphological endings such as *-ed, -ing,* and *-s*. Provided a child has a strong foundation in oral language, he will already have encountered words that possess these morphological endings and will know their meanings. Armed with this knowledge, the young reader will read the words quickly and accurately. Common orthographic patterns also come into play with word families or word neighborhoods. For example, *bake, cake, take,* and *lake* all belong to the same word family because they share the common stem of *-ake*. A child will likely have encountered these words in oral language through word games such as rhyming as well as in emergent literacy activities such as shared book reading. Fluent reading is facilitated through the recognition of these words because the reader does not have to devote cognitive resources to sounding out each word.

In a very broad sense, *vocabulary* can be defined as the words we must know to communi-cate effectively (NICHHD, 2000). It exists in both the oral and written mode. In the oral mode, vocabulary refers to the words we use when speaking or the words we hear when someone else is speaking. In the written mode, vocabulary refers to the words we recognize or use in print (NICHHD, 2000). According to Biemiller (2006), children require both fluent word recognition skills and at least an average vocabulary to achieve adequate reading comprehension. Children learn vocabulary words directly when an adult tells them the meaning of a word or when they look up the meaning of a word in the dictionary. Most vocabulary learning takes place indirectly. Children learn word meanings indirectly through their exposure to adult conversations, through listening to adults read to them, and by reading on their own (NICHHD, 2000).

Proficiency with phonemic awareness, phonics, vocabulary, and reading fluency—four of the five components of effective literacy instruction—is necessary for the final component of *text comprehension*. Reading comprehension develops from a facility with all aspects of spo-ken language: vocabulary or word knowledge (semantics); sound-level knowledge (phonol-ogy); sentence structure (syntax) including root words, endings, and prefixes; and contextual use of language (pragmatics). Adams (2001) relates the process of text comprehension to a continuum. Mental tasks, on one end of the continuum, require a person to invest a maximum amount of mental energy. Mental tasks, on the opposite end of the continuum, require a mini-mum amount of mental energy and are considered automatic. The task for early readers is to develop the foundational literacy skills that allow them to invest a minimal amount of energy on phonemic awareness so they can instead concentrate on text comprehension, a process that requires purposeful and active engagement (NICHHD, 2001).

Reading comprehension—the ultimate goal of reading—is a skill that is highly correlated with listening comprehension in skilled readers (de Jong & van der Leij, 2002). Beginning readers in the early literacy period usually have better listening comprehension skills than reading comprehension skills (Ashby & Rayner, 2006). A strong foundation in phonics and facility with phonemic awareness support automaticity in reading, which in turn helps skilled readers comprehend at a level that is commensurate with their listening comprehension (Ashby & Rayner, 2006). Successful text comprehension depends on more than accurate and automatic word recognition, however. Text comprehension will suffer if the reader encounters words that are not in his oral vocabulary, if the sentence structure is overly complex, or if the topic is so unfamiliar that the reader cannot make the inferences necessary to understanding the material (Snow, Scarborough, & Burns, 1999).

Snow, Scarborough, and Burns (1999) have identified developmental markers of normal written language development for the early preschool period to the early elementary school years. These developmental milestones are useful when considering whether or not a child is at risk for literacy failure.

Three-Year-Olds

- Primary goal: Discover and appreciate the functions and values of written language in environment
- Interested in signs and labels and their visual image
- Recognize books by cover, orient book, and turn pages
- Understand print is a means of communication (notes, memos, lists)

Four-Year-Olds

- Primary goal: Learn more details about print and words (foundation for understanding alphabetic principle)
- Attend to internal structure of words
- Develop phonological awareness skills
  - Perceive, identify, and separate phonemes (sounds)
  - Differentiate and identify letters accurately
- Engage in inventive writing
  - Practice spelling names
  - Mix letters with scribbling

Four-Year-Olds (continued)

- Vocabulary is expanding
  - Reflects amount of language to which child is exposed
  - Access to greater quantities of talk facilitates more rapid vocabulary development

Five-Year-Olds (Kindergarteners)

- Primary goal: Figure out the alphabetic system
  - Example: If shown *hat* and told what it says, may be able to figure out how to exchange letters to spell *bat* and *sat*
- May be able to read regularly spelled words by knowing first and last phonemes
- May be able to recognize very common, familiar sight words
- Able to understand long stories that are read to them
  - Can ask questions about stories read to them

First Graders

- Primary goal: Expected to remember and apply reliable information about sound–letter correspondences to read words
- Should be able to read regular words accurately and automatically
- Should be able to discuss texts they have read or that have been read to them
  - Requires comprehension of new vocabulary terms
  - Requires familiarity and comfort with academic discourse style
- Writing development
  - Both invented and correct spelling
    - Example: "vakashun" but also "the," "said"
  - Writing for different reasons
    - Stories, journals, personal thoughts, lists about topics
  - Punctuation use is inconsistent
  - Story grammar emerges
    - Example: "Once upon a time . . ."

Second Graders

- Primary goals:
  - Become fluent and automatic readers (fluency and automaticity in reading text)
  - Reading without being aware one is decoding text
- Develop comprehension strategies

Second Graders (continued)

- Develop word inferences strategies
- Use writing to deepen understanding of literature
  - Book reports, research reports (short reports)
  - Conventional spelling more consistent

Third Graders and Beyond

- Primary goals:
  - Silent independent reading
  - Reading comprehension across subject areas
- Continued refinement of language skills
  - More sophisticated knowledge of syntax, morphology, semantics
  - Facilitates reading comprehension
- Continued development of reading comprehension strategies

It is necessary to have a thorough understanding of emergent and early literacy development before considering factors that put a child at risk for literacy failure. Through longitudinal studies, researchers have identified characteristics of early spoken language development that put a young child at risk for later reading difficulty. Next, these research findings are tied into the case studies presented in this text.

EARLY IDENTIFICATION OF LATER READING DISABILITIES _____

Understanding the components of both emergent and early literacy is essential to preventing reading failure in young children. The earlier in a child's education that emergent literacy weakness is identified, the more likely that intervention will be successful (Foorman, Breier, & Fletcher, 2003; Snowling & Hayiou-Thomas, 2006). Both Torgesen (1998) and Stanovich (1986) describe the downward spiral that traps young children who get off to a poor start in reading. Weak phonological skills make it difficult for such children to identify new, unknown words, and their efforts to decode new words often yield many errors. Fluent reading, which depends on automatic word recognition, then suffers, with difficulties in this area often discouraging a child from engaging in reading. Limited exposure to vocabulary words affects vocabulary growth and negatively affects reading comprehension. As Torgesen (1998) warns, children who get off to a poor start in reading rarely catch up to their more able peers.

A number of research studies have followed the reading outcomes of preschool children with speech and/or language impairments through school age (Catts, Fey, Tomblin, & Zhang, 2002; Nathan, Stackhouse, Goulandris, & Snowling, 2004; Scarborough, 1990; Scarborough

& Dobrich, 1990). Findings from these studies reveal that such children are either at risk for later reading disability or do, in fact, become disabled readers.

Nathan and colleagues (2004) reported on the early literacy development of preschool children with specific speech difficulties or speech and language difficulties; these children were first examined as preschoolers and followed through kindergarten and first grade. The children were evaluated for receptive language (picture vocabulary, understanding syntactic structure), expressive language (grammar, mean length of utterance [MLU]), output phonology (accuracy of speech production and word repetition), input phonology (auditory discrimination), phonological awareness (rhyme and phoneme manipulation tasks), and literacy skills (letter-name knowledge, word reading, spelling). As compared to a normally developing control group, subjects in both the specific speech difficulty group and the speech and language difficulty group were at high risk for literacy delay (Nathan, Stackhouse, Goulandris, & Snowling, 2004). The subjects with both speech and language delays were most impaired in literacy skills and had difficulty with phonological awareness, spelling, and reading at grade two. Nathan and colleagues (2004) also found that those children with the most severe speech difficulties had the poorest literacy outcomes.

Scarborough has also documented early language deficits in children who go on to be identified with specific reading impairment or developmental dyslexia. In an early study, Scarborough (1990) looked at the oral language proficiency of preschool children at 30 months who later were identified as reading disabled. Scarborough's 52 subjects consisted of 3 groups of 30-month-old children: 20 children from families with a history of dyslexia who later become disabled readers; 12 children from families with a history of dyslexia who went on to become normal readers; and 20 non-impaired (control) children. In this study, language skills were analyzed both formally and naturally. Formal tests were administered to assess vocabulary recognition, naming vocabulary, and speech discrimination. Language samples from mother–child play sessions were analyzed for productive syntax and lexical diversity. At age 60 months, subjects were again evaluated for naming vocabulary and reading achievement (letter identification, letter–sound correspondence, and phonological awareness). Scarborough found that the preschool children at age 30 months who later developed reading disabilities were delayed in the length, syntactic complexity, and pronunciation accuracy of their spoken language. At five years of age, these children were weak in object-naming, phonemic awareness, and letter–sound knowledge.

Catts, Fey, Tomblin, and Zhang (2002) also investigated the reading outcomes in second- and fourth-grade children with language impairments that had been identified while they were in kindergarten. Their sample consisted of children identified with specific language impairment (SLI—that is, language impairment with normal nonverbal IQ) and nonspecific language impairment (NLI—that is, language impairment and nonverbal IQ at least one standard deviation below the mean). These researchers' test battery included tasks that measured language, phonological processing, reading, and nonverbal cognitive ability. Catts, Fey, Tomblin, and Zhang (2002) found that the language-impaired children scored significantly lower than the non-impaired children (i.e., the control group) on tests of word recognition and reading comprehension in second and fourth grades and that the children with NLI scored significantly lower than the SLI subgroup on each measure of reading achievement. Using a stepwise multiple regression analysis, the researchers determined that the best kindergarten predictor of reading outcomes was letter identification; however, the grammar composite, nonverbal IQ, rapid naming, and phonological awareness also contributed unique variance in reading achievement at the second and fourth grades.

These research studies provide a context within which to discuss the three children profiled in the case studies.

CASE STUDIES

JOHNATHON (TD)

Johnathon appears to be a typically developing toddler. His speech-language evaluation revealed age-appropriate expressive and receptive language skills. Although Johnathon does not appear to have any risk factors associated with later literacy failure, it is still important for him to be engaged in early literacy experiences and be provided with appropriate instruction when he begins school. Given such experiences, and in combination with his typically developing language skills, there is no reason to expect that he will develop later difficulties with reading.

JOSEPHINE (LB)

Josephine's profile suggests concern for later literacy difficulty. The results of her speech-language evaluation revealed a mild to moderate delay in expressive language and a moderate delay in speech-sound development. Josephine is younger than the children in the research studies cited earlier; however, she does possess speech and language delays that could put her at future risk for literacy failure. In the study carried out by Nathan, Stackhouse, Goulandris, and Snowling (2004), the children had deficits as preschoolers in either speech or speech and language. The children with both speech and language delays were at greatest risk of deficits in phoneme awareness at six years. If Josephine continues on this path and does not improve and expand her vocabulary knowledge, she may find book reading an unappealing, difficult activity and could enter into in the downward spiral discussed by Torgesen (1998). If she begins school with a speech-language delay, she may be at risk for future academic struggles.

Josephine's background history of early intervention bodes well for her future success. Her continued participation in speech-language therapy that includes early literacy activities such as word games (rhymes, sound–letter matching), shared book-reading, alphabetic activities, and pretend writing will be imperative.

ROBERT (LT)

Of the three children described in the case studies, Robert is at greatest risk for later literacy difficulty. He exhibits delays in expressive language, speech-sound production, and receptive language. In the research studies cited earlier, the children with the most severe delays as preschoolers went on to experience the most severe delays in literacy skills. Given Robert's delays in receptive language as well as play and gesture, his nonverbal language skills may be suspect. The reading outcomes in the Catts and colleagues (2002) study were poorest for those children who had both nonverbal and language deficits. Scarborough's (1990) report of 30-month-old toddlers who later developed reading disabilities revealed that syntactic deficits most closely corresponded with eventual literacy outcomes; phonological production was also substantially impaired in the children who were later identified as poor readers.

To help Robert, it will be especially important to engage him in early intervention that includes a focus on emergent literacy activities. Robert's caretakers should make sure his home is filled with literacy artifacts and engage him in literacy events using these artifacts. It will be important for Robert to develop a solid understanding of the alphabet and sound–letter correspondences in preparation for his entrance into kindergarten. These activities should be included along with his other prescribed goals for speech and language development.

SUMMARY

Children face a formidable task in learning to read. Even so, most children learn how to read successfully without any conscious effort. Armed with a strong foundation in emergent and early literacy skills, children should be able to successfully navigate the academic curriculum and transition from learning to read to reading to learn.

KEY TERMS

Comprehension

Decoding

Fluency

Grapheme

Literacy

Literacy artifacts

Literacy socialization

Orthography

Phonemic awareness

Phonological awareness

Self-teaching hypothesis

Stage theories

Vocabulary

STUDY QUESTIONS

+ Which important events occur during the emergent literacy period that foster literacy development in young children?
+ What are the five key components of effective literacy instruction according to the National Reading Panel?
+ Which factors put a child at risk for later literacy failure?
+ How does language development interact with and facilitate literacy development?

REFERENCES

Adams, M. J. (1994). *Beginning to read: Thinking and learning about print.* Cambridge, MA: MIT Press.

Adams, M. (2001). Alphabetic anxiety and explicit, systematic phonics instruction: A cognitive science perspective. In S. B. Neuman & D. K. Dickinson (Eds.), *Handbook of early literacy research* (Vol. 1, pp. 66–80). New York: Guildford Press.

Ashby, J., & Rayner, K. (2006). Literacy development: Insights from research on skilled reading. In D. K. Dickinson & S. B. Neuman (Eds.), *Handbook of early literacy research* (Vol. 2, pp. 52–63). New York: Guilford Press.

Biemiller, A. (2006). Vocabulary development and instruction: A prerequisite for school learning. In S. B. Neuman & D. K. Dickinson (Eds.), *Handbook of early literacy research* (Vol. 2, pp. 41–51). New York: Guildford Press.

Catts, H. W., Fey, M. E., Tomblin, J. B., & Zhang, X. (2002). A longitudinal investigation of reading outcomes in children with language impairments. *Journal of Speech, Language, and Hearing Research, 45,* 1142–1157.

Catts, H. W., & Kamhi, A. G. (2005). *Language and reading disabilities.* 2nd ed. Boston: Allyn & Bacon.

Chall, J. S. (1983). *Stages of reading development.* New York: McGraw-Hill.

Chall, J. S. (1996). *Stages of reading development.* (2nd ed.) Fort Worth, TX: Harcourt Brace.

Commission on Reading. (1985). *Becoming a nation of readers: The report of the Commissions on Reading.* Washington, DC: National Institute of Education.

de Jong, P. F., & van der Leij, A. (2002). Effects of phonological abilities and linguistic comprehension on the development of reading. *Scientific Studies of Reading, 6,* 51–77.

Ehri, L. C., & Roberts, T. (2006). The roots of learning to read and write: Acquisition of letters and phonemic awareness. In D. K. Dickinson & S. B. Neuman (Eds.), *Handbook of early literacy research* (Vol. 2, pp. 113–131). New York: Guilford Press.

Foorman, B. R., Breier, J. I., & Fletcher, J. M. (2003). Interventions aimed at improving reading success: An evidence-based approach. *Developmental Neuropsychology, 24,* 613–639.

Juel, C. (2006). The impact of early school experiences on initial reading. In D. K. Dickinson & S. B. Neuman (Eds.), *Handbook of early literacy research* (Vol. 2, pp. 410–426). New York: Guildford Press.

Mason, J. M. (1992). Reading stories to preliterate children: A proposed connection to reading. In P. B. Gough, L. C. Ehri, & R. Treiman (Eds.), *Reading acquisition* (pp. 215–243). Mahwah, NJ: Lawrence Erlbaum.

Meyer, M. S., & Felton, R. H. (1999). Repeated reading to enhance fluency: Old approaches and new directions. *Annals of Dyslexia, 49,* 283–306.

Nathan, L., Stackhouse, J., Goulandris, N., & Snowling, M. J. (2004). The development of early literacy skills among children with speech difficulties: A test of the "critical age hypothesis." *Journal of Speech, Language, and Hearing Research, 47,* 377–391.

National Institute of Child Health and Human Development (NICHHD). (2000). *Report of the National Reading Panel: Teaching children to read: An evidence-based assessment of the scientific research literature on reading and its implications for reading instruction: Reports of the subgroups* (NIH Publication No. 00-4754). Washington, DC: U.S. Government Printing Office.

Phillips, B. M., & Torgesen, J. K. (2006). Phonemic awareness and reading: Beyond the growth of initial reading accuracy. In D. K. Dickinson & S. B. Neuman (Eds.), *Handbook of early literacy research* (Vol. 2, pp. 101–112). New York: Guilford Press.

Pullen, P. C., & Justice, L. M. (2003). Enhancing phonological awareness, print awareness, and oral language skills in preschool children. *Intervention in School and Clinic, 39,* 87–98.

Scarborough, H. S. (1990). Very early language deficits in dyslexic children. *Child Development, 61,* 1728–1734.

Scarborough, H. S., & Dobrich, W. (1990). Development of children with early language delays. *Journal of Speech and Hearing Research, 33,* 70–83.

Share, D. L. (1995). Phonological recoding and self-teaching: sine qua non of reading acquisition. *Cognition, 55,* 151–218.

Share, D. L., & Stanovich, K.E. (1995). Cognitive processes in early reading development: Accommodating individual differences in to a model of acquisition. *Issues in Education: Contributions from Educational Psychology, 1,* 1–57.

Snow, C. E., Scarborough, H. S., & Burns, M. S. (1999). What speech-language pathologists need to know about early reading. *Topics in Language Disorders, 20,* 48–58.

Snowling, M. J., & Hayiou-Thomas, M. E. (2006). The dyslexia spectrum: Continuities between reading, speech, and language impairments. *Topics in Language Disorders, 26,* 110–126.

Stanovich, K. E. (1986). Matthew effects in reading: Some consequences of individual differences in the acquisition of literacy. *Reading Research Quarterly, 21,* 360–406.

Teale, W. H., & Sulzby, E. (1986). Emergent literacy as a perspective for examining how children become writers and readers. In W. H. Teale & E. Sulzby (Eds.), *Emergent literacy: Writing and reading* (p. 18). Norwood, NJ: Ablex.

Torgesen, J. K. (1998). Catch them before they fall. *American Educator/American Federation of Teachers,* Spring/Summer, 1–8.

Torgesen, J. K. (2004). Leaving no child behind: What every teacher should know. Retrieved March 21, 2008, from http://www.fcrr.org/science/pdf/torgesen/Aiken_S_C_keynote.pdf

United Nations Educational, Scientific, and Cultural Organization (UNESCO). (2004). The plurality of literacy and its implications for policies and programs. Retrieved September 9, 2007, from http://unesdoc.unesco.org/images/0013/001362/136246e.pdf

van Kleeck, A., & Schuele, C. (1987). Precursors to literacy: Normal development. *Topics in Language Disorders, 7,* 13–31.

Whitehurst, G. J., & Lonigan, C. J. (1998). Child development and emergent literacy. *Child Development, 69,* 848–872.

Whitehurst, G. J., & Lonigan, C. J. (2001). Emergent literacy: Development from prereaders to readers. In S. B. Neuman & D. K. Dickinson (Eds.), *Handbook of early literacy research* (Vol. 1, pp. 11–29). New York: Guildford Press.

CHAPTER 13

Multicultural Perspectives: The Road to Cultural Competence

Luis F. Riquelme, MS, and Jason Rosas, MS

OBJECTIVES

- Define culture and describe its effects on communication and its assessment/treatment.
- Outline best practices for nonbiased assessment of children with suspected communication disorders.
- Outline procedures for the use of interpreters in the clinical practice of a speech-language pathologist.

INTRODUCTION

This chapter introduces the speech-language pathologist (SLP) to the provision of culturally competent clinical services to all children being evaluated or treated for possible communication disorders. The information presented here is also relevant to the researcher in the area of language development and/or disorders.

As population demographics change in the United States, a larger population of ethnoculturally diverse, communicatively impaired persons obligates speech-language pathologists and audiologists to view service delivery with a fresh perspective (Payne, 1997). To provide the highest quality of services and prevent misdiagnosis and/or mistreatment, every clinician must strive to become increasingly competent in providing services in a nonbiased, nonjudgmental, and ethical manner. Today's clinical practice requires awareness of each person's customs, beliefs, and ethnicity. Moreover, cultural sensitivity is a requirement in the practice of speech-language pathology, as per the field's reliance on interpersonal communication. This chapter addresses issues of cultural and linguistic diversity, including those related to bilingualism.

It is important for all SLPs—whether monolingual or bilingual—to develop an understanding of the cultural and linguistic differences that may exist or emerge within the social communities they serve. Clinicians can provide high-quality services to all clients and their families by valuing and integrating a broad understanding of cultural practices, attitudes, and beliefs into the service delivery process. As the American Speech-Language-Hearing Association's (ASHA, 2004) document on providing culturally and linguistically appropriate services states:

> [B]eliefs and values unique to that individual clinician–client encounter must be understood, protected, and respected. Care must be taken not to make assumptions about individuals based upon their particular culture, ethnicity, language, or life experiences that could lead to misdiagnosis or improper treatment of the client/patient. Providers must enter into the relationship with awareness, knowledge, and skills about their own culture and cultural biases. To best address the unique, individual characteristics and cultural background of clients and their families, providers should be prepared to be open and flexible in the selection, administration, and interpretation of diagnostic and/or treatment regimens. When cultural or linguistic differences may negatively influence outcomes, referral to, or collaboration with, others with the needed knowledge, skill, and/or experience is indicated.

Differences in culture and ethno-biological factors are often overlooked when providing services to persons with communication and/or swallowing disorders. Ethnocentrism on the part of the service provider may be displayed during the assessment and/or treatment process. It is not uncommon for the service provider to focus solely on the language barrier issue and to forget all other cultural factors involved in the communication process. To provide the best services possible, the SLP, or any of the members of the caregiving team, must take into account the person as a whole. This includes understanding the influence of assimilation and acculturation on the assessment and treatment process (Riquelme, 2007). *Assimilation* is the process in which someone in a new environment totally embraces the host culture (C2) (e.g., values, beliefs, behaviors). *Acculturation*, in contrast to assimilation, is viewed as positive for new immigrants. It allows individuals to identify with the primary community (C1) in which they have been socialized as well as with the broader majority community or host culture (C2) (Cabassa, 2003; Kohnert, 2008, p. 31).

The United States, as a country inhabited largely by immigrants, has a long history of struggles with assimilation and acculturation. These processes were mostly assimilatory until the middle of the twentieth century. Subsequent to that point, many immigrant groups began to acculturate—that is, balance their native cultures and beliefs with that of the host culture, or "mainstream America."

All service providers experience and practice the processes of assimilation and acculturation within the environments in which they exist (e.g., work, social, educational) (Dikeman & Riquelme, 2002). Think about your own first few weeks in a new job or a new academic setting: It was important to learn the "rules of the game" that were already established, or the "culture" of the new setting.

Increased awareness about acculturation is needed in part to reduce the potential for stereotyping. Clinicians cannot assume that all persons from a particular group or culture are similar in every aspect of everyday life. For example, not all Asians eat raw fish, not all Hispanics see a "curandero" (healer) before seeking help from a physician, and not all gay people like disco music. It is extremely important for the clinician to obtain information about the person with whom he is working, as the client may not be able to provide all the details secondary to her communication impairment. Creating an open communicative environment with the client may allow for this type of exchange (Riquelme, 2006b).

TERMINOLOGY

Clinicians should become well versed in the sociopolitical vernacular denoting various social groups. To begin, the terms *minority* and *majority* should be discussed. In efforts to categorize the general population, the U.S. Bureau of the Census (2000) defines all nonwhite persons as *minorities*. Payne (1997) has commented that lumping individuals together under the label of "minority" suggests inferiority, whereas the designation of "majority" connotes superiority. She argues that neither term is accurate, because neither term accounts for the continuum of cultural experiences within the two categories, and neither term has saliency for the future. Payne also suggests that this classification system reinforces bias and stereotyping, further widening the cultural distance in cross-cultural communication.

Many individuals now use the term *racial/ethnic minority*, in keeping with the U.S. Census designations of minority groups: Hispanic Americans, African Americans, Native American Indians, Asian/Pacific Islanders, and Others. Of course, not all groups designated as such in this system are homo-racial—that is, of a single race/ethnicity. Hispanics, for example, may be of single or mixed race. In fact, many Hispanics self-identify as white, black, or mixed race. For this reason, the U.S. Census Bureau added a question on ethnicity to the 2000 census, so that persons such as Hispanics could self-identify based on country of origin (e.g., Mexico, Puerto Rico, Cuba, Colombia). Despite nonwhite groups being the majority in many towns and cities across the United States, the term "minority" is still applied across the board to these groups.

Other common misconceptions are that all *culturally and linguistically diverse* groups are nonwhite or that *ethnic diversity* refers only to nonwhite persons. This is also true for the use of the terms *multicultural* and *diversity*. Following this logic, how would Russian immigrants be classified? These persons speak a non-English language, come to the United States from a different culture, and are considered racially Caucasian. Are Russians thought of as a culturally and linguistically diverse group? Are they ethnically diverse?

Another example of diversity arises when the patient or the clinician is gay/lesbian/bisexual/transgender (GLBT). While some people believe these are chosen lifestyles, many others disagree. Some believe that there is a "culture" associated with persons who are GLBT. Nevertheless, the clinician is expected to be sensitive to these aspects of culture/diversity and not make assumptions based on cultural misconceptions or heterosexism (Riquelme, 2006b). For example, why should the clinician assume that the child to be evaluated comes from a home with a mother and a father? The child may actually come from a home where both parents are of the same gender, or from a single-parent home.

These examples highlight the fact that cultural and linguistic diversity applies to all clinicians and their patients, regardless of ethnic background, lifestyle, religious beliefs, and other characteristics. The key point is that all individuals have at least one culture and one language, with most having more than one. To broaden perspectives on culture, clinicians need to define it at a personal level.

CULTURE

Before discussing culture and its relationship to assessment and intervention, we should develop a clear definition of *culture* and related terms. The definitions for "culture" vary as dramatically as the sciences that examine culture; the impact of culture on phenomena in the fields of psychology, anthropology, and sociology, among others, is widely documented. Carbaugh (1988) referred to *ethnic culture* as a system of interrelated behavior and belief patterns, "that are a) deeply felt, b) commonly intelligible, and c) widely accessible" and are used to create and share individual identity (p. 38). Clinicians must accept and fully incorporate the notion that everyone has a culture if they are to be able to provide culturally appropriate services. Furthermore, culture goes beyond race and ethnicity. It is up to the practitioner to define culture more broadly and include not only ethnicity, but also religious beliefs, lifestyles, special interests, and other factors (Riquelme, 2004).

For our purposes, *culture* is defined as the behaviors, artifacts, and beliefs adopted by a person or group used to define their social identity. Culture comprises both *explicit* behaviors and artifacts and *implicit* beliefs (see **Table 13-1**). In other words, some behaviors are evident, external, and perceivable (explicit), whereas other behaviors are abstract and internal, and must be inferred (implicit) (Chamberlain & Medinos-Landurand, 1991).

Culture gives shape to ethnicity and cultural heritage. *Ethnicity* is an ever-changing cultural construct that forms the basis for a sense of social cohesion. Those cultural variables that are shared and accepted help an ethnic group to define itself. In other words, our ethnicity is determined by the cultural beliefs and practices we share with others. Deciding which traits are "common" to an ethnic group becomes very difficult because cultural behaviors shift according

TABLE 13-1   Explicit and Implicit Cultural Variables

Explicit Variables: Behaviors and Artifacts	Implicit Variables: Beliefs Inferred from Behaviors and Artifacts
Language	Language-Ego Permeability: degree to which language mixing or code switching is allowed/accepted
Religious practices	
Eating/feeding preferences	Child-rearing expectancies
Manner of celebration	Role of parent/child/teacher in education
Music/dance	Role of parent/professional in health profession
Homework, newspapers, paintings, crafts	Role of males versus females
	Monotheistic versus polytheistic beliefs

Source: Adapted from Chamberlain & Medinos-Landurand (1991).

to historical contexts. For example, an ethnic Neuyorican (New York–Puerto Rican) in the 1970s may have defined himself very differently from a Neuyorican in the twenty-first century due to changes in the social, economic, and political climate. Thus the term *culture* is used here to refer to the general, collective group of persons sharing a set of cultural variables, rather than referring to any specific ethnic group whose cultural traits are difficult to define.

Cultural variables that are most valued and are passed on from generation to generation constitute an ethnicity's *heritage*. For example, a family heirloom that is passed down from mother to daughter over generations could represent a cultural artifact that has heritage value. Similarly, the language a family speaks may have sufficient significance as to be characterized as having heritage value. Because heritage is so intricately related with ethnicity, changes in the ethnic culture may influence which items or behaviors retain value and significance. For example, one generation of people may strongly value language and deem it a necessary cultural variable to pass down to their children. In contrast, in the next generation, the value of that language may diminish to the point where it no longer has significance in helping to define the ethnic group. Consequently, from one generation to the next, a once-prominent heritage variable such as language may be lost or replaced in value.

Race, a far more controversial construct and term, is widely used in sociopolitical circles when discussing individuals and social groups. Race, as a construct that classifies humanity by arbitrary biological or anatomical features and/or nebulous geographical boundaries, is often misinterpreted and forms the basis for social blights, such as racism and discrimination. Making decisions about a group or person based on appearance or place of origin leads to subjective interpretations of families or clients. This approach leaves little room for the development of interpersonal relationships based on cooperation, communication, and shared understanding—all of which are critical to successful clinical outcomes.

To better appreciate the key role played by the client and the family in the clinical process, SLPs should evaluate their own definitions of culture, ethnicity, heritage, and race. Put simply, the clinician who examines his own beliefs and behaviors will be better equipped to understand and interpret others' beliefs and behaviors. Roseberry-McKibbin (1995, 2002) has listed several cultural variables that may affect larger social groups and that may have unique effects on the individual lives of a family or client (see **Table 13-2**). Specifically, cultural factors that affect the collection of data from family members and the child's performance in assessment and treatment should be considered. Several of these cultural factors will be discussed in this chapter. A more thorough review of the literature discussing these variables should also be undertaken to better understand the complexity and depth of their effects on assessment and intervention.

CULTURAL COMPETENCE

Cultural competence is not a skill that is acquired or learned, but rather one that is developed over time. The need for all SLPs to become culturally competent—and not just those from ethnic minority backgrounds or those who are bilingual—is increasingly apparent. All across the United States, demographics show that more persons are from non-mainstream cultures and from homes where English may not be the first language.

In 2004, the American Speech-Language-Hearing Association (ASHA) approved a practice document entitled "Knowledge and Skills Needed by Speech-Language Pathologists and Audiologists to Provide Culturally and Linguistically Appropriate Services," authored by members of its Multicultural Issues Board. This document outlines the knowledge and skills

TABLE 13-2 Cultural Variables Affecting Language Development	
Educational level	Socioeconomic status/upward class mobility
Languages spoken	Religious beliefs/impact on activities of daily living (ADL)
Length of residence in an area	
Country of birth	Neighborhood of residence/peer group
Urban versus rural background	Degree of acculturation
Individual choice within the intrapersonal realm	Generational membership
	Age and gender

Source: Adapted from Roseberry-McKibbin (1995).

that clinicians must strive to develop so as to provide unbiased and culturally appropriate services. It also acknowledges the need for lifelong learning. The ASHA document lists a variety of competencies needed to achieve cultural competence, such as sensitivity to differences, understanding the influence of culture on service delivery, and the need to advocate for and empower consumers, families, and communities at risk for communication, swallowing, or balance disorders. Among the key cultural factors to understand when working with limited-English-speaking patients are increased respect for individual differences within and between groups (e.g., family structure and roles, approach to disability and rehabilitation); separation of the effects of culture from the effects of socioeconomic status; understanding the patient's sociocultural belief system; greater caution in interpreting and generalizing findings; greater caution in the use of formal tests; and awareness of differences in interpersonal relating (ASHA, 2004).

Learning to work effectively with individuals who are culturally or linguistically different from both the personal and professional experiences of the clinician presents formidable challenges, as well as considerable opportunities for personal growth and professional excellence (Kohnert, 2008, p. 35). In her most recent book, Kohnert (2008) describes four essential characteristics of the culturally competent speech-language pathologist:

+ To simultaneously appreciate cultural patterns and individual variation
+ To engage in cultural self-scrutiny
+ To embrace principles of evidence-based practice
+ To seek to understand language disorders within the client's social context

She further states that a deep understanding that there are many different ways of seeing and being in the world is essential for cultural competence.

In discussing speech-language assessment issues within the multicultural context, differentiation must be made between *cultural diversity*, as discussed earlier, and *language diversity*. Embracing the concept that all persons have a culture, including the client and the clinician, requires using nonbiased assessment and treatment practices for all clients receiving speech-language services. In other words, every child—whether mainstream or not—must be treated in a culturally sensitive manner. In the case of language diversity, other clinical factors must be added to the picture. In this scenario, the clinician needs to be familiar with issues regarding second language acquisition and bilingualism. As demographics have changed in the United States, SLPs have begun to see more children who use English as the preferred language for communication, but who are from bilingual homes, and are often bilingual themselves. This presents many challenges to the clinician without experience in bilingualism, as testing such a child as a monolingual speaker of English would be inappropriate and may well result in the child being misdiagnosed with a communication disorder.

BILINGUALISM: PERSPECTIVES IN THE UNITED STATES

A review of the U.S. Census figures from 2000 indicates that approximately 47 million persons in the United States speak a language other than or in addition to English (approximately 18% of the total U.S. population). Of these 47 million people, almost half report speaking English "less than very well." Almost 60% of this group (approximately 28 million) report Spanish as the language they use other than or in addition to English. These figures, of course, include many children who are English language learners (ELLs), previously known as limited-English proficient (LEP) or non-English proficient (NEP). As of 2001, there were an estimated 4.6 million ELLs in U.S. schools, representing a 105% increase from 1990 (Kindler, 2001). Of those children identified as ELLs, 79% (3.6 million) spoke Spanish.

It is also important to briefly discuss how bilingualism is viewed in this country. While bilingualism and multilingualism are viewed as assets in most countries around the world, that is not the case in the United States. According to Ruiz (1988, in Goldstein, 2004), the United States has had three main orientations to language planning:

+ **Language as Problem.** In the 1950s, bilingualism was seen as a problem of modernization—that is, the need to deal with issues such as code selection, standardization, literacy, orthography, language stratification, and so forth. During this time, language issues were linked to the "disadvantaged," similar to other social issues such as poverty, low socioeconomic status, and lack of social mobility. Bilingualism, then, was perceived as a problem to be overcome and was viewed mostly as a deficit.
+ **Language as Right.** In the 1960s, language was recognized as a civil right. This movement was manifested as government forms, ballots, instructional pamphlets, judicial proceedings, and civil service exams being printed in languages other than English.
+ **Language as Resource.** Historically, neither language diversity nor non-English language maintenance has been encouraged in the United States. There is, however, current support on some fronts for the "language as resource" perspective, which advocates the conservation of language abilities of non-English speakers and in increase in language requirements in universities (if for no other reason than the need for linguistic diversity for business purposes). There is, however, a contradiction, because most individuals support foreign-language instruction in schools but ask non-native English speakers to lose their first language.

The rapid growth of ELLs has greatly challenged the present support system for assessing and treating ELL children with communication disorders. As reported in the *23rd Annual Report to Congress on the Implementation of IDEA*, "a significant number of LEP students also have a concomitant disability; those students are at even greater risk for negative educational outcomes" (U.S. Department of Education, 2007). This is the same information reported in the 2001 annual report (p. II-38). Significantly, no figures exist as to the exact number of ELLs who are mandated to receive special education programs and/or speech-language treatment and who have been misdiagnosed with a learning disability or a communication disorder when, in fact, these children may simply require ESL (English as a second language) services. This underscores the need for improved professional training in this area. All speech-language pathologists, psychologists, and educators would benefit from cultural and linguistic diversity training and effort toward achieving cultural competence. This may help in ensuring reduced assessment bias for this population of children, and it may eliminate the incidence of misdiagnosis.

CASE STUDY

To better illustrate these factors, we will use the example of Josefina (previously Josephine), our "late-blooming" language learner. Relevant cultural and language developmental information has been added to her "significant history" so as to illustrate points mentioned previously. This example involves a girl of Puerto Rican culture and the Spanish language. The variables and factors presented here are not intended to be generalized to all Puerto Rican families and children. Instead, the cultural variables are used as exemplars of a broader set of variables that may be adapted by any family given *their* individual definitions of self and community.

JOSEFINA: Adjusted Relevant History

Josefina is a 22-month-old Hispanic female child of Puerto Rican decent who was referred to this appointment due to continued concern of limited expressive vocabulary. Josefina's **prenatal and birth** histories were unremarkable. She was born at term, weighing 7 pounds, 2 ounces. **Medical/health** history was significant for pneumonia at 19 months and two bouts of otitis media (ear infections) since that time. She has known allergies to dust and mold. Josefina's **hearing** was recently evaluated and found to be within normal limits. **Developmental** milestones were reached in a timely manner (e.g., sat at 6 months, walked at 11 months). Josefina's **speech-language** development was remarkable for limited vocalizations during infancy, including little babbling. Her first word was delayed until 15 months, and her mother believed Josefina to have a small vocabulary for her age.

Family history was remarkable for a paternal uncle who was described as "tartamudo"—that is, a stutterer.

Josefina lives with her parents and two older siblings in a bilingual English–Spanish community in Brooklyn, New York. The family rents an apartment in a three-family home, which is also home to Josefina's godparents and paternal aunt and grandmother.

Mrs. X was originally from a rural district of Puerto Rico and moved to the United States with her husband, Mr. X, two years ago. She completed a third-grade level education and was trained as a seamstress. Mrs. X considered herself a monolingual Spanish speaker. Mrs. X suggested that her primary motivation for moving to the United States included better financial opportunities and educational advantage for her children.

Mr. X was born in Puerto Rico and moved to New York at the age of five. He completed high school in Manhattan. Mr. X considered himself a fluent bilingual English–Spanish speaker, who used English in the home when speaking to Josefina. He reported frequent trips to Puerto Rico to visit his family because his parents wished for him to develop and maintain his Spanish-language skills. Mr. X stated that he learned to read and write in Spanish while visiting his family, who encouraged his participation in Sunday Bible study. Mr. X is currently unemployed, although he is attending trade classes with the hopes of opening his own construction business.

CULTURAL VARIABLES AFFECTING THE ASSESSMENT AND INTERVENTION PROCESS

Orientation

Orientation describes the degree to which people orient themselves toward the considerations of a collective body (e.g., a family) or toward individual achievement and motivation. In some cultures, decisions are made for the greater good of the family rather than any one person's achievement. Support may be offered from a large network of relatives and friends. Also, success may be measured by the amount of prestige or honor that is brought to the family. In contrast, cultures that encourage individual performance may de-emphasize the importance of the larger social unit.

In Josefina's case, the extended family lives in the same residence as Josefina's immediate family. Exploring the parents' views and values of kinship and individual achievement may facilitate our clinical understanding of the support network available to Josefina and suggest how she may be encouraged to succeed in the clinical context.

Verbal and Nonverbal Communication

Verbal and nonverbal communication describes the beliefs governing communication between children and adults. *Verbal communication*, or discourse, rules may affect a speech-language pathologist's interactions with parents and the child. Some cultures prefer succinct discourse exchanges and place unspoken limitations on the amount of talking children are allowed with adults. Other cultures allow children to be present in, but not participate in, adult conversations (Heath, 1983). Still other cultures place a high value on the direct role of family as the child's principal model for language form, content, and use. These cultures may emphasize the parent's role as facilitator and instructor in the parent–child dynamic and may encourage a child's increased responsiveness and openness with adults, both familiar and novel.

Nonverbal communication refers to the nonlinguistic behaviors that may accompany verbal interactions. Gestures, proximity, eye contact, and touch may have substantial meaning in social interactions (Chamberlain & Medinos-Landurand, 1991).

+ *Gestures*, such as head nods, head shakes, finger shaking, or other combined body movements, may have substantial meaning independent of the verbal utterances. They may also affect the meaning of a verbal utterance. Consider the meaning transmitted when a mother says, "You are thinking of going outside now?" while shaking her head side-to-side. This could be interpreted as disapproval or a veiled comment suggesting to the child that going out is out of the question.

+ *Proximity* is the degree of "personal space" used or shared during verbal interaction. Some cultures value distance between conversational partners, whereas others may embrace physical closeness. For example, a clinician who leans her body in to hear a speaker may be perceived as rude and aggressive or, conversely, give the impression that she is engaged and sympathetic.

+ *Eye contact* (or eye gaze) is a variable that is used subjectively by clinicians to judge attentiveness and engagement. Averting direct eye contact when speaking may, in fact, be a sign of respect in some cultures. In other cultures, sustaining eye contact with adults when responding to or engaging in discourse demonstrates that the child has confidence, alertness, and honesty.

+ *Touch* may be permitted as a sign of affection or to demonstrate communicative engagement. In some cases, touch is prohibited or restricted to specific persons or for specific meaning. These behaviors may have roots in religious beliefs and practices or may be governed by individual expectations regarding adult–child or adult–adult interaction.

In Josefina's case, it may prove useful to observe the nonverbal behaviors of the family during the interview process. Prolonged eye contact with adults may not be encouraged with adults or figures of authority. Distance and reduced contact with strangers may be promoted. Verbally, the child may be taught to "speak only when spoken to." Each of these factors could affect the child's interaction with the evaluator and, if not considered appropriately, could lead to erroneous judgments regarding the child's pragmatic capabilities.

Play Interactions

The manner in which a child plays is highly influenced by culture. Play dimensions, including self–other relations, symbolic play props, and thematic contexts, are all affected by cultural expectations (Westby, 1990) Some cultures may have finely defined expectations regarding which kinds of play or activities are permissible for a boy versus a girl. Play and gender role factors can influence how a child plays, which types of games chosen, what level of prowess in play the child demonstrates, what the child plays with, and whom the child chooses or is allowed to play with (Farver, Kim, & Lee, 1995; Rubin & Coplan, 1998; Sutton-Smith, 1972).

For example, Josefina's family may feel strongly about which kinds of toys she plays with (i.e., dolls versus trucks). The parents may also engage her, to a limited degree, in adult–child play interactions. This may lead to a difference in play performance owing to lack of experience rather than underdeveloped symbolic (cognitive) play skills.

Illness and Disabilities

Another culturally influenced belief is the perception of disease, illness, and disability. *Disease* refers to the observable disruption of physical or mental processes, whereas *illness* refers to an individual's experience of that condition. (Kleinman, Eisenberg, & Good, 2006). In other words, "illness" is the term used to indicate when a change in physical or mental state is judged abnormal or deficient. This may result in a family's or client's change in social interaction and performance due to insecurities, shame, or other emotional reactions to the individual's condition. In a sociopolitical sense, nomenclature such as "disabled," "handicapped," and "impaired" also has stigmatizing effects for some groups.

Limited research has been conducted in the field of speech-language pathology with regard to cross-cultural beliefs of illness or disability (Bebout & Arthur, 1992; Maestas & Erickson, 1992; Salas-Provance, Erickson, & Reed, 2002). Remaining focused on the notion of individual differences in cultural beliefs may facilitate a clinician's understanding of the needs of the family or parent of a child with communication concerns.

For example, Josefina's parents may have their own views on communication disabilities. These views should be examined, given the existence of an uncle with history of a fluency disorder.

Language–Ego Permeability

Adults may also have beliefs about how language should be used or produced. In other words, they develop a sense of "boundaries" for what is acceptable language use and what is not. They develop a sense for when language output is being degraded or changed and may have varying levels of tolerance for nonstandard forms of the language (e.g., language borrowing, code switching). These implicit beliefs are associated with *language–ego permeability* (Guiora & Acton, 1979; Schumann, 1986). The less flexible or closed the person is to allowing change to occur in the languages spoken, the greater the likelihood that the native language will persevere and be used actively in the home. This bears great significance for sustaining a non-mainstream language (Spanish, in Josefina's case). It may also affect the decision as to in which language to intervene and how active the non-mainstream language remains after the child begins interacting with the mainstream language (for Josefina, English).

LINGUISTIC VARIABLES AFFECTING THE ASSESSMENT AND INTERVENTION PROCESS

The societal manner in which language is used plays an important role in the development of language in a bilingual child. Chamberlain and Medinos-Landurand (1991) reviewed several linguistic factors that influence the assessment process—specifically, language-use patterns, language loss, code switching, and dialectal variance.

Language-use patterns refer to the way that language is used given the context of discourse. The pragmatics of language require that we pay attention to the participants, setting, functions, and topics involved in discourse (Fantini, 1985). In other words, who are the people involved in modeling language to the child? Where do these communicative acts take place? What reasons does the child have for communicating? What is spoken about and what are children expected to talk about? These questions must be answered from the point of view of both parent and child. How does the child seem to interpret the message of how language should be used given the input received from the environment?

Language loss refers to the apparent loss (attrition) of functional vocabulary and utterances in the nondominant language due to reduced exposure. This process may occur in children who undergo a change in the amount, frequency, or perceived relevance for a given language. If Josefina's parents were to stop using Spanish for some reason after months of providing that stimulation to Josefina, that decision may lead to a decrease in productive language in the child, and ultimately a reduced ability to access the language that was learned without external, supporting input. Therefore, a history of inconsistent language input, where one language or the other is not supported, may lead to apparent delays in one or both languages. This assumption is a common diagnostic error leading to misdiagnosis of bilingual children.

Code switching is a rule-governed socially and grammatically constrained communicative behavior, wherein a person alternates between two languages within the same communicative event. This behavior may be socially stigmatized as "improper" use of either language, but may have functional and appropriate uses in a given speech community. Zentella (1997), for example, has provided a detailed account of code switching in an urban Puerto Rican community.

Understanding of the cultural and societal role of code switching and the rules that govern permissible language alternations will reduce the likelihood of misdiagnosis.

Dialectal variance pertains to the non-mainstream production of a language at the sound, word, or syntax level (Sapir, 1921). These variations (also known as social dialects) may arise because of factors such as geographical location, social status, education level, and communicative contexts (Chamberlain & Medinos-Landurand, 1991). Josefina's parents, for example, may speak several dialectal variations of Spanish. Josefina's mother may speak a dialect specific to rural Puerto Rico, just as her father may speak varieties of Puerto Rican Spanish and urban New York English. Similarly, both parents may speak with differing accents. These language differences may be echoed in the Josefina's productions. So long as her productions match the adult model available to her, these language differences are not considered error patterns requiring therapeutic intervention.

An important final consideration: If the child demonstrates adequate language production in one of her languages, the child is not considered language impaired. Such a child may have mastered the linguistic elements of a language and, therefore, may communicate effectively in that language. In other words, a child who is born to bilingual parents, yet who grows up monolingual, is not considered a candidate for treatment. So long as the child's development in that language meets the standards of the linguistic community at some level, the child is judged communicatively within normal limits. However, if there is suspicion that the child is not meeting the communicative demands of her environment in one or either language, it becomes doubly essential that both languages be evaluated thoroughly.

LANGUAGE DEVELOPMENT: BILINGUAL PERSPECTIVES

How does one define the *type* of language learner that the child is becoming, and subsequently how does one define the child's level of *proficiency*? Researchers have attempted to classify dual-language learners into those who have been exposed to two languages—say English and Spanish—from an early age (birth), and those who have become exposed to a second language later in their development (sometime after birth). This distinction has led to the classifications known as *simultaneous-bilingual* and *sequential-bilingual*. The simultaneous-bilingual child has been exposed to two languages from an early age. The sequential-bilingual child is characterized by his exposure to a second language after developing a level of fluency in first language skills. Two additional subcategories within this type—classification as early versus late sequential bilingual—may also be used.

The age range suggested as a reasonable demarcation between simultaneous- and sequential-bilingual children has been the subject of some debate (Bhatia & Ritchie, 1999; de Houwer, 1995; McLaughlin, 1984). The age range for sequential-bilingual learners has been proposed as, at the earliest, one month old to approximately three years of age. Most experts agree that simultaneous-bilingualism requires a balanced input in each language from an early age. In reality, maintaining equal balance of both languages over the lifespan of the child is extremely difficult, if not unlikely (Fishman, 1966). In either case, it appears far more reasonable to define how the child has developed her bilingualism by measuring quantity and quality of input rather than using a criterion based strictly on age. Josefina's background suggests primary exposure to Spanish from her parents, but English-language input may come through television and the neighborhood community. More detailed information would be useful regarding the communicative contexts in which Josefina is engaged.

When addressing the critical period for second language (L2) acquisition, consensus has been reached on three points:

- Adults proceed more quickly through the very early stages of phonological, syntactical, and morphological development.
- When time and exposure are controlled, older children move through the stages of syntactical and morphological development in L2 faster than do younger children.
- Individuals who begin to acquire their L2 as young children usually achieve higher levels of oral proficiency in L2 phonology and syntax than do individuals who begin to develop the L2 as adults. The prepubescent and postpubescent periods have been identified as major markers in this area.

An early theory proposed by Volterra and Taeschner (1978), the *unitary language system view*, suggested that children exposed to two languages simultaneously processed those languages through the same system, only to have the languages be separated over time before the age of three. This view was widely accepted until the *dual- (differentiated-) language system hypothesis* was proposed (Genesee, 1989; Pyke, 1986). According to this hypothesis, which is also referred to as *a fractionated system* view (Kohnert & Bates, 2002; Kohnert, Bates, & Hernández, 1999), a child processes each language through distinct language systems, thereby developing differentiated mental representations of the two languages from the onset of exposure. Modern research appears to support the dual-language system hypothesis given findings across linguistic domains. These studies support the notion that nascent dual-language learners process languages separately (Johnson & Lancaster, 1998; Nicoladis & Secco, 2000; Paradis, Nicoladis, & Genesee, 2000; Pearson, Fernández, & Oller, 1995; Quay, 1995).

It is important to note that the assessment of the child may be conducted at any time along the continuum of acquiring the second language. As a consequence, it becomes possible to see a child whose scores may be depressed in his native language, L1, because he has stopped developing in that area, so as to commence acquiring the second language, L2. Thus, at the time of testing, this child may present with depressed scores for both L1 and L2. Does this imply a communication disorder? No, it does not. The clinician needs to be aware that this phase is part of the typical process of acquiring a second language.

DEVELOPMENTAL SIMILARITIES AND DIFFERENCES BETWEEN SIMULTANEOUS-BILINGUAL AND MONOLINGUAL CHILDREN

Our case study, Josefina, provides an example of a simultaneous-bilingual language learner. Josefina receives Spanish-language input from her mother and English-language input from her father. Researchers examining the development of simultaneous-bilingual children have found specific patterns of behavior across linguistic domains (phonology, morpho-syntax, semantics, pragmatics). Let us consider some of the possible linguistic behaviors we could expect from Josefina as compared to a monolingual child.

First, simultaneous-bilingual children generally produce the morpho-syntactic rules for each language to which they are exposed at approximately the same rate and order as a monolingual child producing each language separately (Meisel, 1989, 1994; Paradis & Genesee, 1996, 1997).

Second, *language mixing* is a common developmental process in simultaneous-bilingual children. Another term used to describe this phenomenon, *language transfer*, refers to the use of a linguistic structure from one language as a replacement for a structure in the other language for a period of time in development (Paradis, Crago, Genesee, & Rice, 2003). In this scenario, one morphological or syntactic system may be favored based on linguistic constraints (avoiding more difficult constructions), or the linguistic environment may shift in favor of one language versus the other.

Third, Vihman's (1985) research on bilingual phonological development suggests that the child's phonemic repertoire will consist of sounds from both languages given their relative salience and ease of production. Phonological transfers may occur just as they would for lexical or morpho-syntactic construction.

Fourth, lexical development is predominantly context specific. That is, the child learns the vocabulary for specific items in a language through naturalistic interactions with the item or exposure to the concept. In some cases, this will lead to the child knowing only one term rather than two terms from each language for a concept. Research suggests that the child's vocabulary size in each language significantly correlates with the amount of vocabulary exposure or input she is given in each language (Marchman & Martinez-Sussman, 2002; Pearson, Fernández, Lewedeg, & Oller, 1997).

Fifth, as the child approaches the age of 36 months (but perhaps earlier), the amount of language mixing/transfer decreases and the child develops greater awareness of the two languages. The use of the languages becomes more discrete, reflecting the environmental context, participants, topic, and other factors. Patterson (1998) suggests that the aggregate vocabulary of a bilingual child will equal that of a monolingual child. That is, if each language is measured separately, the child's total vocabulary in each language will seem deficient and will under-represent the bilingual child's true lexical development.

Sixth, if this behavior is sustained in the environment, simultaneous-bilingual children may demonstrate facility with code switching. Children may develop an understanding of the use constraints for this manner of communication and begin to apply them if supported.

In assessing bilingual children, some clinicians look at *communicative competence*, which comprises the child's ability to communicate messages effectively. When adopting this perspective, the speech-language pathologist should differentiate between the following types of competence:

+ *Grammatical competence*: phonological, syntactic, and lexical skills
+ *Sociolinguistic/sociocultural competence*: the use of language and communication rules appropriate in one's language
+ *Discourse competence*: the skills involved in the connection of a series of utterances to form a conversation and/or narrative
+ *Strategic competence*: the strategies used by the bilingual person to compensate for breakdowns in communication that may result from imperfect knowledge of the rules or fatigue, memory lapses, distraction, and anxiety

Evaluating the child in a variety of communicative contexts may allow the clinician to observe competence in different areas (Riquelme, 2006a).

COLLABORATING WITH INTERPRETERS/TRANSLATORS _____

Regulations on the use of interpreters/translators for speech-language assessment and intervention vary by state. In some states, every bilingual child referred for a speech-language evaluation is required to undergo an assessment that can be performed only by a clinician who is bilingual in the child's native language. Needless to say, this is sometimes quite difficult, as a match between the child's native language and the clinician's bilingual proficiency is not always possible. Indeed, fewer than 2% of ASHA members identify themselves as bilingual or multilingual (ASHA, 2002).

An *interpreter* is a person who is specially trained to transpose oral or signed text from one language to another. A *translator* is a person who is trained to transpose written text from one language to another. Speech-language pathologists most often require the services of an interpreter. Not every bilingual person has the ability to be an interpreter, of course. In addition to proficiency in two languages, other skills needed by the interpreter include (1) the ability to say the same things in different ways; (2) the ability to shift styles; (3) the ability to retain chunks of information while interpreting; and (4) familiarity with medical, educational, and professional terminology (Langdon, 2002). The interpreter should not be a friend or family member, as the information may be misunderstood, relayed inaccurately, or purposely omitted (Kayser, 1995).

Interpreters/translators are often used by the SLP for assessment and intervention purposes. Often the interpreter/translator is hired as support personnel, if the need is great (Kayser, 1995). This point underscores the need for all clinicians to become culturally competent, as even a monolingual/English SLP will likely have bilingual children in his or her caseload. Recall that the bilingual child may be dominant in English; thus the clinician treating this child may be a monolingual/English professional who will need to be sensitive to the cultural and linguistic differences of the child. In any event, it would be inappropriate to measure the bilingual child's communication skills and style against that of a monolingual/English language speaker.

This understanding is particularly important with regard to the translation of testing material for assessment purposes. Translated tests are statistically invalid; the standardized norms associated with the original test are not representative of the translated version. Therefore, performance on the translated version must be evaluated by other measures (e.g., criterion-referenced measures) rather than by relying on the original norms. Likewise, the representation of developmental language milestones on translated tests can present challenges. Standardized tests assume a developmental progression of language skills across domains. However, this progression is language-specific. For example, aspects of English may not emerge in Spanish at an age-equivalent period of development. Therefore, a translated test should be *adapted* to address the developmental expectations for the target language used in the community. Establishing local norms for the translated, adapted test is critical. Also, using multiple measures (e.g., narratives, language samples) will support the clinical impressions derived from using translated, adapted material.

If a professional interpreter is used, training of that person by the SLP will be required. The clinician needs to introduce the interpreter to the goals of assessment and intervention, stressing the importance of accurate/direct interpretation as per the complexity of speech-language diagnostics. This training serves to highlight how the clinician reaches an impression based on what may be interpreted. If a professional interpreter is not available, then another professional may be trained to assist the SLP. As mentioned earlier, the SLP should avoid the use of a family member or friend as an interpreter.

During the session, it is important that the clinician direct his attention and communication attempts to the student/client—not to the interpreter. Other modifications to testing procedures may include the following measures:

+ Reword instructions as needed.
+ Allow for additional response time.
+ Record all responses for later analysis.

- Accept culturally appropriate responses.
- Repeat stimuli as needed.
- Use culturally appropriate pictures and themes.

Langdon (2002) has developed a handbook that contains procedures and training exercises for the interpreter who is collaborating with the speech-language pathologist. Additional guidelines and suggestions are offered by Wallace (1997) and Kayser (1995).

IMPROVING CULTURAL COMPETENCE IN ASSESSMENT

The most powerful weapon that SLPs have in their diagnostic repertoire is information. The more data one collects from colleagues, the community, family, and the child, the more likely one is to diagnose the child correctly. Cultural information may be obtained from several resources. Roseberry-McKibbin (1995) has provided a list of suggestions for improving cultural sensitivity and competence. Among these, three stand out as being essential: analyzing one's own assumptions and values, using cultural informants and interpreters, and considering the child's needs within her linguistic community.

In addition to increasing cultural and linguistic knowledge, SLPs have other diagnostic tools at their disposal for data collection. Language sampling across naturalistic, communicative contexts is essential. In the case of the bilingual child, it is imperative to analyze both languages. The examiner has ethical and legal obligations to fulfill in determining the linguistic potential of a given child, and only by considering all aspects of a child's linguistic and cultural history will the strongest diagnosis take place.

Formal Testing

Given the complexity of cultural and linguistic factors, strict use of standardized tests is not recommended with bilingual children. To appropriately validate an examination and deem its results to be reliable, the standardization sample must be well defined (McCauley, 1996). Unfortunately, the heterogeneity of bilingual populations makes standardization untenable for these groups. Although some sample characteristics are discrete (e.g., age, gender), the sample must also account for continuous variables (e.g., level of bilingualism, language proficiency, language-use patterns, dialect changes, acculturation) that are in constant state of flux. This consideration is also relevant for children who may speak the language used by the examiner and the diagnostic tool, but may differ in cultural terms. For example, vocabulary tests may present stimuli that are specific to a particular geographic region or cultural perspective.

Looking at cultural relevance and the normative sample of a test battery should be a routine procedure for any examiner. Nevertheless, any formal test battery employed inherently carries some sorts of linguistic and cultural biases (Anderson, 2002). Anderson describes *linguistic bias* as the language used during testing and/or the language expected in the child's responses. This decision is often quite subjective, as is the examiner's acceptance of responses from the child being tested. Anderson describes *cultural bias* as "the language used during testing and the language expected in the child's responses" (p.146). She further defines *cultural bias* as referring to "the use of activities and items that do not correspond to the child's experiential base" (p.146).

Another aspect to consider is that most children being tested are bilingual to differing degrees. Norm-referenced tests look at each language as a separate entity and do not assess the relationship between the two languages (Riquelme, 2006a).

Research has shown that formal tests tend to over-identify Hispanic children as language learning disabled (Kayser, 1995; Peña, Quinn, & Iglesias, 1992). Unfortunately, in spite of these findings, many examiners and school districts continue to rely on the results of norm-referenced tests for the identification of children with communication disorders (Kayser, 1995).

Informal Testing

Many examiners consider informal testing to be an important part of the assessment process. When reporting results, however, this type of testing appears to lack objectivity.

Of greater validity are *criterion-referenced procedures*. These procedures provide the examiner with information that cannot be obtained from formal tests. They assess an individual's performance of a particular skill, structure, or concept. The fundamental purpose of criterion-referenced procedures is to distinguish between levels of performance (McCauley, 1996). Examples include measuring the percentage of syllables stuttered during a speech sample, maximum phonation time, percentage of consonants correct, and mean length of utterances (McCauley, 1996).

Criterion-referenced measures are relatively narrow in focus, as they are used to differentiate among levels of performance. Anderson (2002) offers the following example:

> "A criterion-referenced measure may be a child's ability to use episodic structure in a story-telling task. As such, it is developed so that the particular relevant aspects of the episodic structure during a retelling task can be scrutinized. The clinician may establish how many stories the child will retell, how many episodes each story contains, and the expected performance level, such as number of complete episodes produced..." (p. 162).

An obvious advantage of these measures is that they can be tailored to the individual child. Use of familiar tasks and objects can reduce the effects of bias associated with reduced or limited experience and variations in culturally-determined interaction styles. Another diagnostic alternative or adjunct is the use of *ethnographic observations*. This technique allows the examiner to observe the child in a variety of communicative contexts and to determine his competence in those contexts. The examiner is cautioned, however, to observe a variety of settings (e.g., one or more classrooms, playground). Likewise, the examiner must understand that this type of observation is inevitably colored by the examiner's own view of the world. If the examiner interprets the child's behavior incorrectly, it may result in misdiagnosis of the child. To prevent examiner bias to the greatest extent possible, clear objectives/goals for the observation should be established in advance (Anderson, 2002; Kayser, 1995), and a cultural informant should review the results of the assessment.

Language sampling is another available technique for the assessment of bilingual children. This is a well-known technique in our field. For specific suggestions on conducting language sampling with Latino children, the reader is referred to works by Anderson (2002), Kayser (1995), and Restrepo (1997).

Another option for informal testing is *dynamic assessment*. This procedure assesses not only the child's current performance level, but also the child's potential to learn. Because dynamic assessment provides information on the child's ability to learn, it provides the examiner with great insight for both identifying a language disorder and planning intervention. Peña et al. (1992) and Ukrainetz et al. (2000) have documented the benefits of using this procedure. They tested children in a particular task, then taught it to the children, and subsequently retested the children on the task without using cues or other supports. Both studies documented that children who were language impaired failed to demonstrate learning in the same manner as children who had typical language skills. Dynamic assessment certainly appears to be a viable procedure for use by SLPs in assessing the communicative skills of bilingual and/or ELL children.

Background Information

For many SLPs, it is common practice to report a child's history as "background information" related to, but separate from, the linguistic data collected. A "traditional" assessment model imitates the psychological model of assessment. This view suggests that language is a self-contained domain that can be analyzed apart from other domains—namely, the cognitive and emotional domains. In contrast, a *sociological* assessment model attempts to recognize the influences of other domains on language and to observe language in the most authentic contexts possible while capturing the most naturally occurring form, content, and uses of the language as possible.

The cultural information that a family provides is not "background," but rather a central feature of the data needed to improve SLPs' diagnostic and therapeutic decision making. Many parent questionnaires and checklists have been developed to facilitate and streamline the collection of background information. Unfortunately, formal questionnaires or checklists may provide only a superficial understanding of the relevant cultural and linguistic behaviors specific to a family or social group. Although it may seem simple to generalize traits of a given social group to all members of that group, such action will obscure the individual behaviors of smaller units within the group—for example, the family unit. Because the behaviors of individual members of a cultural group can vary widely (Van Kleeck, 1994), it is especially important to hear the "story" of the family unit as unique and incomparable. Generalization may well lead to biases and misconceptions that endanger the diagnostic process and damage the relationship between the clinician and the family being served.

To strengthen the clinician–family relationship, an approach that focuses on the family's values and concerns from the onset of interaction may reduce inadvertent over-generalizations and biases. One such approach suggested by Westby (1990) includes *ethnographic interviewing*. Many parents and caregivers are accustomed to the traditional model of interviewing in which the clinician requests answers to a series of questions designed to obtain the most essential diagnostic information. In contrast, the clinician, when working as an ethnographic interviewer, attempts to gain a more intimate understanding of a family's dynamics and the child's role in that system. One can think of the ethnographic approach as a personalized method of exploration that provides the clinician with an opportunity to obtain a deep, true, and naturalistic understanding of the behavior or culture under study. Through this process, the clinician listens to the behaviors and beliefs reported by the parent or caregiver, as obtained through a systematic and guided dialogue with the caretaker. Essential elements of effective ethnographic interviewing required of the clinician include the following components (Westby, 1990; Wallace, 1997):

+ Establishment of rapport
+ Good listening skills
+ A clear set of goals for information to be obtained
+ Skill in selecting the appropriate types of questions (i.e., grand tour, mini-tour, example, experience, or native-language questions)
+ Skill in framing questions, so that they are open-ended yet targeted to probe into key areas of interest
+ Skill in looking for patterns and common theme expressions as an essential key to detecting critical concerns of interest to the client/patient and family

Ethnographic interviewing allows for the following outcomes:

+ Conveys empathy/acceptance of the world as defined by the informant
+ Collects information necessary for generating appropriate support and clinical practice
+ Helps equalize the power differential between clinician and informant

✦ Provides a means for the professional to discover the culture of the family and their strengths and needs

✦ Provides a means for focusing on the perspective of the informant

✦ Helps reduce potential bias in assessment and intervention

✦ Allows the data to be collected in a more ecologically valid framework (Westby, 1990)

During ethnographic interviewing, the clinician has a general set of questions at the outset, but the flow of questioning is guided by the scope and depth of information obtained as the interview unfolds. The clinician is also advised to pay attention to how questions are worded: Use open-ended rather than closed-ended questions; use presupposition questions effectively; ask one question at a time; make use of preliminary statements; and maintain control of the interview. Saville-Troike (1978) offered additional suggestions for asking questions that are geared to understanding the family's position on several cultural dimensions. In any case, the SLP conducting the interview must realize that her background will affect the kinds of questions to be presented, the way the questions are posed, and the way answers are interpreted.

Hammer (1998) notes the importance of using several resources to develop an understanding of a particular family's cultural beliefs and practices. In addition to interviews and questionnaires, Hammer suggests literature review, examination of written documents (e.g., medical records), and analysis of open observation systems (child interacting in naturalistic contexts) as means to gather evidence. A correlation can then be determined between the anecdotal data of an ethnographic interview and the data collected from direct observations, prior research on that culture or language, and formal assessment procedures.

TREATMENT CONSIDERATIONS

Choice of Language for Treatment

Deciding on the language of treatment for bilingual or non-English-speaking children has been a hotly debated issue in the bilingual education literature, as well as in speech-language pathology. Many questions arise when deciding how to approach remediation of the bilingual child with a language disorder: Will intervention in L1 retard the progression of L2? Should treatment be provided only in L2? Will treatment in both L1 and L2 be too "taxing" to the child? Gutierrez-Clellen (1999) provides an excellent review of these and other issues and their clinical implications. To date, no study has been able to support an "English only" (L2) approach. Instead, most studies have focused on bilingual or monolingual/L1 intervention.

In reviewing the literature, researchers appear to emphasize that children's language learning can be maximized when the language of instruction/treatment matches the child's language(s), and L1 is used as an organizational language framework to facilitate second-language learning (Gutierrez-Clellen, 1999). Language-impaired children who are learning a second language constitute a heterogeneous group. This diversity is evidenced by the various types of deficits presented (e.g., phonological, pragmatic, morpho-syntactic), the severity of the disorders, the modality of the disorders (e.g., receptive, expressive, both), the language experiences of the child in L1 and L2, and the child's position along the second language acquisition continuum. All of these factors will influence the rate of learning each language as well as the child's progress in an intervention program.

Collaborations

Of great importance to the clinician working with bilingual children is the joint work with ESL teachers, classroom teachers, and parents. The SLP's success in treating a language-impaired child hinges on this collaboration and on her ability to develop culturally relevant strategies, tasks, and materials. Application of the previously mentioned culturally and linguistically sensitive considerations is as critical during treatment planning as it is during the assessment process.

Service Delivery

Another factor that influences the success of the language-impaired child is the type of service delivery models available for intervention. This factor is largely determined by the resources of the particular school district, as well as by the school district's underlying philosophy in regard to bilingual and special education. Providing optimal treatment to the bilingual or non-English-speaking child is a multifaceted endeavor that requires commitment to working with families, students as individuals, and school team members to foster success for the child (Roseberry-McKibbin, 2002).

SUMMARY

As speech-language pathologists continue to practice in a multicultural world, and as they continue to provide services to culturally and linguistically diverse children, the need to become culturally competent becomes increasingly obvious. Cultural competence will allow SLPs to provide services to children from all cultural and linguistic backgrounds with as little bias as is humanly and clinically possible.

The impact of language, as a cultural construct, has significance in our conception of children as dual-language learners. In the case study, Josefina's Spanish and English language use will be affected by the contexts of that exposure:

+ Who will the participants in language input be?
+ How does having the mother as model of Spanish versus having the father as model of English influence Josefina's development?

- Where will she obtain her language stimulation?
- Will she spend more time at home, where Spanish will abound, or will she spend more time in the community, where English is a more prominent fixture in daily activities?
- Will Josefina have contact with other caretakers? Will she have contact with other children?
- How will those individuals influence her language development?
- What do people talk to Josefina about?
- Is she privy to adult conversations, or will she be shielded from certain conversational topics?
- What are the contexts that drive Josefina's language use?
- Is she expected to remain a passive observer and listener, or will she be expected to produce language on par with peers or even adults?

The answers to these questions can be obtained by the SLP through observation and analysis of the culturally and linguistically significant behaviors unique to the family. The answers may not be readily accessible or easily learned in every case, but their discovery will result in improved outcomes for the families and children in SLPs' care.

Speech-language pathologists face many challenges ahead, many of them linked to the notion of a culture that originally intended to be homogeneous (e.g., America as a "melting pot"). Providing culturally competent services to children of all cultural backgrounds should be a challenge that all clinicians approach with enthusiasm and passion. Until misdiagnosis because of cultural differences is a thing of the past, speech-language pathologists cannot stop learning and challenging their clinical practices.

KEY TERMS

Acculturation	Discourse competence
Assimilation	Dual- (differentiated-) language system hypothesis
Code-switching	Dynamic assessment
Communicative competence	Ethnic diversity
Criterion-referenced measures	Ethnicity
Cultural bias	Ethnic majority
Cultural competence	Ethnic minority
Cultural diversity	Ethnographic interviewing
Cultural variables	Grammatical competence
Culture	Heritage
Dialectal variance	Illness
Disability	Interpreters

Language diversity

Language–ego permeability

Language loss

Language mixing

Language sampling

Language transfer

Language-use patterns

Linguistic bias

Nonverbal communication

Norm-referenced measures

Orientation

Race

Sequential-bilingual

Service delivery

Simultaneous-bilingual

Sociolinguistic/sociocultural competence

Sociological assessment model

Strategic competence

Traditional assessment model

Translators

Unitary language system view

Verbal communication

STUDY QUESTIONS

+ Define culture, and explain how it affects assessment and treatment practices with all children.
+ Outline a protocol for nonbiased assessment practices.
+ Outline questions you might ask a parent during an evaluation, using ethnographic interviewing constructs.
+ If formal tests currently in use (criterion-referenced) were normed on a population different from that which you are testing, how would you report the results of your assessment with these batteries? Why? Outline other options for assessment.
+ Discuss the decision-making process for providing treatment to a child in L1, L2, or L1 + L2.

REFERENCES

Anderson, R. T. (2002). Practical assessment strategies with Hispanic students. In A. Brice, *The Hispanic child*. Boston, MA: Allyn and Bacon.

American Speech-Language-Hearing Association (ASHA). (2004). Knowledge and skills needed by speech-language pathologists and audiologists to provide culturally and linguistically appropriate services. Available at: http://www.asha.org/NR/rdonlyres/BA28BD9C-26BA-46E7-9A47-5A7BDA2A4713/0/v4K-Scultlinguistic2004.pdf.

American Speech-Language-Hearing Association. (2002). *Communication development and disorders in multicultural populations: Readings and materials*. Available at: http://www.asha.org/about/leadership-projects/multicultural/ readings/OMA_fact_sheets.htm

Bebout, L., & Arthur, B. (1992). Cross-cultural attitudes toward speech disorders. *Journal of Speech-Language-Hearing Research, 35*, 45–52.

Bhatia T. K. & Ritchie, W. C. (Eds.), (1999). The bilingual child: Some issues and perspectives (pp. 457–491). *Handbook of child language acquisition*. San Diego: Academic Press.

Cabassa, L. J. (2003). Measuring acculturation: Where we are and where we need to go. *Hispanic Journal of Behavioral Sciences, 25*(2), 127–146.

Carbaugh, D. (1988). Comments on "culture" in communication inquiry. *Communication Reports, 1*, 38–41.

Chamberlain, P., & Medinos-Landurand, P. (1991). Practical considerations for the assessment of LEP students with special needs. In E. Hamayan & J. Damico, *Limiting bias in the assessment of bilingual students* (pp. 112–129, 131). Austin, TX: Pro Ed.

de Houwer, A. (1995). Bilingual language acquisition. In P. Fletcher & B. MacWhinney (Eds.), *Handbook of child language* (pp. 219–250). Oxford, UK: Basil Blackwell.

Dikeman, K. J., & Riquelme, L. F. (October 2002). Ethnocultural concerns in dysphagia. *Perspectives on Swallowing and Swallowing Disorders*, 31–35.

Fantini, A. (1985). *Language acquisition of a bilingual child: A sociolinguistic perspective.* San Diego: College Hill Press.

Farver, J. M., Kim, Y. K., & Lee, Y. (1995). Cultural differences in Korean- and Anglo-American preschoolers' social interaction and play behaviors. *Child Development, 66*, 1088–1099.

Fishman, J. A. (Ed.). (1966). *Language loyalty in the United States.* The Hague: Mouton.

Genesee, F. (1989). Early bilingual development: One language or two? *Journal of Child Language, 16*, 161–179.

Goldstein, B. (2004). *Bilingual language development and disorders in Spanish–English speakers.* Baltimore: Paul H. Brookes.

Guiora, A. Z., & Acton, W. R. (1979). Personality and language: A restatement. *Language Learning, 29*, 193–204.

Gutierrez-Clellen, V. F. (1999). Language choice in intervention with bilingual children. *American Journal of Speech-Language Pathology, 8*, 291–302.

Hammer, C. S. (1998). Toward a "thick description" of families: Using ethnography to overcome the obstacles to providing family-centered early intervention services. *American Journal of Speech Language Pathology, 7*, 5–22.

Heath, S. (1983). *Ways with words: Language, life, and work in communities and classrooms.* New York: Cambridge University Press.

Johnson, C., & Lancaster, P. (1998). The development of more than one phonology: A case study of a Norwegian–English bilingual child. *International Journal of Bilingualism, 2*(3), 265–300.

Kayser, H. (1995). *Bilingual speech-language pathology: An Hispanic focus.* San Diego, CA: Singular.

Kindler, A. (2001). *Survey of the states' LEP students 2000–2001 summary report.* Washington, DC: National Clearinghouse for English Language Acquisition.

Kleinman, A., Eisenberg, L., & Good, B. (2006). Culture, illness, and care: Clinical lessons from anthropologic and cross-cultural research. *Focus, 4*, 140–149.

Kohnert, K. (2008). *Language disorders in bilingual children and adults.* San Diego, CA: Plural.

Kohnert, K. J., & Bates, E. (2002). Balancing bilinguals II: Lexical comprehension and cognitive processing in children learning Spanish and English. *Journal of Speech-Language-Hearing Research, 45*, 347–359.

Kohnert, K. J., Bates, E., & Hernández, A. E. (1999). Balancing bilinguals: Lexical–semantic production and cognitive processing in children learning Spanish and English. *Journal of Speech-Language-Hearing Research, 42*, 1400–1413.

Langdon, H. W. (2002). *Interpreters and translators in communication disorders: A Practitioner's handbook.* Eau Claire, WI: Thinking Publications.

Maestas, A. G., & Erickson, J. G. (1992). Mexican immigrant mothers' beliefs about disabilities. *American Journal of Speech-Language Pathology, 1*, 5–10.

Marchman, V. A., & Martínez-Sussmann, C. (2002). Concurrent validity of caregiver/parent report measures of language for children who are learning both English and Spanish. *Journal of Speech-Language-Hearing Research, 45*, 983–997.

McCauley, R. J. (1996). Familiar strangers: Criterion-referenced measures in communications disorders. *Language, Speech and Hearing Services in Schools, 29*, 3–10.

McLaughlin, B. (1984). Early bilingualism: Methodological and theoretical issues. In G. Duncan & J. Brooks-Gunn (Eds.), *Consequences of growing up poor* (pp. 35–48). New York: Russell Sage Foundation.

Meisel, J. (1989). Early differentiation of languages in bilingual children. In K. Hyltenstam & L. Obler (Eds.), *Bilingualism across the lifespan: Aspects of acquisition, maturity and loss* (pp. 13–40). Cambridge, UK: Cambridge University Press.

Meisel, J. (1994). *Bilingual first language acquisition: French and German grammatical development.* Amsterdam: John Benjamins.

Nicoladis, E., & Secco, G. (2000). Productive vocabulary and language choice. *First Language, 20*(58), 3–28.

Paradis, J., Crago, M., Genesee, F., & Rice, M. (2003). French–English bilingual children with SLI: How do they compare with their monolingual peers? *Journal of Speech-Language-Hearing Research, 46*, 113–127.

Paradis, J., & Genesee, F. (1996). Syntactic acquisition of bilingual children: Autonomous or interdependent? *Studies in Second Language Acquisition, 18*, 1–15.

Paradis, J., & Genesee, F. (1997). On continuity and the emergence of functional categories in bilingual first language acquisition. *Language Acquisition, 6*(2), 91–124.

Paradis, J., Nicoladis, E., & Genesee, F. (2000). Early emergence of structural constraints on code-switching: Evidence from French–English bilingual children. *Bilingualism: Language and Cognition, 3*(3): 245–261.

Patterson, J. L. (1998). Expressive vocabulary development and word combinations of Spanish–English bilingual toddlers. *American Journal of Speech-Language Pathology, 7*, 46–56.

Payne, J. C. (1997). *Adult neurogenic language disorders: Assessment and treatment—A comprehensive ethnobiological approach.* San Diego, CA: Singular.

Pearson, B. Z., Fernández, S. C., Lewedeg, V., & Oller, D. K. (1997). The relation of input factors to lexical learning by bilingual infants. *Applied Psycholinguistics, 18*, 41–58.

Pearson, B. Z., Fernández, S., & Oller, D. K. (1995). Cross-language synonyms in the lexicons of bilingual infants: one language or two? *Journal of Child Language, 22*, 345–368.

Peña, E., Quinn, R., & Iglesias, A. (1992). The application of dynamic methods to language assessment: A non-biased procedure. *Journal of Special Education, 26*, 269–280.

Pyke, C. (1986). One lexicon or two? An alternative interpretation of early bilingual speech. *Journal of Child Language, 13*, 591–593.

Quay, S. (1995). The bilingual lexicon: Implications for studies of language choice. *Journal of Child Language, 22*, 369–387.

Restrepo, M. A. (1997). Guidelines for identifying primarily Spanish-speaking preschool children with language impairment. *Perspectives on Cultural and Linguistic Diverse Populations, ASHA Special Interest Division 14, 3*, 11–12.

Riquelme, L.F. (13 April 2004). Cultural competence in dysphagia. *The ASHA Leader, 9* (7), 8, 22.

Riquelme, L. F. (2006a). Working with Hispanic/Latino students. In E. H. Gravani & J. Meyer (Eds.), *Speech-language-hearing programs: A guide for students and practitioners,* 2nd ed. (pp. 429–446). Austin, TX: Pro Ed.

Riquelme, L. F. (December 2006b). Working with limited-English speaking adults with neurological impairment. *Perspectives on Gerontology, ASHA SID 15, 11*(2), 3–8.

Riquelme, L. F. (2007). The role of cultural competence in providing services to persons with dysphagia. *Topics in Geriatric Rehabilitation, 25*(3), 228–239.

Roseberry-McKibbin, C. (1995). *Multicultural students with special language needs: Practical strategies for assessment and intervention.* Oceanside, CA: Academic Communication Associates.

Roseberry-McKibbin, C. (2002). Principles and strategies in intervention. In A. Brice (Ed.), *The Hispanic child.* (pp. 199–233). Boston: Allyn and Bacon.

Rubin, K. H., & Coplan, R. J. (1998). Social and nonsocial play in childhood: An individual differences perspective. In S. N. Saracho & B. Spodek (Eds.), *Multiple perspectives on play in early childhood education* (pp. 144–170). Albany, NY: State University of New York Press.

Salas-Provance, M., Erickson, J. G., & Reed, J. (2002). Disabilities as viewed by four generations of one Hispanic family. *American Journal of Speech-Language Pathology, 11,* 151–162.

Sapir, E. (1921). *Language: An introduction to the study of speech.* New York: Harcourt Brace.

Saville-Troike, M. (1978). *A guide to culture in the classroom.* Rosslyn, VA: National Clearinghouse for Bilingual Education.

Schumann, J. H. (1986). Research on the acculturation model for second language acquisition. *Journal of Multicultural Development, 7*(5), 379–392.

Sutton-Smith, B. (1972). *The folkgames of children.* Austin, TX: University of Texas Press.

Ukrainetz, T.A., Harpell, S., Walsh, C., Coyle, C. (2000). A preliminary investigation of dynamic assessment with Native American kindergarteners. *Language, Speech and Hearing Services in Schools, 31,* 142–154.

U.S. Bureau of the Census. (2000). *Statistical abstract of the United States 119th ed.* Washington, DC: U.S. Department of Commerce.

U.S. Department of Education. (2007). *Executive summary OSERS 23rd Annual Report to Congress on the Implementation of the IDEA.* Available at: http://www.ed.gov/about/reports/annual/osep/2001/execsumm.html.

Van Kleeck, A. (1994). Potential cultural bias in training parents as conversational partners with their children who have delays in language development. *American Journal of Speech-Language Pathology, 3,* 67–78.

Vihman, M. (1985). Language differentiation by the bilingual infant. *Journal of Child Language, 12,* 297–324.

Volterra, V., & Taeschner, T. (1978). The acquisition and development of language by bilingual children. *Journal of Child Language, 5,* 311–326.

Wallace, G. L. (1997). *Multicultural neurogenics: A resource for speech-language pathologists.* San Antonio, TX: Communication Skill Builders.

Westby, C. E. (1990). Ethnographic interviewing: Asking the right questions to the right people in the right ways. *Journal of Childhood Communication Disorders, 13*(1), 101–111.

Zentella, A. C. (1997). *Growing up bilingual: Puerto Rican children in New York.* Malden, MA: Blackwell.

CHAPTER 14

Children with Language Impairment

Liat Seiger-Gardner, PhD

OBJECTIVES

+ Differentiate between the various terms (e.g., language impairment, language difference, language delay) used to describe language abilities in children.
+ Understand the difference between primary and secondary language impairments.
+ Explain how language form (phonology, syntax, and morphology), content (semantics), and use (pragmatics) are affected children with primary language impairments.
+ Describe the hallmark characteristics of late talkers, late bloomers, children with specific language impairment (SLI), and children with language learning disability (LLD).
+ Differentiate between a language delay and a language disorder (late bloomers versus late talkers).
+ Describe the language characteristics of children with autism spectrum disorder (ASD) and children with mental retardation (MR).
+ Explore the most commonly used methods for assessing the language abilities of infants, toddlers, preschoolers, and school-age children with primary and secondary language impairments.
+ Identify various treatment methods and strategies for children with primary and secondary language deficits.

INTRODUCTION

A variety of terms are used to describe the language difficulties seen in children whose ages range from infancy to school age. Language impairment/disorder, language disability, language delay, language deviance, and even childhood aphasia are often used interchangeably by nonprofessionals to refer to the same deficits; however, these terms are used to distinguish between and characterize different conditions or states.

Language Disorder/Impairment

According to the American Speech-Language-Hearing Association (ASHA), *language disorder* is defined as "an impairment in comprehension and/or use of spoken language, written, and/or other symbol system. The disorder may involve (1) the form of language (phonologic, morphologic, and syntactic systems), (2) the content of language (semantic system), and/or (3) the function of language in communication (pragmatic system), in any combination" (ASHA, 1993, p. 40). Paul adds that children exhibit a language disorder "if they have a significant deficit in learning to talk, understand, or use any aspect of language appropriately, relative to both environmental and norm referenced expectations for children of similar developmental level" (Paul, 2001, p. 3). Thus, in addition to being noticeably impaired in the ability to use language to communicate, the child has to score significantly below age-expected norms on standardized or norm-referenced tests to be identified as having language impairment and be eligible for speech and language services. A score of one to two standard deviations below the mean for the child's age is typically the criterion used to diagnose a child as having language impairment and qualifies him for services. Fey (1986) has suggested a standard score of 1.25 as a criterion, which places the child below the 10th percentile for his or her expected level of language performance.

Language impairments can be classified as primary or secondary. A *primary language impairment* is present when a language delay cannot be accounted for by a peripheral sensory deficit such as hearing loss; a motor deficit, such as cerebral palsy; a cognitive deficit, such as mental retardation (MR); a social or emotional impairment, such as autism spectrum disorders (ASD); harmful environmental conditions, such as lead poisoning or drug abuse; or gross neurological deficit, such as that associated with traumatic brain injury (TBI) or lesions. This type of delay is often presumed to be due to impaired development or dysfunction of the central nervous system (Leonard, 1998). *Secondary language impairment* refers to a language disorder that is associated with and presumed to be caused by factors such as sensory (hearing loss) or cognitive impairments (mental retardation). This type of language disorder may also be part of a syndrome—that is, the presence of multiple abnormalities in the same individual that are all caused by or originated from same source. For example, in fragile X syndrome or Down syndrome, language impairment is one of many other anomalies present; others may include mental retardation or specific facial characteristics.

Language and Learning Disability

The term *language disability* refers to the consequences language impairment may have on a child's ability to function in the real world, and especially in school. The term *disability* is often used—especially among nonprofessionals—interchangeably with the term *handicap*, which is an impaired condition or behavior that precludes the child from engaging in age-appropriate life activities. The term "language disability" is often used hand in hand with the term *learning disability*, suggesting limitations in the ability to perform certain tasks such as reading, writing, listening, reasoning, spelling, and word recognition. Difficulties in learning how to perform on these tasks are often attributed to deficits in language abilities.

Language Delay

A child is considered to have a *language delay* if he exhibits typical development in all other areas except for language. Language development in a child with a language delay is believed to follow the same patterns seen in children with typical language development; however, the development of language is protracted, with the child reaching the same milestones at a slower pace. Leonard (1998) has noted that the term *delay* suggests a late start and the possibility of making up for lost time (i.e., late bloomers). For many children with language impairment, the early delay involves not only the late emergence of first words and two-word combinations, but also the slow development of linguistic features until the point of mastery (Rescorla, 2005). This slow development can persist until adulthood, opening a gap that widens as children get older, and in turn making it more difficult to "make up" for lost time. At this point the language delay can be viewed as language impairment. A more extended overview of the characteristics that distinguish language delay (i.e., late bloomers) from language impairment (i.e., late talkers) is presented later in this chapter.

Language Deviance

The term *language deviance* suggests that the child's language development is not just slower than the typical but actually different in some qualitative way. This definition does not fit most children with primary language impairments, who tend to follow the same developmental patterns as typical but younger developing children (i.e., those presenting with a language delay). The language profiles of children exhibiting concomitant conditions such as ASD and MR may reveal some idiosyncratic patterns that deviate from typicality.

Language Difference

Paul (2005) defines *language difference* as a rule-governed language form (i.e., dialect) that deviates in some ways from the standard language used by the mainstream culture. Some children from culturally diverse backgrounds who are speaking a dialect may also exhibit language impairment. In such cases, distinguishing between a language difference and true language impairment is one of the challenges faced by the speech-language pathologist. Language remediation by a speech-language pathologist for children exhibiting language differences is not warranted, although it may be offered through educational programs to facilitate communication in the mainstream culture (Paul, 2005).

This chapter focuses on the characteristics of primary and secondary language impairments/disorders in children spanning in age from toddlerhood to school age. It reviews the linguistic characteristics of primary language deficits as in late bloomers and late talkers, preschool children with specific language impairment (SLI), and school-age children with language and learning disabilities, as well as the linguistic characteristics of secondary language deficits as in ASD and MR. In addition, assessment methods and intervention strategies that can be used with all children will be covered in this chapter.

PRIMARY LANGUAGE IMPAIRMENT

Late Talkers and Late Bloomers

Whereas most children acquire language naturally and for the most part without formal instruction, for some children the acquisition of language poses a challenge. The majority of children with primary language impairments are not identified until they reach 24 months of age. In the absence of other significant sensory, cognitive, or motor disabilities, the first evidence for a language delay is the late onset of first-word production and a slow development of vocabulary growth (Leonard, 1998). Typically in the first two years of life, toddlers developing language with no difficulties go through a developmental stage called the *emerging language stage* (Paul, 1995). During this stage they acquire their first words, typically between 12 and 18 months of age; they then produce two-word combinations, typically between 18 and 24 months of age, after they had at least 50 words in their productive lexicon (Nelson, 1973). Children who fail to reach these lexical milestones at the specified ages are referred to as *late talkers* (Rescorla, 1989; Rescorla & Schwartz, 1990).

Delays in phonological development are also characteristic of late talkers (Paul, 1991; Paul & Jennings, 1992; Rescorla & Ratner, 1996; Roberts, Rescorla, Giroux, & Stevens, 1998). They are overall less vocal and verbal compared to their typically developing peers; they exhibit proportionally smaller consonantal and vowel inventories, with their consonantal inventory consisting of primarily voiced stops (/d/, /g/, /z/), nasals (/m/, /n/), and glides (/j/, /w/). They also exhibit a more restricted and less complex array of syllable structures, using predominantly single vowels and consonant–vowel (CV) syllable shapes. The babbling stage in late talkers tends to extend over time, as does the use of phonological processes—that is, strategies children with and without language impairment use to simplify adults' speech.

Delays in morpho-syntactic development are also characteristic of late talkers at age 3;0 (Rescorla & Roberts, 1997). It is during the second and third years of life that new morphological forms such as grammatical morphemes (see **Table 14-1**) and basic sentence forms (see **Table 14-2**) (e.g., subject–verb–object as in *She drinks milk* and subject–copula–complement

TABLE 14-1   Stages of Morpho-Syntactic Development in Typically Developing Children

Stage	Age (months)	Morpho-syntactic Characteristics	Examples
I	12–26	Single-word utterances and multiword combinations based on word-order/semantic-syntactic rules	*Eat cookie*: Action + Object *Daddy shoe*: Possessor + Possession *Doggie bed:* Entity + Locative
II	27–30	The appearance of grammatical morphemes	*Mommy is driving*: Present Progressive -*ing* and Auxiliary *is* *I love dogs*: Regular plural -*s*
III	31–34	Simple sentence forms: • Development within noun and verb phrases with the addition of grammatical morphemes, quantifiers, adjectives, and adverbs • Development of different sentence types (declarative, interrogative, imperative, and negative forms)	*Dave eats banana*: Subject–Verb–Object *This is Mommy's car*: Copula and possessive *Diana has three cats*: Quantifiers *She has a blue cap*: Adjectives *She runs quickly:* Adverbs *I'm eating ice cream*: Declarative *What are you eating?*: Interrogative *Throw me the ball, please*: Imperative *I don't want that*: Negative forms
IV	35–40	The appearance of embedded phrases and subordinate clauses within a sentence. Subordinate clauses are introduced by conjunction words: *after, although, before, until, while, when,* or relative pronouns: *who, which, whom,* and *that.*	*The woman in the blue dress is my teacher*: Embedded phrase *The boy, we met last week, is in my class*: Embedded clause
V	41–46	The appearance of conjoined sentences. Conjoining sentences with conjunction words: *and, if, because, when, but, after, before,* and *so.*	*I play the violin and she plays the piano; She cried because she fell down the stairs; We went to school after we ate breakfast; I like fruit but I don't like vegetables.*

Source: Bernstein, D. & Seiger-Gardner, L. (in press). *An introduction to early childhood special education: Strategies and practices.* Upper Saddle River, NJ: Pearson Education.

TABLE 14-2 The Acquisition of Grammatical Morphemes		
Morpheme	**Example**	**Age of Mastery (in Months)**
Present Progressive –*ing* (no auxiliary verb)	*Mommy driving*	19–28
In	*Ball in cup*	27–30
On	*Doggie on sofa*	27–30
Regular Plural –*s*	*Kitties eat my ice cream*	27–33
Irregular Past	*came, fell, broke, sat, went*	25–46
Possessive '*s*	*Mommy's balloon broke*	26–40
Uncontractible Copula (verb *to be* as main verb)	*He is my teacher*	27–39
Articles	*I see a kitty*	28–46
	I throw the ball to daddy	
Regular Past –*ed*	*Mommy pulled the wagon*	26–48
Regular Third Person –*s*	*Kathy hits*	26–46
Irregular Third Person	*She does like me*	28–50
	He has the ball	
Uncontractible Auxiliary	*He is wearing a hat*	29–48
Contractible Copula	*Daddy's big* (for *Daddy is big*)	29–49
Contractible Auxiliary	*Daddy's drinking juice* (for *Daddy is drinking juice*)	30–50

Source: Adapted with permission from Owens, R. (2005). *Language development: An introduction,* 6th ed. Boston: Allyn & Bacon.

as in *She is pretty*) are evident in typically developing children (Brown, 1973). The difficulties late talkers exhibit in morpho-syntax are apparent in both noun and verb morphology (Paul & Alforde, 1993; Rescorla & Roberts, 2002), with nominal morphemes such as articles (*the, a*) and pronouns (*she, his*) and verbal morphemes such as contractible copulas (*he's a painter*) and auxiliaries (*she is dancing*) being the most difficult. Later pragmatic difficulties are also evidenced in late talkers at age four years (Paul & Smith, 1993); their narratives reflect their difficulties in encoding, organizing, and linking schemes, as well as retrieving precise and diverse words from their lexicons.

Some 75% to 85% of late talkers who are identified at age 2;0 seem to "catch up" to their typically developing peers in their expressive language skills by age 5;0 (Paul, 1996; Rescorla, 2002; Rescorla & Lee, 2001; Rescorla, Mirak, & Singh, 2000; Whitehurst & Fischel, 1994). These children are referred to as *late bloomers* (Thal & Tobias, 1992; Thal, Tobias, & Morrison, 1991). Late bloomers, although they may be slow in developing their productive lexicon in the first 2 years of life, make tremendous amount of progress after their second birthday, and by their third birthday they are very similar to their typically developing peers in terms of their language capabilities (Rescorla et al., 2000). Unfortunately, many toddlers never really "catch up" to their peers and continue to show persistent language difficulties even after the age of 3;0. These children are often identified at age 4 as having *specific language impairment (SLI)*. Children with SLI typically have performance IQs within normal limits, normal hearing acuity, no behavioral or emotional disorders, and no gross neurological deficits. Nevertheless, they present significant deficits in language production and/or comprehension (Leonard, 1998). The language characteristics of children with SLI are reviewed later in this chapter.

Two clinical markers can be used by clinicians to distinguish transient language difficulties (i.e., late bloomers) from persistent language impairments (i.e., late talkers). Specifically, a delay in the development of receptive language (Thal, Reilly, Seibert, Jeffries, & Fenson, 2004; Thal & Tobias, 1992; Thal et al., 1991) and a delay in the use of conventional gestures (e.g., pointing, showing) and symbolic gestures (e.g., panting like a dog, sniffing to indicate a flower) (Thal & Tobias, 1992; Thal et al., 1991) are potential predictors of persisting language delays. Comprehension at 13 months of age has been shown to predict the development of receptive vocabulary and grammatical complexity (i.e., mean length of utterance [MLU]) at 28 months of age in typically developing children (Bates, Bretherton, & Snyder, 1988) and is suggested to play an important role throughout the second year of life in both receptive and expressive language acquisition (Watt, Wetherby, & Shumway, 2006). Similarly, the use of gestures early in the second year of life has been shown to correlate closely with total vocal production at 20 months (Capirci, Iverson, Pizzuto, & Volterra, 1996) and with the development of receptive language at age 3 years (Watt et al., 2006). Typically developing children use conventional and symbolic gestures prior to the use of words to communicate with others (Acredolo & Goodwyn, 1988; Caselli, 1990; see Capone & McGregor, 2004, for a full review). (See **Table 14-3.**) Late bloomers appear to use more communicative gestures compared to their typically developing peers in an effort to compensate for their lack of words, whereas late talkers fail to show an increase in communicative gestures as a compensation for their verbal delay (Thal & Tobias, 1992). Thus compensatory use of communicative gestures is a positive prognostic sign for later typical language development.

The two case studies of Josephine and Robert clearly demonstrate the two clinical markers that distinguish between transient language difficulties (i.e., late bloomers) and persistent

TABLE 14-3   A Timeline of Gesture Development

10–13 Months	12–13 Months	15–16 Months	18–20 Months	2–5 years (School Age)	School Age
Showing Giving Pointing Ritualized request	Representational gestures, play schemes	Gesture or vocal preference	Spoken word preference, gesture-plus-spoken combinations	Speech–gesture integration, beat gestures emerge	Mismatched gesture-plus-spoken combinations
Point predicts first words	First words emerge		Significant increase in words (types, tokens)	Gesture scaffolds spoken expression and comprehension	Mismatches index the transitional knowledge state
Other prelinguistic behaviors include: eye contact, joint attention, and turn-taking	Gesture serves a complementary function to spoken forms		Increased pointing in combination with spoken words	Transition from BPO to IO gestures	Gesture aids in the transition to concept acquisition
			Transition to empty-handed play schemes	Iconic and beat gestures accompany longer utterances	

BPO = body part as object; IO = imaginary object.

Source: Capone, N., & McGregor, K. (2004). Gesture development: A review for clinical and research practices. *Journal of Speech, Language, and Hearing Research, 47,* 173–186.

language difficulties (i.e., late talkers). Josephine exhibits expressive language delays in the presence of age-appropriate receptive skills. For example, she was able to choose one object from a group of five and follow novel and two-step directions. Josephine compensated for her expressive language delay by using prelinguistic gestures (e.g., showing, pointing) and iconic gestures (e.g., hand under cheek to indicate sleeping). Her age-appropriate receptive skills and use of gestures suggest a good prognosis for outgrowing the expressive language delays.

Robert, by contrast, exhibited both expressive and receptive language delays. His receptive skills were appropriate for a 9- to 12-month-old child; hence, those skills are delayed in development by more than a year. Although he was able to respond to requests to say words and to choose two objects from an array of objects, Robert was inconsistent in responding to his name and had difficulty following commands involving two actions with an object. His gesture use was typical of a 9- to 12-month-old child, again reflecting a delay of more than a year. He used prelinguistic gestures such as showing and pointing, and he tended to use them to satisfy basic needs rather than for socialization. Considering the delays in both receptive and expressive language domains and the limited use of gestures, as well as the attention difficulties and the delay in play skills, Robert's prognosis for outgrowing his language delays is poor, suggesting persisting language impairments.

Preschool Specific Language Impairment

Late talkers who are identified at age two as having a language delay, as in the case of Robert, may continue to exhibit language deficits during the preschool years. These children are referred to as having *specific language impairment (SLI)*. SLI affects approximately 7% of all children (Leonard, 1998). It often runs in families and is suggested to have a genetic component (Newbury, Bishop, & Monaco, 2005), although a clear inheritance pattern or specific genes have not yet been identified. In Robert's case, his family history was remarkable for an uncle diagnosed with SLI as a child.

The appearance of subtle irregularities in brain structure suggests some neurological involvement in the disorder. For example, atypical left–right perisylvian area configurations, with a larger than usual right perisylvian area that equal or exceeds the size of the left perisylvian area, are associated with SLI (Leonard, 1998).

The language deficits exhibited by children with SLI can be manifested solely in language production or in both language production and comprehension; they can affect one or more areas of language (i.e., form–phonology, syntax, morphology, content–semantics, and use–pragmatics). Considering his prognosis, it is suspected that Robert, our 27-month-old late talker, will continue to exhibit language difficulties during the preschool years. His linguistic profile as a toddler suggests persisting language impairments in both receptive and expressive language domains.

Limitations in Language Content: Semantics

Children with SLI exhibit a slower rate of vocabulary growth (Windfuhr, Faragher, & Conti-Ramsden, 2002) and have a less diverse and more restricted lexicon (Watkins, Kelly, Harbers, & Hollis, 1995). In language production, their semantic difficulties are apparent in the speech errors they produce, which tend to be semantic in nature—for example, saying *dog* to refer to a *horse* or *clown* to refer to a *circus*. They reveal low performance on lexical comprehension tests (Lahey & Edwards, 1999; McGregor, 1997) and on tasks focusing on multiple levels of noun hierarchy such as superordinate nouns (e.g., *furniture*), coordinate nouns (e.g., *chair*), and subordinate nouns (e.g., *rocking chair*) (McGregor & Waxman, 1998). In addition, preschoolers with SLI may exhibit *word-finding difficulties*—that is, difficulties in generating a specific word for any given situation (Rapin & Wilson, 1978). Their difficulties are manifested in single-word naming tasks as well as in conversational discourse (German & Simon, 1991). Their language is characterized by repetitions, substitutions, reformulations, pauses, and use of nonspecific words such as *stuff* or *thing* (Faust, Dimitrovsky, & Davidi, 1997; German, 1987; McGregor & Leonard, 1989).

Difficulties in lexical comprehension are apparent in the understanding and use of basic concepts that mark spatial relations (e.g., *on, in, above, behind*), temporal relations (e.g., *tomorrow, before, after*), kinship relations (e.g., *grandmother, sister, daughter*), causal relations (e.g., *because, why*), sequential relations (e.g., *first, next, finally*), and physical relations (e.g., *hard/soft, wide/narrow, shallow/deep*).

The difficulties preschoolers with SLI exhibit in semantics are not limited to concepts or nouns; they also extend to verb learning. The verb lexicons of such children are characterized as small and less diverse with heavy reliance on "general all-purpose" (GAP) verbs such as *go, make, do,* and *look* (Conti-Ramsden & Jones, 1997; Rice & Bode, 1993; Thordardottir & Weismer, 2001).

Limitations in Language Form: Phonology, Morphology and Syntax

Children with SLI follow similar patterns of phonological development as typically developing children; however, their development is protracted over time. As a result, they show many of the phonological characteristics seen in younger, typically developing children. Preschoolers with SLI are late in acquiring their consonant inventory, and later-acquired sounds such as /s/ and /v/ tend to remain difficult for children with SLI even into the school-age years. Difficulties in the acquisition of the sound system of the language, for example, are apparent in activities that involve phonological awareness. *Phonological awareness* refers to the explicit awareness that words in the language are composed of syllables and phonemes (i.e., consonants and vowels) (Catts, 1991), and that words can rhyme or begin with the same sound. Children demonstrate phonological awareness by tapping syllables (i.e., segmenting multisyllabic words into their syllable components), recognizing and producing rhymes, segmenting words into their phonemic components, blending and manipulating sounds within words, and understanding letter–sound correspondence. Compared to their typically developing peers, preschoolers with SLI perform more poorly on phonological awareness tasks (Fazio, 1997).

Preschoolers with SLI display extraordinary difficulty with nominal (e.g., noun plural *-s* inflection) and verbial morphology (e.g., third singular *-s*, regular past tense *-ed*, copula *be* forms), with the latter being more challenging for these children (Bedore & Leonard, 1998; Norbury, Bishop, & Briscoe, 2001; Rice, Wexler, & Cleave, 1995). In fact, a delay in acquiring verb morphology is considered to be a clinical marker for language impairment. Similar to the path seen with development of phonology, preschoolers with SLI follow the same morphological patterns as their typically developing peers, but their development is protracted, occurring over a longer period of time (Rice & Wexler, 1996; Rice et al., 1995). Compared to language- and age-matched peers, children with SLI produce verb and noun morphological markers less consistently and with a lower percentage of use in sentence completion tasks and in spontaneous speech (Leonard, Eyer, Bedore, & Grela, 1997; Rice & Wexler, 1996; Rice et al., 1995). For example, they are likely to omit the "be" verb form (i.e., auxiliary) or the present progressive *-ing* form, producing sentences such as *I playing with these dolls* (omitting the auxiliary) or *I'm wear the green pants* (omitting the present progressive). Similarly, they are likely to misuse the "be" verb form, as in the sentence *She were driving the car* (misuse of auxiliary "be" form) or in the sentence *The boy and the girl is sad* (misuse of copula "be" form). In addition, preschoolers with SLI are likely to misuse pronouns in discourse. For example, sentences such as <u>*Him*</u> *not nice*, <u>*Me*</u> *play with the doll*, and *This is not my book, it is <u>her</u>* may be apparent in the language of a child with SLI.

The limitations children with SLI exhibit in syntactic development are manifested in the reduced length and complexity of the syntactic forms they use. Specifically, they produce shorter sentences (Scott & Windsor, 2000), do not elaborate on noun and verb phrases within sentences, and use simple conjunctions (e.g., *and*) to produce compound sentences. Most often, preschoolers with SLI fail to use prepositional phrases, as in the sentence *The house <u>on the corner</u> is mine*, or verb embedded phrases, as in the sentences *He fought <u>with courage</u>* and *The man <u>in the green suit</u> is my father* (Schuele & Dykes, 2005; Schuele & Tolbert, 2001).

Limitations in Language Use: Pragmatics

Many conversational skills are acquired during the preschool years. Preschoolers who are developing language typically exhibit gradual improvement in their ability to respond to their conversational partners, to engage in short dialogues, to adjust their language style to the listener, to self-monitor and self-correct errors produced during conversation, to provide clarifications to their conversational partner, and to introduce or shift to a new topic of conversation. By comparison, preschoolers with SLI exhibit difficulties in the acquisition and implementation of many of these conversational skills. They display difficulties initiating and sustaining conversation beyond a few exchanges (Hadley & Rice, 1991). Their difficulties in auditory comprehension and short-term memory impede their ability to maintain the flow of conversation and follow through with directions. Preschoolers with SLI avoid asking for clarifications or providing clarifications in cases where communication breakdowns occur (Fujiki, Brinton, & Sonnenberg, 1990). They also show difficulty in adapting their speech and language to their listener (Leonard, 1998). Preschoolers with SLI not only engage in fewer peer interactions (Rice, Sell, & Hadley, 1991), but also are less likely to be picked by typically developing peers as potential conversational partners. Their overall language difficulties prevent them from being able to resolve conflicts in a verbal manner, resulting in their withdrawal or expression of aggression (Leonard, 1998).

School-Age Language and Learning Disability

Language learning disability (*LLD*), like SLI and late talking, is an impairment that does not stem from a cognitive deficit, a sensory impairment, a social deficit, or a gross neurological deficit (Paul, 2001). School-age children with LLD experience difficulties not only in speaking and listening, but also in reading and writing. In particular, they exhibit difficulties in reading comprehension, identifying and distinguishing between salient and extraneous information in a story, connecting and sequencing ideas in stories, and using visual and contextual cues to understand the story lines. These difficulties affect the child's ability to acquire knowledge about the world from reading books, magazines, and newspapers, leading to increased gaps in their knowledge base. School-age children with LLD exhibit difficulties writing well-formed and grammatically correct sentences. They have difficulty spelling and perform poorly on tasks that tap into letter–sound correspondence and phonological awareness. As in children with SLI, their difficulties may be manifested in one or more of the areas of language (i.e., content, form, or use).

If Robert, our 27-month-old late talker, were to continue exhibiting language impairments in the preschool years—as suggested by his prognosis—these deficits may persist into his school years, ultimately affecting other skills such as reading and writing. Although Josephine, our 22-month-old late bloomer, has a good prognosis for outgrowing her language delays, research suggests that slow development of language in the first few years of life may place children at risk for slower acquisition of a wide range of language-related skills (e.g., vocabulary, grammar, verbal memory, and reading comprehension) during the middle school years and even into adolescence (Rescorla, 2002, 2005). Despite performance within the normal range on most language measures during the school-age years, late bloomers tend to score on the lower end of the distribution compared to their typically developing peers (Paul, 1996; Rescorla, 2002, 2005). Thus it is important to continue monitoring the development of language and related skills during the school-age years of children who were identified early on as late bloomers. Rescorla (2005) has suggested the delivery of services to these children may improve their language processing, phonological discrimination, verbal memory, and word retrieval, thereby preventing later language weakness.

Limitations in Language Form: Phonology, Morphology, and Syntax

Children with LLD, although usually intelligible, may have experienced phonological deficits as preschoolers. These subtle but often persistent phonological deficits may, in fact, underlie the reading difficulties exhibited during the school years. Such deficits are manifested in these children's poor performance on tasks that require phonological awareness. Phonological awareness is found to be a good predictor of reading ability and is an essential skill for the development of print literacy.

The language output of students with LLD can be characterized as syntactically simple and immature. These children produce fewer complex sentence structures and fewer embedded clauses than their typically developing peers (Marinellie, 2004). They use fewer modifiers (e.g., *Look at the tall, funny-looking clown*), prepositional phrases (e.g., *The car in the driveway is my father's*), embedded clauses (e.g., *The dress I bought last year does not fit me anymore*), and adverbs (e.g., *She ate her hamburger very quickly*). School-age children with LLD interpret passive structures based on the order of appearance of the subject and object in the sentence instead of relying on the meaning of passive forms. For example, children with LLD will interpret the sentence *The cat was chased by the dog* to mean "The cat chased the dog," instead of the other way around. They also exhibit difficulty with grammatical morphemes that are typically acquired later in development, such as comparatives (*small–smaller*) and superlatives (*smallest*), and advanced prefixes and suffixes (*unrelated, rewrite, disinterested, accomplishment,* and *madness*).

Limitation in Language Content: Semantics

The semantic difficulties exhibited by school-age children with LLD are apparent at the word level as well as at the sentence level. At the word level, these children present with a small vocabulary size that is restricted to high-frequency or short words with low phonological complexity. Their knowledge of word meanings is often restricted, revealing limited associations between words and poor categorization skills (Lahey & Edwards, 1999; McGregor, 1997; McGregor & Waxman, 1998; McGregor & Windsor, 1996). They also have difficulty in understanding the meaning of abstract words (e.g., *wonder, thought, postulate, ponder*) and using words that mark temporal relations (e.g., *next week, while, before*), spatial relations (e.g., *behind* and *above*), quantity (e.g., *more* and *a lot*), and order (e.g., *first* and *next*). Finally, school-age children with LLD may exhibit word-finding difficulties (Faust et al., 1997; German, 1987; McGregor & Leonard, 1989)—that is, the momentary inability to retrieve already known words from the lexicon. Their language is characterized by repetitions, substitutions, pauses, and use of non-specific words such as *thing* (Faust et al., 1997).

At the sentence level, school-age children with LLD exhibit difficulty in understanding complex verbal directions and explanations. They struggle to integrate meaning across sentences and paragraphs, revealing their limited ability to process semantic information. Children with LLD also reveal difficulty in understanding and producing figurative language and tend to interpret language literally. For example, a child with LLD may interpret a sentence such as *Break a leg* as an insult, assuming that someone really wants her to get hurt instead of wishing her good luck (Seidenberg & Bernstein, 1986).

Limitations in Language Use: Pragmatics

The limitations that school-age children with LLD exhibit are manifested in their use of language for communication, social development, peer relations, and classroom learning. In most cases, children with LLD have difficulty learning the rules of classroom discourse. They exhibit difficulties initiating conversations with their peers (Liiva & Cleave, 2005), clarifying miscommunications, maintaining the topic of conversations, noticing a shift in the topic of conversation and adjusting accordingly, and contributing relevant information to conversations (Paul, 2005). Due to their language and social difficulties, school-age children with language impairment are less likely to be addressed by their classroom peers and are more likely to have their initiations ignored (Hadley & Rice, 1991; Rice et al., 1991). They tend to experience fewer reciprocal relationships (Conti-Ramsden & Botting, 2004; Fujiki, Brinton, Hart, & Fitzgerald, 1999) and describe themselves as lonelier and less satisfied with their peer relationships compared to their typically developing classmates (Fujiki, Brinton, & Todd, 1996).

Furthermore, children with LLD have difficulty in narrative production. They use fewer cohesive ties (e.g., *after, because, while*) and often use them incorrectly (Liles, 1985a, 1985b, 1987; Ripich & Griffith, 1988). They use a less diverse vocabulary in narration (Paul & Smith, 1993), and their narratives are less informative, lack details, and are short with less overall organization (Scott & Windsor, 2000). In addition, these children have poor understanding of temporal and causal relations and have difficulty answering inferential questions that assess the relationships between the story parts (Merritt & Liles, 1987; Purcell & Liles, 1992).

Expository texts or textbooks present an even greater challenge for children with LLD (Bernstein & Levey, 2002). Expository texts usually contain information that is new to the reader, making it difficult or impossible for the reader to use prior knowledge to comprehend the text. Compared to narratives, textbooks provide very limited contextual support, have no known structure (i.e., the settings, the characters, the main event, and the consequences) to facilitate interpretation, and rely most heavily on children's ability to process linguistic information.

SECONDARY LANGUAGE IMPAIRMENT

Autism Spectrum Disorders

Autism spectrum disorder (ASD) is a childhood disorder involving deficits in social, communication, play, and verbal behavior that was first identified in 1943 by Leo Kanner, an American psychiatrist. Its prevalence in the United States is reported to be 3.4 per 1000 children, or almost 1 in 250 (Yeargin-Allsopp, Rice, Karapukar, Doernberg, Boyle, & Murphy, 2003). The onset of autism usually occurs prior to age three. Twin and familial studies suggest a genetic component as the etiological basis for autism. The disorder is classified as one of the pervasive developmental disorders (PDD), which also include Rett's disorder, childhood disintegrative disorder, Asperger's disorder, and pervasive developmental disorder—not otherwise specified (PDD-NOS).

According to the *Diagnostic and Statistical Manual of Mental Disorders*, Fourth Edition (*DSM-IV*; APA, 1994), the diagnostic criteria for autism are as follows:

1. Impairment in social interaction as manifested by at least two of the following behaviors:
   a. Impairment in the use of nonverbal behaviors such as eye contact, facial expression, body postures, and gestures to regulate social interaction
   b. A lack of spontaneous seeking to share enjoyment, interests, or achievements with other people characterized by a lack of showing, bringing, or pointing out objects of interest
   c. Failure to develop peer relationships appropriate to the child's developmental level.
   d. Lack of social or emotional reciprocity
2. Impairments in communication as manifested by at least one of the following behaviors:
   a. Delay in the development of spoken language or its complete absence with no attempt to compensate through alternative modes of communication such as gestures.
   b. In children developing speech, marked impairment in the ability to initiate or sustain a conversation with others
   c. Stereotyped and repetitive use of language or the use of idiosyncratic language
   d. Lack of varied, spontaneous pretend play or social imitative play appropriate to the child's developmental level.
3. Restricted repetitive and stereotyped patterns of behavior, interests, and activities, as manifested by at least one of the following behaviors:
   a. Preoccupation with one or more stereotyped and restricted patterns of interest that is abnormal either in intensity or focus
   b. Inflexible adherence to specific, nonfunctional routines or rituals
   c. Stereotyped and repetitive motor mannerisms such as hand or finger flapping or complex whole-body movements
   d. Persistent preoccupation with parts of objects

Associated conditions seen in children with autism include mild to profound mental retardation, hyperactivity, short attention span, impulsivity, aggression, and temper tantrums (APA, 1994). Some children with autism may demonstrate over- or under-sensitivity to sensory input; they also may exhibit behaviors such as sensitivities to sounds, tastes, textures, and touch, or visual avoidance or tactile defensiveness. In addition to the atypical motor behaviors of hand flapping, spinning, and jumping, children with autism may experience difficulties in motor planning, manipulation, balance, and coordination. These difficulties are apparent in activities such as speaking, writing, dressing, playing with toys, toilet training, and adapting to changes in routine or environments (Prelock, Dennis, & Edelman, 2006).

The language deficits exhibited by children with autism are not limited to pragmatics. Children with autism may also show evidence of deficits in semantics. Their language is very concrete, lacking abstract thinking. They tend to interpret language literally and lack the understanding of figurative language. Such children also exhibit difficulties with verbal reasoning and problem solving as well. Nonmeaningful, *echolalic speech*—that is, the immediate or delayed imitation of others' speech—occurs very frequently in children with autism disorder.

Recently, the *DSM-IV* (APA, 2000) distinguished between autism disorder and *pervasive developmental disorders not otherwise specified* (*PDD-NOS*), with the latter term being used to describe those children who appear to represent "atypical autism." A child diagnosed with PDD-NOS presents with a pervasive impairment in social interaction and communication skills or stereotyped patterns of behavior, interests, or activities that do not meet the criteria for autistic disorder because of late age at onset, atypical symptoms, or sub-threshold symptoms (APA, 2000).

Despite the existence of tools and checklists to diagnose autism, accurate diagnosis of the disorder remains challenging and relies heavily on clinical experience. Prelock and Contompasis (2006) have summarized some of the early indicators (i.e., "red flags") that can be used by clinicians to diagnose children with autism:

+ Poor social visual orientation and attention
+ Failure to point so as to express interest
+ The use of hand leading or another's body as a tool
+ Mouthing of objects excessively
+ Talking stops after using three or more meaningful words
+ Use of fewer than five meaningful words on a daily basis at age two years or lack of vocalizations with consonants
+ Failure to look at others or abnormal/inappropriate eye contact
+ Failure to show interest in other children, ignoring people, and a preference to be alone
+ Failure to orient to name or a delayed response to name, or lack of attention to voice
+ Lack of symbolic play and conventional play with a variety of toys
+ Unusual hand and finger mannerisms or repetitive movements
+ Aversion to social touch
+ Lack of expressive behaviors and gestures or the presentation of unusual behaviors

+ Failure to share enjoyment or interest
+ Failure to show objects, interest, or joint attention to games for pleasure or connection with others
+ Failure to spontaneously direct another's attention
+ Failure to show warm, joyful expressions with gaze; lack of emotional facial expression and social smile
+ Production of repetitive movements with objects
+ Unusual prosody
+ Failure to respond to contextual cues

Early identification of autism is key to the development of appropriate and effective intervention programs. Because communication deficits are the central feature of the disorder, speech-language pathologists are primarily the professionals treating children with autism. Nevertheless, a variety of other professionals—such as occupational therapists, psychologists, and *applied behavioral analysis (ABA)* therapists—provide important services to children with autism to facilitate their difficulties in other areas of development.

Mental Retardation

Mental retardation (MR) is a condition that is characterized by a significantly lower than average level of intellectual functioning and adaptive behavior. *Adaptive behavior* refers to the skills or abilities needed to live independently and function in one's community—for example, daily living skills (e.g., getting dressed, using the bathroom), communication skills (e.g., understanding spoken language, expressing ideas and thoughts), and social skills. Mental retardation is diagnosed by measuring the individual's intellectual capacity or functioning on an IQ test or by clinical judgment in the case of individuals who cannot take an IQ test. The Individuals with Disabilities Education Act (IDEA) defines mental retardation as "significantly subaverage general intellectual functioning, existing concurrently with deficits in adaptive behavior and manifested during the developmental period, that adversely affects a child's educational performance" [34 *Code of Federal Regulations* §300.7(c)(6)].

According to the *DSM-IV* (APA, 1994), to be diagnosed as having mental retardation, an individual must manifest deficits in at least two of the following areas: communication, health, leisure time, safety, school, self-care, social, taking care of a home, and work. In addition, the onset of impairment must occur before the age of 18 years. An IQ score of at least two standard deviations below the mean signifies the presence of mental retardation. The average IQ score in the normal population is 100, and the standard deviation equals 15; thus an IQ score of 70 or less suggests the existence of mental retardation.

Four degrees of mental retardation are distinguished:

+ Mild: IQ ranging from 50 to70. Approximately 85% of individuals who have mental retardation fall into this category.
+ Moderate: IQ ranging from 35 to 50. Approximately 10% of individuals who have mental retardation fall into this category.
+ Severe: IQ ranging from 20 to 35. Approximately 3–4% of individuals who have mental retardation fall into this category.
+ Profound: IQ less than 20. Approximately 1–2% of individuals who have mental retardation fall into this category.

Many of the language characteristics of children with mental retardation are similar to those seen in children with primary language impairments. In particular, the former children present with deficits in both language comprehension and production, and they show delays in language form, content, and use. Their acquisition of words is much slower, and they exhibit a tendency to rely on concrete word meanings. They use shorter, less complex syntactic structures, with the acquisition of the sound system being protracted over time. The speech intelligibility of children with mental retardation may also be affected owing to involvement of facial traits such as a large protruding tongue and a small oral cavity, as in Down syndrome. For some children with mental retardation, the acquisition of speech and language poses such a challenge that the use of alternative and augmentative communication may be needed.

Among the most common causes of mental retardation are the following:

+ Genetic conditions. Mental retardation can be the result of abnormal genes inherited from parents, as in Fragile X Syndrome, or chromosomal changes, as in Down Syndrome.
+ Problems in fetus development during pregnancy. Mental retardation can be the result of maternal infections during pregnancy, such as rubella or cytomegalovirus (CMV), or the consumption of toxins or chemicals that are hazardous to the fetus, as in the case of Fetal Alcohol Syndrome (FAS).
+ Complications during pregnancy or delivery. Mental retardation can be the result of the fetus not receiving enough oxygen (i.e., anoxia), as in the case of cerebral palsy or the fetus being born premature.
+ Exposure to diseases such as measles and meningitis or to toxins and poisons such as lead and mercury
+ Environmental factors such as neglect, malnutrition, and sensory deprivation (as in the case of prolonged isolation or institutionalization). All of these factors can negatively affect the child's development and result in mental disability.

As in the case of primary language impairments, it is vital to provide remedial programs to children with secondary language deficits as early as possible to help them in overcoming their difficulties related to their speech, language, and communication disorders. Whereas primary language deficits are usually not being identified until the second year of life, secondary language deficits are often identified very early in the first year of life, as soon as the primary deficit (e.g., hearing loss, MR) is recognized. Thus children with secondary language deficits tend to receive speech and language services much earlier compared to children with primary language impairments. Assessment and intervention in these children need to take into account the primary deficit the child exhibits. For example, in the case of a child with MR, the child's mental age, rather than his chronological age, may guide decisions about the appropriate assessment tools and intervention strategies that should be used in the clinic. Similarly, in the case of a child with a hearing loss, other modes of communication (e.g., sign language, alternative and augmentative communication devices) may be used to target the child's language deficits.

The remainder of this chapter reviews the procedures most commonly used to assess the language of children with primary and secondary language deficits from toddlerhood to the school-age years. A review of the most common intervention strategies used by speech-language pathologists for treating children with language deficits follows.

ASSESSMENT PROCEDURES FOR CHILDREN WITH LANGUAGE IMPAIRMENTS

Early identification of children who present with language deficits is vital. A language evaluation, performed by a certified speech-language pathologist (SLP), should be the assessment method of choice when early signs of language impairment are present. The purpose of this kind of language evaluation is twofold: identification and diagnosis.

First, the SLP must either confirm or rule out the existence of language impairment. During the evaluation process, the child's language abilities are compared to norms gathered from age-matched children who are developing language in a typical fashion. This process is used to determine the eligibility of a child for speech and language services.

Next, following the identification process, the SLP diagnoses the child to understand the nature of the language difficulty and confirms the presence of a specific language disorder. The SLP needs to determine whether the language deficit is (1) primary, as in late talkers, preschoolers with SLI, and school-age children with LLD, or (2) secondary, resulting from other deficits (e.g., cognitive deficit, autism, hearing loss). During the course of making a diagnosis, the SLP gathers information about the child's strengths and weaknesses, her needs, the family's concerns and priorities, and the resources available to the child and her parents. Especially in the case of infants and toddlers, it is important to incorporate the caregivers in the evaluation process. It is also important to gather information from multiple sources—for example, pediatricians and other professionals working with the child, as well as other family members who frequently interact with the child and can provide information about her abilities. This information will eventually guide the selection of an intervention and ensure that the intervention will be carried out effectively.

In infants, language assessment and intervention are inseparable processes owing to the rapid rate of development that occurs during the first months of life. The two most commonly used models of communication assessment for very young children are the *traditional (developmental) approach* and the *dynamic approach*. The traditional or developmental approach to assessment relies almost exclusively on age expectations and normative data. It includes checklists of age-expected behaviors to which infants and toddlers are compared or measured against. The dynamic approach advocates for a more naturalistic approach to assessment, in which the SLP examines a child's language and communication skills in natural contexts. It involves the observation of the child in routine activities—for example, interacting with familiar people, manipulating objects, and playing with different toys alone and with others. Play-based assessment is an important component of the dynamic approach. It allows the SLP to collect information about a child's language and communication skills in play-oriented activities. In addition, it allows the SLP to determine the strategies that may optimally stimulate the child to communicate at higher developmental levels.

The evaluation of a preschooler or a school-age child with language deficits involves the use of standardized tests, criterion-referenced measures, or performance assessment procedures.

Standardized tests (also called *norm-referenced measures*) rank the child's abilities against the performance of age-matched children with typical language development. Norms, which summarize the average performance of children in a specific age group, are used to compare a child's score to the scores of his age-matched peers. This comparison allows the SLP to determine whether a child's score falls within the age-expected range or below it, suggesting the presence of language impairment. Obtaining scores on standardized tests is usually necessary to determine the child's eligibility for services. Most standardized tests consist of a set of subtests that are designed to measure various aspects of receptive and expressive language in one or more areas of language (i.e., phonology, syntax, morphology, semantics, and pragmatics). Subtests that require the child to manipulate objects or point to pictures usually measure receptive language skills, whereas subtests that require the child to imitate, complete, or formulate sentences, or provide descriptions, usually measure expressive language skills.

Although standardized tests are the most commonly used method for evaluating a child's language abilities and are often mandated by the board of education as well as other agencies to determine eligibility for speech and language services, they have several limitations. These tests are limited in the content and scope of what is being examined, usually devoting only a few items to assessment of each linguistic form. They provide a cursory overview of the child's linguistic abilities, which minimizes the SLP's ability to use the results to determine the appropriate intervention goals. Furthermore, most standardized tests do not focus on language use, social communicative skills, and play skills.

Criterion-referenced measures are nonstandardized tools that measure the child's language skills in terms of absolute level of mastery instead of comparing the child's skills to those of her age-matched peers so as to determine whether the child differs significantly from the norm. These measures provide more in-depth information about the child's performance in specific domains and, as such, are more appropriate for formulating intervention goals. As opposed to standardized tests, where the SLP evaluates the child's performance quantitatively by computing a standardized score, in criterion-referenced measures the SLP evaluates the child's responses qualitatively by looking for any missing forms that can be targeted in therapy. The results of a child's performance on criterion-referenced measures are summarized as pass/fail scores, percentages correct, or performance rates; these scores indicate the child's level of mastery of a specific linguistic form. For example, if a 5;4-year-old preschooler with language impairment produced the present progressive *-ing* form only 40% of the time, the SLP might target this form as a goal in therapy, with the expectation that the child will eventually reach a mastery level of 90% production.

Performance assessment procedures are methods by which the SLP evaluates a child's language knowledge, abilities, and achievements in a more naturalistic manner. One of the most common procedures is *language sampling*. Language sampling can be used to assess a child's strengths and weaknesses in all language areas: syntax and morpho-syntax (e.g., calculating MLU, examining the length and complexity of utterances), phonology (e.g., phonetic inventory, syllable structure complexity, and phonological processes), semantics (e.g., vocabulary size), and pragmatics (e.g., conversational skills, the use of gestures, maintenance of eye contact). Language sampling can also be used to establish treatment goals and to monitor progress in therapy or assess the effects of intervention by comparing the language samples pre- and post-intervention. Language sampling is performed while the child is engaged in free play with the SLP or the child's caregiver. Alternatively, it can be carried out in more structured situations using predictable contexts (i.e., scripts), which employ familiar toys/activities.

The assessment of *narratives* is another commonly used procedure in the evaluation of language abilities of preschool and school-age children with language impairments (Paul & Smith, 1993). In a narrative, all language components come together to form a cohesive, well-formulated, meaningful story. The analysis of narratives provides information about the child's morphological and syntactic abilities (Scott & Windsor, 2000), the child's ability to use cohesive devices (e.g., *because, after, if*) to relate meanings across sentences (Hesketh, 2004;

Liles, 1985a, 1985b, 1987; Liles, Duffy, Merritt, & Purcell, 1995), and his ability to organize and sequence the story's content in a meaningful way (Liles et al., 1995; Merritt & Liles, 1989; Scott & Windsor, 2000). Similar to the case with language sampling, the analysis of narratives provides a lot of information about a child's language. Narratives can be elicited from children by using sequencing cards, using wordless books, or having children describe routine events and personal experiences.

Another type of assessment that can be used to assess the language skills of preschoolers and school-age children is the *transdisciplinary play-based assessment* (Linder, 2005). This approach to assessment is advantageous in that it allows the assessment of not only language and communication skills, but also social–emotional, cognitive, and sensory–motor abilities. The assessment is implemented by a team that includes the parents and professionals from various disciplines (i.e., SLPs, occupational therapists, physical therapist, psychologist). The context of the assessment is play activities that vary depending on the child and the areas being evaluated. This approach is natural and follows the child's attentional needs. It is less stressful and demanding compared to other assessment tools (e.g., standardized tests), which makes it very useful when assessing the language abilities of children who demonstrate language impairments secondary to other disorders such as ASD or MR. Information gathered during play-based assessment is very useful in developing treatment goals and assessing treatment progress, especially in the areas of pragmatics and discourse, which standardized measures often neglect to assess.

School-age children with language impairments can also be evaluated using *curriculum-based language assessment*. These tools assess a child's ability to use language to learn classroom material (Paul, 2005) and include evaluations of a child's written work for the level of narrative development, grammaticality and complexity, use of diverse vocabulary, and use of figurative language.

Systematic observations may also be used to assess a child's pragmatic skills and ability to adhere to classroom discourse rules and expectations. The SLP can observe the child during classes to assess the demands that classroom activities place on the student and, in turn, the child's ability to handle and manage these demands.

INTERVENTION STRATEGIES FOR CHILDREN WITH LANGUAGE IMPAIRMENTS

Federal law (Part C of Disabilities Education Act [IDEA], 1997) requires that state must provide services to children younger than three years of age if they experience developmental delays, as measured by appropriate diagnostic instruments and procedures, in five areas of development: cognitive, physical, communication, social or emotional, and adaptive behavior. Such services must also be provided if the child has a diagnosed physical or mental condition that has a high probability of resulting in a developmental delay (Sec. 632 (5)).

Early language intervention often provides a means for toddlers with language delays to "catch up" to their typical language-developing peers (Leonard, 1998). Conversely, delayed intervention may lead to adverse academic outcomes later in a child's life. Continuing difficulties in reading comprehension, verbal memory, grammar, and vocabulary have been reported in late bloomers during adolescence (Rescorla, 2005). Studies indicate that many late bloomers who seemed to have "recovered" at age five years later demonstrate inferior performance on language tests when compared to their typically developing age-matched peers (Rescorla, 2002, 2005). Consequently, in cases where early formal intervention is not provided, it is recommended that caregivers expose their children to games and activities that strengthen their abilities in word retrieval, verbal working memory, phonological processing and discrimination, and grammatical processing to support their later academic learning (Rescorla, 2002).

Part H of the Education of the Handicapped Act (1990) requires the development of an *individual family service plan (IFSP)* for each family with an eligible child younger than the age of three years. It recommends the delivery of services in naturalistic environments (e.g., in the child's home or in childcare facilities). The IFSP includes information about the child's physical, cognitive, social, emotional, and communicative development, as well as the child's family and its resources, concerns, and priorities. The plan also provides information about the services needed for the child, their frequency and intensity, and the expected outcomes.

The *Individuals with Disabilities Education Act (IDEA)* requires states to provide all children with a free, appropriate public education. When a school-age child is diagnosed with a language learning disability, the school personnel and the child's parents meet to develop an *individualized education plan (IEP)* that describes the child's strengths and weaknesses, the goals and objectives for therapy, the type of services the child needs, and the amount of time each week that services will be provided. The IEP team must reconvene yearly to review the child's IEP and eligibility for special education services.

Once a child is diagnosed as having a language impairment, the selection of intervention goals and strategies in therapy is guided by the information obtained in the assessment described earlier in this chapter. The goal of early intervention with infants and toddlers is the development of those basic skills that are critical to ongoing language learning. The speech-language assessment is the foundation of intervention planning for infants and toddlers. Intervention may focus on habilitating functional and symbolic play skills, functional and symbolic gestures, production of communicative intents such as initiating conversation, language comprehension, and production of sounds, words, and word combinations (Paul, 2005). The SLP can use the following guidelines when making intervention decisions with young children exhibiting language delays/impairments:

- Examine the frequency with which the child initiates and responds to the communication attempts of others.

+ Examine the variety and frequency of communication attempts (e.g., requesting, protesting, calling, greeting, and showing off) and comments the child makes about objects and events in her environment.
+ Examine the frequency with which the child uses communicative gestures (e.g., giving, showing, reaching, pointing, waving, and nodding).
+ Look for the production of babbling, sequences of consonants and vowels, words, and two-word combinations in an attempt to communicate with others.
+ Examine the child's ability to use eye contact and facial expressions to signal intentions.
+ Examine the child's ability to understand and produce words and sentences.
+ Examine the child's ability to engage in symbolic play.

Preschoolers with language disorders are at risk for developing academic problems as a result of their language difficulties (Catts, 1993; Catts, Fey, Tomblin, & Zhang, 2002; Schuele, 2004; Snowling, Bishop, & Stothard, 2000). The academic challenge most often observed in school-age children with language disorders is the ability to learn to read and write. Exposing preschoolers with language impairments to literacy activities may facilitate the development of literacy. Early literacy activities that may be incorporated into therapy sessions include phonological awareness activities and joint story reading.

Phonological awareness activities include exercises such as sound play tasks, segmentation, blending, and sound manipulation tasks. *Phonological awareness* refers to the explicit awareness that words in the language are composed of syllables and phonemes (i.e., consonants and vowels) (Catts, 1991), and that words can rhyme or begin with the same sound. Preschoolers can demonstrate phonological awareness by tapping syllables (i.e., segmenting multisyllabic words into their syllable components) and by recognizing and producing rhymes.

Joint story reading supports a child's communication and literacy development (Fey, Catts, & Larrivee, 1995). Books selected should be language and age appropriate, highly repetitive, and predictable in both form and content. The SLP should stop periodically to ask the child inferential questions about the story using *wh*-questions (e.g., *why, where, who, when, what*) and expand on the child's descriptions, introducing new linguistic forms. The story should be read to the child multiple times, having the child take turns telling parts of the story.

Language intervention with school-age children can be provided by the SLP on an individual basis or in small groups outside the classroom; this method of service delivery is referred to as *pull out*. To facilitate the child's participation in classroom activities, the SLP may also provide the therapy in the classroom; this method of service delivery is referred to as *push in*. Some of the general strategies SLPs can use to facilitate language in the classroom include simplifying questions in form (using simple sentence structures) and in meaning; simplifying verbal directions by shortening them, using simpler syntactic forms, and using visual cues to facilitate auditory processing; providing the child with extra time to process information; and repeating and/or reformulating questions and directions before concluding a failure on the child's part to execute a direction. Redundancy is crucial and improves comprehension in children with language impairments. It is also important to provide children with cues and additional instructions, teach them how to outline and mark key points in a story or an expository text so that they are able to draw conclusions and inferences about what was read, and provide positive reinforcement for any verbal attempt at class discussion to encourage more participation.

Many facilitative techniques can be incorporated into therapy for children who exhibit language difficulties. These techniques can be used with children spanning in age from infancy to school age and can be modified according to the child's language abilities, his age, and the focus of the therapy. One of the most common techniques used in the clinic is *enhanced milieu teaching*. This intervention, which employs language-facilitating techniques in a naturalistic, conversation-like context (Kaiser, 2000; Kaiser & Hester, 1994), focuses on four types of teaching strategies:

- *Modeling:* a technique in which the targeted linguistic form/behavior is presented to the child by the SLP a naturalistic context.
- *Mand-model procedure:* a technique in which the SLP mands (explicitly directs the child, "Tell me what this is"), or provides the child with a choice ("Is the ball red or blue?") and then provides the child with the model.
- *Time delay procedure:* a technique in which the SLP anticipates the child's needs or desires and intentionally waits for the child to initiate.
- *Incidental teaching procedure:* a technique in which toys are strategically placed to elicit specific linguistic or communicative forms.

Other facilitative techniques that can be used in conjunction with the milieu teaching include *expansion* and *recasting*. These techniques are used when a child incorrectly produces a particular linguistic form; the SLP then reinforces the correct production of the linguistic form by repeating the child's utterance while adding the missing grammatical markers or lexical items (Camarata, Nelson, & Camarata, 1994; Nelson, Camarata, Welsh, Butkowsky, & Camarata, 1996). The difference between the two techniques is that in recasting, the SLP changes the type of utterance—for example, from a statement to a question—or changes the voice or the mood in which the utterance is being produced. In these techniques, the child is not required to respond. Both expansion and recasting are based on the premise that children will be bombarded with the correct linguistic form and will independently produce it when they are ready to do so.

Imitation, another technique used in the clinic, is considered to be less naturalistic than the previously described techniques (Connell, 1987; Haley, Camarata, & Nelson, 1994; Nelson et al., 1996). In the imitation procedure, the child receives a visual prompt (such as a picture or a toy) that provides her with an incentive to verbalize. The SLP then provides a verbal model and asks the child to imitate the target. The child's response is reinforced by verbal praise or by a token (Nelson et al., 1996).

The following exchange demonstrates the use of imitation, modeling, expansion and recasting:

SLP: Look at the girl. The girl is eating! (Modeling)
Child: Girl eat.
SLP: Yes, the girl is eating. (Expansion)
Child: eating.
SLP: The girl is eating, right? (Recasting)
SLP: Say: The girl is eating. (Imitation)

Another method used in the clinic to promote communication and language learning in children with language difficulties is *facilitative play*, also known as *indirect language stimulation*. In this intervention, language is facilitated by using toys or objects that draw the child's interest. It provides multiple opportunities for the child to map the nonlinguistic context onto words and sentences. The SLP arranges the environment such that opportunities for the child to provide target responses occur as a natural part of the play. The SLP may place the desired objects in front of the child and wait until the child initiates labeling, joint action, or eye contact signaling joint attention. The SLP may also purposefully hold back items, hide them, or place them out of reach to force the child to initiate a request. Another way to get the child to interact with and be responsive to the SLP's communicative attempts is by using objects inappropriately or in a funny way. For example, in a play activity of bedtime, the clinician may put the doll to sleep in the tub instead of in a bed just to draw the child's attention and elicit a reaction. While employing this method, the SLP can use self-talk and parallel talk to model language production. In *self-talk*, the SLP describes his or her own actions; in *parallel talk*, the SLP describes the child's actions.

Another method that employs play activities for language teaching is *scripted play*. During a scripted play routine, a child and the SLP enact a play routine based on common scripts with which the child is familiar (Olswang & Bain, 1991). These scripts can range from daily routines such as a morning routine (e.g., waking up, brushing teeth, eating breakfast), to special-occasion scripts (e.g., planning a birthday party). These routines offer conventionalized, predictable contexts in which the SLP can teach turn-taking, conversational skills, new linguistic forms such as vocabulary, grammatical morphology (such as verb tensing), and higher-level functions such as planning and problem solving.

Focused stimulation is another method used in therapy. In this approach, the child is bombarded with the target form in a variety of contexts. The child is exposed to multiple exemplars of a specific linguistic target (e.g., a word, a morpheme) within meaningful communicative contexts. Following exposure, the child is provided with opportunities to produce the targeted linguistic form. The therapy session is arranged with materials that would encourage spontaneous productions of the target forms following the SLP's repeated models. Imitation is not used in this approach; instead, an attempt is made to elicit spontaneous productions of the target form by using naturalistic conversational contexts. This intervention can be used to target form, content, or use and is typically used with toddlers with early language delays (late talkers) and preschool and early-school-age children with language impairments.

SUMMARY

A child's language abilities are the foundation for social and communication success as well as school achievement. Therefore, early identification of children with language impairments and early implementation of language services are vital. The speech-language pathologist plays an important role in the identification of these children and the delivery of remedial programs to them. This chapter discussed the characteristics of primary language impairments in toddlers (i.e., late bloomers and late talkers), preschoolers (i.e., SLI) and school-age children (i.e., LLD), as well as the characteristics of secondary language deficits characteristic of children with MR and ASD. Speech-language pathologists use a variety of assessment methods to evaluate the language of children with primary and secondary language deficits. The information gathered by the speech-language pathologist using the assessment tools is then used to devise intervention plans for supporting communication in infants, toddlers, preschoolers, and school-age children.

Although the characteristics, assessment, and intervention procedures discussed in this chapter focused mainly on primary language impairments such as late talkers and late bloomers, children with SLI, and children with LLD, the strategies outlined are also effective with children with language impairments that occur secondary to another condition, such as children with ASD or MR. These strategies may need to be slightly modified to accommodate the specific deficits or special needs of a child with secondary language impairments.

KEY TERMS

Applied behavioral analysis (ABA)

Autism spectrum disorder (ASD)

Criterion-referenced tests

Curriculum-based language assessment

Dynamic approach to assessment

Expansion

Facilitative play (indirect language stimulation)

Focused stimulation

Imitation

Incidental teaching procedure

Individual family service plan (IFSP)

Individualized education plan (IEP)

Individuals with Disabilities Education Act (IDEA)

Language delay

Language deviance

Language difference

Language disability

Language disorder

Language learning disability (LLD)

Late bloomers

Late talkers

Learning disability

Mand-model procedure

Mental retardation (MR)

Modeling

Parallel talk

Performance assessment procedures

Pervasive developmental disorder not otherwise specified (PDD-NOS)

Phonological awareness

Primary language impairment

Pull out

Push in

Recasting

Scripted play

Secondary language impairment

Self-talk

Specific language impairment (SLI)

Standardized test (norm-referenced measures)

Time delay procedure

Traditional (developmental) approach to assessment

Transdisciplinary play-based assessment

Word-finding difficulty

STUDY QUESTIONS

+ Define the following terms and discuss the differences between them: language impairment, language delay, language deviance, and language difference.
+ What are the two clinical markers that can help differentiate between late bloomers and late talkers? How do they come into play in the two case studies of Josephine and Robert?
+ Describe some of the limitations preschool children with primary language impairments exhibit in language form, content, and use.
+ Our late talker, Robert, is now in first grade and his language skills need to be reevaluated to devise more appropriate school-related intervention goals. What are some of the assessment tools/methods you might use to evaluate his language?
+ Describe some of the characteristics of children with autism spectrum disorder and explain how they may guide your decision regarding the most appropriate assessment and intervention tools/strategies for use with these children.

REFERENCES

Acredolo, L., & Goodwyn, S. (1988). Symbolic gesturing in normal infants. *Human Development, 28,* 40–49.

American Psychiatric Association (APA). (1994). *Diagnostic and statistical manual of mental disorders,* 4th ed. Washington, DC: Author.

American Psychiatric Association (APA). (2000). *Diagnostic and statistical manual of mental disorders* (text revision). Washington, DC: Author.

American Speech-Language-Hearing Association (1993). Definitions of conmunication disorders and variations. Rockville, MD: American Speech-Language-Hearing Association.

Bates, E., Bretherton, I., & Snyder, L. (1988). *From first words to grammar: Individual differences and dissociable mechanisms*. Cambridge, UK: Cambridge University Press.

Bedore, L., & Leonard, L. (1998). Specific language impairment and grammatical morphology: A discriminant function analysis. *Journal of Speech, Language, and Hearing Research, 41*, 1185–1192.

Bernstein, D., & Levey, S. (2002). Language development: A review. In D. K. Bernstein & E. Tiegerman-Farber (Eds.), *Language and communication disorders in children*, 5th ed. (pp. 28–94). Boston: Allyn & Bacon/Pearson Education.

Bernstein, D. and Seiger-Gardner, L. (in press). *An introduction to early childhood special education: Strategies and practices*. Upper Saddle River, NJ: Pearson Education.

Brown, R. (1973). *A first language, the early stages*. Cambridge, MA: Harvard University Press.

Camarata, S., Nelson, K., & Camarata, M. (1994). Comparison of conversational-recasting and imitative procedures for training grammatical structures in children with specific language impairment. *Journal of Speech and Hearing Research, 37*, 1414–1423.

Capirci, O., Iverson, J., Pizzuto, E., & Volterra, V. (1996). Gestures and words during the transition to two-word speech. *Journal of Child Language, 23*, 645–673.

Capone, N., & McGregor, K. (2004). Gesture development a review for clinical and research practices. *Journal of Speech, Language, and Hearing Research, 47*, 173–186.

Caselli, M. (1990). Communicative gestures and first words. In Volterra, V. & C. Erting (Eds.), *From gesture to sign in hearing and deaf children* (pp. 56–67). New York: Springer-Verlag.

Catts, H. W. (1991). Facilitating phonological awareness: Role of speech-language pathologists. *Language, Speech, and Hearing Services in Schools, 22*, 196–203.

Catts, H. W. (1993). The relation between speech-language impairments and reading disabilities. *Journal of Speech and Hearing Research, 36*, 948–958.

Catts, H. W., Fey, M. E., Tomblin, J. B., & Zhang, X. (2002). A longitudinal investigation of reading outcomes in children with language impairments. *Journal of Speech, Language, and Hearing Research, 45*, 1142–1157.

Connell, P. (1987). An effect of modeling and imitation teaching procedures on children with and without specific language impairment. *Journal of Speech and Hearing Research, 30*, 105–113.

Conti-Ramsden, G., & Botting, N. (2004). Social difficulties and victimization in children with SLI at 11 years of age. *Journal of Speech, Language, and Hearing Research, 47*, 145–161.

Conti-Ramsden, G., & Jones, M. (1997). Verb use in specific language impairment. *Journal of Speech, Language, and Hearing Research, 40*, 1298–1313.

Education of the Handicapped Act of 1990, PL 101–476.

Faust, M., Dimitrovsky, L., & Davidi, S. (1997). Naming difficulties in language-disabled children: Preliminary findings with the application of the tip-of-the-tongue paradigm. *Journal of Speech, Language, and Hearing Research, 40*, 1037–1047.

Fazio, B. B. (1997). Learning a new poem: Memory for connected speech and phonological awareness in low-income children with and without specific language impairment. *Journal of Speech, Language, and Hearing Research, 40*, 1285–1297.

Fey, M. (1986). *Language intervention with young children*. San Diego, CA: College-Hill Press.

Fey, M., Catts, H., & Larrivee, L. (1995). Preparing preschoolers for the academic and social challenges of school. In M. Fey, J. Windsor, & S. Warren (Eds.), *Language intervention: Preschool through the elementary years* (pp. 3–37). Baltimore: Paul H. Brookes.

Fujiki, M., Brinton, B., Hart, C.H., & Fitzgerald, A.H. (1999). Peer acceptance and friendship in children with specific language impairment. *Topics in Language Disorders, 19*(2), 49–69.

Fujiki, M., Brinton, B., & Sonnenberg, E. A. (1990). Repair of overlapping speech in the conversations of specifically language-impaired and normally developing children. *Applied Psycholinguistics, 11,* 201–215.

Fujiki, M., Brinton, B., & Todd, C. M. (1996). Social skills of children with specific language impairment. *Language, Speech , and Hearing Services in Schools, 27,* 195–201.

German, D. J. (1987). Spontaneous language profiles of children with word-finding problems. *Language, Speech, and Hearing Services in Schools, 18,* 217–230.

German, D. J., & Simon, E. (1991). Analysis of children's word-finding skills in discourse. *Journal of Speech and Hearing Research, 34,* 309–316.

Hadley, P. A., & Rice, M. L. (1991). Conversational responsiveness of speech- and language-impaired preschoolers. *Journal of Speech and Hearing Research, 34,* 1308–1317.

Haley, K., Camarata, S., & Nelson, K. (1994). Social valence in children with specific language impairment during imitation-based and conversation-based language intervention. *Journal of Speech and Hearing Research, 37,* 378–388.

Hesketh, A. (2004). Grammatical performance of children with language disorder on structured elicitation and narrative tasks. *Clinical Linguistics and Phonetics, 18,* 161–182.

Individuals with Disabilities Education Act [IDEA] of 1997, PL 101–336.

Kaiser, A. (2000). Teaching functional communication skills. In M. E. Snell & F. Brown (Eds.), *Instruction of students with severe disabilities,* 5th ed. (pp. 453–492). Upper Saddle River, NJ: Merrill/Prentice-Hall.

Kaiser, A. P., & Hester, P. P. (1994). Generalized effects of enhanced milieu teaching. *Journal of Speech and Hearing Research, 37,* 1320–1340.

Lahey, M., & Edwards, J. (1999). Naming errors of children with specific language impairment. *Journal of Speech, Language, and Hearing Research, 42,* 195–205.

Leonard, L. (1998). *Children with specific language impairment.* Cambridge, MA: MIT Press.

Leonard, L., Eyer, J., Bedore, L., & Grela, B. (1997). Three accounts of the grammatical morpheme difficulties of English-speaking children with specific language impairment. *Journal of Speech, Language, and Hearing Research, 40,* 741–753.

Liiva, C. A., & Cleave, P. (2005). Roles of initiation and responsiveness in access and participation for children with specific language impairment. *Journal of Speech, Language, and Hearing Research, 48,* 868–883.

Liles, B. Z. (1985a). Narrative ability in normal and language disordered children. *Journal of Speech and Hearing Research, 28,* 123–133.

Liles, B. Z. (1985b). Production and comprehension of narrative discourse in normal and language disordered children. *Journal of Communication Disorders, 18,* 409–427.

Liles, B. Z. (1987). Episode organization and cohesive conjunctives in narratives of children with and without language disorders. *Journal of Speech and Hearing Research, 30,* 185–196.

Liles, B. Z., Duffy, R. J., Merritt, D. D., & Purcell, S. L. (1995). Measurement of narrative discourse ability in children with language disorders. *Journal of Speech and Hearing Research, 38,* 415–425.

Linder, T. W. (2005). *Transdisciplinary play-based assessment: A functional approach to working with young children* (revised). Baltimore: Brookes.

McGregor, K. K. (1997). The nature of word-finding errors of preschoolers with and without word finding deficits. *Journal of Speech and Hearing Research, 40,* 1232–1244.

McGregor, K. K., & Leonard, L. B. (1989). Facilitating word-finding skills of language- impaired children. *Journal of Speech and Hearing Disorders, 54,* 141–147.

McGregor, K. K., & Waxman, S. R. (1998). Object naming at multiple hierarchical levels: A comparison of preschoolers with and without word-finding deficits. *Journal of Child Language, 25*, 419–430.

McGregor, K. K., & Windsor, J. (1996). Effects of priming on the naming accuracy of preschoolers with word-finding deficits. *Journal of Speech and Hearing Research, 39*, 1048–1058.

Merritt, D. D., & Liles, B. Z. (1987). Story grammar ability in children with and without language disorder: Story generation, story retelling, and story comprehension. *Journal of Speech and Hearing Research, 30*, 539–552.

Merritt, D. D., & Liles, B. Z. (1989). Narrative analysis: Clinical applications of story generation and story retelling. *Journal of Speech and Hearing Disorders, 54*, 429–438.

Nelson, K. (1973). Structure and strategy in learning to talk. *Monographs of the Society for Research in Child Development, 38*, 1–2.

Nelson, K., Camarata, S., Welsh, J., Butkowsky, L., & Camarata, M. (1996). Effects of imitative and conversational recasting treatment on the acquisition of grammar in children with specific language impairment and younger language-normal children. *Journal of Speech, Language, and Hearing Research, 39*, 850–859.

Newbury, D. F., Bishop, D. V. M., & Monaco, A. P. (2005). Genetic influences on language impairment and phonological short-term memory. *Trends in Cognitive Sciences, 9*, 528–534.

Norbury, C. F., Bishop, D. V. M., & Briscoe, J. (2001). Production of English finite verb morphology: A comparison of SLI and mild–moderate hearing impairment. *Journal of Speech Language and Hearing Research, 44*, 165–178.

Olswang, L., & Bain, B. (1991). Intervention issues for toddlers with specific language impairments. *Topic in Language Disorders, 11*, 69–86.

Owens, R. (2005). *Language development: An introduction*, 6th ed. Boston: Allyn & Bacon.

Paul, R. (1991). Profiles of toddlers with slow expressive language growth. *Topics in Language Disorders, 11*, 1–13.

Paul, R. (1995). *Language disorders from infancy through adolescence: Assessment and intervention.* St. Louis, MO: Mosby-Year Book.

Paul, R. (1996). Clinical implications of the natural history of slow expressive language development. *American Journal of Speech-Language Pathology, 5*, 5–21.

Paul, R. (2001). *Language disorders from infancy through adolescence: Assessment and intervention.* St. Louis, MO: Mosby-Year Book.

Paul, R. (2005). *Language disorders from infancy through adolescence: Assessment and intervention.* St. Louis, MO: Mosby-Year Book.

Paul, R., & Alforde, S. (1993). Grammatical morpheme acquisition in 4-year-olds with normal, impaired, and late developing language. *Journal of Speech and Hearing Research, 36*, 1271–1275.

Paul, R., & Jennings, P. (1992). Phonological behavior in toddlers with slow expressive language development. *Journal of Speech and Hearing Research, 35*, 99–107.

Paul, R., & Smith, R. L. (1993). Narrative skills in 4-year-olds with normal, impaired, and late-developing language. *Journal of Speech and Hearing Research, 36*, 592–598.

Prelock, P. A., & Contompasis, S. H. (2006). Autism and related disorders: Trends in diagnosis and neurobiologic considerations. In *Autism spectrum disorders: Issues in assessment and intervention* (pp. 3–63). Austin, TX: Pro-Ed.

Prelock, P. A., Dennis, R. E., & Edelman, S. (2006). Sensory and motor considerations in the assessment of children with ASD. In *Autism spectrum disorders: Issues in assessment and intervention* (pp. 303–339). Austin, TX: Pro-Ed.

Purcell, S., & Liles, B. Z. (1992). Cohesion repairs in the narratives of normal-language and language-disordered school-age children. *Journal of Speech and Hearing Research, 35*, 354–362.

Rapin, I., & Wilson, B. (1978). Children with developmental language disability. Neurological aspects and assessment. In M. Wyke (Ed.), *Developmental dysphasia* (pp. 13–41). New York: Academic Press.

Rescorla, L. (1989). The language development survey: A screening tool for delayed language in toddlers. *Journal of Speech and Hearing Disorders, 54*, 587–599.

Rescorla, L. (2002). Language and reading outcomes to age 9 in late-talking toddlers. *Journal of Speech, Language, and Hearing Research, 45*, 360–371.

Rescorla, L. (2005). Age 13 language and reading outcomes in late-talking toddlers. *Journal of Speech, Language, and Hearing Research, 48*, 459–472.

Rescorla, L., & Lee, E. C. (2001). Language impairments in young children. In T. Layton & L. Watson (Eds.), *Handbook of early language impairment in children: Volume I: Nature* (pp. 1–55). Albany, NY: Delmar.

Rescorla, L., Mirak, J., & Singh, L. (2000). Vocabulary growth in late talkers: Lexical development from 2;0 to 3;0. *Journal of Child Language, 27*, 293–311.

Rescorla, L., & Ratner, N. B. (1996). Phonetic profiles of typically developing and language-delayed toddlers. *Journal of Speech and Hearing Research, 39*, 153–165.

Rescorla, L., & Roberts, J. (1997). Late-talkers at 2: Outcomes at age 3. *Journal of Speech and Hearing Research, 40*, 556–566.

Rescorla, L., & Roberts, J. (2002). Nominal versus verbal morpheme use in late talkers at ages 3 and 4. *Journal of Speech, Language, and Hearing Research, 45*, 1219–1231.

Rescorla, L., & Schwartz, E. (1990). Outcome of toddlers with expressive language delay. *Applied Psycholinguistics, 11*, 393–407.

Rice, M. L., & Bode, J. (1993). GAPs in the lexicon of children with specific language impairment. *First Language, 13*, 113–132.

Rice, M. L., Sell, M. A., & Hadley, P. A. (1991). Social interactions of speech and language impaired children. *Journal of Speech and Hearing Research, 34*, 1299–1307.

Rice, M. L., & Wexler, K. (1996). Toward tense as a clinical marker of specific language impairment in English-speaking children. *Journal of Speech and Hearing Research, 39*, 1239–1257.

Rice, M. L., Wexler, K., & Cleave, P. L. (1995). Specific language impairment as a period of extended optional infinitive. *Journal of Speech and Hearing Research, 38*, 850–863.

Ripich, D. N., & Griffith, P. L. (1988). Narrative abilities of children with learning disabilities and nondisabled children: Story structure, cohesion, and propositions. *Journal of Learning Disabilities, 21*(3), 165–173.

Roberts, J., Rescorla, L., Giroux, J., & Stevens, L. (1998). Phonological skills of children with specific expressive language impairment (SLI-E): Outcome at age 3. *Journal of Speech, Language, and Hearing Research, 41*, 374–384.

Schuele, C.M. (2004). The impact of developmental speech and language impairments on the acquisition of literacy skills. *Mental Retardation and Developmental Disabilities Research Reviews, 10*, 176–183.

Schuele, C. M., & Dykes, J. (2005). A longitudinal study of complex syntax development in a child with specific language impairment. *Clinical Linguistics and Phonetics, 19*, 295–318.

Schuele, C. M., & Tolbert, L. (2001). Omissions of obligatory relative markers in children with specific language impairment. *Clinical Linguistics and Phonetics, 15*, 257–274.

Scott, C. M., & Windsor, J. (2000). General language performance measures in spoken and written narrative and expository discourse of school-age children with language learning disabilities. *Journal of Speech, Language, and Hearing Research, 43*, 324–339.

Seidenberg, P., & Bernstein, D. (1986). The comprehension of similes and metaphors by learning disabled and nonlearning disabled children. *Language, Speech, and Hearing Services in Schools, 17,* 219–229.

Snowling, M., Bishop, D.V.M., & Stothard, S.E. (2000). Is preschool language impairment a risk factor for dyslexia in adolescence? *Journal of Child Psychology and Psychiatry, 41,* 587–600.

Thal, D. J., Reilly, J., Seibert, L., Jeffries, R., & Fenson, J. (2004). Language development in children at risk for language impairment: Cross-population comparisons. *Brain & Language, 88,* 167–179.

Thal, D., & Tobias, S. (1992). Communicative gestures in children with delayed onset of oral expressive vocabulary. *Journal of Speech and Hearing Research, 35,* 1281–1289.

Thal, D., Tobias, S., & Morrison, D. (1991). Language and gesture in late talkers: A 1-year follow-up. *Journal of Speech and Hearing Research, 34,* 604–612.

Thordardottir, E. T., & Ellis Weismer, S. (2001). High frequency verbs and verb diversity in the spontaneous speech of school-age children with specific language impairment. *International Journal of Language and Communication Disorders, 36,* 221–244.

Watkins, R. V., Kelly, D. J., Harbers, H. M., & Hollis, W. (1995). Measuring children's lexical diversity: Differentiating typical and atypical learners. *Journal of Speech and Hearing Research, 39,* 1349–1355.

Watt, N., Wetherby, A., & Shumway, S. (2006). Prelinguistic predictors of language outcome at 3 years of age. *Journal of Speech, Language, and Hearing Research, 49,* 1224–1237.

Whitehurst, G., & Fischel, J. (1994). Practitioner review: Early developmental language delay: What, if anything, should the clinician do about it? *Journal of Child Psychology and Psychiatry, 35,* 613–648.

Windfuhr, K., Faragher, B., & Conti-Ramsden, G. (2002). Lexical learning skills in young children with specific language impairment (SLI). *International Journal of Language and Communication Disorders, 37,* 415–432.

Yeargin-Allsopp, M., Rice, C., Karapukar, T., Doernberg, N., Boyle, C., & Murphy, C. (2003). Prevalence of autism in a U.S. metropolitan area. *Journal of American Medical Association, 289,* 49–55.

CHAPTER 15

Communication Development in Children with Multiple Disabilities: The Role of Augmentative and Alternative Communication

Melissa A. Cheslock, MS, Andrea Barton-Hulsey, MA, Rose A. Sevcik, PhD, and Mary Ann Romski, PhD

OBJECTIVES

- Describe the communication profiles of children with multiple disabilities.
- Explain the role of augmentative and alternative communication (AAC) in communication development.
- Explain the components of an AAC system.
- Discuss the challenges that children with multiple disabilities face when using AAC.
- Discuss the foundations of augmented language intervention and assessment.

INTRODUCTION

The inability to speak, or the inability to communicate one's own words fluently, is the greatest disability a person can have in the social circle of life...

—Tony Diamanti, "Get to Know Me" (2000)

Communication is the very essence of human life. It forms the foundation for everyday learning, social relationships with friends and family, and participation in familial and societal events. Put simply, it affects quality of life for all individuals. Children with multiple disabilities who have difficulty learning to communicate effectively often lack the same opportunities for participation that same-aged children without disabilities are offered. They also face challenges in the form of social and educational isolation and significant frustration because they are unable to adequately convey their necessities, desires, knowledge, and emotions to their parents, siblings, extended family members, peers, friends, and teachers (Romski & Sevcik, 2005).

It is the philosophy of the National Joint Committee (NJC) for the Communication Needs of Persons with Severe Disabilities (2002), as well as the authors of this chapter, that all children can and do communicate. Speech-language pathologists (SLPs) who interact with children with significant communication disabilities recognize these children's natural communication behaviors and seek ways to promote the functionality and effectiveness of their communication (NJC, 2002). Augmentative and alternative communication (AAC) is a multimodal intervention approach (Glennen, 2000) that uses forms of communication such as manual sign language, picture communication boards, and computerized/electronic devices that produce speech called speech-generating devices (SGDs), with the goal of maximizing the functional language and communication abilities of individuals who have severe communication impairments and little to no speech (ASHA, 2002). It incorporates their full communication abilities, including any existing vocalizations, gestures, sign language, pictures, and/or SGDs.

In this chapter, we describe the communicative development of children with multiple disabilities, and more specifically the role AAC can play in that development. The many challenges these children face on a daily basis are discussed, followed by a description of foundational principles necessary for the successful implementation of AAC as a means to navigate those challenges.

Multiple disabilities is a general term that indicates a combination of two or more impairments occurring at the same time and can apply to children with a broad range of impairment in cognitive development, expressive and receptive communication, and physical ability. Children with multiple disabilities may be born with a complex congenital disorder that hinders their development, or they may experience an acquired injury or illness early in life that substantially affects their development. While some children with multiple disabilities may need little to no support, most will require extensive supports to fully participate in daily life activities (e.g., social, educational, personal). Primary diagnoses for these children may include cerebral palsy, a specific genetic syndrome, intellectual disability, autism, or even a stroke at or near birth (Romski, Sevcik, & Forrest, 2001). Other concomitant impairments may include diagnoses such as seizure disorder, scoliosis, speech and language disorders, or sensory impairment. It is important to recognize that each child with multiple disabilities is unique in his individual communication patterns, motor ability, and cognitive ability.

Multiple factors must be considered when describing, assessing, or intervening in the communication development of children with multiple disabilities. *Communication* is defined as "any act by which one person gives to or receives from another person information about that person's needs, desires, perceptions, knowledge, or affective states" (NJC, 1992, p. 2). It includes speech as well as other forms of expression such as body gestures, eye gaze, symbols, and the printed word. Children with multiple disabilities may demonstrate one or any combination of difficulties with communication.

This chapter introduces three children with multiple disabilities—Sam, Amber, and Oscar—each of whom requires individualized and specific communication intervention and supports for his or her development. You will see that all of these children with multiple disabilities, regardless of the type and level of their individual impairment, can develop their communication.

COMMUNICATIVE PROFILES OF CHILDREN WITH MULTIPLE DISABILITIES_____

Sam

Sam is an 8-year-old boy whose multiple diagnoses include spastic quadriplegia cerebral palsy, cleft lip/palate, severe intellectual disability, and severe receptive and expressive language delay. He enjoys playing with toys and reading books, just like any other 8-year-old boy. Sam is severely physically limited. He is unable to walk and uses a wheelchair. He has difficulty initiating and terminating muscle activity throughout his body, including his legs, torso, arms, and facial muscles, due to his diagnosis of cerebral palsy.

Receptively, Sam is able to eye gaze to familiar named objects to show his comprehension of specific words and is reported to understand some words from a variety of categories, including words for animals, body parts, clothing, and food and drink; action words; descriptive words; words about time; and question words. His receptive language is difficult to characterize accurately using standardized assessments partially owing to his significant physical limitations; however, his abilities in this area have been estimated to be scattered across a developmental range of 16 to 32 months.

Although his receptive language skills are delayed, Sam is able to understand more than he is able to speak. He primarily communicates by pointing or reaching toward an item or picture of interest. He also uses focused eye gaze to communicate specific interest in one item over another when interacting with someone. Sam produces vocalizations consisting of mostly vowel sounds and few consonants to approximate less than 10 words for verbal communication.

Given Sam's limitations in terms of his current expressive and receptive communication skills, his learning and social development are at risk for being affected by his disabilities. Without effective communication skills, a child with multiple disabilities is unable to have a reciprocal conversation, share his knowledge, and improve upon his comprehension by asking further questions. (See **Appendix 15-A: Case Study 1** for more detailed information on Sam.)

Amber

Amber is a 12-year-old girl with moderate intellectual disability and delays in receptive and expressive language development with extreme word-finding difficulties. In addition to her intellectual disability and subsequent language deficits, Amber exhibits speech production deficits characterized by low oral motor tone, frequent drooling, articulation errors, and low volume. She uses vocalizations, limited single-word and two- to three-word phrases, gestures, facial expression, and pictures to communicate. Amber's immediate family understands her when she uses these communicative forms, but unfamiliar people and other communication partners rarely understand her.

Amber often has behavioral problems when at school. When she does not want to participate in classroom activities, she will often cry, vocalize strongly to protest the activity, or refuse to comply with activities presented to her by pushing away or throwing items she is given. Unlike Sam, Amber is able to walk and communicate through limited speech. Similar to Sam, Amber comprehends much more than she is able to expressively produce. (See **Appendix 15-B: Case Study 2** for more information on Amber.)

Oscar

Oscar is a 3-year, 10-month-old little boy who has a diagnosis of schizencephaly, a rare neurological disorder characterized by abnormal clefts in the cerebral hemispheres of the brain. His gross and fine motor development has been delayed as a result of his condition. Oscar is unable to walk independently and uses a wheelchair.

Oscar's play skills, social skills, and overall receptive language skills appear to be age appropriate as assessed through standardized language and vocabulary assessments and observations during play with his family. His cognitive, receptive language, and social abilities are areas of strength. In contrast, his motor limitations in producing expressive speech appear to be his greatest barrier to communication. Oscar uses mostly vowel sounds and some consonants to approximate short words that only close family members who are very familiar with him understand. He is rarely understood by anyone unfamiliar to him. He often uses focused eye gaze and pointing combined with vocalizations to expressively communicate. (See **Appendix 15-B: Case Study 3** for more information on Oscar.)

Constructing a Communicative Profile

For children like Sam, Amber, and Oscar, a thorough communicative profile must be constructed to fully understand the child's language development thus far, and to perceive how the child may continue to develop further communication skills. A *communicative profile* is a complete description of a child's strengths and needs in a variety of settings as related to the child's language comprehension and expression (e.g., vocabulary, grammar, social use of language), speech, oral–motor skills, and ability to communicate using nonconventional forms of communication such as gestures or sign language. Four factors that contribute to a child's unique communicative profile are the child's cognitive development, communicative experiences, vocal and gestural production skills, and comprehension skills (Romski, Sevcik, Hyatt, & Cheslock, 2002).

Cognitive Development

The cognitive skills of a child with multiple disabilities can vary from no evidence of intellectual and developmental disabilities to severe/profound intellectual and developmental disabilities. A child who exhibits an intellectual disability will have limitations in both intelligence and adaptive behavior skills. The *intelligence* of a child refers to her general mental capability and involves her ability to reason, plan, problem-solve, think abstractly, understand complex ideas, learn quickly, and generalize information from one context to another. *Adaptive behavior* refers to a child's conceptual (e.g., language understanding and use, money concepts), social (e.g., interpersonal skills, following community rules), and practical (e.g., eating, dressing) skills (Luckasson et al., 2002). Significant limitations in these skills affect the child's ability to fully function in everyday activities and routines.

Knowledge of where a child falls within this range of development affects where a child will begin along the continuum of communication intervention strategies. Nevertheless, cognitive development should never be the sole factor that determines whether a child actually receives intervention services (NJC, 2002). For example, Sam was diagnosed as having a severe intellectual disability, while Oscar was assessed as having no intellectual disability. Regardless of their differences in cognitive ability, both Sam and Oscar achieve success in improving in their communication development.

Communicative Experiences

The communicative experiences of a child with multiple disabilities are highly variable and will ultimately depend on factors such as the age of the child and his communication partners. Ideally, an older child will have had a greater number of opportunities for communicating, which may in turn positively affect his or her comprehension and production skills. For example, Amber, who is 12 years of age, is reported to make herself understood by her immediate family using limited verbal expression, facial expressions, and gestures. Through intervention, her family has learned to give Amber multiple opportunities to communicate in a variety of familial situations and then allow her the time needed to successfully respond communicatively. In contrast, Amber is rarely understood by unfamiliar communication partners, who typically limit their interactions with her owing to her unintelligibility. Amber's limited expressive communication ability reduces her opportunity to interact with new people and, therefore, constrains her ability to develop further communication skills in a variety of contexts.

Amber demonstrates how others' communicative interaction styles may ultimately affect a child's communicative experiences and profile. Among typically developing children, children whose parents are more responsive to their communication attempts have better language outcomes than children whose parents are less responsive (Baumwell, Tamis-LeMonda, & Bornstein, 1997; Snow, 1991). For children with disabilities, the literature suggests that a communication partner's communicative input tends to be different in quality and quantity than the input received by their typically developing peers. Specifically, input to children with disabilities may be more adult directed (Davis, Stroud, & Green, 1988; Girolametto, Weitzman, Wiigs, & Pearce, 1999) and less frequent in nature (Blackstone, 1997; Calculator, 1997). For children with multiple disabilities, their interaction with a variety of communication partners and in a variety of settings should be taken into consideration when identifying their strengths and areas of needed intervention for developing their communication.

Vocal and Gesture Ability

Children with multiple disabilities may have a wide range of vocalizations and gestures they use for producing communication. Many children with multiple disabilities are described as having extensive natural vocal skills, albeit being unintelligible, prior to the onset of intervention (Romski, Sevcik, Reumann, & Pate, 1989). Abbeduto (2003) reports that most children with multiple disabilities will develop functional spoken communication skills. The amount of functional spoken communication they develop will vary, however, based on factors such as cognitive development and/or underlying oral motor weakness or dysfunction. Some children with multiple disabilities will not develop functional spoken communication skills.

Sam, Amber, and Oscar provide examples of different levels of functional speech. Sam uses gross vowel sounds for vocalizations combined with occasional consonant sounds and focused eye gaze, and some gestures. The vowel sounds he uses are not easily discriminated and are not used to refer to a set of specific items. By comparison, Oscar uses mostly vowel sounds, with changes in intonation that refer to specific items. Amber uses two- to three-word short phrases combined with facial expression and gestures to communicate.

The differences in communication patterns across each individual child also vary greatly, such that not every child who lacks functional communication skills as a toddler will be nonspeaking into adolescence and adulthood. Amber, for example, did not begin speaking real words and word approximations until she was 3 years of age, and at age 12 uses two- to three-word phrases. It is important to remember that a child with multiple disabilities may have a changing vocal or gestural profile over the course of her development. This change over time should be monitored so that the intervention directed at that child's communication development can evolve accordingly.

Language Comprehension

Speech and language comprehension skills are also incorporated into the communicative profiles of children with multiple disabilities. Their comprehension may range from no or minimal comprehension to comprehension skills that are appropriate to their chronological age (Nelson, 1992). Children who do comprehend some speech show that they have knowledge about the relationship between words and their referents in the environment (Sevcik & Romski, 2002). Children who do not understand spoken words must establish conditional relationships between words or symbols to be learned and their real world referents.

As mentioned earlier, each child with multiple disabilities presents with a unique pattern of development that contributes to his or her overall communicative profile. There is no one specific course of communication development that children with multiple disabilities will follow. Each child's communication development reflects his or her stage of cognitive development, communication experiences, ability to vocalize and gesture, and language comprehension skills. Many of these children will be able to use functional speech for communication; however, for children who are unable to develop functional expressive speech, or who have difficulty using or understanding language, *augmentative and alternative communication* (AAC) may be used to successfully enhance their communication development (Beukelman & Mirenda, 2005; Goossens, 1989; Romski & Sevcik, 1996).

THE ROLE OF AUGMENTATIVE AND ALTERNATIVE COMMUNICATION IN LANGUAGE DEVELOPMENT

What Is AAC?

As mentioned at the beginning of this chapter, AAC is a multimodal intervention approach (Glennen, 2000) that uses forms of communication such as manual sign language, communication boards, or computerized/electronic devices that produce speech called *speech-generating devices* (*SGDs*) with the goal of maximizing the functional language and communication abilities of individuals who have severe communication impairments and little to no speech (ASHA, 2002). Communication boards and SGDs typically display pictures that represent what the child wants to say or express. When a specific picture is pressed on a SGD, it generates speech in a digitized (recorded) or synthesized (computerized) form for the communication partner to hear. AAC intervention approaches take into account a child's total communication abilities, including more conventional forms such as existing speech, vocalizations, gestures, facial expressions, body language, eye gazing, and/or posturing.

What Are the Components of an AAC System?

AAC does not comprise one single component, but rather is an integrated system of components, working in concert to provide the maximum amount of support needed for a child to fully communicate in all situations. The four primary components of an *AAC system* are aids, symbols, strategies, and techniques. A child's unique needs, skills, preferences, and learning characteristics, along with the family's preferences, concerns, resources and learning styles, should all be taken into account when developing an AAC system and intervention program (Hurth, Shaw, Izeman, Whaley, & Rogers, 1999; Paul, 2001). The following paragraphs describe the components of an AAC system for a child with multiple disabilities.

Aids or Modes of Communication

The first component of an AAC system is the mode of communication or the way in which an individual communicates. As previously defined, AAC is a multimodal intervention approach, encompassing all available communicative methods including behaviors, gestures, eye gaze, pictures, SGDs, written communication, or extant vocalizations or speech. The term *communication aid* itself is defined as "a device, whether electronic or non-electronic, that is used to transmit or receive messages" (ASHA, 2004). Aids can range from simple devices, such as a choice board with objects or pictures or a single-message SGD, to a very high technology, such as a SGD with multiple pictures and text capabilities. (The Web sites, http://www.augcominc.com and http://www.aactechconnect.com, provide extensive information on a variety of communication aids and vendors.) The modes or aids that a child uses to communicate with others at any given point in time will vary depending on a variety of factors and circumstances, such as the child's developmental abilities, child/family preference, and communication partners. For example, a child such as Sam with cerebral palsy and significant physical involvement may benefit from use of a SGD by directly pressing the pictures during morning activities, but due to physical fatigue may benefit from use of a communication board via eye gaze for afternoon activities.

Romski and Sevcik (1996) contend that the use of a SGD as a mode for communication may be more beneficial for children with multiple disabilities than are other modes such as sign language and picture boards alone, because the "voice" of a SGD allows a child to immediately be understood by communication partners. This aspect of SGDs is particularly important when children are integrated within the general community and need to interact with unfamiliar communicative partners. Research with individuals with severe disabilities who use SGDs (Schlosser, Belfiore, Nigam, Blischak, & Hetzroni, 1995) has also suggested that the synthetic speech of the SGD can contribute to more efficient learning of the pictures used to represent concepts and ideas.

Vocabulary and Symbols

The vocabulary available on an AAC system plays a vital role: It provides the foundation on which communicative interaction is built (Romski, Sevcik, Cheslock, & Barton, 2006). Regardless of the aid or mode of communication used, the child's communication partners identify what the child needs to say to achieve functional communication during daily activities and routines and then select appropriate vocabulary words to target in intervention. When possible, the child should also be given opportunities to indicate preferred vocabulary.

After the vocabulary targets are chosen, *symbols* are selected to represent the vocabulary. A variety of symbol types may be used with children with multiple disabilities, not limited to the modality of an SGD alone. Symbols can be unaided (e.g., signs, manual gestures, and facial expressions) when there is no need for any extrinsic support, or aided (e.g., actual objects, pictures, line drawings, and printed words) when the individual must rely on supports beyond those that are available naturally (ASHA, 2004). For example, when sign language is used as the mode of communication, vocabulary is represented through the use of manual signs (unaided). When a non-electronic communication board or an electronic SGD is used as the mode of communication, vocabulary is typically represented on the board or SGD in the form of visual-graphic symbols (aided). Children with visual impairments may benefit from the use of auditory symbols (aided) or tactile/textured symbols (aided).

A number of symbol sets are available for use, ranging from arbitrary to transparent (refer to the following websites for extensive examples of symbols and available symbol sets: http://www.augcominc.com and http://www.aactechconnect.com). *Arbitrary symbols* do not resemble the vocabulary they represent (e.g., printed words), whereas *transparent symbols* do resemble, in varying degrees, what they represent (e.g., a photograph of a concrete object). In clinical practice, easily depicted vocabulary items (e.g., nouns) are often chosen for children with cognitive and/or multiple disabilities, limiting their available vocabulary for communication interactions. The rationale underlying this decision is that these words are concrete and more easily learned than less easily depicted abstract words (e.g., verbs, adjectives, social-regulatives) (Rosmki et al., 2006). Research, however, has shown that when social-regulative symbols are placed on a SGD, children with cognitive disabilities can readily use them appropriately in context (Adamson, Romski, Deffebach, & Sevcik, 1992). Sevcik, Romski, and Wilkinson (1991) and Fuller and Lloyd (1997) provide further discussion regarding issues surrounding symbol representation and symbol set selection.

Young preliterate children with multiple disabilities who use AAC must rely on others to select vocabulary for them. For use of the AAC system to be successful, the targeted vocabulary should be meaningful, motivating, functional, and individualized (Fried-Oken & More, 1992). Individualized factors to consider include the child's age, gender, and experiences; developmental appropriateness of vocabulary; and child/family preferences. Vocabulary is identified by using various selection techniques (e.g., environmental inventories, standard word lists, and communication diaries) and involving multiple communication partners (Fallon, Light, & Paige, 2001; Morrow, Mirenda, Beukelman, & Yorkston, 1993).

Techniques

An *AAC technique* consists of the various ways in which messages can be transmitted (ASHA, 2004). Selection techniques can be classified into two broad categories: direct selection and scanning.

Direct selection allows the AAC user to communicate specific messages from a large set of options and includes techniques such as pointing, signing, gesturing, and touching. Some children with significant physical disabilities may benefit from the use of a head pointer or eye pointing (eye gaze) to select pictures or objects.

Scanning is a technique in which the messages are presented to the AAC user in a sequence by either a person or a SGD. The individual specifies his or her choice by responding "yes" or "no" to the person presenting the messages or by pressing a switch that is connected to the SGD. Scanning techniques include linear scanning, group-item scanning, directed scanning, and encoding (ASHA, 2004).

Strategies

The last, and perhaps the most important component, of an AAC system comprises the strategies used to implement the system. Strategies are specific ways in which AAC aids, symbols, and techniques are used to develop and/or enhance communication efficiency and effectiveness (e.g., language stimulation strategies, augmented input, aided language stimulation, communication-partner instruction, rate of communication enhancement strategies). A strategy includes the intervention plan for facilitating a child's ability to actively participate and communicate in all environments (ASHA, 2004).

How Does AAC Facilitate the Development of Children with Multiple Disabilities?

AAC can play many important roles in the language and communication development of a child with multiple and severe disabilities that may not be as obvious as providing an outlet for expressive communication. The roles will vary depending on each individual child's unique needs and abilities. AAC intervention can augment existing natural speech, provide a primary output mode for communication (i.e., expressive use), provide input and output modes for language and communication (i.e., understanding and expressive use), and serve as a language intervention strategy (Romski & Sevcik, 2005).

The most well-known role is to provide an expressive output mode for communication. For example, Oscar's attempts at speech are somewhat unintelligible to family members and highly unintelligible to everyone other than his family members owing to his diagnosis of schizencephaly and his oral–motor limitations for expressive communication. Oscar understands everything spoken to him—his understanding of language and cognitive abilities are within normal limits for his age. Oscar could use AAC as either a primary communication output mode or to supplement his existing speech in his interactions with family, teachers, and friends in a variety of settings.

The other roles of AAC interventions are also important, especially for a young child who is just beginning to develop communication skills. Consider Amber, who is 12 years old and has cognitive and language delays. She also has some challenging behaviors (i.e., tantrums, throwing) related to her communicative profile. Amber understands concrete words and concepts and has approximately 200 words in her expressive vocabulary. She is learning to use AAC in the form of activity-specific picture boards to indicate her wants and needs and to comment during daily activities and routines. AAC provides Amber with a visual system that (1) allows her to express what she already comprehends but may not be able to readily recall for communication and (2) facilitates her comprehension and learning of new vocabulary words. Amber's family and teachers also use the picture board and spoken words when communicating with her (aided language stimulation) to demonstrate an acceptable means of communication and to help Amber increase her understanding of unknown words by pairing them with pictures. In Amber's case, AAC serves very different roles than it did for Oscar, functioning as an input–output mode and a language intervention strategy. In this context, AAC interventions can be viewed as tools that foster the development of early language skills and set the stage for later vocabulary development regardless of whether the child eventually talks.

In addition to facilitation of language and communication development, AAC plays an important role in the social development and well-being of a child. The ability to communicate is paramount to being able to interact with others and to establish friendships and social closeness. In some cases, the content of the message being communicated is less important than the social interaction itself (Beukelman & Mirenda, 1992, p. 8). Sam, for example, has diagnoses of severe intellectual disability and spastic quadriplegia cerebral palsy. He attends regular education classes for portions of his school day. His understanding of language is significantly affected, as he understands names of familiar personal objects such as his favorite sunglasses and some of his favorite toys. Although Sam understands context-based directions such as "Let's go to the bus," he has more difficulty understanding nonconcrete vocabulary such as shapes, colors, and complex action and descriptive words. His expressive speech is limited to the production of vowel sounds, isolated consonant sounds, consonant–vowel (C-V) combinations, and a few C-V combinations that sound like words. At school, Sam's teachers programmed his

Step-by-Step SGD (Ablenet Company), one of the aids in his AAC system, so that Sam can tell age-appropriate jokes to his peers before class starts in the mornings. While Sam has difficulty fully understanding the complex language involved in telling jokes, the social interaction that ensues by making his peers laugh may facilitate further social initiation by Sam and his peers as well as further develop Sam's overall communication ability.

Continual advances in technology provide new opportunities for facilitating language and social learning for children with multiple disabilities. A young child does not need to have age-appropriate language comprehension abilities in place before initiating the use of technological AAC devices if one considers the range of devices available. In social situations, AAC can be a means to increase participation and interactions during daily activities and routines and to enhance intellectual credibility as perceived during social interactions with peers, friends, and family (Cheslock, Barton-Hulsey, Romski, & Sevcik, in press).

CHALLENGES FOR SUCCESSFUL AAC COMMUNICATION IN DEVELOPING LANGUAGE

For all individuals, communication forms the foundation for learning, social relationships, and participation in familial and societal events and affects quality of life. Children who have great difficulty learning to communicate face social and educational isolation as well as significant frustration because they are unable to adequately convey their necessities, desires, knowledge, and emotions to their parents, siblings, extended family members, peers, friends, and teachers (Romski & Sevcik, 2005). Children with multiple disabilities face many challenges in successfully accessing communication on a daily basis, whether it be natural or augmented communication. These challenges may be internal to the child and his or her disability characteristics, or they may be externally oriented, deriving from the child's environment and those providing communication supports. The challenges children with multiple disabilities face are often rooted in myths about the roles that AAC can play in their communication and language development instead of in empirical research. This section discusses these factors as they relate to communicative success, and particularly as they apply to AAC.

Internal Challenges

Medical Needs

Sustaining health and nutrition often do, and naturally should, take priority early on for children with multiple disabilities. Medical complications during infancy, surgeries during the toddler years, and chronic feeding difficulties often take precedence over communicative development and intervention and may be some reasons why there are delays in providing access to

AAC for very young children. After intervention with AAC is initiated, children with multiple disabilities may continue to have chronic medical needs requiring recurring hospitalizations and/or surgeries that interfere with consistent experience and practice with augmented communication. Progress may be slowed, but intervention should be continued.

Physical Ability

A wide variety of motoric difficulties present significant challenges for some children with multiple disabilities in physically accessing an AAC system. Motoric difficulties are often caused by injury to the parts of the brain that control our ability to use our muscles and bodies, as in the case of cerebral palsy; they can be mild, moderate, or severe. Their effects may be seen in one part of the body, such as the right arm, or they may be more widespread, affecting the arms, legs, torso, and facial muscles (see www.nichcy.org for a more in-depth discussion of motoric difficulties and presentation in children). Other diagnoses that may contribute to children's impairments in motor difficulty include Rett's syndrome, mitochondrial disorder, stroke, and traumatic brain injury.

Regardless of the motoric difficulty's etiology, motor function in a child is dependent on and influenced by multiple factors, including emotional state, level of arousal, comfort, motivation or attitude, attention, and understanding (Treviranus & Roberts, 2003). Certainly, these motor challenges can contribute to a child's ability to directly or indirectly access symbols on an AAC system. Nevertheless, these challenges should not be used as an excuse for failing to provide AAC to the child with physical disabilities. The National Joint Committee for the Communication Needs of Persons with Severe Disabilities (NJC, 2002) asserts that everyone has the right to access AAC technology (electronic or non-electronic) and states that physical ability or the lack thereof should not be used as a prerequisite to the implementation of AAC intervention. Accommodations using switches for scanning, head pointers, keyguards, and other specific modifications can all be used to ensure a child's most appropriate access to an AAC system (Campbell, Milbourne, & Wilcox, 2008).

When working with children who have motor difficulties, it is important to remember that complex interactions are involved in learning motor control for access to an AAC system. Continued practice with a consistent mode of access is often necessary for a child with significant motoric challenges to achieve his fullest ability in accessing AAC (Treviranus & Roberts, 2003).

Learned Helplessness

Some older children with multiple disabilities have a long history of being unable to successfully control their environment independently either physically or through communication (Beukelman & Mirenda, 2005). This lack of control over one's environment may lead to what is known as *learned helplessness*, an attitude of dependence on others to speak for the person and to make decisions for the individual.

Support teams working with children with multiple disabilities can provide an intervention plan to establish multiple opportunities for children and their caregivers or other communication partners to successfully communicate and participate in natural daily activities and routines. Technology such as adapted toys and adapted controls called *environmental controls* can be utilized to help the child interact with his or her environment where he or she was previously unable to interact (Beukelman & Mirenda, 2005; Campbell et al., 2008). Children with multiple disabilities can be taught early that they have a voice, and that their voice can influence their environment and the people around them. This understanding is important to their ability to advocate for themselves throughout their lives.

Challenging Behavior

Some children with severe multiple disabilities engage in *challenging behaviors*, such as biting, tantrums, screaming, task refusal, or self-injurious behaviors that constitute barriers to their receiving appropriate communication services, including AAC. For example, the child's behavior may present a barrier to her access of an appropriate AAC system if her service providers cannot resolve or do not know how to resolve the behaviors. In the case study, Amber's challenging behaviors have been cited in the past as a barrier to her access of an AAC system. Because Amber has some functional speech, her need for an AAC system to enhance her communication has been overlooked as her behaviors have escalated.

Many researchers view these challenging behaviors as a form of unconventional communication (Carr & Durand, 1985; Carr, Levin, McConnachie, Carlson, Kemp, & Smith, 1994; Durand & Merges, 2001) in which the child attempts to express wants and needs related to objects and activities (Sigafoos & Mirenda, 2002) or social interaction (Hunt, Alwell, & Goetz, 1988), to refuse objects/activities (Sigafoos, O'Reilly, Drasgow, & Reichle, 2002), or to indicate pain and discomfort. It is quite difficult and frustrating for clinicians, parents, and caregivers to interpret and manage such socially inappropriate behaviors. It is, therefore, important to determine and understand the underlying message or function that the problem behavior is serving. This goal can be achieved through a process known as *functional behavior assessment* (Bopp, Brown, & Mirenda, 2004), which should be conducted prior to determining appropriate intervention strategies. AAC is often included as an intervention strategy for children with challenging behaviors as it can replace their unacceptable forms of communication with more conventional forms (Romski & Sevcik, 2005).

Amber's behavior was determined to be caused partially by her difficulty in understanding verbal communication. AAC was then implemented as an input strategy to enable her to comprehend communication efforts directed at her; it was successful in reducing the amount of challenging behaviors she exhibits. Amber has also used AAC expressively to replace some of her challenging behaviors and better communicate her needs.

External Challenges

Attitudes and Lack of Knowledge

A number of negative attitudes influence the access of AAC to children with disabilities, most often resulting in low expectations and limited opportunities for these children's participation in activities in which children without disabilities readily participate (Beukelman & Mirenda, 2005). Professional and familial attitudes, philosophy, and beliefs about the use of AAC during the early childhood years continue to evolve, however. The literature supports the idea that even very young children with severe disabilities can use and benefit from AAC, specifically SGDs. Nevertheless, some SLPs continue to believe that AAC is a "last resort" measure, to be used only after intensive spoken language intervention has failed. Others believe that the use of an SGD will hinder the child's development of spoken language. Still others think that children must have a certain set of skills—such as the ability to point, identify pictures, or understand causal relationships—to use AAC. **Table 15-1** details a list of common myths and the reality behind each one as it relates to the use of AAC in language intervention.

The lack of knowledge about available AAC technology and the roles AAC can play in the life of a young child with severe communication difficulties poses great barriers to the child's participation and enhanced communication development.

Environmental Barriers

Environmental barriers may be locations in the community, school, and/or home that create physical segregation between the child and his ability to communicate using the AAC system effectively. Beukelman and Mirenda (2005) discuss space/location adaptations and physical structure adaptations of the environment that can be made to eliminate barriers. For example, Sam, who has a SGD mounted on his wheelchair, wants to participate in an art class activity but cannot because there is no accessible route for him to navigate his chair through the aisles of tables and chairs within the classroom while taking his SGD with him. A simple modification—rearranging the furniture—can allow Sam to easily enter the classroom with his SGD so that he can communicate during art class activities.

Opportunities for Participation

Beukelman and Mirenda (2005) indicate that the first step to increasing communication is to increase children's meaningful participation in natural activities and routines. Unfortunately, many children with multiple disabilities lack the same participation opportunities as their typically developing peers, both in school and through community activities. Because of motor and/or intellectual impairments, these children may be segregated from participation in activities such as baseball, dance classes, physical education at school, cooking activities, and art

TABLE 15-1 Myths and Realities in AAC Intervention	
Myth	**Reality**
AAC is a last resort in speech-language intervention.	AAC can play many roles in early communication development including the development of natural speech (Cress & Marvin, 2003; Reichle, Buekelman, & Light, 2002; Romski, Sevcik, Adamson, Cheslock, Smith, Barker, & Bakeman, in press).
AAC hinders or stops further speech development.	A number of empirical studies suggest that AAC actually improves speech skills and provides for greater gains in verbal speech development than does spoken intervention alone (Beukelman & Mirenda, 1998; Romski & Sevcik, 1996; Romski et al., in preparation).
Children must have a certain set of skills to benefit from AAC.	There is a continuum of AAC systems that can be used to develop language skills (NJC, 1992). Access to these systems is critical if the individual is expected to make cognitive gains. Early communication behaviors including spontaneous and nonintentional behaviors support the development of later symbolic communication (Siegel & Cress, 2002).
Speech-generating devices are only for children with intact cognition.	A broad range of speech-generating devices are available to use with children along the continuum of communication development. Children as young as two years of age with cognitive delays have been taught to use basic speech-generating devices for communication (Romski et al., in preparation).
Children have to be a certain age to benefit from AAC.	There is no evidence to support this myth. Infants, toddlers, and preschoolers with a variety of disabilities have benefited from the use of AAC (Cress, 2003; Romski, Sevcik, & Forrest, 2001; Romski et al., in preparation).
There is a representational hierarchy of symbols from objects to written words that children must master in sequence.	Namy, Campbell, and Tomasello (2004) have found that children as young as 13 to 18 months have been able to learn symbol–referent relationships regardless of the iconicity of the symbol. Preschool-age children with developmental disabilities have been able to learn symbol–referent relationships regardless of symbol iconicity (Barton, Sevcik, & Romski, 2006).

Source: Adapted from Romski and Sevcik (2005).

lessons. This lack of participation in natural activities is primarily attributable to lack of effort or knowledge on the part of these children's teachers, SLPs, or caregivers, who all too often do not find ways to engage them.

Sam, for example, is engaged in many activities at school, including music, art, computer time, lunch, and speech, physical, and occupational therapies. He is also involved in private therapies, frequently attends doctor appointments, and participates in church activities. One of his favorite daily activities is riding the bus to and from school. Because of his multiple diagnoses involving severe motor impairment and limited speech ability, Sam's participation and communication interaction with others would be significantly limited without the use of AAC technology. Sam requires others to acknowledge the need for him to continue participation in activities he enjoys and to successfully use and learn to use his AAC system. Without responsive communication partners in real environments at home, in school, and in the community, Sam would have no opportunity to communicate and thus learn communication.

Like Sam, many children with multiple disabilities encounter participation barriers in daily activities when those around them do not allow the appropriate modifications for their participation. To achieve full and optimal participation for children with disabilities, their natural environments and the communication opportunities within those environments should first be addressed through comprehensive AAC assessment or diagnostic intervention. Then intervention strategies, such as increasing opportunities for communication and using adaptive toys, SGDs, and environmental controls, can be implemented.

NAVIGATING THE CHALLENGES: FOUNDATIONS FOR IMPLEMENTATION OF AUGMENTED LANGUAGE INTERVENTION

Several foundational principles that address the previously discussed challenges must be acknowledged for the successful implementation of AAC with children with multiple disabilities. These principles are based on research, values and perspectives, policy, clinical knowledge of early language and communication development, and clinical expertise and can be used as guides in providing effective services and supports. **Table 15-2** summarizes the research base and provides a broad overview of practical strategies for implementation of foundational principles in using AAC to facilitate the communication and language development of children with multiple disabilities.

Philosophical Beliefs

Central to the SLP's ability to facilitate a child's ability to communicate within his or her environment is the philosophical belief that all children can and do communicate (NJC, 2002). While the effectiveness and efficiency of that communication may vary from child to child, communication inevitably begins at birth, starting with non-symbolic forms such as crying, vocalizations, facial expressions, eye gazing, or natural gestures, and then, as the child grows and develops, evolves into more symbolic forms, such as words, pictures, or sign language. In addition, some children with severe disabilities develop unconventional and socially inappropriate

TABLE 15-2   Practical strategies for implementation of AAC

Foundations	Research Bases	Strategies for Implementation
Philosophical beliefs	All children can and do communicate (www.asha.org/njc). Intervention with young children with multiple disabilities requires a collaborative service-delivery model (ASHA, 2008).	Read more information about these philosophies and working with children with multiple disabilities on the NJC Web site.
AAC assessment	Assessment is a critical component of AAC service delivery and provides the foundation for basing intervention decisions (Romski, Sevcik, Hyatt, & Cheslock, 2002). AAC assessment focuses on the AAC user, various communication partners, environments, and the AAC system (Beukelman & Mirenda, 2005; NJC, 1992; Peck, 1989; Seigel-Causey & Bashinski, 1997; Wasson, Arvidson, & Lloyd, 1997).	Conduct a comprehensive, team-based assessment to determine child's strengths and needs. Conduct diagnostic AAC intervention when needed.
Begin AAC intervention early	Children are likely to make the greatest gains when services begin early in development (Girolametto, Wiigs, Smyth, Weitzman, & Pearce, 2001). A number of empirical studies report increases in speech skills following AAC intervention (Beukelman & Mirenda, 2005).	Supplement early language and communication intervention with AAC strategies, as opposed to using AAC as a last resort.
Knowledge of language comprehension and production	For young children to develop functional language and communication skills, they must be able to comprehend and produce language so that they can take on the roles of both listener and speaker in conversational exchanges (Sevcik & Romski, 2002).	Integrate goals focused on language development, including comprehension, production, and literacy, into AAC intervention plans.

Systematic language-based instruction	Research has indicated successful outcomes for young children in AAC intervention integrated with existing naturalistic language interventions (Schepis, Reid, Behrmann, & Sutton, 1998; Yoder & Stone, 2006).	Systematically and consistently implement AAC strategies within existing language intervention. Establish functional, language-based goals.
Teaching through natural communicative activities and routines	Implementation of AAC in home and community (e.g., daycare center, local park) settings emphasizes functional language, facilitates generalization, and increases spontaneous communication (Romski et al., 2002).	Implement AAC into the child and family's existing routines and activities. Use the child's own toys, books, and personal items.
Communication-partner instruction and education	Education and training is a dynamic process of joint discoveries, problem solving, and guided practice (Buyse & Wesley, 2005). Training of AAC systems is essential to its long-term use; conversely, lack of training is associated with abandonment (Johnson, Inglebret, Jones & Ray, 2006; Smith, 2002).	Acknowledge the family's pre-existing knowledge, values, beliefs, perspectives, and experiences. Consider adult learning styles and provide materials and/or feedback appropriately (e.g., video feedback, Internet, books, articles, written instructions).
Ongoing monitoring	AAC intervention is a dynamic process; abilities change over time, albeit sometimes very slowly. The system for use at one age may need to be modified as a young child grows and develops (Beukelman & Mirenda, 2005). Continuous updating of AAC systems has been identified as a factor contributing to long-term use (Smith, 2002).	Regularly observe the child's participation in targeted daily routines and document abilities and needs. Establish formal and informal ways of gaining information from family members, such as journals, e-mails, and teleconferencing.

Source: Adapted from Cheslock, Romski, Sevcik, & Barton-Hulsey (2007).

means to communicate, including aggressive behaviors toward themselves or others. Speech-language pathologists who interact with individuals with severe disabilities must develop skills in recognizing all communication behaviors produced by those children and diligently seek ways to promote the effectiveness of their communication (NJC, 2002). Bopp, Brown, and Miranda (2004) identify a number of ways that SLPs can facilitate the communication of children with challenging behaviors, such as undertaking a thorough assessment of their communication abilities, designing visual schedules and picture boards/SGDs, selecting appropriate symbol representation for AAC systems, and implementing parent/caregiver instruction. The NJC also provides a series of frequently asked questions highlighting the fact that all children can and do communicate, indicating how to look for signs of that communication regardless of level and type of disability, and ultimately answering questions about the multiple issues revolving around AAC intervention (see www.asha.org/njc).

Successful implementation of AAC for children with multiple disabilities also requires a philosophical focus on collaborative service delivery models that embrace inclusive practices and services delivered in natural environments and focus on functional communication during the child and family's natural daily activities and routines (ASHA, 2008). Consistent and positive communicative interaction among the child's family, caregivers, teachers, and the SLP is an important factor in the provision of collaborative service delivery. This model is critical to the belief that children can learn language and communication skills in the natural environment with communication supports to bolster achievement (Romski, Sevcik, Cheslock, & Barton, 2006).

AAC Assessment

Assessment is a critical component of AAC service delivery and provides the foundation for making intervention decisions for all individuals who require AAC intervention. The focus of *AAC assessment* is typically not to determine the need for AAC but rather to explore the range of appropriate AAC strategies, adaptations, devices, and services that may help children fully participate in their environment and enhance their functional communication with a variety of communication partners within multiple environments (Romski et al., 2002).

AAC assessment is conducted within a comprehensive, team-based assessment framework, often in a variety of environments and with several team members providing essential information. A comprehensive AAC assessment includes assessment of the AAC user, various communication partners, environments, and the AAC system (Beukelman & Mirenda, 2005; NJC, 1992; Peck, 1989; Seigel-Causey & Bashinski, 1997; Wasson, Arvidson, & Lloyd, 1997). **Table 15-3** outlines these assessment areas in more detail. Because they have specialized knowledge of typical and atypical language, communication, cognitive, and early literacy devel-

TABLE 15-3   Comprehensive AAC Assessment Areas

I. Person Using AAC	II. Communication Partners
• Language comprehension • Language production • Cognitive abilities • Play behaviors • Motor functioning, including oral–motor development • Literacy skills • Sensory acuity and processing ability, including vision, hearing, and tactile skills • Motivation to communicate • Present communication needs • Future communication needs	• Identify critical partners in each of the child's daily environments • Measure communication opportunities and other acts that may or may not facilitate the communicative development of the child provided by identified partners • Assess the child's responses to the communication partners
III. Environments	**IV. AAC System**
• Identify multiple locations and activities the child attends • Identify opportunities for participation in those environments • Identify barriers or challenges to participation • Identify communication opportunities and needs within the environments • Identify communicative functions that may be useful in the identified environments	• Device(s) or aid(s) • Vocabulary • Symbols • Techniques used to access the system • Strategies for effective and efficient use • Ability of system to meet multiple communication needs of child • Cultural appropriateness of the system

Sources: NJC (1992) and Wasson, Arvidson, & Lloyd (1997).

opment, SLPs usually lead AAC assessment teams. Because of the depth of knowledge needed in so many developmental areas pertaining to the child, other team members also play crucial roles in the assessment, including the child, family, and other caregivers or family friends, as well as the physical therapist, occupational therapist, psychologist, teacher(s) and/or educational specialist, and medical doctor.

Because of the various motor, behavioral, or other developmental factors involved, making a valid determination of the developmental abilities of a child with multiple disabilities can be quite challenging. Information, however, is obtained using multiple methods, including standardized and nonstandardized tests, informal observations during authentic activities and routines (e.g., playtime, meals, story reading, diaper changing/toileting) with multiple communication partners (e.g., parents, grandparents, childcare workers, friends) within the child and family's natural environments, and family/caregiver questionnaires. Standardized and non-standardized tests can be useful for identifying specific developmental abilities, communicative strengths, and areas of need in a structured manner. Some children may benefit from standard-assessment adaptations, where permissible, to enhance their ability to understand and respond to test directives. When adapting a standardized assessment, the validity of norm-referenced scoring is reduced; even so, valuable information may be gained about the child's language ability in the process.

Table 15-4 lists some adaptation needs and methods that are often used with children having multiple disabilities so that a standardized assessment may be administered. Wasson, Arvidson, and Lloyd (1997) provide further details on test adaptation. Beukelman and Mirenda (2005) describe specific assessment tests that may be easily adapted for use with children with multiple and severe disabilities. Because the goal of AAC is to enhance an individual's functional communication and language abilities within his natural environment, observations and family/caregiver interviews may actually provide more valuable information than administration of tests (Blackstone, 1994). This information may, for example, support standardized and nonstandardized test information; provide qualitative information regarding everyday communicative strengths, opportunities, and needs; identify critical communication partners; and help determine internal and external challenges that affect the child's participation in play, cognitive, communication, physical, and self-help activities.

TABLE 15-4   Adapting Standardized Assessments

Adaptation Need	Method
Simplification of lengthy test instructions	Paraphrase the test instructions by using less complex directions that the child understands
Child needs consistent feedback to sustain performance	Give positive feedback instead of only neutral feedback, as most tests instruct
Physical adaptation: The child cannot physically point to a picture choice	Read the test question and then ask the child to give a yes/no response while you scan through the picture choices
	Picture choices may be placed in four corners of an eye-gaze board for the child to use eye gaze to make a choice
Testing material is too small	Enlarge the test materials manually and/or with color to meet the child's visual needs

Source: Adapted from Lloyd, Fuller, and Arvidson (1997).

Although the assessment provides a rationale for AAC service delivery to the specific child, it should not delay the beginning of intervention services in its absence. Some children may be on long waiting lists to receive an AAC assessment. For others, the extent of their disability and, therefore, their ability to participate in assessment activities may preclude the full completion of valid assessment in a more timely fashion. In these cases, *diagnostic intervention* may be warranted. Goossens (1989), for example, described a six-year-old child with cerebral palsy who participated in naturalistic augmented language intervention utilizing spoken language stimulation coupled with pictures, referred to as *aided language stimulation*. Because of the child's physical limitations and lack of spoken communication, her cognitive skills were originally estimated to be at a 16- to 20-month age level. After 7 months of intervention, the child developed a viable method of communication using AAC (i.e., eye gaze to pictures) and her cognitive abilities were found to be within normal limits. Goossens's study demonstrates the need for diagnostic AAC intervention with some children and reinforces the idea that AAC assessment should be viewed as a continual process.

Beginning AAC Intervention as Early as Possible

Beginning intervention as early as possible not only improves the life and functioning of a child, but also reduces the stress on the family, which in turn improves the family environment (Guralnick, 2000). Despite the trend toward early intervention, many young children with multiple disabilities are not introduced to AAC until they are 3 or 4 years of age, or even older (Light, 2003). One reason for this delay, as previously discussed, may be the medical challenges faced by the child. However, the justification most commonly cited by interventionists and parents for not using AAC is that it may hinder speech development. In reality, a modest number of empirical studies have actually reported improvement in natural speech skills after AAC intervention (see Beukelman & Mirenda, 2005, for a review; Sigafoos, Didden, & O'Reilly, 2003). Just as important, there are no studies that support the idea that AAC hinders speech development (Romski, Sevcik, Adamson, Cheslock, & Smith, 2007).

AAC is a multimodal communication intervention strategy that is incorporated into a child's program to enhance both expressive and receptive communication skills and should incorporate a child's full communication abilities, including any existing vocalizations, gestures, manual signs, and aided communication (ASHA, 2002). For young children for whom AAC may function to facilitate speech, monitoring and encouraging the emergence of intelligible speech are integral parts of the AAC intervention process (Romski et al., 2002). While children are likely to make the greatest gains when services begin during the early stages of development (Girolametto, Wiigs, Smyth, Weitzman, & Pearce, 2001), AAC can be successfully implemented beginning at any age.

Knowledge of Language Comprehension and Production

Implementation of AAC requires a belief that language and communication development focuses on a child's comprehension and production skills. *Language comprehension* is the ability to understand what is said so that one can function as a listener in conversational exchanges. *Language production* is the ability to express information so that one can function as a speaker in conversational exchanges. For young children to develop functional language and communication skills, they must be able to comprehend and produce language so that they can take on the roles of both listener and speaker in conversational exchanges (Sevcik & Romski, 2002).

To function as a listener, an individual must be able to understand the information that is conveyed to him or her by a variety of communicative partners. In practice, children with multiple disabilities are often asked to produce communication with the assumption that they have an adequate foundation of understanding on which to build AAC productions. This may have occurred for a variety of reasons—for example, lack of knowledge of the importance of language comprehension in AAC interventions, incorrect assumptions about the child's communication abilities, or even a lack of methods for adequately assessing comprehension in children with significant disabilities (Cheslock, 2004). For children with multiple disabilities, including cognitive and/or comprehension difficulties, this sole focus on production may make learning to communicate via an AAC system a slow or extremely difficult process.

The language comprehension skills of children with multiple disabilities vary widely, and this individual variance may determine how a child will respond to a particular AAC device or intervention strategy. If a symbols-based AAC system (e.g., a communication board or SGD) is used, a child must heavily rely on the visual modality to understand the symbolic relationship between words and their picture referents (Romski & Sevcik, 1996; Romski, et al., 2002).

For example, Sam was provided with an eight-picture, level-based SGD at the age of 3 years while he was continuing to develop language comprehension skills. He learned the meaning of visual-graphic symbols and their object referents or actions to expressively communicate. His development of language comprehension relied heavily on visual symbols at an early age.

In contrast, Amber developed language comprehension primarily through spoken words (no visual-graphic symbols) until the age of 12, when she was first provided with picture communication boards for multiple activities. She understood that a visual-graphic symbol had meaning for communication of basic wants and needs, just as a spoken word did. In her case, AAC was used to further enhance her expressive language ability.

It is critical to understand where children fall along the continuum of language comprehension if SLPs are to adequately construct their communication profiles and intervene in their communication development using developmentally appropriate AAC devices or intervention strategies. Speech-language pathologists must, therefore, incorporate their knowledge of early language development, both comprehension and production, into AAC intervention practices so that the end goal of enhanced and functional language and communication can be achieved for each child.

Systematic Language-Based Intervention

AAC intervention should be integrated within a framework of individualized language interventions. Research has indicated successful communication outcomes for young children with multiple disabilities in AAC intervention integrated with existing evidence-based naturalistic language interventions and strategies (Schepis, Reid, Behrmann, & Sutton, 1998; Yoder & Stone, 2006; see Romski et al., 2002, for a review), such as milieu teaching, functional communication training, and prompting. Intervention approaches are carefully planned and systematically implemented by identifying valid goals, outlining procedures for teaching skills to children and caregivers, consistently implementing the procedures, and evaluating effectiveness of the intervention based on data (Gresham, Beebe-Frankenberger, & MacMillan, 1999).

Language and communication goals and objectives for AAC intervention should be functional in nature and derived from knowledge obtained as part of the comprehensive, team-based AAC assessment, as described earlier. Seigel-Causey and Bashinski (1997) describe a tri-focus framework, in which intervention goals focus not only on the child's communicative development (e.g., language, literacy, natural speech), but also on the communication environment and communication partners. For example, at an early age Oscar was provided with a SGD to use in his natural communication environments at home. When he was first introduced to an SGD, his goals focused on providing increased opportunities for communication in multiple environments and teaching communication enhancement strategies to multiple communication partners. One strategy his mother was taught to use was *augmented communication input* to teach Oscar how the symbols on his SGD were to be used for communication. His mother modeled the use of the SGD during natural communication interactions with him, and Oscar ultimately used the SGD himself to communicate to her.

With some children, it may also be necessary to establish goals and objectives related to their use and access of the AAC system. It is important to remember that AAC systems are tools to achieve functional language and communication goals and not the goal in and of itself (Romski et al., 2002).

Teaching through Natural Communicative Activities and Routines

The literature strongly advocates the use of natural, integrated settings as the preferred environments for intervention for children with multiple disabilities (Beukelman & Mirenda, 2005; Romski et al., 2002). The implementation of AAC interventions within these natural settings maximizes teaching and learning opportunities throughout the day (Woods & Wetherby, 2003), emphasizes the functional nature of language, facilitates the generalization of communicative routines to diverse contexts, and increases the spontaneity of communication interactions (Bruder, 1998; Romski et al., 2002). Natural environments for consideration include home and community settings (e.g., a neighborhood park, church or synagogue, library story time, grocery store) in which typically developing children of the same age would participate. However, the provision of AAC intervention in natural environments goes beyond the consideration of location alone, to also integrate services within natural and authentic activities and routines of the child within those locations (e.g., feeding, diapering, book reading, washing hands, dressing).

Communication-Partner Instruction and Education in Language Intervention

Family members are the most stable, influential, and valuable people in a child's life (Iovannone, Dunlap, Huber, & Kincaid, 2003) and are the young child's primary *communication partners*. Immediate family members include parents, siblings, and perhaps grandparents. Extended family members might include aunts, uncles, or cousins. As a child becomes older and is involved in more activities, other communication partners become influential as well; they could potentially include teachers (e.g., child care, preschool, Sunday school), child and family friends, people in the community (e.g., librarians, athletic coaches, dance/art instructors), and other caregivers.

Family members and other caregivers in a child's life have unique expertise and insight to offer relative to that child that cannot be obtained through assessment by professionals. For the SLP, it is important to consider their perspectives because they can positively or negatively affect AAC outcomes. In recent years, many researchers and practitioners have explicitly acknowledged the importance of family/caregiver participation in AAC service delivery (Bruno & Dribbon, 1998; Culp, 2003; Culp & Carlisle, 1988; Romski & Sevcik, 1996). Research has indicated that the inclusion of instructing caregivers in the use of AAC systems in the intervention process is essential to its long-term use and that lack of instruction is associated with abandonment of the use of AAC (Johnson, Inglebret, Jones, & Ray, 2006). Research has also demonstrated that interventions implemented by parents are just as effective at facilitating expressive language as clinician-implemented interventions (Law, Garrett, & Nye, 2004; Romski et al., 2007). Communication partner instruction and education can be viewed as a dynamic process of problem-solving and reflective-learning opportunities that can involve a variety of activities ranging from ongoing hands on support/coaching for implementing AAC intervention devices and strategies, sharing resources, and advocacy training (Culp, 2003; Romski et al., 2007).

Professionals may first work with families and communication partners by providing educational information and support. McWilliams and Scott (2001) have described three types of support necessary to offer to communication partners: informational support, material support, and emotional support. Provision of informational support focuses on child development, disabilities, research-based interventions and strategies, and area resources. Material support may involve helping the family to find requested resources, a SGD, or picture symbols for a communication board; adapt toys or books for enhanced participation and communication; or locate funding for purchase of equipment. Emotional support can be provided by listening to and talking with families and communication partners in a positive and friendly manner, and by acknowledging their concerns.

Speech-language pathologists also work with communication partners to identify and implement AAC techniques and strategies that can be easily integrated into the child's natural activities and routines. For example, the SLP may teach strategies such as modeling language, augmented input, environmental arrangement, or pausing by providing the partner with in-depth and multiple examples of targeted strategies during hands-on activities; the SLP may then provide feedback to the partner as he or she implements those strategies with the child. Throughout the communication partner instruction and education process, it is important to respect each child's and family's values, beliefs, customs, cultural identification, and preferences. Speech-language pathologists should also consider the various adult learning styles and provide materials and/or feedback appropriately (e.g., video feedback; information via the Internet, books, or journal articles; written instructions).

Ongoing Monitoring

AAC intervention is a dynamic and ongoing process, reflecting the fact that children's abilities change over time, albeit sometimes very slowly. The system that is appropriate at one age may need to be modified as a young child grows and develops (Beukelman & Mirenda, 2005). Given this potential for flux, it is important to consider the child's success as falling along a continuum rather than as being an all-or-nothing phenomenon (Romski et al., 2006).

Systematic plans for periodic assessment of intervention progress along the continuum should be in place to monitor intervention successes or challenges. Wolery (2004) has suggested that such monitoring serves three broad functions of monitoring:

+ To validate the conclusions from the initial assessment
+ To develop a record of progress over time
+ To determine whether and how to modify or revise intervention plans

For AAC service delivery, ongoing monitoring should focus on the effectiveness and efficiency of the communication mode(s), vocabulary development and use, communication interactions with all partners, developmental abilities of the child including understanding and use of language, use of strategies in multiple environments, challenges that may impede communication, and, if appropriate, development of speech (ASHA, 2004). This continuous updating of an AAC system has been identified as a factor contributing to long-term successful use (Johnson et al., 2006).

The SLP, in conjunction with family and other team members, monitors the child's progress toward goals and outcomes on a regular basis, revising and establishing new goals and outcomes as appropriate to meet the changing needs of the child. Various options are available for monitoring progress, including structured and informal observations during targeted daily routines and activities, caregiver/parent perception surveys (Romski et al., 2007), questionnaires, and traditional progress reports tracking behavior for a set period of time. Speech-language pathologists can establish multiple methods to obtain information from family members and other caregivers, such as journals, periodic face-to-face meetings, e-mail, and teleconferencing.

SUMMARY

First and foremost, children with multiple disabilities are children who enjoy similar activities as children without disabilities, such as social interaction games with caregivers, playing with toys, and listening to stories. Children with multiple disabilities, however, have unique impairments in two or more developmental areas, including communication, physical, or cognitive skills, that typically affect their ability to fully participate in daily activities.

This chapter focused on the communicative development of children with multiple disabilities and, more specifically, on the role AAC can play in that development. There is no one pattern of development that leads to certain communication strengths and needs. Instead, each child presents with a unique pattern, regardless of his diagnoses, that becomes his own personal communicative profile. Important factors to consider include a child's cognitive development, communication experiences, ability to vocalize and gesture, and ability to understand the world around himself.

Most children with multiple disabilities will be able to functionally communicate, to varying degrees, via spoken language (Abbeduto, 2003). For other children, the severity of their disability may preclude their ability to expressively communicate with speech, despite intensive spoken language intervention. For these children, AAC intervention approaches have proved successful in enhancing their overall ability to communicate with family, friends, and other communication partners. The roles AAC can play in communicative language intervention for children with multiple disabilities are broader than just providing an expressive means of communication, however: AAC can also be used to supplement existing natural speech, enhance understanding and use of speech, serve as a language intervention strategy, replace unacceptable behaviors that are being used as communication, and facilitate the social development of friendships and closeness with others through communication.

Children with multiple disabilities face many challenges in accessing successful communication to convey their wants and needs, knowledge, and emotions. These challenges are often rooted in philosophical beliefs about what children with multiple disabilities can and cannot achieve and in myths about how an intervention approach such as AAC can facilitate communicative development. When implemented using sound research and principles, values, stakeholder perspectives, policy, and clinical knowledge, AAC can be a means to navigating the many challenges that children with multiple disabilities face on a daily basis.

KEY TERMS

AAC assessment

AAC strategy

AAC system

AAC technique

Aided language stimulation

Augmentative and alternative communication (AAC)

Augmented communication input

Communication

Communication aid

Communication partners

Communicative profile

Diagnostic intervention

Environmental controls

Language comprehension

Language production

Multiple disabilities

Speech-generating device (SGD)

Symbols

STUDY QUESTIONS

+ Describe the primary components of an augmentative communication system.
+ Discuss three roles that AAC can play in the language development of children with multiple disabilities.
+ Explain two internal and two external challenges that children with multiple disabilities may face when using an AAC system. How could these challenges be navigated with their families', teachers', or speech-language pathologist's help?
+ There are at least six myths associated with introducing AAC to children younger than the age of three years. List three of these myths and discuss the evidence against them.
+ Which factors contribute to a child's individual communicative profile? Why are these factors important to consider when planning an appropriate AAC intervention?
+ Discuss two adaptations of a standardized assessment that would make it accessible for children with multiple disabilities. What scoring outcomes should be considered when making these adaptations?

- Discuss in detail the areas that should be addressed when conducting a comprehensive AAC assessment.
- What does it mean to provide ongoing monitoring of a child's use of an AAC system? Why should a child's use of AAC be continually monitored?
- Discuss the role of AAC as a language intervention strategy rather than an external means of communication alone.
- Describe the role of the communication partner in AAC intervention with children with multiple disabilities. Why are they so important?

RECOMMENDED READINGS

Augmentative and Alternative Communication: Management of Severe Communication Impairments (Beukelman & Mirenda, 2005)

Exemplary Practices for Beginning Communicators: Implications for AAC (Reichle, Beukelman, & Light, 2002)

REFERENCES

Abbeduto, L. (2003). *International review of research in mental retardation: Language and communication.* New York: Academic Press.

Ablenet. (2008). Step-by-step communicator. Available at: http://www.ablenetinc.com.

Adamson, L. B., Romski, M. A., Deffebach, K., & Sevcik, R. A. (1992). Symbol vocabulary and the focus of conversations: Augmenting language development for youth with mental retardation. *Journal of Speech and Hearing Research, 35,* 1333–1343.

American Speech-Language-Hearing Association (ASHA). (2002). Augmentative and alternative communication: Knowledge and skills for service delivery. *ASHA Supplement, 22,* 97–106.

American Speech-Language-Hearing Association (ASHA). (2004). *Roles and responsibilities of speech-language pathologists with respect to augmentative and alternative communication: Technical report.* Available at: www.asha.org/policy.

American Speech-Language-Hearing Association (ASHA). (2008). *Roles and responsibilities of speech-language pathologists in early intervention: Guidelines.* Available at: www.asha.org/policy.

Barton, A., Sevcik, R. & Romski , M. A. (2006). Exploring visual-graphic symbol acquisition by pre-school age children with developmental and language delays. *Augmentative and Alternative Communication, 22,* 10–20.

Baumwell, L., Tamis-LeMonda, C. S., & Bornstein, M. H. (1997). Maternal verbal sensitivity and child language comprehension. *Infant Behavior and Development, 20,* 247–258.

Beukelman, D., & Mirenda, P. (1992). *Augmentative and alternative communication: Management of severe communication disorders in children and adults.* Baltimore: Paul H. Brookes Publishing Co.

Beukelman, D., & Mirenda, P. (1998). *Augmentative and alternative communication: Management of severe communication disorders in children and adults.* Baltimore: Paul H. Brookes Publishing Co.

Beukelman, D., & Mirenda, P. (2005). *Augmentative and alternative communication: Management of severe communication impairments,* 3rd ed. Baltimore: Paul H. Brookes Publishing Co.

Blackstone, S. (1994). The purpose of AAC assessment. *Augmentative Communication News, 7*(1), 2–3.

Blackstone, S. (1997). The intake's connected to the input. *Augmentative Communication News, 10*(1), 1–6.

Bopp, K. D., Brown, K. E., & Mirenda, P. (2004). Speech-language pathologists' roles in the delivery of positive behavior support for individuals with developmental disabilities. *American Journal of Speech-Language Pathology, 13,* 5–19.

Bruder, M. B. (1998). A collaborative model to increase the capacity of childcare providers to include young children with disabilities. *Journal of Early Intervention, 21*(2), 177–186.

Bruno, J., & Dribbon, M. (1998). Outcomes in AAC: Evaluating the effectiveness of a parent training program. *Augmentative and Alternative Communication, 14,* 59–70.

Buysse, V., & Wesley, P.W. (2005). *Consultation in early childhood settings.* Baltimore: Paul H. Brookes.

Calculator, S. (1997). Fostering early language acquisition and AAC use: Exploring reciprocal influences between children and their environments. *Augmentative and Alternative Communication, 13,* 149–157.

Campbell, P. H., Milbourne, S., & Wilcox, M. J. (2008). Adaptation interventions to promote participation in natural settings. *Infants & Young Children, 21,* 94–106.

Carr, E. G., & Durand, V. M. (1985). Reducing behavior problems through functional communication training. *Journal of Applied Behavior Analysis, 18,* 111–126.

Carr, E. G., Levin, L., McConnachie, G., Carlson, J. I., Kemp, D. C., & Smith, C. E. (1994). *Communication-based intervention for problem behavior: A user's guide for producing positive change.* Baltimore: Paul H. Brookes.

Cheslock, M. A. (2004). Issues of language input and output in AAC with young children. *Perspectives on Augmentative and Alternative Communication, 13,* 3.

Cheslock, M. A., Barton-Hulsey, A., Romski, M. A., & Sevcik, R. A. (in press). Using a speech-generating device to enhance communicative abilities and interactions for an adult with moderate intellectual disability: Case report. *Intellectual and Developmental Disabilities.*

Cheslock, M. A., Romski, M. A., Sevcik, R. A., & Barton-Hulsey, A. (2007). *Providing quality AAC intervention services to young children and their families.* Poster session presented at the annual meeting of the American Speech-Language Hearing Association, Boston, MA.

Cress, C. (2003). Responding to a common early AAC question:"Will my child talk?", *Perspectives on Augmentative and Alternative Communication, 12,* 10–11.

Cress, C. & Marvin, C. (2003). Common questions about AAC services in early intervention. *Augmentative and Alternative Communication, 19,* 254–272.

Culp, D. (2003). "If mama ain't happy, ain't nobody happy": Collaborating with families in AAC interventions with infants and toddlers. *Perspectives on Augmentative and Alternative Communication, 12,* 5.

Culp, D. M., & Carlisle, M. (1988). *Partners in augmentative communication training: A resource guide for interaction facilitation training for children.* Tucson, AZ: Communication Skill Builders.

Davis, H., Stroud, A., & Green, L. (1988). Maternal language environment of children with mental retardation. *American Journal of Mental Retardation, 93,* 144–153.

Diamanti, T. (2000). Get to know me. In M. B. Williams & C. J. Krezman (Eds.), *Beneath the surface: Creative expressions of augmented communicators* (p. 98). Toronto, Ontario: International Society for Augmentative and Alternative Communication.

Durand, V. M., & Merges, E. (2001). Functional communication training: A contemporary behavior analytic technique for problem behavior. *Focus on Autism and Other Developmental Disabilities, 16,* 110–119.

Fallon, K. A., Light, J. C., & Paige, T. K. (2001). Enhancing vocabulary selection for preschoolers who require augmentative and alternative communication (AAC). *American Journal of Speech-Language Pathology, 10,* 81–94.

Fried-Oken, M., & More, L. (1992). An initial vocabulary for nonspeaking preschool children based on developmental and environmental language sources. *Augmentative and Alternative Communication, 8,* 41–56.

Fuller, D. R., & Lloyd, L. L. (1997). AAC model and taxonomy. In L. Lloyd, D. R. Fuller, & H. H. Arvidson (Eds.), *Augmentative and alternative communication: A handbook of principles and practices* (pp. 27–37). Needham Heights, MA: Allyn & Bacon.

Girolametto, L., Weitzman, E., Wiigs, M., & Pearce, P. (1999). The relationship between maternal language measures and language development in toddlers with expressive vocabulary delays. *American Journal of Speech-Language Pathology, 8,* 364–374.

Girolametto, L., Wiigs, M., Smyth, R., Weitzman, E., & Pearce, P. S. (2001). Children with a history of expressive vocabulary delay: Outcomes at 5 years of age. *American Journal of Speech-Language Pathology, 10,* 358–369.

Glennen, S. (January 2000). AAC assessment myths and realities. Paper presented at the ASHA SID 12 Leadership Conference on Augmentative and Alternative Communication, Sea Island, GA.

Goossens, C. (1989). Aided communication intervention before assessment: A case study of a child with cerebral palsy. *Augmentative and Alternative Communication, 5,* 14–26.

Gresham, F. M., Beebe-Frankenberger, M. E., & MacMillan, D. L. (1999). A selective review of treatments for children with autism: Description and methodological considerations. *School Psychology Review, 28,* 559–575.

Guralnick, M. J. (2000). Early childhood intervention: Evolution of a system. *Focus on Autism and Other Developmental Disabilities, 15*(2), 68–79.

Hunt, P., Alwell, M., & Goetz, L. (1988). Acquisition of conversation skills and the reduction of inappropriate social interaction behaviors. *Journal of the Association for Persons with Severe Handicaps, 13,* 20–27.

Hurth, J., Shaw, E., Izeman, S. G., Whaley, K., & Rogers, S. J. (1999). Areas of agreement about effective practices among programs serving young children with autism spectrum disorders. *Infants and Young Children, 12,* 17–26.

Individuals with Disabilities Education Improvement Act of 2004, 20 U.S.C. §1400 *et seq.*

Iovannone, R., Dunlap, G., Huber, H., & Kincaid, D. (2003). Effective educational practices for students with autism spectrum disorders. *Focus on Autism and Other Developmental Disabilities, 18*(3), 150–165.

Johnson, J. M., Inglebret, E., Jones, C., & Ray, J. (2006). Perspectives of speech language pathologists regarding success versus abandonment of AAC. *Augmentative and Alternative Communication, 22*(2), 85–99.

Law, J., Garrett, Z., & Nye, C. (2004). The efficacy of treatment for children with developmental speech and language delay/disorder: A meta-analysis. *Journal of Speech, Language, and Hearing Research, 47,* 924–943.

Light, J. C. (2003). Shattering the silence: Development of communicative competence by individuals who use AAC. In J. C. Light, D. R. Beukelman, & J. Reichle (Eds.), *Communicative competence for individuals who use AAC: From research to effective practice* (pp. 3–38). Baltimore: Paul H. Brookes.

Lloyd, L., Fuller, D. R., & Arvidson, H. H. (1997). *Augmentative and alternative communication: A handbook of principles and practices.* Needham Heights, MA: Allyn & Bacon.

Luckasson R., Borthwick-Duffy, S., Buntinx, W. H. E., et al. (2002). *Mental retardation: Definition, classification, and systems of supports,* 10th ed. Washington, DC: American Association on Mental Retardation.

McWilliams, P. A., & Scott, S. (2001). A support approach to early intervention: A three-part framework. *Infants and Young Children, 13,* 55–66.

Morrow, D., Mirenda, P., Beukelman, D., & Yorkston, K. (1993). Vocabulary selection for augmentative communication systems: A comparison of three techniques. *American Journal of Speech-Language Pathology, 2*(2), 19–30.

Namy, L., Campbell, A., Tomasello, M. (2004). The changing role of iconicity in non-verbal symbol learning: A u-shaped trajectory in the acquisition of arbitrary gestures. *Journal of Cognition and Development, 5,* 37–56.

National Joint Committee for the Communication Needs of Persons with Severe Disabilities (NJC). (1992). *Guidelines for meeting the communication needs of persons with severe disabilities.* Available at: www.asha.org/policy; www.asha.org/njc.

National Joint Committee for the Communication Needs of Persons with Severe Disabilities (NJC). (2002). Access to communication services and supports: Concerns regarding the application of restrictive eligibility criteria. *Communication Disorders Quarterly, 23,* 145–153.

Nelson, N. (1992). Performance is the prize: Language competence and performance among AAC users. *Augmentative and Alternative Communication, 8,* 3–18.

Paul, R. (2001). *Language disorders from infancy through adolescence,* 2nd ed. St. Louis, MO: Mosby.

Peck, C. A. (1989). Assessment of social competence: Evaluating environments. *Seminars in Speech and Language, 10,* 1–16.

Reichle, J., Beukelman, D. R., & Light, J. C. (2002). *Exemplary practices for beginning communicators: Implications for AAC.* Baltimore: Paul H. Brookes.

Romski, M. A., & Sevcik, R. A. (1996). Breaking the speech barrier: Language development through augmented means. Baltimore: Paul H. Brookes.

Romski, M. A., & Sevcik, R. A. (2005). Augmentative communication and early intervention: Myths and realities. *Infants & Young Children, 18*(3), 174–185.

Romski, M. A., Sevcik, R. A., Adamson, L. B., Cheslock, M., & Smith, A. (2007). Parents can implement AAC interventions: Ratings of treatment implementation across early language interventions. *Early Childhood Services, 1*(4), 249–259.

Romski, M. A., Sevcik, R. A., Adamson, L. B., Cheslock, M., Smith, A., Barker, R., & Bakeman R. (in press). Comparison of parent-implemented augmented and non-augmented language interventions for toddlers with developmental delays.

Romski, M. A., Sevcik, R. A., Cheslock, M. A., & Barton, A. (2006). The system for augmenting language: AAC and emerging language intervention. In R. McCauley & M. Fey (Eds.), *Treatment of language disorders in children* (pp. 123–147). Baltimore: Paul H. Brookes.

Romski, M. A., Sevcik, R.A., & Forrest, S. (2001). Assistive technology and augmentative communication in early childhood inclusion. In M. J. Guralnick (Ed.), Early childhood inclusion: Focus on change (pp. 465–479). Baltimore: Paul H. Brookes.

Romski, M. A., Sevcik, R. A., Hyatt, A. M., & Cheslock, M. A. (2002). A continuum of AAC language intervention strategies for beginning communicators. In J. Reichle, D. R. Beukelman, & J. C. Light (Eds.), *Exemplary practices for beginning communicators: Implications for AAC* (pp. 1–23). Baltimore: Paul H. Brookes.

Romski, M. A., Sevcik, R. A., Reumann, R., & Pate, J. L. (1989). Youngsters with moderate or severe spoken language impairments I: Extant communicative patterns. *Journal of Speech and Hearing Disorders, 54,* 366–373.

Schepis, M., Reid, D., Behrmann, M., & Sutton, K. (1998). Increasing communicative interactions of young children with autism using a voice output communication aid and naturalistic teaching. *Journal of Applied Behavioral Analysis, 31,* 561–578.

Schlosser, R., Belfiore, P. J., Nigam, R., Blischak, D., & Hetzroni, O. (1995). The effects of speech output technology in the learning of graphic symbols. *Journal of Applied Behavior Analysis, 28,* 537–549.

Seigel, A., & Cress, C. (2002). Overview of the Emergence of Early AAC behaviors. In Riechle, J., Beukelman, D., & Light, J. (Eds.). *Exemplary practices for beginning communicators: Implications for AAC* (pp. 25–57). Baltimore: Paul H. Brookes.

Seigel-Causey, E., & Bashinski, S. M. (1997). Enhancing initial communication and responsiveness of learners with multiple disabilities: A tri-focus framework for partners. *Focus on Autism and Other Developmental Disabilities, 12*(2), 105–120.

Sevcik, R. A., & Romski, M. A. (2002). The role of language comprehension in establishing early augmented conversations. In J. Reichle, D. R. Beukelman, & J. C. Light (Eds.), *Exemplary practices for beginning communicators: Implications for AAC* (pp. 453–474). Baltimore: Paul H. Brookes.

Sevcik, R. A., Romski, M. A., & Wilkinson, K. (1991). Roles of graphic symbols in the language acquisition process for persons with severe cognitive disabilities. *Augmentative and Alternative Communication, 7*, 161–170.

Sigafoos, J., Didden, R., & O'Reilly, M. (2003). Effects of speech output on maintenance of requesting and frequency of vocalizations in three children with developmental disabilities. *Augmentative and Alternative Communication, 19*(1), 37–47.

Sigafoos, J., & Mirenda, P. (2002). Strengthening communicative behaviors for gaining access to desired items and activities. In J. Reichle, D. Beukelman, & J. Light (Eds.), *Exemplary practices for beginning communicators: Implications for AAC* (pp. 123–156). Baltimore: Paul H. Brookes.

Sigafoos, J., O'Reilly, M., Drasgow, E., & Reichle, J. (2002). Strategies to achieve socially acceptable escape and avoidance. In J. Reichle, D. Beukelman, & J. Light (Eds.), *Exemplary practices for beginning communicators: Implications for AAC* (pp. 157–186). Baltimore: Paul H. Brookes.

Smith, G. (2002). *Users' perspectives of factors related to long-term use or abandonment of augmentative and alternative communication systems.* Unpublished master's research project. Washington State University, Spokane, WA.

Snow, C. E. (1991). The language of the mother–child relationship. In M. Woodhead, R. Carr, & P. Light (Eds.), *Becoming a person* (pp. 195–210). New York: Routledge.

Treviranus, J., & Roberts, V. (2003). Supporting competent motor control of AAC systems. In J. C. Light, D. R. Beukelman, & J. Reichle (Eds.), *Communicative competence for individuals who use AAC: From research to effective practice* (pp. 199–240). Baltimore: Paul H. Brookes.

Wasson, C. A., Arvidson, H. H., & Lloyd, L. L. (1997). AAC assessment process. In L. L. Lloyd, D. R. Fuller, & H. H. Arvidson (Eds.), *Augmentative and alternative communication: A handbook of principles and practices* (pp. 169–198). Needham Heights, MA: Allyn & Bacon.

Wolery, M. (2004). Monitoring children's progress and intervention implementation. In M. McLean, M. Wolery, & D. Bailey (Eds.), *Assessing infants and preschoolers with special needs* (pp. 545–584). Baltimore: Paul H. Brookes.

Woods, J. J., & Wetherby, A. M. (2003). Early identification of and intervention for infants and toddlers who are at risk for autism spectrum disorders. *Language, Speech and Hearing Services in Schools, 34*, 180–193.

Yoder, P., & Stone, W. (2006). A randomized comparison of the effect of two prelinguistic communication interventions on the acquisition of spoken communication in preschoolers with ASD. *Journal of Speech, Language, and Hearing Research, 49*, 698–711.

APPENDIX 15-A

CASE STUDY 1: Speech-Language Evaluation

Name: Sam
Sex: Male
Age: 8 years

SIGNIFICANT HISTORY

Sam is an 8-year-old boy whose mother requested this assessment to receive recommendations regarding his use of a recently acquired dynamic display speech-generating augmentative communication device (SGD) that could enhance Sam's overall communication abilities throughout his functional, daily routines and activities.

Sam's *prenatal and birth histories* were unremarkable. He was born at full term weighing 7 pounds, 6 ounces.

Sam's m*edical/health history* is remarkable. Sam is diagnosed as having spastic quadriplegia cerebral palsy, a cleft lip and palate, and severe intellectual disability. He is able to eat some foods, but also has a G-tube to support adequate nutrition intake.

Hearing and vision are reportedly within normal limits.

Developmental milestones are delayed for motor, speech-language, and cognitive development. His physical abilities are a direct result of his diagnoses, as Sam is unable to walk and uses a wheelchair. He has difficulty initiating and terminating muscle activity throughout his body, including his legs, torso, arms, and facial muscles, as a result of his cerebral palsy. He is unable to communicate functionally using verbal speech.

Sam's expressive *speech-language development* is significantly delayed. He also has difficulty learning language, generalizing language concepts to a new context, and problem solving. Nevertheless, his receptive language and cognitive skills have bypassed his ability to expressively communicate. Sam has received speech/language therapy since infancy to improve his oral motor skills, with gains being noted in his increased ability to chew and swallow foods and produce some consonants.

Sam began receiving weekly speech/language intervention using an eight-location voice output augmentative communication system at the age of three years through his state's *early intervention* program. He transitioned to services through his local public school system and also receives private speech/language therapy.

Family history for Sam is negative for speech disorders.

CLINICAL PROCEDURES

Assessment Tests
Peabody Picture Vocabulary Test—III (PPVT-III, Form B)
MacArthur Commutative Development Inventory: Words and Gestures
Sequenced Inventory of Communication Development, Revised (SICD-R)

Other
Informal observations at home

CLINICAL FINDINGS

General Observations
Sam is an 8-year-old boy who enjoys music, playing ball, and reading books. Sam's mother reported that one of Sam's favorite daily activities is riding the bus to and from school. He enjoys interactions with friends, family, and teachers; however, his ability to interact with others is significantly limited as a result of his lack of verbal communication ability.

Nonverbal Communication
Sam has successfully used an eight-location speech-generating device to communicate in multiple environments, including home and private speech/language therapy. Vocabulary has been represented using Boardmaker Picture Communication Symbols (Mayer-Johnson), and Sam uses his hand to directly access the device. He typically has had six to eight pictures available per activity overlay (playtime, book reading, snacktime). Although Sam fully understands the concept of using this communication device, his functional communication has been somewhat limited owing to his inconsistent ability to access it given his physical limitations and the limited vocabulary/memory capabilities of the augmentative communication device. By report and observation, Sam is able to directly hit the appropriate picture for voice output with no difficulties. At other times—and especially later in the day as the result of fatigue—Sam has many mishits or accidental hits to inappropriate pictures as he attempts to directly access the appropriate pictures. Sam primarily communicates nonverbally by pointing/reaching, focused eye gaze, laughing, and vocalizations. His family has recently purchased a dynamic display SGD. This device has the capability for Sam to use an external switch to access the device using his head when his hand becomes fatigued.

Receptive Language
Sam's understanding of vocabulary was formally assessed using the PPVT-III. Adaptations were made by cutting out the four pictures per test item and mounting them

farther apart onto a rectangular-shaped, clear Lexan board. Sam responded accurately to test items by looking at his selected picture and then looking back to the examiner. In addition, he often reached for the correct picture with his hand. Incorrect items were noted when there was a much shorter eye gaze time to a particular picture accompanied with random looks to other pictures. Sam received a raw score of 12, a standard score of 40, a percentile rank of less than 1, and an age equivalent of less than 21 months. Sam was quite accurate in identifying familiar pictured objects, but had more difficulty with conceptual pictured vocabulary such as shapes and body parts and pictured actions.

To get a broader picture of Sam's understanding of vocabulary in typical daily routines, his mother was asked to fill out the *MacArthur Commutative Development Inventory: Words and Gestures*, a parent questionnaire of vocabulary comprehension and use. Out of a possible 396 words, Sam's mother indicated that he understands 311 words and uses 0. Sam was reported to functionally understand vocabulary in a variety of categories, including words for animals, body parts, clothing, food and drink; action words; descriptive words; words about time; and question words.

On the Receptive Language Portion of the SICD-R, Sam received 100% accuracy at the 16- and 20-month age levels. He readily identified some color-pictured body parts, identified color-pictured objects, and responded to the question type "where" by looking toward the person. He achieved 25% accuracy at the 28-month age level, primarily due to his physical limitations. Accuracy at the 32-month age level increased to 75%, as Sam was able to discriminate noise makers, demonstrate function of objects through pictures, and understand turn-taking.

Expressive Language

Sam's expressive language skills were formally assessed using the *Sequenced Inventory of Communication Development, Revised* (SICD-R). Item administration was achieved through parent report, direct child participation, and informal clinical observations. As Sam's chronological age is outside the limits of this test, any scores reported should be used with great caution. Sam received an expressive language age equivalent of eight months of age. He was reported to produce vowel sounds, consonant sounds, consonant–vowel (C-V) combinations, and C-V combinations that sound like words, and to inconsistently imitate sounds. He was unable to imitate motor acts because of his physical skills. During informal activities, Sam was observed to vocalize with intent, reach, and eye gaze toward desired objects, and laugh often.

Oral–Motor Examination

Sam has received speech/language therapy since infancy to improve his oral motor skills, with gains being noted in the form of his increased ability to chew and swallow foods and produce some consonants. However, his oral–motor deficits related to his medical diagnosis of cerebral palsy are such that there will most likely be no improvement for effective and functional speech production purposes, despite intervention. His lack of speech production has, and will continue to have, a significant impact on his ability to communicate his wants and needs, to tell if and how he may be hurt, to comment on his environment, and to socially interact with peers, teachers, doctors, and family.

DIAGNOSIS AND PROGNOSIS

Sam's prognosis for functional communication is good given the use of an appropriate augmentative communication system using a SGD along with adequate and consistent assistive technology services and supports.

RECOMMENDATIONS

It is recommended that Sam be seen for a minimum of one time per week for approximately 8 to 12 weeks to facilitate his communications skills and use of the dynamic display speech-generating augmentative communication device. Intervention services should focus on customizations of vocabulary within activity-based pages; helping Sam to use the device throughout his functional communication environments, routines, and activities (e.g., home, school, community activities); helping Sam to communicate with a variety of communications partners (e.g. family, friends, therapists); and conducting communication partner training on a variety of communication enhancement techniques. The SGD should be used in all environments and during all parts of the day with Sam. Sam's need for additional services will also be monitored on a quarterly basis, as his vocabulary and communication needs will most likely change over time. Sam's mother will primarily be responsible for the care, programming, and troubleshooting of the SGD.

It will be very important for Sam's family and other communication partners to receive training for the SGD so that they may become proficient in its usage. Sam's family and communication partners should consistently and systematically utilize a variety of communication enhancement strategies, including aided input, modeling, expansion, and environmental arrangement, to teach Sam to independently use features of the SGD and to provide multiple opportunities for communication during natural everyday activities and routines.

Sam should continue his school- and private-based speech/language interventions. The goals of these interventions should focus on functional communication skills, understanding and use of language, oral–motor skills, and early literacy skills. It will be important for current therapies to be coordinated and to address use of the SGD in Sam's natural and functional activities and routines.

Given that Sam will most likely need to rely on technology throughout his lifetime, it is recommended that he have consistent access to technology that will allow him control over his environment. Most notably, the dynamic display communication device will allow Sam to control his environment through communication. The device also features a universal remote control so that Sam can learn to control common household appliances and develop his play/social/language/cognitive skills though play with infrared toys. Once set up, all of these devices can be controlled with the communication device. Environmental controls are also commercially available to allow Sam to independently participate in other daily activities, such as cooking, playing, music, and art.

APPENDIX 15-B

CASE STUDY 2: Speech-Language Evaluation

Name: Amber
Sex: Female
Age: 12 years

SIGNIFICANT HISTORY

Amber's *prenatal and birth histories* were unremarkable. She weighed 8 pounds and was the product of a full-term pregnancy.

Amber's *medical/health* history was significant for ear infections and having her adenoids removed at age three years. Amber also experienced a seizure at the age of six years.

Amber's *hearing* was evaluated in school and found to be within normal limits.

Her *developmental milestones* have generally been slow. Amber walked unassisted at 19 months and began speaking when she was 3 years old. Her mother reported that she had problems coordinating the oral–motor movements required for breastfeeding, bottle feeding, and chewing and swallowing food until she was 2½ years old, which resulted in frequent choking and drooling.

Amber's *speech-language development* is severely delayed, as evidenced by receptive language scores indicating a 6½-year delay and an expressive language delay of 4 to 5 years. Her speech, although within normal limits for sounds in words, is moderately unintelligible in conversation. Her mother reported that she and Amber's immediate family understand Amber about half the time, but unfamiliar people and other communication partners rarely understand her.

In terms of *early intervention,* Amber attended a preschool readiness program from age four through five and has received language therapy, physical therapy, and sensory integration therapy.

Family history was negative for speech-language disorders.

CLINICAL PROCEDURES

Assessment Tests
Expressive Vocabulary Test (EVT)
Peabody Picture Vocabulary Test–III (PPVT-III)
Sequenced Inventory of Communication Development (SICD) *for Adolescents and Adults*

Other
Educational placement and intervention history
Informal observations at home

CLINICAL FINDINGS

General Observations
Amber is a female, 12 years old, who has a medical diagnosis of moderate intellectual disability. Amber experiences expressive and receptive language deficits and has received speech/language therapy since she was 4 years old. Her mother reported that Amber shows overall delays in cognitive and language development. She expressed the belief that Amber receptively understands much more than she is able to communicate.

Amber is observed and reported to have extreme word-finding difficulties. In addition to her intellectual disability and subsequent language deficits, Amber exhibits speech production deficits characterized by low oral–motor tone, frequent drooling, articulation errors, and low volume. She uses vocalizations, limited speech, gestures, facial expression, and pictures to communicate. Her mother reported that she and Amber's immediate family understand Amber about half the time when she uses the previously mentioned communicative forms, but unfamiliar people and other communication partners rarely understand her.

Amber's teachers reported that she often has behavioral problems when at school and she does not want to participate in classroom activities. She often cries, vocalizes strongly to protest the activity, or refuses to comply with activities presented to her by pushing away or throwing items she is given.

Amber has received only spoken communication language intervention until now. She has recently been introduced to an activity-based static display picture communication board by her speech-language pathologist. The SLP has noted a reduction in her negative behaviors and increase in verbal and symbolic expressive communication since the introduction of this form of AAC.

Nonverbal Communication

As reported by her mother, Amber most often uses facial expression, gestures, and telegraphic speech to communicate. Her ability to spontaneously express her wants and needs is extremely limited by her word-finding difficulties. Amber's mother reported that she understands Amber using these forms of communication approximately 50% of the time, and others understand Amber about 20% of the time they are communicating with her.

Receptive Language

On the *Peabody Picture Vocabulary Test* (PPVT), an assessment of Amber's receptive vocabulary requiring her to point to the picture named from an array of four, Amber's score fell below the first percentile. The age-equivalent score given to her performance was 6 years, 0 months (6;0).

The *Sequenced Inventory of Communication Development* (SICD) for adolescents and adults was given to Amber to further assess her receptive and expressive language. The SICD is an assessment with items on it that require the individual to process multiple directions, descriptive vocabulary, and numbers. During this assessment, Amber was able to follow two-step directions and identify coins (penny, dime, nickel). She had difficulty though following three-step directions, often doing only the last step in the sequence.

Expressive Language

On the *Expressive Vocabulary Test* (EVT), Amber's scores fell below the first percentile; in other words, less than 1% of peers her age scored below her. Amber's standard score was 40, and she was assessed as having an age equivalent of 4 years, 1 month. She demonstrated the ability to speak the labels of highly familiar pictures such as colors, animals, and body parts. However, she often took in excess of one minute to verbally label the picture. Her mother reported that Amber comprehends many of the pictures presented to her, but Amber was not able to expressively generate a label for them (examples: leaf, octopus).

Amber's lack of word finding was further demonstrated when she was asked to give synonyms for familiar words. She was unable to give many appropriate synonyms, but instead used a word to describe it. For example, when asked to give a synonym for road, she said, "this way." When asked to give a synonym for steps, she said, "down."

Amber is estimated to use approximately 200 consistent words for expressive communication. She is learning to use augmentative and alternative communication in the form of activity-specific picture boards to indicate her wants and needs and to comment during daily activities and routines.

Phonology

In general, Amber's speech was moderately unintelligible. Administration of the Goldman Fristoe Test of Articulation, however, revealed substitution of only two sounds (g/d, t/thumb), with other sounds being within normal limits for sounds in words. That is, Amber's unintelligibility is in connected speech rather than on the phonemic level.

Oral–Motor Examination

An oral peripheral examination revealed a tooth growing approximately one centimeter within the tooth arch or the hard palate. Lip pursing appeared distorted, with the obicularis muscle appearing weaker on the right side. Amber was able to implode air, lateralize, and raise and lower her tongue. Her diadochokinetic rates were slow and labored.

DIAGNOSIS AND PROGNOSIS

As Amber has developed, her cognitive and receptive language skills, while delayed, have bypassed her ability to expressively communicate. Her difficulty producing functional verbal speech will continue to have a significant impact on her daily routines. This communication may consist of explanations of why she may be hurt, comments about the environment around her, and social interaction with peers during everyday activities such as going out into the community, interacting with peers, and communicating her medical needs to her family.

Amber's speech production deficits and word-finding difficulty hinder her ability to effectively and efficiently express herself to others. This inability to express herself has become very frustrating for both Amber and her communication partners. For example, when Amber becomes frustrated because she cannot effectively communicate her intended message, she was observed to sigh and say, "I just forgot." Her psychosocial and physical well-being are clearly affected by her poor expressive communication ability.

RECOMMENDATIONS

It is very important that Amber's communication partners use the symbols on her picture communication board to communicate to her through the use of aided input to teach Amber the meaning of symbols. To use this strategy effectively, the communication partner participates in an activity with Amber and uses the communication board to describe and expand upon ideas. Through modeling of the use of symbols in this way, Amber will be able to expand her language system and develop ways to organize her vocabulary to efficiently increase the quality and rate of her communication.

It is also suggested that a visual schedule be used with Amber at school to prepare her for the events of the day. If Amber is prepared using pictures, she may better understand what is expected of her and refrain from some of her negative behaviors.

Other strategies that could be used to facilitate Amber's language development include recasts of her communication to correct forms, and expansion of Amber's limited utterances using the picture communication board. Both of these strategies can be incorporated into natural interactions with Amber.

Amber should be continually assessed during intervention to see if the combination of the picture communication board and her verbal speech is meeting her communication needs. She should continue to see a speech-language pathologist to facilitate her use of the communication board for expressive language. The SLP should also continually monitor her use of an appropriate vocabulary and symbol set for functional communication. Intervention services should focus on helping Amber learn to use symbols for communication. The use of a voice output speech-generating device should not be ruled out, even though Amber currently uses some functional speech. Considerations should be made for Amber to use a voice output communication device to further enhance her language comprehension and the amount of vocabulary available to her at one time.

APPENDIX 15-C

CASE STUDY 3: Speech-Language Evaluation

Name: Oscar
Sex: Male
Age: 3 years, 10 months

SIGNIFICANT HISTORY

Oscar's *prenatal and birth histories* are remarkable, as he was born prematurely at 28 weeks.

His *medical/heath history* is remarkable for asthma and ear infections. PE tubes were placed when he was two and a half. Oscar is diagnosed as having schizencephaly, an extremely rare developmental birth defect characterized by abnormal slits, or clefts, in the cerebral hemispheres of the brain.

Hearing and vision appear to be within normal limits. However, Oscar has not been formally tested for problems in these areas since birth.

Developmental milestones are delayed for motor and speech-language development. Oscar's physical abilities are a direct result of his diagnosis—Oscar is unable to walk and uses a wheelchair. He is unable to communicate functionally using verbal speech.

While Oscar's expressive *speech-language development* is significantly delayed, his receptive language and cognitive skills appear to be developing typically. Oscar has received speech/language therapy since infancy in an attempt to improve his oral–motor skills, with gains being noted in his increased ability to approximate some consonant sounds; this therapy was conducted through his state's *early intervention* program. Oscar's attempts at speech are somewhat unintelligible to family members and highly unintelligible to everyone other than his family members. He is currently using a 32-location voice output augmentative communication device. He receives speech/language therapy and music therapy once a week and occupational therapy and physical therapy twice a week.

There is no *family history* for speech-language disorders.

CLINICAL PROCEDURES

Assessment Tests
Mullen Scales of Early Development
Vineland Adaptive Behavior Scales

MacArthur Communicative Development Inventory (MCDI)
Clinical Assessment of Language Comprehension (CALC)
Sequenced Inventory of Communication Development (SICD-R)

Other
Informal observations at home

CLINICAL FINDINGS

General Observations
Oscar is a three-year-old boy who enjoys social interaction with others, playing with toy trains, and reading books. He uses gestures, vocalizations, and eye gaze to communicate. Oscar enjoys interactions with friends, family, and teachers. His ability to interact with others is significantly limited, however, owing to his lack of verbal communication ability.

Play
Oscar's functional play and social skills appear age appropriate. Both his cognitive skills and his social abilities appear to be areas of strength for Oscar, and they may continue to help his communication skills develop. Oscar exhibits extraordinary curiosity and perseverance when playing with toys. His manipulation and explorations of age-appropriate toys appear to be compromised only by his motor capabilities.

Nonverbal Communication
Oscar has successfully used 9-location and 32-location voice output augmentative communication devices to communicate in multiple environments, including home and private speech/language therapy. He uses his hand to directly access the device. He has progressed from using only 8 picture communication symbols available per activity overlay (playtime, book reading, snacktime) to having as many as 32 picture communication symbols available per activity. Oscar appears to fully understand the concept of using a communication device. He primarily communicates nonverbally by pointing, focused eye gaze, laughing, and vocalizations.

Receptive Language
When given the *Peabody Picture Vocabulary Test—III* (PPVT-III), Oscar received a standard score of 92, a percentile rank of 30, and an age equivalent of 38 months. He understands a range of vocabulary, including nouns, pronouns, shapes, and action and descriptive words. Overall, as reported by the SICD, Oscar demonstrates receptive language skills within the 48-month age range.

Expressive Language

Oscar demonstrates expressive language skills within the 12-month age range as reported by the SICD. He makes mostly vowel sounds, with some occasional consonants. He will occasionally imitate an "mmm" sound (to approximate "more"). Oscar's oral motor limitations due to his diagnosis of schizencephaly contribute to his expressive speech delay.

Oral–Motor Examination

Oscar is able to imitate a pucker, open his mouth, and smile (lip spread) when asked. He can slightly move his tongue forward. He has some drooling and pooling of saliva. He is beginning to make his vowels distinguishably long and short, yet shows difficulty with high/low pitch and producing the alveolar sounds /m, n, d/.

DIAGNOSIS AND PROGNOSIS

Oscar's prognosis for improved communication skills is excellent with ongoing speech-language therapy.

RECOMMENDATIONS

It is recommended that Oscar continue to use a voice output SGD for expressive communication. Intervention services should focus on customization of vocabulary within a language-based strategy to build upon his comprehension of words and appropriate syntax.

Oscar may quickly become limited with 32 words per activity setting. He will require continual evaluation during intervention sessions to see if a more advanced dynamic display communication device would best meet his expressive language needs.

Oscar should continue to use his device consistently throughout daily routines and activities (e.g., home, school, community activities) and with a variety of communication partners (e.g., family, friends, therapists).

Oscar's family and other communications partners should provide consistent feedback on his communication needs as he grows so that the vocabulary available to him on his communication device grows with him over time.

Oscar should continue his school- and private-based speech/language interventions, with goals focusing on understanding and use of syntax in making sentences, early literacy skills, and speech production abilities. It will be important for current therapies to be coordinated and for therapists to be cognizant of Oscar's rapidly changing communication needs.

GLOSSARY

Acculturation   The process by which someone identifies with both the primary community (C1) in which he or she as been socialized and the broader majority community or host culture (C2).

Acoustic immittance measures   Also known as tests of middle ear function; they include both tympanometry and acoustic reflex testing. These procedures, which give information about the presence or absence of middle ear pathology, are used in conjunction with the remainder of the audiometric test battery.

Acoustic reflex   Part of the immittance test battery. This test involves the recording of the stapedius muscle activity.

Action words   Words used to describe or demand an action. A class of words that refers to verbs.

Aided language stimulation   An augmentative and alternative communication (AAC) intervention strategy in which the intervention facilitator (e.g., clinician, parent, teacher) points to picture symbols on a child's picture communication display in conjunction with ongoing spoken language stimulation.

American Sign Language   A manual set of language symbols that are akin to spoken language symbols (e.g., semantics, grammar).

American Speech and Hearing Association (ASHA)   The professional, scientific, and credentialing association for more than 130,000 members who are speech-language pathologists, audiologists, and speech, language, and hearing scientists in the United States and internationally.

Applied behavior analysis (ABA)   A behavioral system of intervention that is utilized to teach skills in humans, from toilet training to language; a combination of psychological and educational techniques that are utilized based on the needs of each individual child to measure behavior, teach functional skills, and evaluate progress. ABA therapists provide important services to children with autism to facilitate their difficulties in various areas of development.

Articulation   The process of producing speech sounds.

Assessment   The process of determining an individual's development, as well as his or her strengths and weaknesses, by interpreting his or her performance on formal tests, formal analyses, and informal observations within the context of his or her background history and reason for referral.

Assimilation   The process by which someone in a new environment adopts and embraces the values, beliefs, and behaviors of the host culture (C2).

Attachment   The bond or affective tie of infants to their parents.

Attention   The ability of the child to focus in on listening long enough to complete a task, such as understanding the content and meaning of what is said.

Attunement   The ways in which internal emotional states are brought into communication within infant–caregiver interactions.

Auditory brain stem response audiometry   A reliable, noninvasive, objective procedure that records neuroelectrical activity in response to sound. It is an indirect measure of hearing sensitivity.

Auditory closure   The ability to fill in a missing or misspoken part of a word or message.

Auditory memory   A type of memory that includes attention, listening, and recall. It is an essential ingredient for a child at the identification level and for the overall perception and processing of speech in general.

Augmentative and alternative communication (AAC)   A multimodal intervention approach that uses forms of communication such as manual sign language, picture communication boards, and *speech-generating devices*, with the goal of maximizing the functional language and communication abilities of individuals who have severe communication impairments and little to no speech (ASHA, 2002).

Augmentative and alternative communication (AAC) assessment   A critical component of AAC service delivery that can provide the foundation for basing intervention decisions for individuals requiring AAC intervention. It is conducted within a comprehensive, team-based assessment framework, often within various environments, and includes assessment of the AAC user, communication partners, environments, and the AAC system. The goal is to explore the range of appropriate AAC strategies, adaptations, devices, and services that may help a child fully participate in their environment(s) and enhance his or her functional communication with a variety of communication partners.

Augmentative and alternative communication (AAC) strategy   The specific way or method in which AAC aids, symbols, and techniques are used to develop and/or enhance communication efficiency and effectiveness (e.g., language stimulation strategies, augmented input, aided language stimulation, communication-partner instruction, rate of communication enhancement strategies).

Augmentative and alternative communication (AAC) system   An integrated set of components, including communication aids, symbols, strategies, and techniques, all working in concert to provide the maximum amount of support needed for an individual to fully communicate in all situations.

Augmentative and alternative communication (AAC) technique   The way in which communicative messages are transmitted, such as direct selection or scanning.

Augmented communication input   An augmentative and alternative communication (AAC) intervention strategy in which the intervention facilitator or communication partner uses both picture symbols and speech output produced by a speech-generating device (SGD) when the symbols are activated, in conjunction with ongoing spoken language during naturalistic and authentic daily activities. This strategy provides spoken and augmented language input to the child, models functional use of the SGD, and demonstrates to the AAC user that the SGD is an acceptable form for communicative interactions.

Autism spectrum disorder (ASD)   A childhood disorder involving deficits in social, communication, play, and verbal behavior; first identified in 1943 by Leo Kanner, an American psychiatrist.

Baby signs   See *representational gestures.*

Background history   An inventory of the child's past and current events and characteristics (e.g., reason for referral, events surrounding gestation and birth, medical and health status, points at which

developmental milestones were met, genetic factors).

Basic-level terms   The most general (or intermediate-level) terms in the hierarchy of semantic organization. These terms are generally acquired before other terms in the hierarchy. Also referred to as ordinate-level terms.

Beat gestures   Manual movements that are produced with the rhythm of speech but do not convey semantic or deictic reference.

Behavioral (procedure)   A procedure that requires a volitional response from a person.

Bottom-up approach   An approach that is directed and planned, and typically employs a linear presentation in the sequence of easiest to most difficult. The therapist focuses on the child mastering one skill or skill level completely and then moves on to the next, more difficult level.

Bound morpheme   A unit of language that is meaningful but must be combined with a free morpheme.

Central executor   The component of working memory that allocates processing resources and attention to other components (visuo-spatial sketchpad, phonological working memory, episodic buffer).

Child-directed speech   Patterns of speech directed to babies and young children that are characterized by utterances that are shorter in length, simpler in grammatical complexity, slower in rate of speech, contextually redundant, and perceptually salient than speech directed to older persons. Researchers suggest that the vocal and grammatical parameters of the primary linguistic data that are provided by the caretaker make semantic, syntactic, phonological, and pragmatic information more accessible to the young infant, who is innately wired to receive this information.

Classical conditioning   Paradigm described by Pavlov, who discovered that dogs could be conditioned to salivate in response to a bell after pairing the bell with the presentation of food. Many concepts (e.g., stimuli, response, paired association, stimulus generalization) are derived from this paradigm.

Cochlea   A snail-shaped structure in the inner ear. It houses the sensory end organ of hearing (i.e., the organ of Corti).

Code switching   The juxtaposition within the same speech exchange of passages belonging to two different grammatical systems. The switch can be intrasentential, within a sentence (Spanish–English switch: *Dame a glass of water. "Give me a glass of water."*), or it can be intersentential, across sentence boundaries (Spanish–English switch: *Give me a glass of water; tengo sed. "Give me a glass of water; I'm thirsty."*). The switches are not random, but rather are governed by constraints such as the free morpheme constraint and the equivalency constraint. Many people who are bilingual

and/or bidialectal are self-conscious about their code switching and try to avoid it with certain interlocutors and in particular situations. In informal speech, it is a natural and powerful feature of a bilingual's/ bidialectal's interactions.

Cognition   In developmental psychology, a term used to refer to multiple processes such as memory, attention, perception, action, problem-solving, and imagery. In child development, a term used to refer to children's emerging ability to make sense of the world around them by interpreting input, integrating this information, and then producing planned actions.

Cognitive-constructivist   Referring to the theoretical paradigm introduced by Jean Piaget, who described the developing human as being grounded in action—both observable and mental. The human infant was said to actively construct its knowledge through the use of invariant mechanisms, including the establishment of mental constructs or schemas, while engaging in sensory and motor activities.

Communication   An act in which one person gives to or receives from another person information about that person's needs, desires, perceptions, knowledge, or affective states and includes speech, as well as other forms of expression such as body gestures, eye gaze, picture symbols, and printed words.

Communication aid   A device used to transmit or receive messages during communicative exchanges. Aids range from simple non-electronic devices, such as picture symbol choice boards and head pointers, to high-technology electronic aids, such as dedicated speech-generating devices and laptop computers with speech synthesis software.

Communication partners   Those individuals with whom the augmentative and alternative communication (AAC) user interacts; could include family, friends, peers, clinicians, teachers, and/or community workers.

Communicative competence   The ability to use language(s) and/or dialect(s) and to know when and where to use which and with whom. This ability requires grammatical, sociolinguistic, discourse, and strategic competence. It is evidenced in a speaker's unconscious knowledge (awareness) of the rules/factors that govern acceptable speech in social situations.

Communicative profile   A complete and individualized description of a child's strengths and needs in a variety of settings regarding the child's understanding and use of language, speech, oral–motor skills, and ability to communicate using nonconventional forms of communication such as gestures or sign language. It may be influenced by factors such as the child's cognitive development, communicative experiences, vocal and gestural production abilities, and comprehension skills.

Comprehension   The process of turning an often highly complicated set of linguistic or nonlinguistic (or both) cues (e.g., signs, signals, or word combinations) into a meaningful message.

Comprehension (reading comprehension)   The successful connection of statements and ideas in a text that leads to forming a coherent mental representation of the text; the reader is required to use prior knowledge to interpret information in the text and to construct a coherent mental representation or picture of what the text is about (Kendeou et al., 2005).

Comprehension level   The comprehension of sound and its meaning; the final and most complicated stage of auditory development.

Conditioned play audiometry   A method used to complete a hearing test on a young child. This method turns the hearing test into a listening game for the child; almost any toy or game will do. The idea is to condition the child to do something each time a sound is heard; this action can be dropping a block, putting a ring on a stick, or putting a piece in a puzzle, for example.

Conductive hearing loss   A hearing loss that is the result of damage in the outer and/or middle ears. It is usually characterized by a decrease in the loudness of sound, but the clarity of speech typically remains intact. Conductive hearing loss is very often medically and/or surgically treatable. When it is caused by a condition such as otitis media, it fluctuates in severity, with some days much better or much worse than others.

Conductive mechanism   The combination of the outer and middle ears. In its normal state, it is an air-filled environment. The conductive system as a whole (that is, the outer and middle ear together) has the job of gathering the sound (acoustic energy) from the environment, converting the sound (acoustic energy) into mechanical energy, and then delivering this mechanical energy to the inner ear.

Consonants   Sounds produced by partially or totally constricted vocal tract; classified by manner (degree and type of obstruction), place (location of obstruction), and voicing (whether vocal folds are vibrating).

Coordination/coregulation   Ongoing mutual social referencing of the participants involved in social interactions.

Criterion-referenced measures   Measures used to differentiate among levels of performance where no standardized measure of performance has been established.

Criterion-referenced tests   Tests in which the speech-language pathologist evaluates the child's responses qualitatively, looking for any missing forms that can be targeted in therapy. The results of a child's performance on criterion-referenced measures are summed up as pass/fail

scores, percentage correct, or performance rates; these scores indicate the child's level of mastery of a specific linguistic form.

Cultural bias   Reduced or absent consideration of the examinee's experiential base as evidenced by the use of activities and items that do not correspond to the examinee's experiential base. This may lead to unfavorable performance on tasks and failure to represent the examinee's true skill or performance capabilities.

Cultural competence   A person's knowledge and awareness of cultural and/or linguistic differences that may affect both the personal and professional experiences of the clinician with his or her clients.

Cultural diversity   The exposure or immersion of an individual or group in more than one set of cultural beliefs, values, and attitudes. These beliefs, values, and attitudes may be influenced by race/ethnicity, sexual orientation, religious or political beliefs, or gender identification.

Cultural variables   Shared and accepted factors that help a group define itself.

Culture   The *explicit* behaviors and artifacts and *implicit* beliefs adopted by a person or group to define their social identity.

Curriculum-based language assessment   Assessment of a child's ability to use language to learn classroom material (Paul, 2005). It includes assessing a child's written work for the level of narrative development, grammaticality and complexity, use of diverse vocabulary, and use of figurative language.

Cycles phonological approach An intervention developed for use with children who have highly unintelligible speech. The child is given quick but limited exposure to a target, and the speech-language pathologist typically returns to the pattern after a period of time. This allows for the child to internalize, sort, experiment with, and do self-rehearsal as a typically developing child does. Through this process, the child's sound system is reorganized. The child learns new rules to use in producing the sounds of the words of his language.

Deaf culture The culture of the Deaf community, which has its own language (sign language) and its own accepted cultural norms. Hearing-impaired individuals who are members of the Deaf community are, for the most part, isolated from the "hearing world." It is not surprising, therefore, that they are a separate and unique culture.

Decoding The ability to translate letters into sounds and blend them to produce words; the core skill required in learning to read an alphabetic language.

Decontextualization The gradual distancing of a symbol from the original referent or learning context.

Deictic gestures Gestures that make reference to something in the environment (i.e., *showing, giving, pointing,* and *ritual request*). Also referred to as prelinguistic gestures because they emerge before the child speaks his or her first word.

Detection level The most basic level of sound awareness; it refers to the baby being able to detect the presence or absence of sound in the environment. In the normal-hearing infant, this is a clear-cut and uncomplicated process.

Development A gradual change in maturation over time that is described in terms of its typicality by comparisons with a normative sample.

Diagnostic intervention An informal means of assessing abilities when formal assessment (or diagnostic) measures are ineffective, invalid, or unable to be conducted in a timely fashion. The process involves implementation of intervention strategies and informal observation to determine the individual's strengths and needs and to determine the most appropriate course of intervention.

Dialect A neutral term used to describe a language variation. Dialects are seen as applicable to all languages and all speakers. All languages are analyzed into a range of dialects, which reflect the regional and social background of their speakers.

Dialectal variance The non-mainstream production of a language at the sound, word, or syntactic level.

Disability   A social construct perceived by those with an illness or disease.

Discourse competence   The skills involved in the connection of a series of utterances to form a conversation and/or narrative.

Discrimination level   The next higher level in difficulty in sound awareness beyond the detection level. With the discrimination level, children first master discrimination of the suprasegmental aspects of language before they master the segmental aspects.

Distributed neural network   The connection of nodes of information across modalities that are represented throughout the brain.

Dual (differentiated) language system hypothesis   The assumption that children process individual languages through distinct language systems, thereby developing two differentiated mental representations of the languages from the onset of exposure.

Dynamic approach to assessment   A more naturalistic approach to assessment, in which the speech-language pathologist examines a child's language and communication skills in natural contexts. It involves the observation of the child in routine activities, interacting with familiar people, manipulating objects, and playing with different toys alone and with others.

Dynamic assessment   Assessment of not only what the child's current performance level is, but also how the child can learn. Because dynamic assessment provides information on the child's ability to learn, it provides the examiner with great insight for both identifying a language disorder and planning intervention.

Early communicative gestures   Gestures that are part of routines, such as hand waving to say *good-bye* or nodding the head to say *no*.

Electrophysiologic (procedure)   A procedure that does not require any active participation from the child. Such tests are unaffected by any degree of sleep or arousal and are not negatively affected by sedation. Further, they can be performed on anyone, aged pediatric through geriatric. These tests are the procedures of choice for screening hearing in the newborn infant population.

Emblems   Conventional symbols such as the *high-five* to convey camaraderie, *okay* or *thumbs up* gestures to signal agreement, and the *hand across the throat* to signal stop. They are language-like in that they are abstract symbols.

Emergentist coalition model   A theory of word learning that proposes children take advantage of multiple environmental cues as well as innate cognitive biases to learn new words. With experience, these cues and biases work together and become more efficient in helping the child learn language.

Emotion   A mental and physiological state associated with a wide variety of feelings, thoughts, and behaviors.

Encoding Basic and essential skill whereby the ear and auditory pathway (in a bottom-up fashion) physically receive and code sound, then send it upward toward the brain for eventual interpretation. Sound encoding is necessary and allows, for example, the perception and analysis of the acoustics of speech. In essence, children learn that sound has meaning and that they can produce sound for the purpose of communication in their environment.

Endogenous factors Factors within the child.

Engagement The human infant's ability to interact with others by utilizing joint attention, reciprocity, and intentionality.

Environmental controls Items that can be utilized to help an individual interact with his or her environment where he or she was previously unable to interact; examples include adapted toys and remote controls.

Episodic buffer The component of working memory that integrates newly processed phonological, visual, and other modalities of information with old information from long-term memory prior to its storage in long-term memory.

Episodic memory Links that connect the emotional experience of an event with the what, when, and how of the event. This type of memory makes it possible for individuals to recollect happenings and events from their past and to use this information to project anticipated events into the future (Tulving, 1993). Episodic memory enables the individual to make predictions and, therefore, to infer in social interactions and in text comprehension.

Ethnic diversity Similar to *cultural diversity*; differences within and between groups of people already categorized by ethnicity.

Ethnic majority According to the U.S. Census Bureau (2000), those who identify as "white," connoting superiority.

Ethnic minority According to the U.S. Census Bureau (2000), all "nonwhites," suggesting inferiority.

Ethnicity An ever-changing cultural construct that forms the basis for a sense of social cohesion.

Ethnographic interviewing A personalized method of exploration that provides the clinician with an opportunity to obtain a deep, true, and naturalistic understanding of the behavior or culture under study. Through this process, the clinician listens to the behaviors and beliefs reported by the parent or caregiver, as obtained through a systematic and guided dialogue with the caretaker.

Evaluation See *assessment*.

Exogenous factors Factors in the environment.

Expansion An intervention used when a child incorrectly produces a particular linguistic form; the speech-language pathologist then reinforces the correct production of the linguistic form by repeating the child's utterance, adding the missing grammatical markers or lexical items.

Expressive children   Those children for whom general nominals account for less than 50% of their lexicon.

Extended optional infinitive hypothesis   The hypothesis that the central deficit in specific language impairment (SLI) is in the part of grammar responsible for tense marking. According to this account, children with SLI go through an extended stage of mistakenly treating tense marking in main clauses as optional.

Facilitative play (indirect language stimulation)   An intervention in which language is facilitated by utilizing toys or objects that draw the child's interest. It provides multiple opportunities for the child to map the nonlinguistic context onto words and sentences.

Fast mapping   The process of linking a new word with its referent after a brief exposure.

Feedback   "That annoying whistling" from hearing aids, which relatives and close friends of the hearing-impaired person may complain about.

Fine motor skills   Movements involving smaller body muscles, such as the fingers and the muscles of the face that are used in speech (e.g., lip, tongue, and jaw movements). Mastering control of these muscles takes years. For example, it takes children at least age five years or later to learn to use all of the sounds of English correctly.

Fluency   The ability to read words without a conscious effort to sound out or blend them; it includes the ability to group words into meaningful phrases and to read with prosody, intonation, and stress.

Focused stimulation   An intervention in which the child is bombarded with the target form in a variety of contexts. The child is exposed to multiple exemplars of a specific linguistic target (e.g., a word, a morpheme) within meaningful communicative contexts. Following exposure, the child is provided with opportunities to produce the targeted linguistic form. The therapy session is arranged with materials that would encourage spontaneous productions of the target forms following the speech-language pathologist's repeated models.

Formal testing   One type of procedure used to evaluate the child's development. The child's performance is summed to a raw score and often statistically converted to a standard score or percentile so that the child's performance can be compared to a normative or criterion-referenced data set. Some formal tests evaluate a particular developmental domain (e.g., vocabulary); others contain a variety of subtests that sample several developmental domains (e.g., PLS-3).

Free morpheme   The smallest unit of language that carries meaning and can exist independently.

Function words   Words referring to items that serve a grammatical function in relating to other content words (e.g., *what, is, for, to*).

Functional ability As it relates to hearing, a consequence of *many* factors; "degree" of loudness loss is just one of them. Other factors involved in determining the person's level of function include pre- or post-lingual onset of hearing loss, age of onset for post-lingual losses, speech-understanding ability, successful use of a hearing aid, speech reading skills, and cognitive abilities.

Functional communication context The discourse contexts in which the child communicates that are part of daily living activities (e.g., conversation, explaining an academic topic, defending a position, communicating needs in the classroom).

Functional core hypothesis A hypothesis stating that words are overextended to novel exemplars based on the shared actions or functions of objects rather than the perceptual features of the referents.

General nominals Words referring to all members of a category. They include word classes such as objects, substances, animals, people, letters, numbers, pronouns, and abstractions.

Gesture–spoken language match combination A situation in which gesture and spoken language are produced at the same time, and each modality conveys the same information.

Gesture–spoken language mismatch combination A situation in which gesture and spoken language are produced at the same time and each modality conveys different information. Mismatch combinations are often produced when children talk about concepts that they are still in transition of learning.

Give gesture A deictic gesture in which the child hands off an object to a communicative partner.

Government binding—Principles and parameters A theory developed by Chomsky in 1981 that describes the idiosyncratic parameters of particular languages as well as universal principles across languages.

Grammatical competence Knowledge and awareness of phonological, syntactic, and lexical skills.

Grammatical specific language impairment (SLI) A distinct subtype of language impairment characterized by persistent receptive and expressive language impairments that are restricted to core grammatical operations.

Grapheme A written symbol (letter) that represents a phoneme (sound).

Gross motor skills Movements involving large muscles of the body, such as the arms and legs. Examples include rolling over, sitting unsupported, and walking. Acquisition of these skills occurs in an orderly, predictable process that usually precedes mastery of fine motor skills.

Heritage Cultural variables that are most valued and are passed on from generation to generation.

Hierarchical organization of the lexicon
The systematic organization of the lexicon such that the relationship between members of a category can be characterized as superordinate (e.g., animal), ordinate (e.g., dog, cat, pig, cow), and subordinate (e.g., collie, poodle).

High-frequency sensorineural hearing loss   A hearing loss in which the person's ability to hear high frequencies is not merely "somewhat poorer," but rather "a lot poorer." At the same time, hearing for the lower frequencies is often intact.

Horizontal development   The range of abilities or communicative functions within a particular developmental level.

Iconic gesture   See *representational gestures*.

Identification level   The point at which the child is able to identify or label an item; this can be by naming the item or pointing to it.

Illness   An individual's *experience* of that condition.

Imitation   An intervention in which the child receives a visual prompt (such as a picture or a toy) that provides him or her with an incentive to verbalize. The speech-language pathologist then provides a verbal model and asks the child to imitate the target form. The child's response is reinforced by verbal praise or by a token.

Impedance   Resistance or opposition to the flow of energy.

Impedance mismatch   The difference in the resistance properties of the air-filled middle ear and of the fluid-filled inner ear.

Incidental teaching procedure   An intervention in which toys are strategically placed to elicit specific linguistic or communicative forms.

Independent (individualistic)   A cultural orientation that stresses independence, self-reliance, and individual liberty; one's personal goals take priority over the goals of the group.

Indeterminate errors/responses   A type of word retrieval error that provides no discernable relationship with the target (e.g., "I don't know" or "thing").

Index of Productive Syntax (IPSyn)   A method of evaluating the grammatical complexity of language in preschool children. Language development is assessed in four separate areas of language knowledge and structure: noun phrases, verb phrases, questions/negations, and sentence structures. IPSyn requires the identification of 56 specific language structures in a corpus of 100 child utterances.

Individual family service plan (IFSP)   A plan that recommends the delivery of services in naturalistic environments (e.g., in the child's home or in childcare facilities). It includes information about the child's physical, cognitive, social, emotional, and communicative development, and about his or her family, including its resources, concerns, and priorities. The IFSP also provides information about the services needed for the child, their frequency and intensity, and the expected outcomes.

Individualized education plan (IEP)   A plan that states the child's strengths and weaknesses, the goals and objectives for therapy, the type of services the child needs, and the amount of time each week that services will be provided.

Individuals with Disabilities Education Act (IDEA)   Federal legislation that requires states to provide children with a free, appropriate public education.

Information processing   A theoretical perspective that explains the human acquisition of information in a way that is analogous to the working of a computer, in that information is considered to be processed serially and/or simultaneously.

Information processing speed   The speed or efficiency with which the brain performs basic cognitive operations; in effect, how quickly a person can react to incoming information.

Initiating behavior request (IBR)   A type of protoimperative in which the infant uses eye contact and gestures to initiate attention coordination with another person to elicit aid in obtaining an object or event. IBR is used less for social purposes, but more for instrumental purposes.

Initiating joint attention (IJA)   A type of protodeclarative in which the infant uses eye contact and/or deictic gestures (pointing or showing) to spontaneously initiate coordinated attention with a social partner. The infant is seeking interaction with another simply for the sake of sharing an experience.

Innate biases   Intrinsic tendencies or preferences that children use to pair a newly heard word with the referent in their environment. Also referred to as *constraints* or *principles* of word learning.

Intentionality   Purposive motivation that drives language acquisition.

Intentionality model   Bloom and Tinker's (2001) model of the interaction between two domains of development—affect and cognition—in the young child. In this model, the development of the form, content, and use of language is embedded in engagement (i.e., the social–emotional development of the child) and effort (i.e., the cognitive development of the child).

Interactionist perspective   A perspective derived from a range of perspectives that are either cognitive or social, placing equal emphasis on preexisting information that the child brings to learning and the role of environmental input on the child.

Interdependent (collective)   A cultural orientation that stresses interdependence among members of a group or society and the importance of the goals/desires of the group over the goals/desires of the individual.

Interpreter   A person specially trained to transpose oral or signed text from one language to another.

Intervention   The process of facilitating development to age-appropriate or developmentally appropriate levels.

Joint attention   The process of sharing one's experience of observing an object or event by following gaze or pointing gestures.

Language   (1) A complex and dynamic rule system of conventional symbols that is used in various modes for thought and communication (e.g., spoken, signed, written) and is generative. Rules govern five separable domains: pragmatics, phonology, morphology, semantics, and syntax. At the same time, these domains evolve within specific historical, social, and cultural contexts. (2) A socially shared code of symbols—written, spoken, or signed—that serve a communicative function. The symbols incorporated into a language have no inherent meaning but instead are arbitrary. Because competent users of the same language share a grammatical (rule-governed) system for generating new and allowable sentences, regardless of mode, it is presumed that they can meaningfully communicate with one another.

Language comprehension   The ability to understand what is said so that the person can function as a listener in conversational exchanges. It provides an essential foundation on which individuals can build language production.

Language delay   A situation in which a child exhibits typical development in all other areas except for language.

Language deviance   A situation in which the child's language development is not just slower than that of the typically developing child but is different in some qualitative way.

Language difference   A rule-governed language form (i.e., dialect) that deviates in some way from the standard language used by the mainstream culture.

Language disorder (impairment)   An impairment in comprehension and/or use of spoken language, written language, and/or some other symbol system. The disorder may involve (1) the form of language (phonologic, morphologic, and syntactic systems), (2) the content of language (semantic system), and/or (3) the function of language in communication (pragmatic system), in any combination" (ASHA, 1993, p. 40).

Language diversity   Patterns of linguistic differences inherent within and across populations, including second language acquisition processes, dialects, and bilingualism, where an individual or group has had significant exposure to more than one language or dialect.

Language ego–permeability   Beliefs about how language should be used or produced; a sense of 'boundaries" for what is acceptable language use and what is not; a sense for when language output is being degraded or changed. Individuals may have varying levels of tolerance for nonstandard forms of the language (e.g., language borrowing, code switching).

Language loss   The apparent loss (attrition) of functional vocabulary and/or utterances in a language due to reduced exposure.

Language mixing   Use of a linguistic structure from one language in place of a structure in another language; observed in the production of early bilinguals during periods in their development.

Language production   The ability to express information so that the person can function as a speaker in conversational exchanges.

Language sampling   A technique for the assessment of bilingual children whereby naturalistic utterances are collected, transcribed, and analyzed.

Language transfer   The use of a linguistic rule from one language that affects the production of structures in the other language for a period of time in development.

Language-use patterns   The way that language is used given the context of discourse.

Late bloomers   Children with slow expressive vocabulary growth during the toddler years who catch up to their typically developing peers by the end of their preschool years.

Late talkers   Children with slow expressive vocabulary growth during the toddler years who do not catch up to their typically developing peers. Their delays eventually transcend vocabulary to difficulty with grammar.

Lexical bootstrapping   The notion that lexical and grammatical development are inseparable. Children use their accumulating knowledge of individual words to construct the grammar of their language.

Lexical representation   The word form stored in memory; a sequence of phonemes that make up the lexeme.

Lexical–semantic network   The connection of nodes of phonological, lexical, and semantic information across modalities that are represented throughout the brain.

Linguistic bias   Reduced or absent consideration of the examinee's linguistic differences during testing; typically a result of prescriptive beliefs of language development and production.

Linguistic construction   A syntactic template that is paired with a conventionalized semantic and pragmatic content. Constructions are often associated with specific speech acts, such as asking a question or making a promise. Constructions vary with respect to their complexity, ranging from single words to complex sentences.

Literacy   The ability to identify, understand, interpret, create, communicate, and compute using printed and written materials associated with varying contexts. Literacy involves a continuum of learning in enabling individuals to achieve their goals, to develop their knowledge and potential, and to participate fully in their community and wider society.

Literacy artifacts   Representations of print that enrich a child's environment.

Literacy socialization   The social and cultural aspects of reading that a child acquires by being a member of a literate society.

Localization   The location of the sound source in the environment.

Mand-model procedure   A technique in which the speech-language pathologist mands (explicitly directs the child, "Tell me what this is"), or provides the child with a choice ("Is the ball red or blue?") and then provides the child with the model.

Mastery   The threshold when a child uses a particular linguistic form (e.g., the *-ing* morpheme) consistently and accurately 90% of the time when it is required or expected to be used.

Mean length of utterance (MLU)   A measure of linguistic productivity in children. It is usually calculated by collecting 100 utterances from a child and dividing the number of morphemes by the number of utterances. A higher MLU is taken to indicate a higher level of language proficiency.

Mental representation   Knowledge that is stored, or represented, in memory.

Mental retardation (MR)   A condition characterized by a significantly lower than average level of intellectual functioning and adaptive behavior.

Middle ear transformer function   Functionality in which the ear is able to overcome the impedance mismatch.

Milestones   Expected ages or time frames during which certain skills emerge or are acquired.

Minimalist program   The most recent version of Chomsky's theory, in which the description of the language faculty includes only a representation of meaning and a recursive element called "merge" that provides the mechanism for joining words and phrases.

Mixed hearing loss   A hearing loss that results from simultaneous damage to both the conductive and the sensorineural pathways.

Modeling   An intervention technique in which the targeted linguistic form/behavior is presented to the child by the speech-language pathologist in a naturalistic context.

Modifiers   Words referring to properties or qualities of things or events, such as attributes, states, locations, or possessives.

Morpheme   The smallest unit of language that carries meaning.

Morphology   A domain of language that encompasses the rules of the smallest unit of language that expresses meaning (e.g., plural *-s*, root word).

Multiple disabilities   A general term for a combination of two or more impairments occurring at the same time; it can apply to children with a broad range of impairment in cognitive development, expressive and receptive communication, and physical ability.

Naming insight   See *vocabulary spurt.*

Naming explosion   See *vocabulary spurt.*

Natural partitions hypothesis   A hypothesis proposing that concrete nouns promote more rapid learning than other word classes, particularly verbs, because they allow for greater transparency of the mapping between lexical and semantic information.

Nature perspective   A perspective derived from rationalist philosophy that emphasizes the internal wiring of the child for perception and learning.

Nominal insight   See *vocabulary spurt.*

Nonverbal communication   The nonlinguistic behaviors that may accompany verbal interactions. Gestures, proximity, eye contact, and touch, for example, may have substantial meaning in social interactions.

Norm-referenced measures   Standardized tasks that compare individual performance to performances of a defined population. These measures tend to examine the languages of a bilingual speaker as a separate construct, and they provide limited information as to the relationship between the two languages.

Novel–name–nameless category (N3C)   Principle stating that a novel word will be taken as the name for a previously unnamed object.

Nurture perspective   A perspective derived from empiricist philosophy that relies primarily on observable phenomena to explain learning.

Obligatory context   The context in which a particular language form is expected to occur. For example, if a child is referring to more than one object, the plural *-s* morpheme would be considered obligatory in that it must be used to convey the meaning of "more than one."

Operant conditioning   Paradigm described by B. F. Skinner, who discovered that a rat's behavior could be shaped by systematically presenting a reinforcing stimulus to the successive approximations until ultimately the target behavior is produced. Concepts such as reinforcement, punishment, and schedule of reinforcement are derived from this paradigm.

Ordering of word classes   The order of nouns, in subject (S) and object (O) positions, and verbs (V).

Ordinate terms   See *basic-level terms.*

Organ of Corti   The end organ of hearing.

Orientation   The degree to which a person orients himself or herself toward the considerations of a collective body (e.g., a family, ethnic group) or toward individual achievement and motivation.

Orthographic   Referring to print.

Otitis media   An inflammation of the middle ear; a middle ear infection.

Otoacoustic emissions (OAE)   An electrophysiologic procedure that is based on the principle that a normal and healthy cochlea not only hears sound, but can also produce sound. OAEs can be spontaneously present or evoked. An *evoked* OAE occurs when a sound has been sent into the ear, and in response the ear produces a sound and sends it back out; this response can be recorded. *Spontaneous* OAEs are spontaneously present.

Overextension   A type of word retrieval error that is characterized by a word being used too broadly to refer to referents that may be similar in perceptual feature or function.

Overgeneralization errors   Errors that involve children's use of words in grammatical constructions in ways that are not conventional in their language community. Children may overgeneralize morphological patterns, for example, by saying *goed* instead of *went*, and they may overgeneralize syntactic patterns, for example, by saying *She broomed the floor.*

Parallel talk   An intervention in which the speech-language pathologist describes the child's actions.

Performance assessment procedures   Methods by which the speech-language pathologist evaluates a child's language knowledge, abilities, and achievements in a more naturalistic manner. One of the most common procedures is language sampling.

Perseverative errors   A type of word retrieval error that is characterized by the repetition of a previously said word within a relatively short time interval.

Personal–social words   Words that express affective states and social relationships, such as assertions (e.g., *no, yes, want*) and social expressive words (e.g., *please, ouch*).

Pervasive developmental disorder not otherwise specified (PDD-NOS)   A classification used to account for those children who appear to represent "atypical autism." A child diagnosed with PDD-NOS presents with a pervasive impairment in social interaction and communication skills or stereotyped patterns of behavior, interests, or activities that do not meet the criteria for autistic disorder because of late age at onset, atypical symptoms, or subthreshold symptoms.

Phoneme   The smallest arbitrary unit of sound in a given language that can be recognized as being distinct from other sounds in the language.

Phonemic awareness   The ability to consciously reflect on and manipulate the sounds in words.

Phonetically consistent forms (PCF)   Stable vocalizations used to reference a specific event, object, or situation; not true words.

Phonological awareness   An individual's knowledge or sensitivity to the sound structure of words (Pullen & Justice,

2003); the explicit awareness that words in the language are composed of syllables and phonemes (i.e., consonants and vowels) (Catts, 1991). At the emergent literacy level, it is reflected in activities such as rhyming, word play, and phonological corrections (van Kleeck & Schuele, 1987).

Phonological development Acquisition of the speech sounds and patterns of a language.

Phonological deviations Speech sound changes, including omissions, substitutions, assimilations, and syllable-structure/context-related changes.

Phonological errors A type of word retrieval error that is characterized by similar phonological make-up to that of the target lexeme (e.g., *chicken* for *kitchen* or *miracleride* for *merry-go-round*).

Phonological intervention A remediation process that focuses on reorganizing the child's phonological system by helping the child learn to produce and acquire phonological patterns.

Phonological loop The component of working memory where speech-based input is encoded, maintained, and manipulated.

Phonological patterns Accepted groupings of sounds and word structures within an oral language.

Phonology A domain of language that encompasses the rules of the sound system of the language; one of the five components of language. It is important for morphology, syntax, and semantics.

Point gesture A deictic gesture that is characterized by an extension of the arm from the body and the index finger from the hand in the direction of a target (e.g., object, picture, event).

Pragmatics (1) A domain of language that encompasses the rule system for the use of language form and content. (2) The ability to get things done with gestures and words; the use of language in a social context.

Prelexical forms See *phonetically consistent forms (PCF)*.

Preschool specific language impairment (SLI) An impairment in which the child typically has a performance IQ within normal limits, normal hearing acuity, no behavioral or emotional disorders, and no gross neurological deficits, but presents with significant deficits in language production and/or comprehension (Leonard, 1998).

Primary intersubjectivity Infants' ability to use and respond to eye contact, facial affects, vocal behavior, and body posture in one-to-one interactions with caregivers; it occurs early in life (0–6 months).

Primary language impairment A language deficit that cannot be accounted for by a peripheral sensory deficit (e.g., hearing loss), a motor deficit (e.g., cerebral palsy), a cognitive deficit (e.g., mental retardation), a social or emotional impairment (e.g., autism spectrum disorders), harmful environmental conditions (e.g., lead poisoning or drug abuse), and gross neurological deficit (e.g., traumatic brain injury or lesions). It is often presumed to be due to impaired development or dysfunction of the central nervous system (Leonard, 1998).

Principle of conventionality   A word learning bias that the child uses in word learning; it states that there are culturally agreed-upon names for things and these do not change.

Principle of extendibility   A word learning bias that the child uses in word learning; it states that a word does not refer to only one object. Rather, a word refers to a category of objects, events, or actions that share similar properties.

Principle of mutual exclusivity   A word learning bias that the child uses in word learning; it states that if an object already has a name, it cannot be referred to by another name.

Principle of reference   A word learning bias that the child uses in word learning; it states that words but not other sounds label objects, actions, and events.

Principles of word learning   See *innate biases*.

Probabilistic patterns   Correlations between co-occurring linguistic elements, such as speech sounds, syllable sequences, and word combinations. Language learners are highly sensitive to recurrent patterns in the speech they hear, and they more readily process highly frequent patterns. Probabilistic patterns may involve either adjacent elements (see *sequential dependency*) or non-adjacent elements.

Procedural memory system   The neural system underlying long-term memory of skills and procedures, or "how to" knowledge. Procedural memory is not easily verbalized and can be used without consciously thinking about it. This system supports statistical learning of complex patterns learned over time, such as sequences of linguistic elements.

Protowords   See *phonetically consistent forms (PCF)*.

Pull out   A language intervention used with school-age children can be provided by the speech-language pathologist on an individual basis or in small groups outside the classroom.

Pure tone   An individual frequency of sound.

Push in   A language intervention in which, to facilitate the child's participation in classroom activities, the speech-language pathologist may provide the therapy in the classroom.

Quick incidental learning (QUIL)   Learning that occurs when children learn the meaning of a new word with minimal overt support (no direct teaching of the new word) but multiple cues available to guide learning.

Race   A construct that classifies humanity based on arbitrary biological or anatomical features and/or nebulous geographical boundaries. It is often misinterpreted and forms the basis for social blights such as racism and discrimination.

Recasting   An intervention that is similar to expansion but in which the speech-language pathologist changes the type of utterance (e.g., from a statement to a question) or changes the voice or the mood in which the utterance is being produced.

Referencing   (1) The act of labeling; (2) an individual's ability to interpret other persons' attitudes toward what they are attending to.

Referential children   Those children for whom general nominals account for more than 50% of their lexicon.

Representational gestures   Iconic gestures that convey some aspect of the referent's meaning. The meaning conveyed by representational gestures might be the form of an object, the function of an object, the path or quality of an action, or the spatial relationship between two objects expressed by a preposition.

Resonance properties   The physical properties of an object that result in a natural tendency for it to vibrate at a particular frequency.

Responding to joint attention (RJA)   A situation in which the infant follows the direction of gaze, head turn, and or point gesture of another person.

Ritual request   A deictic gesture that conveys an infant's want or need for something by reaching with open hand or moving an adult's hand to the referent of interest.

Scaffolds   A teaching tool consisting of "help" that a child is given during learning (e.g., a model of a target behavior, cues, prompts).

Scripted play   An intervention which a child and the speech-language pathologist enact a play routine based on common scripts with which the child is familiar (Olswang & Bain, 1991). These scripts can range from daily routines such as a morning routine (e.g., waking up, brushing teeth, eating breakfast) to special-occasion scripts (e.g., planning a birthday party). These routines offer conventionalized, predictable contexts in which the speech-language pathologist can teach turn-taking, conversational skills, new linguistic forms such as vocabulary, grammatical morphology (such as verb tensing), and higher-level functions such as planning and problem solving.

Secondary intersubjectivity   A triadic pattern of communication in which the infant relates to another person in relation to an object or event.

Secondary language impairment   A language disorder that is associated with and presumed to be caused by factors such as sensory (hearing loss) or cognitive impairments (mental retardation). The language disorder can be part of a syndrome, which is the presence of multiple abnormalities in the same individual that are all caused by or originated from the same source.

Segmental   Referring to such speech elements as phonemes, morphemes, and syllables.

Self-talk   An intervention in which the speech-language pathologist describes his or her own actions.

Self-teaching hypothesis   A situation in which "each successful decoding encounter with an unfamiliar word provides an opportunity to acquire the word-specific orthographic information that is the foundation of skilled word recognition. A relatively small number of [successful] exposures appear to be sufficient for acquiring orthographic representations . . . [in] this way, phonological recoding acts as a self-teaching mechanism or built-in teacher enabling a child to independently develop both [word]-specific and general orthographic knowledge" (Share, 1995).

Semantic errors   A type of word retrieval error that is characterized by a taxonomic/hierarchical or thematic relationship with the target lexeme (e.g., *pig* for *cow*, or *animal* for *cow*).

Semantic feature hypothesis   A hypothesis that states children classify and organize referents in terms of perceptual features such as size, shape, animacy, and texture.

Semantic representation   The meaning information about a lexeme stored in memory. Semantic representations are multimodal and encompass learning from all sensory systems.

Semantics   A domain of language that encompasses the rule system for the meaning of language

Sensori-motor morphemes   See *phonetically consistent forms (PCF)*.

Sensorineural hearing loss   A hearing loss that is the result of damage to the inner ear and/or auditory nerve.

Sensorineural mechanism   A function of the body that involves both the inner ear and the auditory nerve.

Sequential-bilingual   A person characterized by exposure to a second language after developing a level of fluency in the first language skills. Different linguistic components are believed to be affected by differing ages of acquisition (example: phonological representations in adults). Also known as successive bilingualism.

Sequential dependency   The likelihood that one linguistic element will follow another in sequence. Language learners form expectations about which linguistic elements are likely to follow others.

Service delivery   A factor that influences the success of the language-impaired child; determined by the resources of the particular school district, as well as by the school district's underlying philosophy regarding bilingual and special education.

Shape bias   The tendency to extend words based on shared perceptual features of the original referent and novel exemplar.

Show gesture   A deictic gesture in which a child holds an object in view of his or her partner to engage him in an interaction but does not hand over the object.

Simultaneous-bilingual   A person characterized by concurrent exposure to two languages from an early age before the person has achieved a high level of fluency, dominance, or proficiency in either language; highly sensitive to the age of the language learner, as well as amount and quality of input provided in each language.

Slow mapping   The extended period of word learning that enriches the lexical–semantic representation of a word after it has been fast mapped.

Social-cognitive perspectives   Approaches to language acquisition that emphasize the interaction between the child's innate skills and his or her social experiences with others. In contemporary views, the child's requisite cognitive abilities allow him or her to process information, while pre-formed concepts for entities in the world serve as the basis for word learning and language development. The child's ability to infer the referential intentions of others is key to the language-learning process.

Social–emotional development   An aspect of development that concerns a child's interest in bonding with others in the environment. It is related to language development in that a child who is related to others, and therefore engaged with others in meaningful activities, is ready to respond to stimuli and learn.

Social-pragmatic perspectives   Approaches to language acquisition that focus on the child's development of the communicative functions or intentions of language, speaker-listener roles, the conversational rules of discourse, nonlinguistic means of communication, and the way that form and content shift based on the linguistic and nonlinguistic aspects of the context.

Sociolinguistic/sociocultural competence   The use of language and communication rules appropriate in one's language and cultural group.

Sociological assessment model   A process of assessment that considers that language learning is a complex process interrelated with personal, cultural, and experiential rules and expectations. Assessment must consider all of these factors to better inform the examiner as to the language experiences, motivations, and skills of the individual client.

Sound system development   Acquisition of the sounds of language.

Specific nominals   Words referring to a specific exemplar of a category, whether or not it is a proper name (e.g., *mommy*, *daddy*, pet's name).

Speech-generating device (SGD)   A computerized/electronic communication aid that produces speech. It displays pictures that represent what the individual wants to say or express. When a specific picture is pressed on the SGD, it generates speech in a digitized (recorded) or synthesized (computerized) form for the communication partner to hear.

Speech-language pathologist (SLP)   A professional who is trained in the assessment and treatment of disorders in the areas of speech (articulation, voice, fluency), language, cognition and eating/swallowing.

Speech mechanism   The six major organs/subsystems that are used in the production of speech.

Speech recognition score   A score that represents the percentage of speech that is understood when a speech signal is made sufficiently loud for the child; it is a measure of the clarity of speech.

Speech recognition threshold   The softest level at which the child can recognize speech 50% of the time.

Speech sound disorders   Problems producing the sounds of a language.

Spontaneous language sampling   The process of eliciting and recording discourse-level communication from an individual for formal analysis.

Stage theories   Theories that are useful in understanding the developmental changes children go through as they become proficient readers.

Standardized (norm-referenced) tests   Tests that rank the child's abilities against the performance of age-matched children with typical language development.

Statistical learning   The ability of infants to track statistics in the language they hear, such as the distribution of sounds in words, and the order of words in phrases. Statistical learning is supported by domain-general associative learning mechanisms and enables the child to discover the building blocks of linguistic structure.

Strategic competence   The strategies used by the bilingual person to compensate for breakdowns in communication that may result from imperfect knowledge of the rules, fatigue, memory lapses, distraction, and anxiety.

Subordinate terms   Specific exemplars of ordinate terms (e.g., *collie* is a subordinate term in relation to *dog*).

Superordinate terms   The broadest class of basic terms (e.g., *animal*, *transportation/vehicles*).

Suprasegmental   Referring to such speech elements as pitch, prosody, rhythm, stress, and inflection.

Suprathreshold   A level that is louder than the "barely detectable" threshold level.

Surface Account   The notion that, due to processing limitations, children with specific language impairments have difficulties perceiving inflections of brief duration, such as the past tense *-ed* and the third person singular *-s*. Incomplete processing of morphemes of low perceptual salience means that fewer of these morphemes are fully processed, which leads to a delay in the acquisition of these forms.

Symbols Items used to represent vocabulary. Symbols may be either unaided (e.g., signs, manual gestures, and facial expressions) or aided (e.g., actual objects, pictures, line drawings, and printed words); they range from arbitrary to transparent.

Syntactic bootstrapping The idea that children use the syntactic knowledge they have acquired to help them learn what words mean. For example, a child might use the constructions in which a novel verb is used to make inferences about the possible meaning of the verb.

Syntactic productivity Knowledge that the grammatical constructions of a language may be extended to new vocabulary. Children may demonstrate syntactic productivity by using a newly introduced word in a construction that they have never heard it used with, or by using the grammatical structure of a sentence to make inferences about the meaning of a newly introduced word.

Syntax A domain of language that encompasses the rule system for the sentence-level structure of language that marks relationships between words and ideas.

Temperament The combination of mental, physical, and emotional traits of children that affect their behavior.

Theory of mind The ability to attribute mental states—beliefs, intents, desires, pretending, knowledge, and so on—to oneself and others, and to understand that others have beliefs, desires, and intentions that are different from one's own.

Threshold The softest level required for a person to just be able to detect the presence of the sound, half of the time; that is, the level where 50% of the time the person hears the sound and 50% of the time he or she does not.

Time delay procedure An intervention technique in which the speech-language pathologist anticipates the child's needs or desires and intentionally waits for the child to initiate an action.

Traditional (developmental) approach to assessment An assessment technique that relies almost exclusively on age expectations and normative data. It includes checklists of age-expected behaviors to which infants and toddlers are compared to or measured against.

Traditional assessment model An imitation of the psychological model of assessment. This view suggests that language is a self-contained domain that can be analyzed apart from other domains (i.e., cognitive and emotional domains).

Transdisciplinary play-based assessment The assessment of not only language and communication skills, but also social–emotional, cognitive, and sensory–motor abilities. The assessment is implemented by a team that includes the parents and professionals from various disciplines (i.e., speech-language pathologists, occupational therapists, physical therapist, psychologist). The context of the assessment is play activities that vary depending on the child and the areas being evaluated. This approach is natural and follows the child's attentional needs.

Transformational Generative Grammar The original 1957 theory put forth by Chomsky, which described the innate knowledge of the native speaker-hearer of a language as including knowledge in the three main components of language—syntax, semantics, and phonology.

Translator A person trained to transpose written text from one language to another.

Treatment See *intervention*.

Tympanic membrane The eardrum.

Tympanometry An assessment method that provides an objective look at middle ear function (or middle ear *dysfunction*, as the case may be). During this test, a graph known as a tympanogram is created; it provides information that helps determine if middle ear pathology is present (e.g., an ear infection or punctured eardrum).

Underextension Use of a word to refer to only one exemplar of a referent (e.g., *dog* refers only to the family dog, not to other dogs).

Unilateral hearing loss A hearing loss that affects one ear only. It may be the result of conductive, sensorineural, or mixed pathology.

Unitary language system view A perspective suggesting that children exposed to two languages simultaneously process those languages through the same system, only to have the languages become separated over time.

Verbal communication Discourse; the use of spoken utterances as means for relaying ideas.

Verbal working memory capacity The limited capacity of the language processing system. The human information processing system has a limited pool of resources available to perform linguistic computations; performance deteriorates when processing demands exceed the available resources.

Vertical development Increasing hierarchical development associated with increasing age and cognitive understanding.

Visual misperception errors A word retrieval error that shares perceptual features with the intended target but has no semantic or phonological relationship with the intended target (e.g., *lollipop* for a *balloon*).

Visual reinforcement audiometry (VRA) An assessment method that combines sound with toys that light up and relies on the child's localization behaviors. The procedure involves conditioning the child to search for the sound when it is heard. When the child hears the sound and localizes it, he or she is rewarded with the toy lighting up.

Visuo-spatial sketchpad   The component of working memory that manipulates visual information for visual recognition and orientation of stimuli.

Vocabulary   The words people must know to communicate effectively; exists in both oral and written modes.

Vocabulary spurt   A discernable rapid increase in the number of words a child is learning and using; typically occurs after the child has acquired his or her first 50 words, between 18 and 24 months of age.

Vowels   Sounds in which the tongue typically does not come in contact with any of the other articulators during production. Vowels are always voiced and typically are not nasalized. Additionally, they are created with a relatively open vocal tract and have no point of constriction.

Whole-object bias   A word learning bias that the child uses in word learning; it guides the child to infer that the word label refers to the entire object and not just a part, an attribute, or its motion.

Word-finding difficulty   The momentary inability to retrieve already known words from the lexicon.

Word learning constraints   See *principles of word learning*.

Word retrieval errors   Production of the wrong lexeme when naming a referent; such errors are often logically related to the word that was targeted.

Word-specific formulae   Rote-learned combinatory patterns that are tied to specific lexical items.

Word spurt   See *vocabulary spurt*.

Working memory   The memory system that is involved in active, online processing of information. It allows for temporary storage of information while it is being manipulated or processed.

REFERENCES

American Speech-Language-Hearing Association (1993). Definitions of communication disorders and variations. Rockville, MD: American Speech-Language-Hearing Association.

American Speech-Language-Hearing Association. (2002). *Communication development and disorders in multicultural populations: Readings and materials.* Available at: http://www.asha.org/about/leadership-projects/multicultural/ readings/OMA_fact_sheets.htm

Bloom, L., & Tinker, E. (2001). The intentionality model and language acquisition. *Monographs of the Society for Research in Child Development, 66*(4), 267.

Catts, H. W. (1991). Facilitating phonological awareness: Role of speech-language pathologists. *Language, Speech, and Hearing Services in Schools, 22,* 196–203.

Leonard, L. (1998). *Children with specific language impairment.* Cambridge, MA: MIT Press.

Kendeou, P., Lynch, J. S., van den Broek, P., Espin, C., White, M., & Kremer, K. E. (2005). Developing successful readers: Building early narrative comprehension skills through television viewing and listening. *Early Childhood Education Journal, 33,* 91–98.

Olswang, L., & Bain, B. (1991). Intervention issues for toddlers with specific language impairments. *Topic in Language Disorders, 11,* 69–86.

Paul, R. (2005). *Language disorders from infancy through adolescence: Assessment and intervention.* St. Louis, MO: Mosby-Year Book.

Pullen, P. C., & Justice, L. M. (2003). Enhancing phonological awareness, print awareness, and oral language skills in preschool children. *Intervention in School and Clinic, 39,* 87–98.

Share, D. L. (1995). Phonological recoding and self-teaching: sine qua non of reading acquisition. *Cognition, 55*(2), 151–218.

Tulving, E. (1993). What is episodic memory? *Current Directions in Psychological Science, 2,* 67–70.

United States Bureau of the Census (2002). *U.S. Census of Population and Housing.* Washington, DC: GPO.

van Kleeck, A., & Schuele, C. (1987). Precursors to literacy: Normal development. *Topics in Language Disorders, 7,* 13–31.

INDEX

A

A Boy, a Dog, and a Frog, 167
AAC. *See* Communication development in
    children with multiple disabilities
ABA (applied behavior analysis), 71, 395
ABR (auditory brain stem response), 110–111
Accommodation, adaptation process, 37
Acculturalization, 350–351
Acoustic immittance testing, 111
Acoustic reflex testing, 111
Acting-out tasks, 317
Action words, 202t, 203
Adaptation process, 36–37
Advanced, logical thinking stages of cognitive
    development, 37
Affect expression, 199
Affect sharing device (AFS), 138–139
Affricates, 227
Affrication, 234
Ages and Stages Questionnaires, 160
Aided language stimulation, 435
Alphabetic principle, 334
Alphabetic stage of literacy development, 334
Alveolars, 229
Amber, 415–416, 417, 418, 423, 436
    speech language evaluation
        clinical findings
            diagnosis and prognosis, 454
            expressive language, 453–454
            general observations, 452–453
            nonverbal communication, 453
            oral-motor examination, 454
            phonology, 454
            receptive language, 453
            recommendations, 455
        clinical procedures, 452
        significant history, 451–452
American Sign Language (ASL), 179
American Speech-Language-Hearing Association
    (ASHA), 109

definition of language, 1–2
document on providing culturally and
    linguistically appropriate services, 350,
    354–355
responsibilities of SPLs with respect to
    reading and writing, 239
Anatomy and physiology of the peripheral
    auditory system
the conductive mechanism
    external ear canal, 97, 97f
    middle ear
        impedance mismatch, 99
        and inner ear compared, 96
        main objective of, 99
        structures, 98–99, 99f
        transformer function, 99–100
    outer ear
        acoustic functions, 97–98
        cerumen (ear wax), 98
        localization, 98
        nonacoustic functions, 98
        resonance properties of, 98
    pinna (auricle), 96–98, 97f
    tympanic membrane (eardrum), 97, 97f,
        99f
the sensorial mechanism, 100–102
    cochlea, 100–101, 101f
    organ of Corti, 100, 102
    outer, middle, and inner ear, 101f
    summary of the conductive mechanism,
        100, 101f
Anderson, R.T., 368
*Annual Report to Congress on the Implementation
    of IDEA,* 356–357
Applebee's System of Scoring Narrative Stages,
    12
Applied behavior analysis (ABA), 71, 395
Arizona Articulation Proficiency, 243t
Articulation, 225, 226
ASD. *See* Autism spectrum disorder (ASD)

ASHA. *See* American Speech-Language-Hearing Association (ASHA)

ASL (American Sign Language), 179

Asperger's disorder, 393

Assessment of hearing in the pediatric population
  birth to six months of age, 108–111
    behavioral procedures, 109
    electrophysiological procedures
      acoustic immittance testing, 111
      acoustic reflex testing, 111
      auditory brain stem response (ABR), 110–111
      auditory steady-state response (ASSR), 110–111
      otoacoustic emissions (OAE), 109–110
      tympanometry, 111
    JCIH position statement (2000), 109
    NIH consensus statement (1993), 109
  children from 7 months to 24-30 months, 111–112
  children from 30 months to 5 years of age, 112
  conditioned play audiometry (CPA), 112
  overview, 108
  speech recognition assessment, 112–113
  speech recognition score, 112
  speech recognition threshold, 112
  visual reinforcement audiometry (VRA), 111–112

Assessment of narratives, 399–400

Assessment protocols, from a nurture perspective, 70–71

Assessment tools
  Battelle Developmental Inventory, 2nd ed. (BDI-2), 49–50
  Communication and Symbolic Behavior Scales (CSBS), 47–48
  Hawaii Early Learning Profile (HELP), 49
  Learning Accomplishment Profile (LAP) system, 49
  MacArthur-Bates Communicative Development Inventories, 2nd ed. (CDIs), 48–49
  Receptive-Expressive Emergent Language Test, 3rd ed. (REEL-3), 48
  Rossetti Infant-Toddler Language Scale (RITLS), 48

Assimilation, 37, 350–351

Associationistic accounts of lexical-semantic representations, 210–211

ASSR (auditory steady-state response), 110–111

Attachment, social competence, 136, 141

Attention, auditory skills development, 107

Audiologists, 9

Auditory behavioral development, 103–104

Auditory brain stem response (ABR), 110–111

Auditory Comprehension subtest (PLS-IV), 14

Auditory processing programs, 74

Auditory skills development
  attention, 107
  auditory closure, 107–108
  auditory memory, 107
  bottom-up approach to language learning, 106

Auditory steady-state response (ASSR), 110–111

Auditory system. *See* Anatomy and physiology of the peripheral auditory system

Augmentative and alternative communication (AAC). *See* Communication development in children with multiple disabilities

Augmented communication input, 437

Aural rehabilitation, 122–123

Autism spectrum disorder (ASD), 80
  ASD and PDD-NOS compared, 394
  associated conditions, 393–394
  diagnostic criteria for (*DSM-IV*), 393
  early indicators, 394–395
  first described, 392–393
  language deficits, 394
  onset of, 393
  pointing impairments, 192
  prevalence in the United States, 393
  social dysfunction in ASD children, 155–156

Automatic word definition, 334–335

Automaticity, 338

Avoidant attachment, 141

B

Baby signs, 178–179

Baby talk, by caregivers, 142

Background history of child, 10–11, 11t

Backing, 234

Bankson-Bernthal Test of Phonology (BBTOP), 243

Basal level of performance, 12

Basic-level terms, 212
Basilar membrane, 100, 101f, 102
Battelle Developmental Inventory, 2nd ed. (BDI-2), 49–50
Beat gestures, 179, 181
Behavioral hearing assessment procedures, 109
Behind-the-ear (BTE) style hearing aid, 119, 120f
Belief emotion, 166
Bilabials, 229
Bilingualism. *See* Cultural competence
Bishop, D., 312–313
Black children in Piedmont region of N.C., cultural variations in caregiver-child interactions, 144
Blank slate philosophy of John Locke, 68
Bloom, L., 64, 81–82
Bloom, Paul, 77
Boardmaker Picture Communication Symbols, 448
Bootstrapping, 204, 277, 278, 280, 281–282, 308–309
Bottom-up approach to language learning, 106
Bound morphemes, 3–4, 256, 257t
Briggs, M.H., 157
Broccoli effect, 332
Brown's 14 stages of morphological development
    grammatical morphemes
        characteristics of, 263–264
        list of, 263t
        process of acquiring, 264–265
        rule-governed morphological system, 265
        uses for, 264
    morphological development
        application of the information, 261
        refinements in sentence complexity, 261
        summary of grammatical morpheme production, 262t
        syntactic specificity, 260–261
        telegraphic, 260
Bruner, J., 77

C

CALC (Clinical Assessment of Language Comprehension), 457
Canonical babbling stage of vocal development, 232

CAS (childhood apraxia of speech), 225, 226
Case studies. *See* Amber; Johnathon (TD); Josephina; Josephine (LB); Oscar; Robert (LT); Sam
Catts, H.W., 334, 342–343
Ceiling level of performance, 12
Central executor, 215
Cerumen (ear wax), 98
Chall, J.S., 333–334
Challenging behaviors, 426
Chapman, K., 302–303, 306–309
Child development
    assessment of young children (*See also* Assessment tools)
        factors
            how, 47
            when, 46–47
            where, 46
            who, 46
        strategies
            direct elicitation, 47
            interview, 47
            observation, 47
    cognitive development, 36–40
        definition of, 36
        Piaget's theories
            accommodation, 37
            assimilation, 37
            disequilibrium (adaptation), 36–37
            four factors of cognitive development, 36
            stages of cognitive development, 37–38, 38t
            stages of the sensorimotor period, 38, 39t, 40
        theories of, 36
    introduction, 35–36
    linguistic development, 43–45, 44t
    motor development, 40–41, 41t
    objectives, 35
    social-emotional development
        achieve and maintain self-regulation, 42–43
        connectedness with the world, 41–42
        development of imitation skills, 43
Child-directed speech (CDS), 79–80
Childhood apraxia of speech (CAS), 225, 226

Childhood disintegrative disorder, 393
Children's Communicative Checklist-2, 160
Chomsky, Noam, 4
    Extended Standard Theory, 65
    Minimalist Program, 65–66
    Principles and Parameters theory, 64–65
    Transformational Generative Grammar,
        60–61
CIC (completely in-the-canal style hearing aid),
    119, 120f
Classical conditioning, 68–69
Classification ability, 40
Clausal embedding, 261
Clinical Assessment of Language Comprehension
    (CALC), 457
Closed syllable, 230
Coalescence, 235
Cochlea, 100–101, 101f, 110
Cochlear implants, 122, 123f
Code switching, 361–362, 365
Cognates, 229
Cognitive-constructivist models, 74–76
Cognitive development, 36–40
    definition of, 36
    Piaget's theories
        accommodation, 37
        assimilation, 37
        disequilibrium (adaptation), 36–37
        four factors of cognitive development, 36
        stages of cognitive development, 37–38, 38t
        stages of the sensorimotor period, 38, 39t,
            40
    theories of, 36
Communication and Symbolic Behavior Scales
    (CSBS), 47–48, 160
Communication development in children with
    multiple disabilities
    augmentative and alternative communication
        (AAC)
        challenges for successful AAC
            external challenges
                attitudes and lack of knowledge, 427
                environmental barriers, 427
                myths and realities in ACC
                    intervention, 428t
                opportunities for participation,
                    427–429

internal challenges
    challenging behavior, 426
    learned helplessness, 425–426
    medical, 424
    physical ability, 425
components of an ACC system
    aids or modes of communication, 420
    strategies, 422
    techniques, 422
    vocabulary and symbols, 421–422
described, 419
roles of ACC intervention
    facilitation of language and
        communication development, 423
    provide an expressive output mode for
        communication, 423
    social development and well-being of a
        child, 423–424
communicative profiles (*See also* Amber;
    Oscar; Sam)
constructing
    adaptive behavior, 417
    cognitive development, 417
    communicative experiences, 417–418
    definition of communicative profile,
        416–417
    intelligence, 417
    language comprehension, 419
    vocal and gesture ability, 418
foundations for implementation of AAC
    intervention, 429–440, 430–431t
AAC assessment
    adaptation needs and methods, 434,
        434t
    aided language stimulation, 435
    assessment areas, 432–433, 433t
    diagnostic intervention, 435
    standardized and nonstandardized tests,
        433–434
augmented communication input, 437
beginning AAC intervention as early as
    possible, 435
communication-partner instruction and
    education in language intervention,
    438–439
knowledge of language comprehension and
    production, 436–437

ongoing monitoring, 439–440
philosophical beliefs, 429, 432
systematic language-based intervention, 437
teaching through natural communicative activities and routines, 437–438
introduction, 413–415
all children can and do communicate, 414
communication and quality of life, 413–414
communication defined, 414
primary diagnoses of these children, 414
term multiple disabilities, 414
ways to promote functionality and effectiveness of communication, 414
objectives, 413
speech-generating devices (SGDs), 414, 419, 420, 421, 423–424, 437, 448, 450, 451
summary, 440–441
Communication-partner instruction, 438–439
Communicative competence, 365
Communicative profiles, constructing
adaptive behavior, 417
cognitive development, 417
communicative experiences, 417–418
definition of communicative profile, 416–417
intelligence, 417
language comprehension, 419
vocal and gesture ability, 418
Completely in-the-canal (CIC) style hearing aid, 119, 120f
Comprehension level of auditory development, 108
Comprehension of language. See also Comprehension of language, measuring
case studies, 323–325
introduction, 297
measuring
acting-out tasks, 317
identification tasks, 317
judgment tasks, 317
nonstandardized comprehension probes
advantage of, 323
probe for Wh-questions, 322–323, 322t
question comprehension, adequacy of, 321–322
standardized assessment
aspects of test giving, 318

assessing infants and toddlers
MacArthur-Bates Communicative Development Inventories, 319–320
Rosetti Infant-Toddler Language Scale (RITLS), 318–319
vocabulary comprehension data, 320
testing procedures for older preschool-age children
identifying pictures, 320–321
Peabody Picture Vocabulary Test-4 (PVVT-4), 321
Test for Auditory Comprehension of Language-3 (TACL-3), 321
summary of caveats, 317–318
objectives, 297
study of in young children
challenge of, 298
example: 5-year-old with age-appropriate language abilities, 298–300
summary, 325
what is language comprehension?
assistance from the environment: nonlingusitic context, 304–305
comprehension of semantic relationships and syntax
addition of prepositions, 314–315
consideration of comprehension strategies, 314
production of two-word combinations, 313–314
use of adverbial connectors, 315
comprehension of single words
development of word category hierarchies, 312
expressive vocabularies, 311
fast mapping, 313
overextensions/underextensions, word meaning boundaries, 311
receptive vocabularies, 311
word language mechanisms: links between phonology and semantics, 312–313
development and use of comprehension strategies

comprehension strategy use in the
    linguistic period
    bootstrapping, 308–309
    order of mention strategy, 309
    word-order strategy, 308
    world knowledge, 309–310
  examples of comprehension strategies,
    307–308
  guessing, a good strategy for learning,
    310–311
  reliance on nonlinguistic or context
    information, 306–307
does language comprehension exceed
    production
  considering whether comprehension
    deficits really exist, 315
  question comprehension: accurate,
    appropriate, or both, 316
interactions between context and
    comprehension of meaning
  clinicians and caregivers disagreements
    about, 302–303
  incorporating information into clinical
    work, 303–304
  types of competencies being developed,
    304
  what we know about development of
    language comprehension, 304
quality of input and context: helping
    children map language
  adult-infant/toddler speech and
    language compared, 305
  how to map language input to the
    context, 305–306
terms used, 300
understanding the role of context
  role of world knowledge in
    comprehension, 300–301
  role played by nonlinguistic information
    (context), 301
Conceptual information, 4
Concrete stage of cognitive development, 37, 38t
Conditioned play audiometry (CPA), 112
Conductive hearing loss, 113–114. See also Otitis
    media
Congenital causes of sensorineural hearing loss,
    114, 116

Connectionistic model of information processing,
    73
Consonants, 227–229
  cluster, 234
  sequence, 234
Context. See Comprehension of language
Conversational protocol, understanding of, 79
Coo and Goo stage of vocal development, 232
Coordination/coregulation, 169–170
Coordination of reaction stage, sensorimotor
    period, 39t
CPA (conditioned play audiometry), 112
Criterion-referenced measures, 13, 368–369, 399
Cross-sectional study, 230
CSBS (Communication and Symbolic Behavior
    Scales), 47–48, 160
Cultural bias, 350
Cultural competence
  bilingualism: perspectives in the United States
    English language learners (ELLs) in the
      U.S., 356
    language as problem, 356
    language as resource, 356
    language as right, 356
    LEP students with a concomitant
      disability, 356–357
  case study: Josephina: adjusted relevant
    history, 357–358
  collaborating with interpreters/translators
    interpreter defined, 365
    modifications to testing procedures,
      366–367
    skills needed by the interpreter, 365–366
    state regulations, 365
    training of an interpreter by the SLP, 366
    translated tests, 366
    translator defined, 365
  culture
    cultural variables affecting language
      development, 354, 354t
    cultural variables: heritage, 353
    definition of, 352
    ethnic culture, 352
    ethnicity, 352–353
    explicit behaviors and implicit beliefs, 352,
      353t
    race, 353–354

development of cultural competence
    ASHA practice document, 354–355
    cultural diversity and language diversity,
        differences between, 355
    essential characteristics of the competent
        SLPs, 355
    need for SLPs to become culturally
        competent, 354
improving cultural competence in assessment
    background information
        ethnographic interviewing, 370–371
        sociological assessment model, 369–370
        traditional assessment model, 369
    formal testing, 367–368
    importance of cultural information, 367
    informal testing
        criterion-referenced procedures,
            368–369
        dynamic assessment, 369
        ethnographic observations, 369
        language sampling, 369
language development: bilingual perspectives
    critical period for second language (L2)
        acquisition, 363
    dual-(differentiated-) language system
        hypothesis, 363
    fractionated system view, 363
    proficiency, defining, 362
    sequential-bilingual child, 362–363
    simultaneous-bilingual child, 362–363
    time of assessment, 363–364
    unitary language system, 363
linguistic variables affecting the assessment
    and intervention process
    the bilingual child, 362
    code switching, 361–362
    dialectal variance, 362
    language loss, 361
    language-use patterns, 361
objectives, introduction
    ASHA document on providing culturally
        and linguistically appropriate
        services, 350
    assimilation and acculturalization, 350–351
    demographic changes in the United States,
        349
    ethnocentrism by the provider, 350
    understanding the cultural and linguistic
        differences, 349–350
simultaneous-bilingual and monolingual
    children compared
    communicative competence, 365
    decrease in amount of language mixing/
        transfer, 364–365
    facility with code switching, 365
    language mixing, 364
    lexical development, 364
    morpho-syntactic rules for each language,
        364
    phonological transfers, 364
summary, 372–373
terminology
    culturally and linguistically diverse groups,
        351
    diversity, 351
    ethnic diversity, 351
    gay/lesbian/bisexual/transgender
        (GLBT), 352
    minority and majority, 351
    multicultural, 351
    racial/ethnic minority, 351
treatment considerations
    choice of language, 371–372
    collaborations, 372
    service delivery, 372
variables affecting the assessment and
    intervention process
    illness and disabilities, 360
    language-ego permeability, 360–361
    orientation, 358
    play interactions, 360
    verbal and nonverbal communication,
        358–359
Cultural diversity, 355
Cultural variables, 353, 354, 354t
Culturally and linguistically diverse groups, 351
Curriculum-based language assessment, 400
Cycles phonological remediation approach,
    245–247

D

Deaf culture, 129
Deaffrication, 234

DEAP (*Diagnostic Evaluation of Articulation and Phonology*), 243
Decoding, 335
Decontextualization, 183, 206
Deictic gestures, 178, 180, 183
Deictic terms, 77
Depalatalization, 234
Derivational morphemes, 4
Descartes, Rene, 59
Detection level of auditory development, 106–107
Developmental psycholinguistics, 63–64
Diagnostic and Statistical Manual of Mental Disorders, 4th ed. (DSM-IV)
   diagnosis of mental retardation, 395
   diagnostic criteria for autism, 393
Diagnostic Evaluation of Articulation and Phonology (DEAP), 243
Diagnostic intervention, 435
Dialectal variance, 362
Diamanti, Tony, 413
Diminutive, 236
Diphthongs, 229
Discourse competence, 365
Discrimination level of auditory development, 107
Disequilibrium (adaptation), 36–37
Disorganized-disoriented attachment, 141
Distributed neural network, 210
Diverse desires, 165
Diversity, 351
Domains of language, 3–6
   morphology, 3–4
   phonology, 3
   pragmatics, 5–6
   semantics, 4–5
   syntax, 4, 5t
Dore, John, 79
Down syndrome, gesture use by children with, 191–192
DSM-IV. *See Diagnostic and Statistical Manual of Mental Disorders, 4th ed.* (DSM-IV)
Dual-(differentiated-) language system hypothesis, 363
Duchan, J., 80
Dunn, C., 236, 236t
Dynamic assessment, 369, 398

E

Early communicative gestures, 180
Early Identification of Hearing Impairment in Infants and Young Children, 109
Early lexical-semantic development
   associationistic accounts of lexical-semantic representations, 210–211
   decontextualization, 206
   emergentist coalition model, 208–209
   expressive *vs.* referential word learners, 205–206
   the first word: locutionary stage, 199–202
      development assessment, 201–202
      mean age of a 50-word vocabulary, 200
      notion of a true word, 200
      vocabulary milestones, importance of, 201
      word spurt, 200–201
   innate biases make word learning efficient, 206–208
      novel name-nameless category principle (N3C), 206–207
      principle of conventionality, 207
      principle of extendibility, 207
      principle of mutual exclusivity, 206
      principle of reference, 206
      shape bias, 207–208
      size of an object, 208
      whole-object bias, 206
   intent to communicate: illocutionary stage, 198–199
   introduction, 197–198
   later lexical development, 216–217
   learning a word
      fast mapping, 209
      quick incidental learning (QUIL), 209
      repeated exposure to words, 210
      slow mapping, 209–210
   naming errors
      functional core hypothesis, 212
      overextension, 211
      phonotactic probability, 212
      semantic feature hypothesis, 211
      underextension, 211
   naming errors in word retrieval
      frequency of word exposure, 214–215
      indeterminate errors, 213
      naming practice, 214

perseverative errors, 213
phonological errors, 213
phonotactic probability words, 213–214
relation to their targets, 212
richness of semantic representation, 214
semantic errors, 213
shape/function, and control, 215
during the word spurt period, 213
objectives, 197
preparing the first year: perlocutionary stage,
    198
a preponderance of nouns, 202–205
    bootstrapping, 204
    classification system of words, 202–203,
        202t
    environment and the developing lexicon,
        204
    influence of maternal language on child's
        early vocabulary, 204
    noun preferences in early lexicons, 203
    ordering of word classes in a sentence,
        203–204
    pattern of noun learning over word-class
        learning, 205
summary, 217
working memory
    central executor, 215
    episodic buffer, 215–216
    online processing, 215
    phonological loop, 215, 216
    visuo-spatial sketchpad, 215, 216
Early representational thought, sensorimotor
    period, 39t
Early Social Communication Scales, 159
Echolalia, 80
ECM (emergentist coalition model), 208–209
Ecologically based programs
    common assumptions, 168
    goals of, 169
    interrupted behavior chain, 168
Education of the Handicapped Act (1990), 401
Effort, intentionality model, 81–83, 83f
Electrophysiologic hearing assessment
    procedures, 109–111
ELLs (English language learners in the U.S.), 356
Emblem gestures, 179, 181
Emergence, 258

Emergentist coalition model (ECM), 208–209
Emotional support, 439
Emotions, 165–167
Empiricist theories, 68
Endogenous factors, social competence, 137
Endolymph, 101
Engagement, intentionality model, 81–83, 83f
English- and Korean-speaking children, early
    vocabularies of, 204
English language learners (ELLs) in the U.S., 356
Entrenchment, 278
Environmental barriers, 427
EOI (Extended Optional Infinitive Hypothesis),
    284
Epenthesis, 236
Episodic buffer, 215–216
Episodic memory, 170
Equilibrium, progression toward, cognitive
    development and, 36
Ethnic culture, 352
Ethnic diversity, 351
Ethnic majority, 351
Ethnic minority, 351
Ethnicity, 352–353
Ethnocultural considerations in speech sound
    disorders, 241
Ethnographic interviewing, 370–371
Ethnographic observations, 369
Eustachian tube, 99, 99f
EVT. See Expressive Vocabulary Test (EVT)
Exogenous factors, social competence, 137
Expansion, 403–404
Experience-sharing, social competence, 136
Explicit behaviors and implicit beliefs, 352, 353t
Explicit false belief, 166
Exploration and expansion stage of vocal
    development, 232
Expressive Communication subtest (PLS-IV), 14
Expressive language and gesture, 182, 189
Expressive vocabularies, 311
Expressive Vocabulary Test (EVT), 14, 453
Expressive vs. referential word learners, 205–206
Extended Optional Infinitive (EOI) Hypothesis,
    284
Extended Standard Theory (Chomsky), 65
External cause of emotion, 165
Eye contact, 198, 359

F

Facilitative play, 404
Fast ForWord, 74
Fast mapping, 209, 313
Feedback
    from hearing aids, 119, 120f
    as a scaffolding tool, 20
Fine motor skills, 40
First word stage, 233
Fluency, 337–338
Focused auditory input/stimulation, 247–248
Focused stimulation, 404–405
Formal stage of cognitive development, 38t
Free morphemes, 3–4, 256
Fricatives, 227
Fronting, 234
Function words, 202t
Functional ability, 116
Functional core hypothesis, 212

G

G-SLI. *See* Grammatical SLI
Gay/lesbian/bisexual/transgender (GLBT), 352
General nominals, 202t, 203
Gesture development
    children with language learning impairments
        gesture as compensation for limited
            spoken language, 190–191
        studies
            at-risk quadruplets, 191
            children with autism spectrum disorder,
                192
            children with Down syndrome, 191–192
            children with SLI, 191
    child's readiness to learn and, 184–187
        analysis of gesture-spoken language
            combinations, 187
        conservation of quantity, 184–185
        gesture-spoken language match
            combinations, 185
        gesture-spoken language mismatch
            combinations, 185–186
        transitional learning state, 186–187
    cultural variables in, 359
    defining gesture types
        American Sign Language (ASL), 179

        beat gestures, 179
        deictic (prelinguistic) gestures, 178
        emblem gestures, 179
        representational gestures (iconic, baby
            signs), 178–179
    emergence of gesture
        beat gestures, 181
        deictic gestures, 180
        emblem gestures, 181
        gesture-word combinations, 181
        pointing, 78, 180
        representational gestures, 180–181
        ritual request, showing, then giving, 180
        summary, 181–182
    final thoughts for the clinician, 192
    function of gesturing, 189–190
    gesture input to the child
        cross-cultural study of, 187
        gesture and spoken language
            combinations, 188–189
        gesture cues, 188
        gesture input by adults, 187–188
        mothers' gestures, 187
        summary, 189
    introduction, 177–178
    mental representations
        decontextualization, 183
        deictic gesture sequence and, 183
        gesture and spoken language, relationship
            between, 183–184
        representational gesture of toddlers and,
            183
    mental representations and, definition of the
        term, 182–183
    summary, 193
GFTA-2 (*Goldman-Fristoe Test of Articulation,
    2nd ed.*), 14–15, 243t, 454
Give gestures, 180
GLBT (Gay/lesbian/bisexual/transgender), 352
Glides (speech sounds), 227
Gliding, 234
Glottal /h/, 229
Goldin-Meadow, S., 78
Goldman-Fristoe Test of Articulation, 2nd ed.
    (GFTA-2), 14–15, 243t, 454
Government binding—principles and
    parameters—Chomsky, 64–65

Grammar development
in children with specific language impairment
(SLI)
the *Extended Optional Infinitive (EOI)*
Hypothesis, 284
impaired statistical learning
in the learning of probabilistic patterns
and sequential dependencies, 287
in the procedural memory system, 287
serial reaction time (SRT) testing,
287–288
information-processing speed and limited
verbal working memory capacity,
285–286
performance accounts of grammatical
difficulties: the Surface Account,
285
remediation of syntactic difficulties, 288
representational deficits and grammatical
SLI (G-SLI)
correlation between vocabulary and
grammar acquisition, 284
difficulties with reversible active-voice
sentences, 283
types of grammatical difficulties,
282–283
SLI described, 281
syntactic bootstrapping and knowledge of
constructions, 281–282
introduction, 271
in late talkers
index of productive syntax (IPSyn), 280
Language Development Survey results,
280
longitudinal study: late talkers and
children with typical development
compared, 280
mean length of utterance (MLU), 279–280
objectives, 271
summary, 289
in typically developing children
acquiring word-specific formulae
child's first constructions, 275–276
transitive and intransitive verb
constructions, 275
acquisition of verbs, 272–273
content words, 272

erroneous syntactic operations, 279
linguistic constructions, 272
semantic roles of nouns in a sentence, 273
statistical learning
beginnings of, 273–274
phonological features and, 274
role in acquisition of word classes, 274
syntactic overgeneralizations
onset of syntactic productivity, 277–278
overgeneralization errors, 278–279
syntactic bootstrapping, 278
verb acquisition and its influence on
grammatical structures
grammar acquisition, 276–277
lexical bootstrapping, 277, 280
order of verb acquisition, 276
transitive subject-verb-object, 276
Grammatical competence, 365
Grammatical SLI (G-SLI)
correlation between vocabulary and grammar
acquisition, 284
difficulties with reversible active-voice
sentences, 283
types of grammatical difficulties, 282–283
Grammatical specifications, 209
Grapheme, 336
Gross motor skills, 40
Guide to Analysis of Language Transcripts, 12

H

Halliday, Nigel, 79
Hammer, C.S., 371
Handicap, 380–381
Hawaii Early Learning Profile (HELP), 49
Hearing aids, 115, 116
basic components of, 119
feedback, 119, 120f
one hearing aid or two, 119
problems with, 118–119
selecting the most appropriate one, 120
styles of, 119, 120f
Hearing and language development. *See also*
Anatomy and physiology of the peripheral
auditory system; Assessment of hearing
in the pediatric population; Hearing
impairment

auditory behavioral development, 103–104
auditory skills development
    attention, 107
    auditory closure, 107–108
    auditory memory, 107
    bottom-up approach to language learning,
        106
    components of
        comprehension level, 108
        detection level, 106–107
        discrimination level, 107
        identification level, 107–108
    comprehension of linguistic and
        nonlinguistic sounds, 105–106
    case studies (*See also* individual names)
        Johnathon (TD), 129–130
        Josephine (LB), 130–131
        Robert (LT), 131
    introduction, 95–96
    normal auditory development
        postnatal
            background noise and reverberation,
                104
            encoding, 103
            selective listening, 103–104
        prenatal, 102–103
    objectives, 95
    speech sound disorders and, 240
    summary, 131
Hearing impairment, 9. *See also* Language
    development of the hearing-impaired
    population
    conductive hearing loss, 113–114
    interventions for hearing loss, 117–123
        aural rehabilitation, 122–123
        cochlear implants, 122, 123f
        hearing aids, 116, 118–120, 157
            basic components of, 119
            feedback, 119, 120f
            one hearing aid or two, 119
            problems with, 118–119
            selecting the most appropriate one, 120
            styles of, 119, 120f
        mixed hearing loss, 116–117
        otitis media, 113–114
        sensorineural hearing loss, 114–116
            causes of, 114

    functional ability, 116
    hearing impaired and deaf, difference
        between, 115–116
    high-frequency hearing loss, 115
    loss of sensitivity and speech distortion,
        114–115
    speech clarity problems, 116
    unilateral hearing loss (UHL), 117
Helicotrema, 101, 101f
HELP (*Hawaii Early Learning Profile*), 49
Heritage, 353
Hiding emotions, 166
High-frequency hearing loss, 115
High vowels, 229
Hodson, B., 245, 246, 247
Hodson Assessment of Phonological Patterns, 3rd
    ed., 243t, 246
Home program, 21
Horizontal development
    communicative functions in preschool
        children, 148, 150t
    discourse level, 148
    early communicative events, 148, 149t
    social level, 148
    utterance level, 147

I

IBR (initiating behavior request), 137–138, 145,
    156
Iconic gestures, 178–179
IDEA. *See* Individuals with Disabilities
    Education Act (IDEA)
Identification level of auditory development,
    107–108
Identification tasks, 317
IEP (individual education plan), 401
IFSP (individual family service plan), 401
IJA (initiating joint attention), 137–138, 156
Illinois Test of Psycholinguistic Abilities
    (ITPA), 73–74
Illness and disabilities, cultural variables in, 360
Illocutionary stage of communication, 7, 78–79,
    145, 198–199
Imitation, 403–404
Impedance/impedance mismatch, 99
In-the-canal (ITC) style hearing aid, 119, 120f

In-the-ear (ITE) style hearing aid, 119, 120f
Incidental teaching, 71, 403
Incus (anvil), 97f, 99, 99f
Independent/individualist, 143
Indeterminate errors, 213
Index of productive syntax (IPSyn), 280
Indicating, joint referencing and, 77
Indicating expression, 199
Individual education plan (IEP), 401
Individual family service plan (IFSP), 401
Individuals with Disabilities Education Act
    (IDEA)
    definition of mental retardation, 395
    legislation, 70–71
    on public education for all children, 401
Infant engagement tools, 138–139
Inflectional morphemes, 4
Information processing models, 72–74
Information-processing speed and limited verbal
    working memory capacity, 285–286
Informational support, 439
Initiating behavior request (IBR), 137–138, 145,
    156
Initiating joint attention (IJA), 137–138, 156
Innate biases and word learning, 206–208
Instrumental expression, 199
Instrumental social actions, 136
Intentionality, 136–137
    development of, 78–79
    implications from the intentionality model,
        83–84
    inference of intentionality by children, 78
    intentionality model, 81–83, 83f
        linguistic development, 45
    intentionality model: engagement and
        effort, 45
    interpretation of intentionality, 78
    stages of
        illocutionary stage, 145
        initiating behavior request (IBR), 145, 156
        locutionary stage, 145
        perculocutionary stage, 144
        protodeclarative (IJA), 145
Interactionist theories
    cognitive interactionist paradigm, 72–84
        cognitive-constructivist models, 74–76
        information processing models, 72–74

intentionality model, 81–84, 83f
interactionist paradigm
    implications from, 80–81
    social-cognitive models, 77–78
    social-pragmatic models, 78–80
Interdentals, 229
Interdependent/collectivist, 143
Interpreters/translators
    interpreter defined, 365
    modifications to testing procedures, 366–367
    skills needed by the interpreter, 365–366
    state regulations, 365
    training of an interpreter by the SLP, 366
    translated tests, 366
    translator defined, 365
Intervention (treatment), definition of, 1
Interviews, 47, 162, 164t, 165
Intervocalic, 227
IPSyn (index of productive syntax), 280
ITC (in-the-canal style hearing aid), 119, 120f
ITE (in-the-ear style hearing aid), 119, 120f
ITPA (Illinois Test of Psycholinguistic
    Abilities), 73–74

J

JA (joint attention), 137–138, 167–170, 198
Jackendorf, R., 66
JCIH (Joint Commission on Infant Hearing),
    109
Johnathon (TD), 21–24
    developmental assessment, 50
    expressive language and gesture, 182, 189
    hearing and language development, 129–130
    language assessment and intervention
        clinical findings
            expressive language, 23
            general observations, 22
            nonverbal communication, 23
            oral-motor examination, 24
            phonology, 23–24
            play, 23
            receptive language, 23
        clinical procedures, 22
        diagnosis and prognosis, 24
        recommendations, 24
        significant history, 22

language comprehension, 323–324
literacy development, 343
morphosyntactic aspect of language
    development using Brown's stages,
    266–267
semantic development, 201–202
speech sound assessment, 248
Joint attention (JA), 137–138, 167–170, 198
Joint Commission on Infant Hearing (JCIH),
    109
Joint story reading, 402
Josephina
    adjusted relevant history, 357–358
    nonverbal behaviors of the family and, 359
    simultaneous-bilingual learner, 364
Josephine (LB), 21, 24–28, 385–387
    developmental assessment, 51
    expressive language and gesture, 182, 189
    hearing and language development, 130–131
    language assessment and intervention
        clinical findings
            diagnosis and prognosis, 27
            expressive language, 26
            general observations, 25
            nonverbal communication, 26
            oral-motor examination, 27
            phonology, 27
            play, 26
            receptive language, 26
            recommendations, 27–28
        clinical procedures, 25
        significant history, 24–25
    language comprehension, 324–325
    literacy development, 343–344
    morphosyntactic aspect of language
        development using Brown's stages,
        266–267
    semantic development, 201–202
    skills and use of gestures, 386
    speech sound assessment, 248
Judgment tasks, 317

K

Kanner, Leo, 392–393
Khan-Lewis Phonological Analysis, 2nd ed., 243t
Klein, M.D., 157

Knowledge access, 165
Kohnert, K., 355
Korean- and English-speaking children, early
    vocabularies of, 204

L

Labeling and requesting, 143. *See also*
    Referencing and requesting
Labiodentals, 229
Lahey, M., 81
Language acquisition, paradigms of, 59–60
Language acquisition device (LAD), 61
Language as problem, 356
Language as resource, 356
Language as right, 356
Language assessment and intervention. *See also*
    Speech-language pathologists; Speech-
    language pathology
    formal testing
        basal level of performance, 12
        ceiling level of performance, 12
        of language domains, 14–15
        normative scoring systems: standard score
            and percentile, 12–13
    intervention (treatment), 1
    introduction, 1–2
    language assessment (evaluation), 1
    language defined
        ASHA definition of, 2–3
        domains, 3–6
            morphology, 3–4
            phonology, 3
            pragmatics, 5–6
            semantics, 4–5
            syntax, 4, 5t
        rules, 3
        symbols, 3
    milestones, 1–2
    receptive *vs.* expressive language, 6–7
    relationship between skills, 2
    spontaneous language sampling, 11–12
    stages of communication, 7–8
Language awareness, literacy and, 331
Language comprehension, children with multiple
    disabilities, 419
Language delay, 381

Language development of the hearing-impaired
      population
   conductive/otitis media population, 123–125
      auditory processing deficits (list), 125
      inconsistent behaviors and responses to
            sound, 123–124
      otitis media with effusion (OME) and
            poor language abilities, 124
      temporary and fluctuating hearing loss, 124
   Deaf culture, 129
   sensorineural population, 125–128
      children with high-frequency sensorineural
            hearing loss
         effect on phonological development,
               126–127
         speech recognition difficulties, 127
      children with mild deficits, 126
      children with moderate impairment, 126
      children with severe to profound hearing loss
         cochlear implantation, 127, 128
         comprehension and production of
               complex sentences, 128
         intelligibility, 127
         language skills, 127–128
      introduction, 125
      phonology and speech intelligibility,
            variability of, 126
      unilateral hearing loss (UHL), 128
Language deviance, 381
Language difference, 381–382
Language disability, 380–381
Language disorder/impairment, 380
Language-disordered children, identification
      of, 81
Language diversity, 355
Language domains, formal testing and, 14–15
Language-ego permeability, 360–361
Language impairment in children
   assessment procedures
      infants
         dynamic approach, 398
         traditional (developmental) approach,
               398
      language evaluation by certified SLP
         diagnosis of the language deficit,
               397–398
         identification, 397

      preschooler or school-age child
         assessment of narratives, 399–400
         criterion-referenced measures, 399
         curriculum-based language assessment,
               400
         language sampling, 399
         performance assessment procedures, 399
         standardized tests (norm-referenced
               measures), 398–399
         transdisciplinary play-based assessment,
               400
   intervention strategies
      academic challenges, 402
      early intervention, 400–401
      enhanced milieu teaching, 403
      facilitative play (indirect language
            stimulation), 404
      facilitative techniques, 402–403
      federally mandated services, 400–401
      focused stimulation, 404–405
      imitation, modeling, expansion and
            recasting, 403–404
      incidental teaching procedure, 403
      individual education plan (IEP), 401
      individual family service plan (IFSP), 401
      joint story reading, 402
      mand-model procedure, 403
      phonological awareness activities, 402
      pull out service delivery, 402
      push in service delivery, 402
      scripted play, 404
      selection of intervention goals and
            strategies, 401–402
      self-talk/parallel talk, 404
      time delay procedure, 403
   introduction
      chapter focus, 382
      disability, 380–381
      handicap, 380–381
      language delay, 381
      language deviance, 381
      language difference, 381–382
      language disability, 380–381
      language disorder/impairment, 380
      learning disability, 380–381
      primary language impairment, 380
      secondary language impairment, 380

objectives, 379
primary language impairment
    definition of, 280
    language learning disability (LLD) in
        school-age children
        limitations in language content:
            semantics, 391–392
        limitations in language form: phonology,
            morphology, and syntax, 391
        limitations in language use: pragmatics,
            392
        specific difficulties described, 390
    late bloomers
        case studies of Josephine and Robert,
            385–387
        described, 385
        distinguishing from late talkers, 385–
            387
        timeline of gesture development, 385,
            386t
    late talkers, 382–385
        acquisition of grammatical morphemes,
            384t
        characteristics of late talkers, 382
        delays in phonological development, 382
        emerging language stage, 382
        morpho-syntactic development, 382,
            383t, 384
    specific language impairment (SLI) in
        preschoolers
        limitations in language content:
            semantics, 387–388
        limitations in language form
            nominal and verbial morphology,
                389
            phonological awareness, 388
            syntactic development, 389
        limitations in language use: pragmatics,
            389–390
secondary language impairment
    autism spectrum disorder (ASD)
        ASD and PDD-NOS compared, 394
        associated conditions, 393–394
        diagnostic criteria for (DSM-IV), 393
        early indicators, 394–395
        first described, 392–393
        language deficits, 394

onset of, 393
    prevalence in the United States, 393
    definition of, 380
    mental retardation (MR)
        adaptive behavior, 395
        causes of, 396
        definition of, 395
        degrees of, 395–396
        diagnosis of, 395
        early remedial programs, 396–397
        language characteristics of children
            with, 396
    summary, 405
Language loss, 361
Language sampling, 369, 399
Language transfer, 364–365
Language-use patterns, 361
LAP (Learning Accomplishment Profile (LAP)
    system), 49
Late bloomers (LB), 201. See also Josephine (LB)
    case studies, 385–387
    described, 385
    distinguishing from late talkers, 385–387
    timeline of gesture development, 385, 386t
Late talkers (LT), 202, 207, 382–385. See also
    Robert (LT)
    acquisition of grammatical morphemes, 384t
    characteristics of late talkers, 382
    delays in phonological development, 382
    emerging language stage, 382
    grammar development in
        index of productive syntax (IPSyn), 280
        Language Development Survey results,
            280
        longitudinal study: late talkers and
            children with typical development
            compared, 280
    morpho-syntactic development, 382, 383t,
        384
Law of effect, 69
Lax vowels, 229
Learned helplessness, 425–426
Learning Accomplishment Profile (LAP) system,
    49
Learning disability, 380–381
Left-to-right probabilistic models, 70
Lexeme, 209

Lexical bootstrapping, 277, 280
Lexical information, 4
Lexical-semantic development. *See* Early lexical-semantic development
Lexical-semantic networks, 210–211
Lexicalization of phonological recoding, 336
Limited-English proficient (LEP) students with a concomitant disability, 356–357
Linguistic awareness, literacy and, 333
Linguistic biases, 350
Linguistic competence, 61
Linguistic constructions, 272
Linguistic creativity, 61
Linguistic development, 43–45, 44t
Linguistic skills, 7–8
Liquids (speech sounds), 227
Literacy development
  case studies, 343–344
  definition of, 329
  early identification of later reading difficulties
    preventing reading failure in young children, 341
    research studies
      Catts et al., 342–343
      Nathan et al., 342
      Scarborough, 342
  early literacy: the transition to school
    areas of reading instruction (NPR)
      automaticity, 338
      fluency, 337–338
      phonemic awareness, 337
      phonics, 337
      text comprehension, 338–339
      vocabulary, 338
    developmental markers
      3-year-olds, 339
      4-year-olds, 339–340
      5-year-olds (kindergartners), 340
      first graders, 340
      second graders, 340–341
      third graders and beyond, 341
    reading comprehension: the ultimate goal, 336, 339
  emergent literacy period, 330–333
    developmental progression in questioning and commenting, 331–332
    foundations of literacy, 330
    language awareness, 331
    linguistic awareness, 333
    literacy artifacts, 331
    literacy events and functions, 331
    literacy knowledge, 332
    literacy socialization, 330–333
    oral language skills and reading achievement, 333
    phonological awareness, 332–333
    term, 330
  introduction, 329–330
  objectives, 329
  the self-teaching hypothesis
    fluent word recognition, 336
    lexicalization of phonological recoding, 336
    orthographic representation of a word, 336
    phonological recoding (decoding), 335
  stages of reading development
    alphabetic principle, 334
    alphabetic stage, 334
    automatic word definition, 334–335
    Chall model, 333–334
    logographic stage, 334
    orthographic stage, 334
  summary, 344–345
Localization, 98
Locke, John, 59, 68
Locutionary stage of communication, 7–8, 78, 79, 145, 199–202
Logographic stage of literacy development, 334
Longitudinal study, 230
Lovaas, O.I., 71
Low vowels, 229

M

MacArthur-Bates Communicative Development Inventories, 2nd ed. (MCDIs), 48–49, 319–320, 457
  Words and Gestures, 449
Malleus (hammer), 97f, 99, 99f
Mand-model procedure, 403
Mands (commands), 69
Manner, 227
Mapping
  fast, 209, 313
  slow, 209–210

Mastery, 258
Material support, 439
Maturation, cognitive development and, 36
MCDIs. *See MacArthur-Bates Communicative Development Inventories, 2nd ed.* (MCDIs)
Mean length of utterance (MLU), 12, 67
  computation of
    calculating MLU for an entire sample, 260
    rules for assigning morphemes to utterances, 259t, 260
    grammar development in late talkers, 279–280
    as a predictor of language complexity, 258
    stages of morphosyntactic development, 257, 258t
    terminology related to morphemes, 257–258
Mediational models, 70
Medical needs, of children with multiple disabilities, 424
Medical-surgical treatment for otitis media, 117–118
Mental retardation (MR)
  adaptive behavior, 395
  causes of, 396
  definition of, 395
  degrees of, 395–396
  diagnosis of, 395
  early remedial programs, 396–397
  language characteristics of children with, 396
Metalinguistic knowledge/skills, 8, 237
Metaphonological awareness, 237
Metathesis, 235
Mid vowels, 229
Middle ear transformer function, 99–100
Milestones, developmental, 1–2
Milieu teaching, 71
Mind Reading, 167
Minimalist Program—Chomsky, 65–66
Minority and majority groups, 351
Mixed hearing loss, 116–117
MLU. *See* Mean length of utterance (MLU)
Modeling, 403–404
Modifiers, 202t, 203
Morphemes, 3–4. *See* Morphology
Morpho-syntactic development, late talkers, 382, 383t, 384

Morpho-syntactic rules, bilingual children, 364
Morphology, 3–4
  bound morphemes, 256, 257t
  clinical applications: case studies
    Johnathon, 266–267
    Josephine, 267
    Robert, 268
  definition of morpheme, 256
  free morphemes, 256
  introduction, 255
  morphological development, 256–265
    Brown's 14 grammatical morphemes
      characteristics of, 263–264
      list of, 263t
      process of acquiring, 264–265
      rule-governed morphological system, 265
      uses for, 264
    form-content-use model of linguistic development, 257
    mean length of utterance (MLU)
      computation of
        calculating MLU for an entire sample, 260
        rules for assigning morphemes to utterances, 259t, 260
      as a predictor of language complexity, 258
      stages of morphosyntactic development, 257, 258t
      terminology related to morphemes, 257–258
    stages of morphological development
      application of the information, 261
      refinements in sentence complexity, 261
      summary of grammatical morpheme production, 262t
      syntactic specificity, 260–261
      telegraphic, 260
    stages of syntactic development, 257
  obligatory morphemes, 263
  summary, 268
Motherese, 79
Motor development, 40–41, 41t
Mullen Scales of Early Development, 456
Multicultural, defined, 351

N

Naming, joint referencing and, 77
Naming errors
    functional core hypothesis, 212
    overextension, 211
    phonotactic probability, 212
    semantic feature hypothesis, 211
    underextension, 211
    in word retrieval
        frequency of word exposure, 214–215
        indeterminate errors, 213
        naming practice, 214
        perseverative errors, 213
        phonological errors, 213
        phonotactic probability words, 213–214
        relation to their targets, 212
        richness of semantic representation, 214
        semantic errors, 213
        shape, function, and control, 215
        during the word spurt period, 213
Naming explosion, 200
Naming insight, 200
Naming practice, 214
Nasals, 227
Nathan, L., 342
National Council on the Developing Child, 84
National Institute of Health (NIH), statement
    on hearing impairment in young children
    (1993), 109
National Research Council & Institute of
    Medicine, science of child development in
    2008: broader perspectives, 84–86
Natural communicative activities and routines,
    437–438
Natural Language Paradigm and Pivotal
    Response Treatment, 71
Naturalistic observations, 161–162, 163t
Nature-nurture debate
    descriptively adequate theories, 59
    interactionist: cognitive interactionist
        paradigm, 72–84
        cognitive-constructivist models, 74–76
        information processing models, 72–74
    interactionist: intentionality model, 81–84, 83f
    interactionist: social interactionist paradigm
        social-cognitive and social-pragmatic
            models: implications from, 80–81

        social-cognitive models, 77–78
        social-pragmatic models, 78–80
    introduction
        assessment of the child with developmental
            needs, 57–58
        the communicating child and the
            noncommunicating child,
            distinguishing between, 56–57
        continuum of the debate, 55–56
        developmental derailments, 56
        experience affects brain architecture, 58
        the nature-nurture debate in 2008, 58–59
    nature: rationalist paradigm
        biological bases, properties of, 62
        a contemporary view—Pinker and
            Jackendoff, 66
        developmental psycholinguistics, 63–64
        evidence for a critical period for language
            learning, 62–63
        government binding—principles and
            parameters—Chomsky, 64–65
        growth and development of the central
            nervous system and, 63
        implications from a nature perspective,
            67–68
        Minimalist Program—Chomsky, 65–66
        recent arguments for, 62
        Transformational Generative Grammar
            (Chomsky), 60–61
    nurture: behaviorist paradigm, 68–72
        classical conditioning, 68–69
        empiricist theories, 68
        implications from a nurture perspective
            assessment protocols, 70–71
            speech-language interventions, 71–72
        mediational models, 70
        operant conditioning, 69
    objectives, 55
    paradigms of language acquisition, 59–60
    science of child development in 2008: broader
        perspectives
        brain architecture and skills built "from
            the bottom up," 85–86
        cognitive, emotional, and social capabilities
            are intertwined throughout the life
            course, 86

conclusion: using this information as a student of speech-language pathology

Timmy, comprehensive approach to intervention, 87–88

understanding diversity in profiles of the children, 86–87

interactive influences of genes and experience, 85

National Council on the Developing Child, 84

need for earlier intervention programs, 85

theoretical adequacy of theories, 59

NDW (number of different words), 12

New Mexican Hispanic/Mexican American cultures, variations in caregiver-child interactions, 143–144

NIH. See National Institute of Health (NIH)

Nominal insight, 200

Nonlinguistic communication, 79, 80

Nonlinguistic vocalizations, 7

Nonreflexive vocalizations, 231

Nonverbal behaviors, pragmatic rules for, 6

Nonverbal communication, cultural variables in, 359

Norm-referenced measures, 398–399

Normative scoring systems: standard score and percentile, 12–13

Nouns, in early lexical-semantic development, 202–205

bootstrapping, 204

classification system of words, 202–203, 202t

environment and the developing lexicon, 204

influence of maternal language on child's early vocabulary, 204

noun preferences in early lexicons, 203

ordering of word classes in a sentence, 203–204

pattern of noun learning over word-class learning, 205

Novel name-nameless category principle (N3C), 206–207

Number of different words (NDW), 12

Nurture debate. See Nature-nurture debate

O

OAE. See Otoacoustic emissions (OAE)

Obligatory contexts, 258, 261

Obstruents, 227

Oller, D.K., 232

One Frog Too Many, 167

Online processing, 215

Onset-rime awareness, 237–238

Open syllable, 230

Operant conditioning, 69

Oral language skills and reading achievement, 333

Order of mention strategy, 309

Ordering of word classes in a sentence, 203–204

Organ of Corti, 100, 102

Orientation, 358

Orthographic representation of a word, 336

Orthographic stage of literacy development, 334

Oscar, 416, 418, 423, 437

speech language evaluation

clinical findings

diagnosis and prognosis, 458

expressive language, 458

general observations, 457–458

nonverbal communication, 457

oral-motor examination, 458

play, 457

receptive language, 457

recommendations, 458

clinical procedures, 456

significant history, 456

use of a voice output SGD, 458

Osgood, C., 73

Ossicular chain, 99, 100

Otitis media, 113–114, 116–117

language development and, 123–125, 240

auditory processing deficits (list), 125

inconsistent behaviors and responses to sound, 123–124

otitis media with effusion (OME) and poor language abilities, 124

temporary and fluctuating hearing loss, 124

medical-surgical treatment for, 117–118

Otoacoustic emissions (OAE), children from birth to six months of age, 109–110

Overextension, 211

Overextensions/underextensions, word meaning
    boundaries, 311
Overgeneralization errors, 278–279

P

Paden, E., 245
Palatalization, 234
Palatals, 229
Paradigms of language acquisition, 59–60
Parallel processing of language, 73
Parallel-talk, 404
Parent training, 21
Parnell, M., 316
Participation barriers in natural activities and
    routines, 427–428
Pavlov, I.P., 68–69
PCF (phonetically consistent forms), 199
PDD (pervasive developmental disorders), 393
Peabody Picture Vocabulary Test, 4th ed.,
    (PPVT-IV), 14, 321
Peabody Picture Vocabulary Test—III (PPVT-
    III, form B), 448, 453, 457
"Peanut Butter Protocol," 160
Percentile score, 12–13
Performance assessment procedures, 399
Perilymph, 101
Perlocutionary stage of communication, 7, 78,
    144, 198
Perseverative errors, 213
Personal-social words, 202t, 203
Personal space (proximity), cultural variables in,
    359
Pervasive developmental disorder—not
    otherwise specified (PDD-NOS), 393,
    394
Pervasive developmental disorders (PDD), 393
Phonation stage of vocal development, 232
Phonemes, 227–230, 228t. *See* Speech sound
    disorders
    consonants, 227–229
    vowels, 229–230
Phonemic awareness, 337
Phonetically consistent forms (PCF), 199
Phonics, 337
Phonological awareness, 332–333, 388, 402. *See
    also* Speech sound disorders

Phonological constancy, 304
Phonological errors, 213
Phonological loop, 215, 216
Phonological patterns, 236t, 246–247
Phonological processes/deviations. *See* Speech
    sound disorders
    assessment of, 243, 243t
    glottal stop replacement, 235
    major assimilations, 235
    omissions, 234
    substitutions, 234–235
    syllable-structure/context-related changes,
        235
Phonological recoding (decoding), 335
Phonological transfer, 364
Phonology, 3, 225–226. *See* Speech sound
    disorders
Phonotactic probability words, 212–214
Photo Articulation Test, 3rd ed., 243t
Phrasal embedding, 261
Physical disabilities, 425
Physical experience, cognitive development
    and, 36
Piaget's model of functional invariants
    accommodation, 75
    adaptation, 74
    assimilation, 74
    children direct their own learning, 75
    critics of Piagetian theory, 75
    language development, 75
    schemas, 74
Piaget's theories of cognitive development
    accommodation, 37, 75
    adaptation, 36–37, 74
    assimilation, 37, 74
    four factors of cognitive development, 36
    stages of cognitive development, 37–38, 38t
    stages of the sensorimotor period, 38, 39t, 40
Pinker, S., 66
Pinna (auricle), 96–98, 97f
Plato, 59
Play, role of in therapy, 76
Play interactions, cultural variables in, 360
PLS-IV (*Preschool Language Scale, 4th ed.*), 14
Pointing gestures, 78, 180
Postnatal auditory development
    background noise and reverberation, 104

encoding, 103
selective listening, 103–104
Postvocalic, 227
PPVT-III, form B (*Peabody Picture Vocabulary Test—III*), 448, 453, 457
PPVT-IV (*Peabody Picture Vocabulary Test, 4th ed.*), 14, 321
Pragmatics, 5–6
 assessment of pragmatic behaviors, 160
 limitations in language use: pragmatics, 389–390, 392
 social-pragmatic models, 78–81
Prelexial forms, 199
Prelinguistic gestures, 178
Prelinguistic skills, 7
Prelogical cognitive development, 40
Prenatal auditory development, 102–103
Preoperational stage of cognitive development, 37, 38t, 40
Preparatory, prelogical stages of cognitive development, 37
Preschool Language Scale, 4th ed. (PLS-IV), 14
Presupposition knowledge of children, 79
Preverbal stage of cognitive development, 37
Prevocalic, 227
Primary circular reaction stage, sensorimotor period, 39t
Primary intersubjectivity, social competence, 137
Primary language impairment. *See* Language impairment in children
Principle of conventionality, 207
Principle of extendibility, 207
Principle of mutual exclusivity, 206
Principle of reference, 206
Principles and Guidelines for Early Hearing Detection and Intervention Program, 109
Principles and Parameters theory (Chomsky), 64–65
Prizant, B., 80
Probabilistic patterns, 287
Procedural memory system, 287
Propositional content, 82
Protodeclarative stage, 145
Protoimperative stage, 145
Protowords, 199, 233
Proximity (personal space), cultural variables in, 359

Psycholinguistics, developmental, 63–64
Psychological attitudes, 82
Pull out service delivery, 402
Pure tone, 104
Push in service delivery, 402
PVVT-4 (*Peabody Picture Vocabulary Test-4*), 321

Q

Quick incidental learning (QUIL), 209

R

Race, 353–354
Racial/ethnic minority, 351
Reading development. *See* Literacy development
Recasting, 403–404
Receptive-Expressive Emergent Language Test, 3rd ed. (REEL-3), 48
Receptive vocabularies, 311
Receptive *vs.* expressive language, 6–7
Recognition of emotion, 165
Reduplication, 235–236
Referencing and requesting, 145–147
 challenges to adult's refusal of a request, 148
 indirect and nonconventionalized requests, 148
 necessary aspects of requests, 147–148
 types of early requests, 147
 verbal requests, 147
Reflexive stage, sensorimotor period, 39t
Reflexive vocalizations, 231
Regulation of emotion, 166
Reissner's membrane, 100, 101f
Representational gestures (iconic, baby signs), 178–179
Requesting and labeling, 143. *See also* Referencing and requesting
Resistant-ambivalent attachment, 141
Resonance properties, 98
Responding to joint attention (RJA), 137–138, 156
Retroflex/rhoticized /r/, 228
Rett's disorder, 393
Reversibility, 40
RITLS. *See Rossetti Infant-Toddler Language Scale* (RITLS)

Ritual request gestures, 180
Robert (LT), 21, 28–33, 385–387
   developmental assessment, 51–52
   expressive language and gesture, 182, 189
   hearing and language development, 131
   language assessment and intervention
      clinical findings
         diagnosis and prognosis, 31
         expressive language, 30
         general observations, 29
         nonverbal communication, 29
         oral-motor examination, 31
         phonology, 30–31
         play, 29
         receptive language, 30
         recommendations, 31–33
      clinical procedures, 29
      significant history, 28
   language comprehension, 325
   literacy development, 344
   morphosyntactic aspect of language
      development using Brown's stages,
      266–267
   prognosis, 390
   semantic development, 201–202
   specific language impairment (SLI), 387
   speech sound assessment, 248–249
Rossetti Infant-Toddler Language Scale (RITLS),
   14, 48, 160, 181, 318–319
Rules of language, 3

S

Sam, 415, 418, 428–429, 436
   speech language evaluation
      clinical findings
         diagnosis and prognosis, 450
         expressive language, 449
         general observations, 448
         nonverbal communication, 448
         oral-motor examination, 449–450
         receptive language, 448–449
         recommendations, 450–451
      clinical procedures, 448
      significant history, 447
   use of a SGD, 420, 423–424, 447, 448,
      450, 451

Scaffolds/scaffolding, 16–17, 20–21, 77
Scala media, 100, 101f
Scala tympani, 101, 101f
Scala vestibuli, 100–101, 101f
Scanning techniques, 422
Scarborough, H.S., 342
Science of child development in 2008: broader
     perspectives
   brain architecture and skills built "from the
     bottom up," 85–86
   cognitive, emotional, and social capabilities
     are intertwined throughout the life
     course, 86
   conclusion: how to use this information as a
     student of speech-language pathology
     Timmy, comprehensive approach to
     intervention, 87–88
     understanding diversity in profiles of the
     children, 86–87
   interactive influences of genes and experience,
     85
   National Council on the Developing Child,
     84
   need for earlier intervention programs, 85
Scripted play, 404
Secondary circular reaction stage, sensorimotor
   period, 39t
Secondary intersubjectivity, social competence,
   137
Secondary language impairment. *See* Language
   impairment in children
Secure attachment, 141
Segmental aspects of language, 107
Selection techniques, 422
Self-talk, 404
Self-teaching hypothesis
   fluent word recognition, 336
   lexicalization of phonological recoding, 336
   orthographic representation of a word, 336
   phonological recoding (decoding), 335
Semantic feature hypothesis, 211
Semantic Generativists, 64
Semantic representation, 209
Semantics, 4–5
Sensorimotor stage of cognitive development, 37,
   38t, 39t, 40

Sensorineural hearing loss, 114–116
  causes of, 114
  functional ability, 116
  hearing impaired and deaf, difference
    between, 115–116
  high-frequency hearing loss, 115
  language development and, 125–128
    children with high-frequency hearing loss
      effect on phonological development,
        126–127
      speech recognition difficulties, 127
    children with mild deficits, 126
    children with moderate impairment, 126
    children with severe to profound hearing
      loss
      cochlear implantation, 127, 128
      comprehension and production of
        complex sentences, 128
      intelligibility, 127
      language skills, 127–128
    introduction, 125
    phonology and speech intelligibility,
      variability of, 126
  loss of sensitivity and speech distortion,
    114–115
  speech clarity problems, 116
Sentence types, 5t
*Sequenced Inventory of Communication
  Development, Revised* (SICD-R), 448, 449,
  452, 453, 457
Sequential-bilingual child, 362–363
Sequential dependencies, 287
Serial processing of language, 73
Serial reaction time (SRT) testing, 287–288
Seriation ability, 40
Service delivery, 372
SGDs. *See* Speech-generating devices (SGDs)
Shape, function, and control, 215
Shape bias, 207–208
Share, D.L., 335, 336
Shared attention, 78
Show gestures, 180
Sibilants, 228–229
SICD-R (*Sequenced Inventory of Communication
  Development, Revised*), 449, 453, 456, 457
Simultaneous-bilingual child, 362–363
Size of an object, bias and, 208

Skills, developmental, 2
Skinner, B.F., 69
Slow mapping, 209–210
SLPs. *See* Speech-language pathologists (SLPs)
Social-cognitive models, 77–78, 80–81
Social-emotional bases of communication
  development
  assessment
    caregiver-child interaction
      caregiver behaviors to observe, 157
      patterns of social interaction, 157, 158t
    interviews, 162, 164t, 165
    of theory of mind and emotion
      understanding, 165–167
  assessment of children's communicative
    behaviors
    formal/standardized assessment
      Early Social Communication Scales, 159
      language tools, 160
      of pragmatic behaviors, 160
    naturalistic observations, 161–162, 163t
  communicating with others
    development of emotional understanding,
      150–151
    horizontal development
      communicative functions in preschool
        children, 148, 150t
      discourse level, 148
      early communicative events, 148, 149t
      social level, 148
      utterance level, 147
    vertical development
      intentionality
        Illocutionary stage, 145
        initiating behavior request (IBR),
          145, 156
        locutionary stage, 145
        perculocutionary stage, 144
        protodeclarative (IJA), 145
      referencing and requesting, 145–147
        challenges to adult's refusal of a
          request, 148
        indirect and nonconventionalized
          requests, 148
        necessary aspects of requests,
          147–148
        types of early requests, 147

verbal requests, 147
conclusion, 170
elements of social competence and language
    attachment, 136
    endogenous and exogenous factors, 137
    experience-sharing, 136
    instrumental social actions, 136
    intentionality, 136–137
    joint attention (JA), 137–138
    primary/secondary intersubjectivity, 137
    theory of mind (TOM), 137
emergence of language
    what caregivers bring to interactions
        cultural variations in caregiver-child
            interactions
            black children in Piedment region of
                N.C., 144
            independent/individualist, 143
            interdependent/collectivist, 143
            New Mexican Hispanic/Mexican
                American cultures, 143–144
            requesting and labeling, 143
        mainstream caregivers, 141–143
    what the child brings to interactions
        affect sharing device (AFS), 138–139
        attachment, 141
        infant engagement tools, 138–139
        temperament, 139–141
factors affecting
    within the child, 152–156
        autism spectrum disorders (ASD),
            155–156
        blindness, 153–154
        deafness and theory of mind, 154
        specific language impairment (SLI),
            154–155
    environmental
        alignment, 151–152
        attunement, 151, 152
introduction: components of language
    acquisition, 135–136
objectives, 135
philosophy of intervention, 167–170
    deficits that underlie joint attention,
        167–170
    ecologically based programs
        common assumptions, 168

goals of, 169
interrupted behavior chain, 168
encourage coordination/coregulation,
    169–170
episodic memory, 170
language intervention programs, 167–168
Social-emotional development
    achieve and maintain self-regulation, 42–43
    connectedness with the world, 41–42
    development of imitation skills, 43
Social interaction, cognitive development and, 36
Social-pragmatic models, 78–81
Sociolinguistic/sociocultural competence, 365
Sociological assessment model, 369–370
Sonorants, 227
Specific language impairment (SLI), 67, 154–
    155, 191
    grammar development of children with
        the Extended Optional Infinitive (EOI)
            Hypothesis, 284
        impaired statistical learning
            in learning probabilistic patterns and
                sequential dependencies, 287
            in the procedural memory system, 287
            serial reaction time (SRT) testing,
                287–288
        information-processing speed and limited
            verbal working memory capacity,
            285–286
        performance accounts of grammatical
            difficulties: the Surface Account,
            285
        remediation of syntactic difficulties, 288
        representational deficits and grammatical
            SLI (G-SLI)
            correlation between vocabulary and
                grammar acquisition, 284
            difficulties with reversible active-voice
                sentences, 283
            types of grammatical difficulties,
                282–283
        SLI described, 281
        syntactic bootstrapping and knowledge of
            constructions, 281–282
    in preschoolers
        limitations in language content: semantics,
            387–388

limitations in language form
  nominal and verbial morphology, 389
  phonological awareness, 388
  syntactic development, 389
limitations in language use: pragmatics,
  389–390
Specific nominals, 202, 202t
Speech acts, primitive, 79
Speech clarity problems, with hearing loss, 116
Speech Correction: Principles and Methods, 245
Speech-generating devices (SGDs), 414, 419,
  420, 421, 423–424, 437, 448, 450, 451,
  458
Speech-language interventions, from a nurture
  perspective, 71–72
Speech-language pathologists (SLPs)
  assessment protocol, 9
  background history of child, 10–11, 11t
  evaluation protocol, 9–10
  initial meeting with parents and child, 8–9
  referrals to, 8
  training for, 8
Speech-language pathology
  assessment
    knowledge of developmental milestones
      and, 17
    other areas of concern, 17
    planning of the language evaluation, 15–16
    profile of child's strengths and weaknesses,
      16
    prognostic statements, 18
    scaffolds, 16–17
    trial treatment activities, 16
    types of goals to be set, 17–18
  introduction, 15
  setting goals and the intervention process, 18
    intervention process
      accuracy measurement, 21
      the activity, 20
      feedback, 20
      the goal, 19–20
      overview, 19
      parent training and home program, 21
      tactile cues, 20
      therapeutic scaffolding, 20–21
      verbal cues, 20
    introduction, 18

long-term goals, 18–19
session objective goals, 19
short-term goals, 19
Speech recognition score, 112
Speech recognition threshold, 112
Speech sound disorders
  acquisition
    first word stage, 233
    later stages, 233
    prelinguistic stages
      nonreflexive vocalizations, 231
      Oller's stages of vocalization, 232
      reflexive vocalizations, 231
      speech perception, 230–231
    protowords, 233
  case studies, 248–249
  evaluation of children with
    assessment
      overview, 241
      tests
        assessment of phonological
          processes/deviations, 243,
          243t
        continuous speech sample, 243
        hearing, 244
        intelligibility, 244
        oral mechanism, 244
        phoneme-oriented tests, 242, 243t
        stimulability, 243
    major etiological factors
      ethnocultural considerations, 241
      hearing, 240
      oral mechanism, 240
      personal factors, 241
    reporting, 244
  introduction
    approaches to addressing speech sound
      disorders, 226
    articulation, 225, 226
    childhood apraxia of speech (CAS), 225,
      226
    phonology, 225–226
    term speech sound disorders, 225
  objectives, 225
  phonemes, 227–230, 228t
    consonants, 227–229
    vowels, 229–230

phonological awareness
    exposure to alphabetic knowledge and
        print referencing activities, 239
    factors influencing, 238–239
    onset-rime, 237–238
    phonemic awareness, 238
    responsibilities of SPLs with respect to
        reading and writing, 239
    syllable awareness, 237
    term, 237
phonological deviations
    glottal stop replacement, 235
    major assimilations, 235
    omissions, 234
    substitutions, 234–235
    syllable-structure/context-related changes,
        235
the speech mechanism, 226–227
speech sound system development
    ages at which phonemes occur, 230
    cross-sectional study, 230
    longitudinal studies, 230
summary, 249
suppression of phonological processes
    age of acquisition of phonological
        patterns/phonemes, 236t
    age of suppression, 236t
treatment, 245–246
    cycles phonological remediation approach,
        245–247
        patterns that should be targeted,
            246–247
        principles of, 245–246
        strength of this approach, 246
        structure of the treatment session, 247
    focused auditory input/stimulation,
        247–248
    phoneme-oriented approaches, 244–245
Spontaneous language sampling, 11–12
Standard score, 12–13
Standardized tests (norm-referenced measures),
    398–399
Stapedius muscle activity, 111
Stapes (stirrup), 99, 99f
Step-by-Step SGD, 423–424
Stimulus-response psychology model, 71
Stoel-Gammon, C., 236, 236t

Stopping, 234
Strategic competence, 365
Stridents, 228–229
Structured elicited production task, 265
Subordinate terms, 212
Superordinate terms, 212
Supra threshold, 105
Suprasegmental aspects of language, 107
Surface Account, 285
Syllabics, 229–230
Syllable awareness, 237
Symbols expressing language, 3
Syntactic bootstrapping, 278
Syntactic productivity, 277–278
Syntactic specificity, 260
Syntax, 4, 5t

T

Tactile cues, 20
Tacts (naming behaviors), 69
Telegraphic words, 260
Temperament, of child, 139–141
Tense (long) vowels, 229
Tertiary circular reaction stage, sensorimotor
    period, 39t
Test for Auditory Comprehension of Language-3
    (TACL-3), 321
Text comprehension, 338–339
Theory of mind (TOM)
    deafness and, 154
    emotion understanding and, 165–167
    social competence and language and, 137
Therapeutic scaffolding, 20–21
Threshold, 104–105
Timmy, comprehensive approach to intervention,
    86–88
Tinker, E., 80–81
Tomasello, M., 78
Touch, cultural variables in, 359
Traditional assessment model, 369
Traditional (developmental) approach to
    assessment, 398
Transdisciplinary play-based assessment, 400
Transformational Generative Grammar
    (Chomsky), 60–61

Transitive and intransitive verb constructions, 275
Translators. *See* Interpreters/translators
Treatment (intervention), 1
Turn-taking, 198
Tympanic membrane (eardrum), 97, 97f, 99f
Tympanometry, children from birth to six months of age, 111
Typical language developmental (TD) case. *See* Johnathon (TD)

U

Underextension, 211
Unilateral hearing loss (UHL), language development and, 128
Unitary language system, 363
United Nations Educational, Scientific, and Cultural Organization (UNESCO), definition of literacy, 329

V

Van Riper, Charles, 244–245
Variegated babbling stage of vocal development, 232
Velars, 229
Verbal communication, cultural variables in, 358–359
Verbal cues, 20
Verbal working memory capacity, 285–286
Verbs
    transitive and intransitive verb constructions, 275
    verb acquisition and its influence on grammatical structures
        grammar acquisition, 276–277
        lexical bootstrapping, 277, 280
        order of verb acquisition, 276
        transitive subject-verb-object, 276
Vertical development
    intentionality
        Illocutionary stage, 145
        initiating behavior request (IBR), 145, 156

locutionary stage, 145
perculocutionary stage, 144
protodeclarative (IJA), 145
protoimperative (IBR), 145
referencing and requesting, 145–147
    challenges to adult's refusal of a request, 148
    indirect and nonconventionalized requests, 148
    necessary aspects of requests, 147–148
    types of early requests, 147
    verbal requests, 147
Vigil, D., 157, 158t
Vineland Adaptive Behavior Scales, 456
Visual reinforcement audiometry (VRA), 111–112
Visuo-spatial sketchpad, 215, 216
Vocabulary, 338
Vocabulary spurt, 200
Vocalizations, 7, 231–232
Voiced consonants, 229
Voiceless consonants, 229
Vowelization, 234
Vowels, 229–230
VRA (visual reinforcement audiometry), 111–112
Vygotsky, L.S., 77

W

Wallace, G.L., 370
Westby, C.E., 157, 158t, 370, 371
Wh-questions, probe for, 322–323, 322t
Whole-object bias, 206
Word category hierarchies, development of, 312
Word-gesture combinations, 181
Word language mechanisms: links between phonology and semantics, 312–313
Word-order strategy, 308
Word-specific formulae, 275–276
Word spurt, 197, 200–201, 213
World knowledge, comprehension and, 300–301, 309–310
Wug Test, 265